Diagnostic Radiology

Satish K Bhargava
MD (Radiodiagnosis), MD (Radiotherapy)
DMRD, FICRI, FIAMS, FCCP, FUSI, FIMSA, RAMS
Formerly, Head Dept. of Radiology and Imaging
University College of Medical Sciences
(Delhi University) and GTB Hospital
Delhi

Peepee Publishers and Distributors (P) Ltd.®

Diagnostic Radiology

Published by
Pawaninder P. Vij and Anupam Vij

Peepee Publishers and Distributors (P) Ltd.
Head Office: 160, Shakti Vihar, Pitam Pura
Delhi-110034 (India)

Correspondence Address:
7/31, First Floor, Ansari Road, Daryaganj
New Delhi-110002 (India)
Ph: 41512412, 9811156083
e-mail: peepee160@yahoo.co.in
e-mail: peepee160@gmail.com
www.peepeepub.com

First Edition: 2021

ISBN : 978-81-8445-2853

Dedicated to
My Loving Late Wife
Kalpana
whose inspiration and sacrifice
have made possible to bring out
this book

Preface

The branch of Radiology has shown a revolution in terms of development and advancement and almost 60-70% of diagnosis depends on imaging techniques. This has also offered many therapeutic guided procedures. All these are not available in a concise form at one place. The purpose of this book is to give comprehensive detail of some of the important topics, which will be helpful to Residents and Postgraduate students of MD, DMRD and Diplomate National Board in their course of study and examination. The book has dealt the complex and varied clinical presentation by disease processes and also the accompanying technical consideration, aids to clinch the diagnosis have been dealt with, all at one place in the most plausible and lucid manner with illustrations and tables. I am sure this book will definitely be helpful to the Residents and Postgraduate students.

Satish K Bhargava

Contributors

Dr. Anubhav Sarikwal
Ex. Senior Resident, Dept of Radiology and Imaging
University College of Medical Sciences and Associated G.T.B.Hospital, Delhi

Dr. Anupama Tandon
Sr. Assistant Professor, Dept of Radiology and Imaging
University College of Medical Sciences and Associated G.T.B.Hospital, Delhi

Dr. Anurag Agarwal
Ex. Senior Resident, Dept of Radiology and Imaging
Maulana Azad Medical College and Associated Lok Nayak Jai Prakash Narain Hospital, Delhi

Dr. Ashish Verma
Ex. Senior Resident, Dept of Radiology and Imaging
University College of Medical Sciences and Associated G.T.B.Hospital, Delhi

Dr. Avneesh Kumar Singh
Resident, Dept of Radiology and Imaging
University College of Medical Sciences and Associated G.T.B.Hospital, Delhi

Dr. Mamta Motla
Ex. Senior Resident, Dept of Radiology and Imaging
University College of Medical Sciences and Associated G.T.B.Hospital, Delhi

Dr. Manish Goel
Ex. Senior Resident, Dept of Radiology and Imaging
University College of Medical Sciences and Associated G.T.B.Hospital, Delhi

Dr. Meenakshi Prakash
Resident, Dept of Radiology and Imaging
University College of Medical Sciences and Associated G.T.B.Hospital, Delhi

Dr. Pardeep Bansal
Ex. Resident, Dept of Radiology and Imaging
University College of Medical Sciences and Associated G.T.B.Hospital, Delhi

Dr. Parul Garg
Ex. Senior Resident, Dept of Radiology and Imaging
University College of Medical Sciences and Associated G.T.B. Hospital, Delhi

Dr. Puneet Singh Kocher
Ex. Senior Resident, Dept of Radiology and Imaging
University College of Medical Sciences and Associated G.T.B. Hospital, Delhi

Dr. Pushpender Gupta
Ex. Resident, Dept of Radiology and Imaging
Ex. Senior Resident, Postgraduate Institute of Medical Sciences, Chandigarh

Dr. Rahul Gera
Ex. Senior Resident, Dept of Radiology and Imaging
University College of Medical Sciences and Associated G.T.B. Hospital, Delhi

Dr. Rajul Rastogi
Ex. Senior Resident, Dept of Radiology and Imaging
University College of Medical Sciences and Associated G.T.B. Hospital, Delhi

Dr. Satish Kumar Bhargava
Head, Dept of Radiology and Imaging
University College of Medical Sciences and Associated G.T.B. Hospital, Delhi

Dr. Sandeep Goyal
Resident, Dept of Radiology and Imaging
University College of Medical Sciences and Associated G.T.B. Hospital, Delhi

Dr. Sapna Maheshwari
Ex. Senior Resident, Dept of Radiology and Imaging
University College of Medical Sciences and Associated G.T.B. Hospital, Delhi

Dr. Shuchi Bhatt
Associate Professor, Dept of Radiology and Imaging
University College of Medical Sciences and Associated G.T.B. Hospital, Delhi

Dr. Sumeet Bhargava
Ex. Resident, Dept of Radiology and Imaging
University College of Medical Sciences and Associated G.T.B. Hospital, Delhi

Contents

3. RESPIRATORY SYSTEM

Intraparenchymal Hemorrhagic Lesions in Brain

Hemorrhagic lesions in brain can be broadly categorized into:

- Non-traumatic.
- Traumatic.

NON-TRAUMATIC LESIONS

On Computed Tomography

- Acute hemorrhage (0-72 hours): It appears hyperdense to human brain because of high globin content in the clotted blood. Unretracted semiliquid clot appears hypodense within the hyperdense acute hematoma, giving rise to the so-called ***swirl sign***.
- Subacute hemorrhage (4-16 days): Subacute hemorrhage becomes virtually isodense with the adjacent brain parenchyma. They may sometimes show a peripheral postcontrast enhancement due to breakdown of blood brain barrier.
- Chronic hemorrhage (>2 weeks): It appears hypodense to the adjacent brain. High attenuation within chronic hematomas is usually secondary to the rebleeding. Rim enhancement around a resolving hematoma typically appears within a few days and disappears between 2-6 months. A target sign on post-contrast images can be seen if rehemorrhage takes place within an organizing hematoma; if rebleeding occurs outside an organized hematoma it can resemble a tumoral hemorrhage.

On magnetic resonance imaging

Stage	Time	Compartment	Hemoglobin	T1	T2
Hyperacute	<24 hrs	Intracellular	Oxyhb	Iso	Hyper
Acute	1-3 days	Intracellular	Deoxyhb	Hypo	Hypo
Subacute					
• Early	3+ days	Intracellular	Methb	Hyper	Hypo
• Late	7+ days	Extracellular	Methb	Hyper	Hyper
Chronic					
• Centre	14+ days	Extracellular	Hemichromes	Iso	Hyper
• Rim		Intracellular	Hemosiderin	Hypo	Hypo

Causes of Non-traumatic Hemorrhage

- Hypertension.
- Aneurysm and vascular malformation (AVM, cavernous angioma).
- Perinatal hemorrhage.
- Hemorrhagic infarction (reperfusion or venous).
- Neoplastic.
- Miscellaneous:
  a. Amyloid angiopathy.
  b. Coagulopathies and blood dyscrasias.
  c. Drug abuse.
  d. Eclampsia.
  e. Infections (vasculitis, encephalitis, abscess, endocarditis with septic emboli).

Hypertensive ICH (HICH)

- Most common non-traumatic cause in adults.
- Most are associated with systemic hypertension and in some, ruptured microaneurysms are implicated.
- Common location include:

1.	Putamen/external capsule	60-65%
2.	Thalamus	15-25%
3.	Pons	05-10%
4.	Cerebellum	02-05%
5.	Subcortical white matter	01-02%

- Late CT manifestations include round or slit like cavities, particularly in the putamen and external capsule but calcification in uncommon.

Aneurysm and Vascular Malformation (AVM, Cavernous Angioma) ICH

- Ruptured aneurysms are associated with either intraparenchymal subarachnoid hemorrhage.
- Acute SAH is characterized by hyperdensity in the subarachnoid spaces (basal cisterns, fissures, sulci).
- Although SAH tends to be diffused; more focal cisternal or parenchymal hematomas can be due to ruptured aneurysms and are helpful in localizing the bleeding source:
  - Blood in the sylvian fissure – Aneurysm on the I/L ICA.
  - Focal interhemispheric blood – Anterior communicating artery aneurysm.
  - Blood in the 4th ventricle – PICA aneurysm.
- Subsequent angiography either CT or MR based or DSA are helpful in making the ultimate diagnosis of aneurysms.
- ICH secondary to AVM are usually seen in children or normotensive young adults.
- AVM are usually associated with gliotic and encephalomalacic changes.
- Cavernous angioma typically has popcorn like appearance with calcification and mixed signal foci inside a hemosiderin ring.

Perinatal Hemorrhage

- In term infants it is usually the result of hypoxic-ischemic insult.
- Areas of hemorrhage are typically seen in the posterolateral lentiform nuclei and ventral thalamus.
- Although the cortex can be involved in profound asphyxia, it is relatively spared compared to the deep grey matter.
- In premature infants, germinal matrix hemorrhage (GMH) is the most common form of ICH followed by intraventricular and intraparenchymal hemorrhage that are usually secondary to the former.
- Although CT and MR accurately depict GMH, most are currently evaluated by transcranial

ultrasound. Regions of hyperechogenicity, particular in the caudate nuclei, are typical with time the ICH becomes sonolucent.

- Germinal matrix hemorrhage is divided into four grades:
  - Grade I : Hemorrhage confirmed to one or both germinal matrices
  - Grade II : Hemorrhage ruptured into a normal sized ventricle
  - Grade III : Intraventricular hemorrhage with hydrocephalus
  - Grade IV : Hemorrhagic extension into the adjacent hemispheric white matter.

Hemorrhagic Infarction (Reperfusion or Venous)

- Hemorrhagic infarction is usually the result of lysis of embolus/opening of collaterals/ restoration of normal blood pressure following hypotension/hypertension/anticoagulation causing extravasation in reperfused ischemic brain.
- It is seen in approximately 6% of brain infarcts and is usually at the corticomedullary junction.
- CT will show the hyperdensity within a previously imaged hypodense acute ischemic infarct. MR will show the hypo intensity on T2WI and hyper intensity on TIWI.
- Venous infarctions are usually hemorrhagic, bilateral and occur primarily in the white matter and are most often associated with cortical vein and dural sinus thrombosis.
- CT demonstrates patchy foci of edema and petechial hemorrhage with or without signs of dural sinus thrombosis.

Neoplastic

- The incidence of hemorrhage in intracranial neoplasms has been estimated to be around 1-15%.
- Common brain tumors that are commonly associated with hemorrhage include pituitary adenomas, high-grade gliomas, PNET, epidermoid and metastases from bronchogenic, renal, chorio and melanocarcinoma.
- Points of benign versus malignant hemorrhage:
  - No absolute criteria.
  - Tumors are complex and heterogenous.
  - Benign lesions usually have a complete hemosiderin ring.
  - Non hemorrhagic area of the tumor enhance on post contrast images.
  - Hemorrhage evolution is disordered or delayed in tumoral lesions in contrast to a orderly evolution seen in benign hemorrhage.
  - Edema/mass effect resolve with resolution of hematoma in benign lesions while it persist with malignant lesions.
  - Hemorrhagic metastatic deposits will be multifocal.

MISCELLANEOUS

1. Amyloid Angiopathy

- This is probably the most common cause of recurrent bleeding in normotensive elderly and the incidence increases with advancing age.
- Hemorrhages are characteristically multiple, spare the basal ganglia and brainstem, and are located at the corticomedullary junction.
- CT and MR findings of multiple peripherally located hemorrhages of different ages in an elderly normotensive patient strongly suggest the cause as amyloid angiopathy.

Chapter 1

2. Inflammatory Diseases and Vasculitis

- Hemorrhage in immunocompetent persons in uncommon but immunocompromised individuals are at increased risk of developing hemorrhage in infectious lesions.
- Such lesions include infective endocarditis with septic emboli, fungal vasculitis and necrotising lesions as herpes encephalitis.
- Aspergillosis and the fungal infections may directly invade the vessel wall and cause thrombosis, hemorrhage or cerebral infarction.
- Type II herpes simplex encephalitis is most prone to develop hemorrhage especially in neonatal herpes.

3. Drug Abuse

- Drugs related ICH occurs more commonly than the ischemic changes.
- Drugs like cocaine can induce an hypertensive episode in which case the location of ICH is similar to that in hypertensive ICH.
- Cocaine also promotes arterial and dural sinus thrombosis producing venous infarction and ischemic infarction with subsequent hemorrhage.
- Vasculitis with hemorrhage is seen commonly with amphetamines and phenylpropanolamine and less commonly with cocaine.

4. Blood Dyscrasias and Coagulopathies

- Common causes of non-iatrogenic coagulopathy include vitamin K deficiency, hepatocellular disease, antibodies that react to clotting factors and DIC. Iatrogenic causes include mainly anticoagulants as heparin, warfarin, thrombolytic agents as streptokinase, antiplatelet agents as aspirin etc.
- Imaging findings in most coagulopathies are similar.
- Although bleeding can occur at any location, the most common site is supratentorial and intraparenchymal with multifocal lesions with fluid-fluid levels within the hematomas.

5. Eclampsia

- Posterior circulation is particularly prone.
- Lesions are commonly seen at cortico-medullary junction and within external capsule and basal ganglia.
- The occipital lobes are a frequent location of cortical and subcortical lesions.
- CT scans will reveal multiple hypoattenuating foci or hemorrhages in the subcortical white matter or basal ganglia.
- MR scans in severe preeclampsia often show non-specific foci or increased signal in the deep cerebral white matter on T2WI. Eclamptic patients show multifocal cortical and subcortical white matter edema, primarily in the occipital lobes.

TRAUMATIC

Diffuse Axonal Injury (DAI)

- It is the most common form of the intra-axial primary traumatic lesion.
- It tends to occur in the lobar white matter, corpus callosum and dorsolateral aspect of the brainstem.
- Nearly two thirds are seen at the grey white matter junction, most often in the fronto-temporal region, splenium and posterior body of the corpus callosum.
- Early CT scans may be unremarkable. Delayed scans in acute DAI may reveal petechial hemorrhages in the location mentioned above.

- MR scans show hyperintense lesions on T2WI in any of the above-described locations.

Cortical Contusions

- It is second most common form of the intra-axial primary traumatic lesion.
- Majority involve the temporal lobes followed by the frontal lobes and other sites as the cerebellar hemispheres.
- Early findings include patchy, ill-defined, frontal or temporal hypodense lesions that may be mixed with smaller hyperdense foci of petechial hemorrhage.
- Delayed scan at 24-48 hours may reveal hemorrhages developing in the previously hypodense regions.
- MR is such more sensitive in detecting the cortical contusions especially in the subacute stage.

Deep Cerebral and Brainstem Lesions

- CT is often normal in these patients.
- Petechial hemorrhages are sometimes seen in the dorsolateral brainstem, periacqueductal region and deep grey matter nuclei.
- MR depicts these lesions with much higher conspicuity and accuracy.

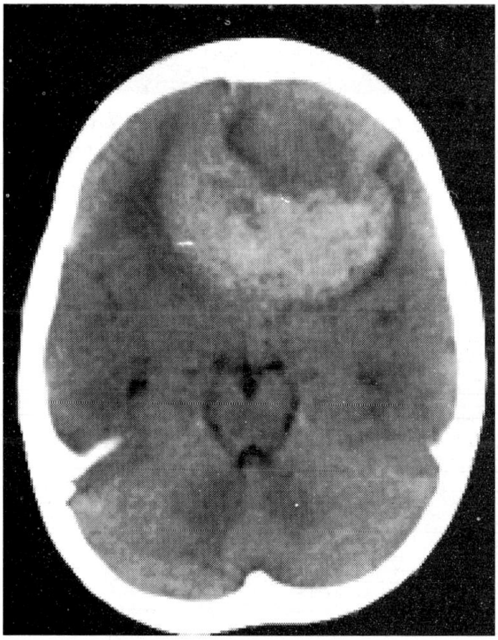

Fig. 1.1: Axial CT image shows hemorrhage in a large tumor in the basifrontal region of the brain

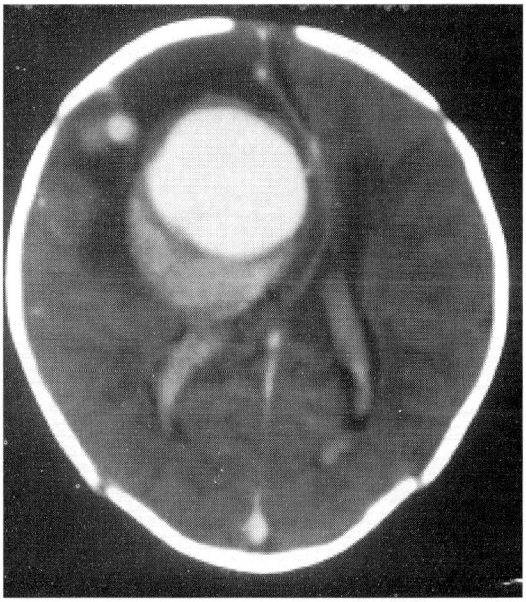

Fig. 1.2: Axial CT image shows intraparenchymal and intraventricular hemorrhage in a case of arteriovenous malformation in the right frontal lobe

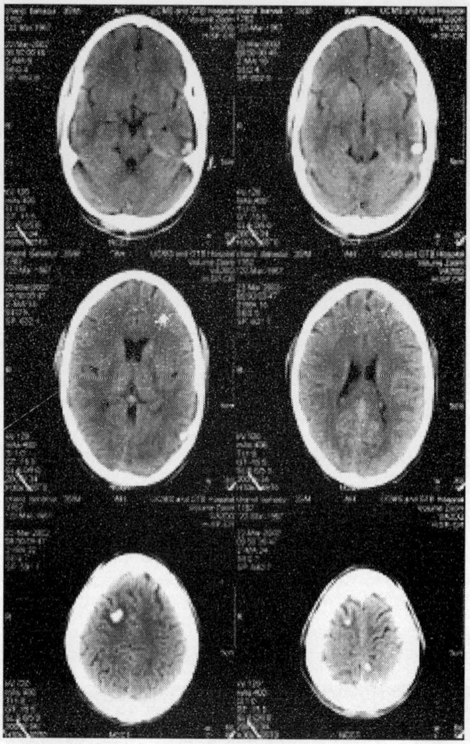

Fig. 1.3: Serial axial non-contrast CT images show post-traumatic hemorrhagic contusions in the rain parenchyma at several locations

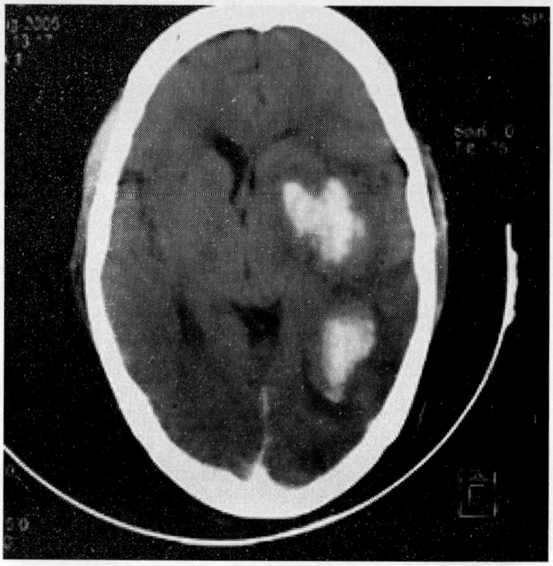

Fig. 1.4: Axial CT image shows intraparenchymal hemorrhage in left ganglionic region with subdural bleed along posterior part of the interhemispheric fissure

(a)

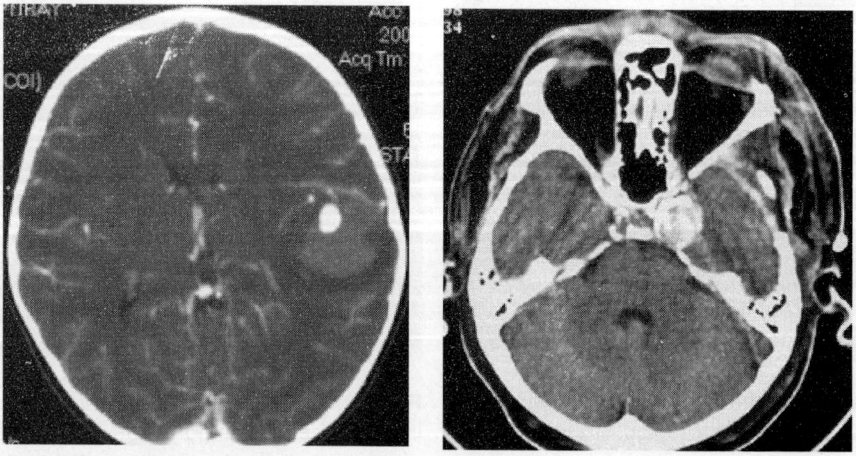

(b)

Fig. 1.5: (a) Axial scan shows a middle arterial intracranial aneurysm (large white spot on right). The light gray area around the aneurysm represents bleeding. (b) Calcified giant aneurysm of the left internal carotid artery in its intracavernous segment

Section 1—Central Nervous System

Chapter 2

Stroke

Definition

- It is defined as a new often-acute loss of neurological function secondary to parenchymal ischemia or hemorrhage.

Term

- Terminal ischemia – Sudden neurological deficit persisting atleast (TIA) <15 min with complex resolution by 24 hours.
- Reversible ischemia – Sudden neurological deficit more than stroke (RIND) 24 hours with resolution in 3 weeks.

Complete stroke (Cerebral infarction): Sudden neurological deficit lasting more than 21 days.

PATHOPHYSIOLOGY OF CEREBRAL ISCHEMIA

- Major cerebrovascular territories to be considered include those supplied by the anterior, middle and posterior cerebral arteries supratentorially and the superior cerebellar and anterior and posterior inferior cerebellar arteries infratentorially.
- The border or watershed zones are the areas between the terminal capillary beds of these major arterial territories.
- Terminal arterial branches of both the anterior and middle cerebral arteries supply the anterior border zone whereas the terminal arterial branches of the middle and posterior cerebral arteries supply the posterior border zone.
- Cerebral ischemia can be defined as the diminution of CBF to all or a portion of the brain, below the level needed to maintain normal cerebral function. The effects of ischemia are determined by the amount of flow reduction, the volume and location of tissue rendered ischemia and the duration of the event creating the ischemia state.
- Infarction results when the threshold level of ischemia has been exceeded resulting in tissue death.
- White matter is more resistant to ischemia than grey matter because of higher metabolic rate of white matter.
- Global cerebral ischemia is the diffuse diminution of cerebral blood flow that occurs with profound systemic hypotension, cardiac arrest or cerebral hypertension.
- With global ischemia, the most vulnerable neurons and the border zone are most subject to ischemic injury leading to cell death. The hippocampal pyramidal neurons, the cerebellar purkinjee cells, the striatal neurons and the

pyramidal neocortical neuron are the most vulnerable to ischemic injury.

- Ischemic penumbra is a team utilized to indicate the area of vulnerable, but potentially salvageable ischemic brain tissue that will return to normal function following restoration of cerebral blood flow.

Development of Edema

- In areas of ischemia, not only is there loss of autoregurgitation but there is also dysfunction of the ion transport and ATP pumps. The disordered transport at the cell membrane leads to water accumulation within the cell, referred to the cytotoxic edema.
- At 3 to 6 hours following the onset of ischemia, cytotoxic edema is evident within endothelial cells even though they are more resistant to ischemic injury than either glia or neurons. Ischemia leads to endothelial cell neurons and compromise to blood brain barrier with resultant leakage of water and plasma proteins into the extracellular space, referred to as vasogenic edema.
- Vasogenic edema begins to develop at 3 to 6 hours following the onset of significant ischemia and becomes maximal between 1 and 3 days following vascular occlusion.

Evolution of Stroke

- At 24 to 48 hours following the onset of ischemia leading to infarction, hemorrhagic transformation of an initially blank infarction may occur.
- Ischemia causes disturbances in the auto regulatory function of the formerly occluded vessel.
- The tissue appears hyperaemic because of rapid cerebral reperfusion. Reperfusion, superimposed on endothelial and parenchymal tissue damage created by the ischemia, results in parenchymal hemorrhage.

IMAGING BASIS IN STROKE

Hyperacute Infarction

- Within the first few hours after icterus, the stroke may be referred to as hyperacute.
- This stage correspond with the earlier cellular changes of cytotoxic edema and early neurotrophilic infiltration.

Signs

1. **Loss of gray-white differentiation**
   - It is attributed to cellular changes resulting from ischemia and secondary edema within a given territory.
   - It can be identified as early as 3 to 6 hours following the icterus particularly when the infarction involves a large vascular territory.
   - The area of hypodensity is initially ill defined, becoming progressively hypodense and better defined during the subsequent 24 to 48 hours.
2. **Early sulcal effacement**
   - Cytotoxin edema, identified within neurons and astrocytic possess within hours of the onset of ischemia and the subsequent influx of protein free fluids into the extracellular space, vasogenic oedema, results in early sulcal effacement.
   - This sign may be evident even before significant loss of grey white differentiation has occurred.
3. **Loss of insular ribbon**
   - It indicates early MCA infarction.
   - The insular ribbon refers to the gray and white matter tracts of the most lateral aspect of the insula, the claustrum, the extreme capsule and island of reil.
   - The claustral arteries and other insular branches of the MOA supply the insula.

- With impaired insular vascular supply, potential collateral are available from the adjacent lentiform nucleus, via the lenticulo striate arteries and the recurrent artery of keubner.
- When there is occlusion of the MCA distal to the lenticulostriate arteries, the insula is isolated from these potential sources of collateral supply and thus is essentially a border zone.
- Focal loss of gray-white differentiation with hypodensity on CT involving the insular ribbon is one of the contrast imaging manifestations of MCA infarction.

4. The hyperdense artery sign

- There is association between the increased density of the middle cerebral artery and the presence of intraluminal thrombus.
- The hyperdense MCA must be of higher density than both the surrounding brain and the contralateral MCA, unlike calcification, the hyperdense vessel should not be visible on bone windows.

5. Obscuration of the lentiform nucleus or loss of definition of the internal capsule

- It is an indication of early MCA infarction, resulting from occlusion of the lenticulo striate arteries.
- There is loss of grey-white differentiation between the lentiform nucleus and the internal and extreme capsule, such that its margins blend imperceptability with the internal capsule medially and the external capsule laterally and is said to "disappear".

ACUTE TO SUB ACUTE INFARCTION

- The subtle loss of gray-white differentiation and/or sulcal effacement on CT scan in the hyperacute stage of infarction, progress to more extensive hypodensity within the cortex and adjacent white matter between 8 and 24 hours following icterus:
- Over the next several days, the hypodense infarct becomes increasingly well defined and assumes a wedge shaped distribution with the base at the cortical surface. These well-defined margins develop because of the presence of intracellular (cytotoxic) oedema.
- The area of hypodensity is limited to the major vascular territory rendered ischemic.
- Between the 3rd and the 5th days following icterus, CT evidence of mass effect increases as cytotoxic and vasogenic edema increases.
- Mass effect may be most severe with larger infarcts particularly with those complicated by hemorrhage.
- Ventricular effacement with or without subfalcine or transtentorial herniation may be present.
- With transtentorial herniation, secondary PCA territory infarctions may result from compression of the PCA against the tentorium with compromise of the arterial flow.
- In the first week, the mass effect diminishes with resolution over the next 2 to 3 weeks.
- As the mass effect resolves, the density of the infarct become more heterogenous, particularly along the cortex, often characterized by iso or slightly hyperdense bands and nodular regions.
- Endothelial proliferation, capillary in growth and the development of collateral flow, each contribute the the heterogeneity which appears in the region of ischemic penumbra.

CHRONIC INFARCTS, LATE SEQUELAE OF CEREBRAL INFARCTION

- As the infarct progresses to a more chronic stage during the period from 4 weeks to 3 months, it returns to a more homogenous, well

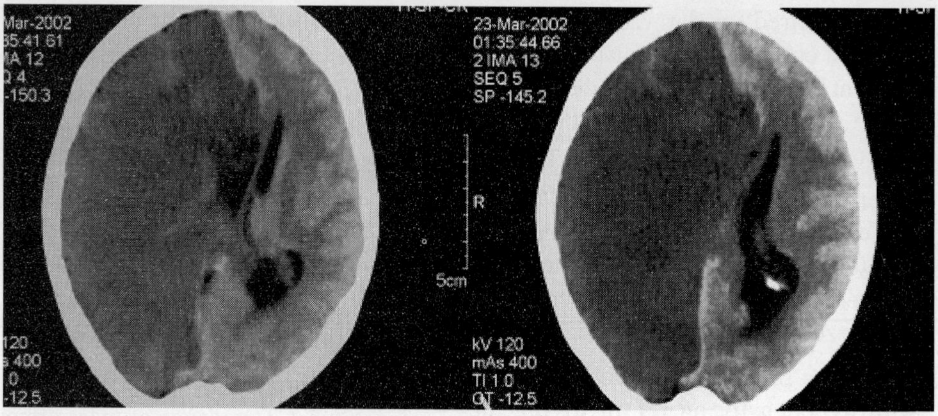

Fig. 2.1: Axial CT images show a large right cerebral infarct with mass effect and hydrocephalus

defined region of hypodensity. This corresponds to cavitation of the infart, with macrophage phagocytosis of necrotic tissue, lipid disposition and glial scar formation (Figures 2.1 and 2.2).

- As the infarct ages, the density approaches that of CSF.
- The greatest hypodensity and cystic change ensure in the central zone of the infarct, where ischemia is maximal.
- Adjacent cortical atrophy often results and may occasionally be only visible residue of infection.
- With larger infarcts, the volume loss may result in ex vacuo dilatation of the ipsilateral ventricle and sometimes, a shift of the contralateral hemisphere towards the side of the infarct.

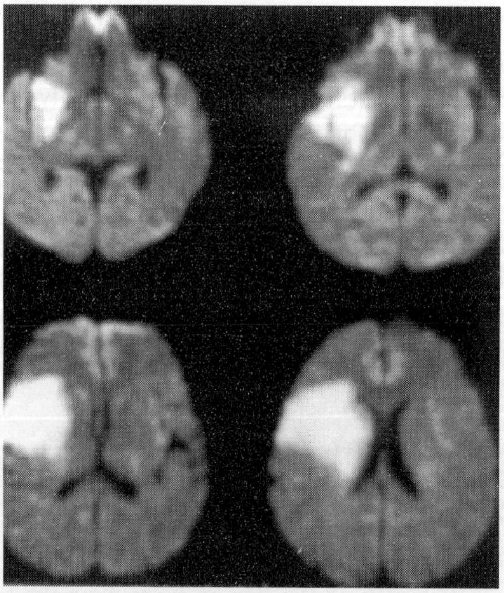

Fig. 2.2: Axial diffusion weighted images showing hyperacute infarct in right frontal lobe

CT CONTRAST ENHANCEMENT

- Infarcts reveal contrast enhancement in the subacute phase, which usually appears during the 2nd week after the onset of symptoms.
- Occasionally one of hypodensity become isodense with the surrounding brain following contrast enhancement and the infarction can be missed in a non-contrast examination if not obtained.
- The mechanism of CECT is the breakdown of the blood brain barrier mechanism of the capillary endothelium. Cerebral capillaries, with their tight junction between endothelial cells restrict the passage of most large molecules through their walls. Cerebral ischemia damages the blood brain barrier, thus permitting passage of these large molecules into the extracellular space.

- The limited circulation in the area of the hyperacute infarction prevents sufficient contrast from arriving at the site of capillary leakage.
- At 7 to 10 days cerebral edema is resolving and collateral circulation improves enough to allow capillary leakage and infarct enhancement to be visualized on CT.
- Enhancing infarcts are usually heterogenous owing to the presence of coagulation necrosis, capillary in growth and variable collateral circulation.
- Enhancement may be homogenous when there is incomplete necrosis and better reperfusion of the infarct.
- The cortex usually enhance more than the white matter on CT.
- With infarction most of the mass effect resolves by the time enhancement appears and the lesion confirm to a wedge shaped distribution with its base at the cortex within a single vascular territory.

MAGNETIC RESONANCE IMAGING IN INFARCTION

- The earliest signs of cerebral ischemia on MRI imaging are those that reflect abnormal blood flow to the affected area.
- Two signs have been described, the absence of a normal arterial flow void and the presence of intravascular enhancement following I.V. Gd compound administration.
- When the vessel is occluded, the low intensity flow void is replaced by increased signal intensity.
- Following contrast administration when flow is slowed within a vessel intravascular contrast is seen as high intensity signal similar to that seen in normal, slowly flowing veins.
- Angiographically, these findings have been correlated with occlusion or arterial slowing.
- The 1st parenchymal sign of acute stroke on spin echo MRI is anatomic distortion secondary to brain swelling. It is frequently manifested as sulcal effacement. Swelling is best appreciated on T1W1 within 2 hours of icterus. The pathophysiologic correlate in the stage of cytotoxic (intracellular) edema. Ed signal on T2W1 has been observed within 2 to 3 hours following icterus.
- The temporal onset of T2W1 abnormality corresponds with the development of vasogenic (extracellular) edema. With vasogenic edema, the T1W1 shows decreased signal intensity in the affected area.
- Meningeal enhancements following I.V. administration of good contrast agents may be seen in large infarcts by 1 to 3 days following icterus. It may represent reactive hyperemia or associated with venous engorgement.
- When enhancement is present early (within the first 3 days) and the area of enhancement exceeds the area of T2W1. High signal intensity, the patients usually suffer a minimal or reversible neurologic deficit consistent with partial ischemia.
- When enhancement appears late (within 1 to 2 weeks) and the area of T2WI high signal intensity equal or exceeds the area of enhancement, the patient usually has a fixed neurologic deficit consistent with infarct. This type of enhancement corresponds with capillary ingrowth and collateral development or luxury perfusion and may be demonstrated angiographically as a blush.
- The mass effect increases, becoming maximal at 2 to 4 days following the event and subsequently declines.

WALLERIAN DEGENERATION

- Cerebral infarcts may cause injury to the proximal axons of neurons in the cortico spinal tracts.
- At 4 to 14 weeks after infarction, hypointense signal is seen on T2WI.

- After 14 weeks, the signal becomes hyperintense on T2WI.

DIFFUSION WEIGHTED MRI

- DWI is sensitive to the random motion (Brownisn motion) of water molecules moving over distance with approximate the diameter of a cell (Figure 2.3).

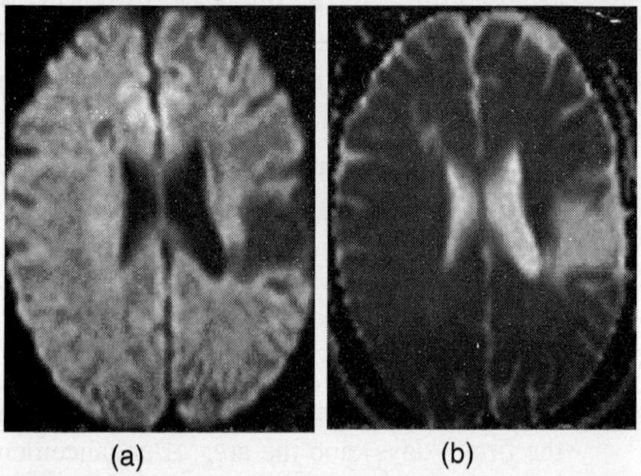

Fig. 2.3: (a) Diffusion-weighted MR image (b = 1000 sec/mm^2) shows areas of decreased signal intensity in the left frontal lobe. (b) ADC map shows increased ADC values in the white matter of the right frontal lobe. These features are suggestive of chronic infarction

- In bulk water and CSF, this motion is unhindered, thus the diffusion is high. The high diffusion tends to decrease signal thus areas of high diffusion have low signal intensity on DWI.
- Parenchymal diffusion decreases within minutes to hours following infarction. This reduction in diffusion has been referred to as restricted diffusion. It corresponds to the development (induction) of cytotoxic edema. The reduction in diffusion within areas of infarction, seen on DCO1 as increased signal intensity.
- In the days following icterus, the diffusion rises until it is increased compared with normal brain. This increases in diffusion II the increase in vasogenic edema and reflects the motion of the increased H_2O within the extracellular space. As edema resolves and encephalomalacia ensures, chronic infarcts develop high diffusion CSF.
- Two important clinical application of DWI in the setting of cerebrovascular disease is:
  1. The detection of early infarction.
  2. Differentiation of acute from subacute and chronic infarction.

DCO I show acute infarcts as high signal (restricted diffusion) subacute infarcts as areas of isointense to low signal and chronic infarcts as areas of low signal high definition.

PERFUSION WEIGHTED MRI

- From these imaging sequences, areas of decreased brain perfusion can be identified (Figure 2.4).
- The central zone of an acute infarct will show little or no perfusion while the ischemic penumbra will show decreased perfusion as compared to normal brain parenchyma. Comparison of DWI and perfusion images can better define the ischemic penumbra.
- In acute strokes, the area of perfusion abnormality is often larger than the corresponding diffusion abnormality and more closely approximates the area of the final infarcts.
- This perfusion/diffusion mismatch delineates the ischemic penumbra.

MAGNETIC RESONANCE ANGIOGRAPHY

- It is a non-invasive imaging that allows evaluation of the vascular anatomy both of the intra and extra cranial cerebral vessels.
- This imaging technique when combined with color duplex sonography has a very high accuracy in detecting vascular abnormality in neck vessels.
- In those instances where there is a discrepancy between the two imaging studies, conventional catheter cerebral angiography often resolves the presence or absence of stenosis or other vascular abnormalities.

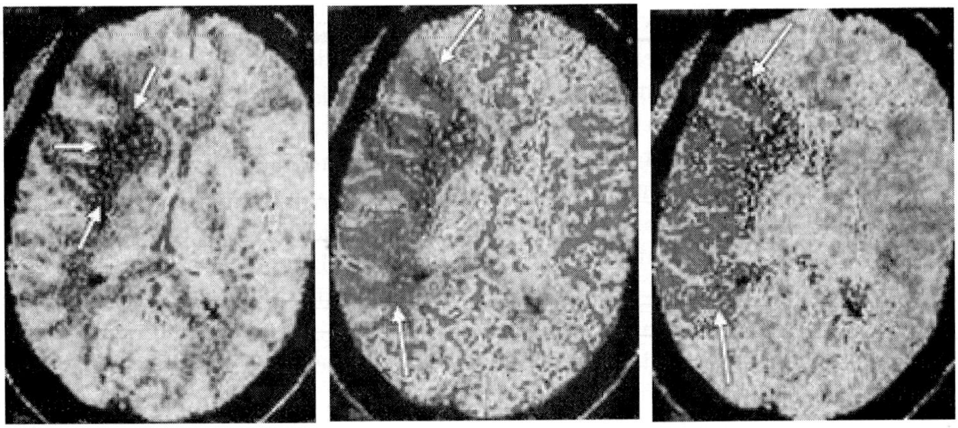

(a) (b) (c)

Fig. 2.4: Acute stroke in an old man with left hemiparesis. (a) CT perfusion maps of cerebral blood volume, (b) cerebral blood flow, and (c) mean transit time, show mismatched abnormalities (arrows) that imply the presence of a penumbra. The area with decreased blood volume represents the ischemic core, and that with normal blood volume but decreased blood flow and increased mean transit time is the penumbra

- The non-invasive intracranial vascular abnormalities associated with stroke are best evaluated with 3D TOF or 3D PC imaging.
- Limitation of either of these two imaging sequences is the lack of clear visualization of medium and small vessels (Figure 2.5).

WHITE MATTER ISCHEMIC CHANGES

- Ischemic changes in the white matter can involve the periventricular region, the deep white matter of the subcortical regions of the brain.
- On CT they are seen as areas of hypodensity and may be difficult to detect unless there is confluence.
- On MR imaging they are seen as bright signals on T2WI in the periventricular regions usually beyond the age of 60 years and usually represent glial or ependymal scarring.

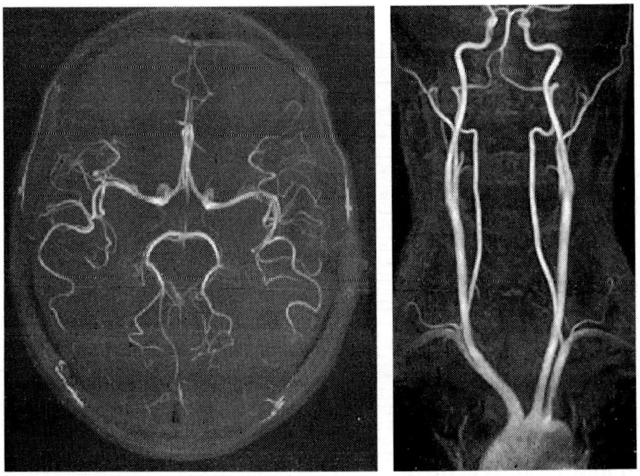

Fig. 2.5: MRA show the vessels known as the Circle of Willis in the brain and neck vessels

- Hyperintense signal within the subcortical white matter and deep white matter resulting from ischemia is not uncommon as part of the ageing process, present in nearly 30 to 60% of older population. They are more common in a variety of neurodegenerative diseases and as a consequence of hyperintensive disease. These foci of bright signal may represent lacunar infarcts.
- They are located in the basal ganglia and thalamus, regions supplied by long single penetrating end arteries.
- In patients under age 40, demyelinating disease is the more common etiology whereas infarction is more likely in the immuno-comprromised.
- Enlarged perivascular (Virrshow-Robin) space may be seen at any age, but have increased prevalence in-patient over age 60. These are most commonly seen in the anterior perforated substance accompanying the lenticulo striate arteries, but may also be seen extending into the centrum semiovale. Virchow Robin spaces follow the signal intensity of CSF on all sequences.
- Periventricular hypertensities correspond pathologically to myelin pallor. They are best seen on short TE, long TR (PDWI) sequences and FLAIL sequences where they appear hyperintense to both brain and CSF.

SPECIFIC DISEASE PROCESSES IN STROKE

Ischemic Infarction

- The typical stroke occurs secondary to occlusive disease involving the large arteries, most commonly atherosclerotic carotid stenosis.
- Thrombosis of the proximal internal carotid artery or distal embolisation from friable thrombus at the carotid bifurcation may result in cerebral ischemia and progress to infarction depending on the duration and degree of ischemia.
- Duplex sonography, MRA and more recently, CTA are all non-invasive techniques capable of imaging the extra cranial carotid to image the degree of stenosis.
- Duplex sonography is the least invasive and least costly screening test with a long, excellent track record in the detection of carotid stenosis.
- MRA is a more expensive screen test than duplex sonography and tends to be more utilized more frequently than cranial MRI for patient's diagnostic evaluation. MRA can demonstrate extracranial stenosis but may overestimate the degree of stenosis.
- CTA requires as a contrast bolus and requires significant post processing time, yet it has the ability to provide quantification of the degree of stenosis.
- The gold standard for assessment of carotid stenosis remains carotid arteriography. It is invasive and requires intracranial contrast injection.
- Angiography permits assessment of tandem and B/L lesions as well as the extent of collateral flow through the circle of willis, leptomeningeal and external carotid collaterals.
- Mechanisms leading to cerebral infarctions in patients with atherosclerotic extracranial carotid stenosis include thrombosis with stenosis or occlusion, embolus formation, fragmentation and migration from the site of the atherosclerotic plaque and information due to intracranial hypoperfusion (decreased CBF) associated with a critical stenosis.
- Thrombosis may occur suddenly, as when there is sub intimal hemorrhage under a plaque or may ensure more gradually often allowing for the development of collateral vascular supply to the tissue at risk.
- The pattern or distribution of infarction following internal carotid artery occlusion may vary from a large, almost holohemispheric infarctions to a small cortical infarct in the periphery of the vascular territory at risk.

Hemorrhagic Infarction

- Revascularization after vascular occlusion

results in hemorrhagic transformation of the infarction.

- The ischemic, initially bland infarctions may develop variable amount of hemorrhage, often potential within 2 hours to 2 weeks following vascular occlusion.
- Hemorrhagic infarction occurs most commonly with stroke caused by emboli from carotid or other sources; atherosclerotic thrombotic infarcts in patients with coagulation disorders or in those on anticoagulant therapy and in hypertension.
- Hemorrhagic infarction is characterized pathologically by potential hemorrhages spread diffusely throughout the infarcted tissue predominating in the grey matter. The cortex at the depth of the sulci is particularly vulnerable to hemorrhagic transformation.
- The longer the period of ischemia before reperfusion occur, the greater the tissue injury and greater the risk of hemorrhagic transformation.
- On CT, hemorrhage may be seen at the depths of sucli as a diffuse ribbon of increased density following the gyri or may extend into the adjacent white matter, mimicking a primary parenchymal hematoma. There is residual hypo-density in the adjacent white matter.
- On MRI, the cortical hemorrhage is initially isointense to slightly hypointense of T1WI and hypointense on T2WI. By the end of the 1st week following hemorrhagic transformation, the T1W1 frequently demonstrated gyriform cortical hyperintensity whereas on T2WI there is cortical hyperintensity. Peripheral contrast enhancement may be identified surrounding the areas of hemorrhage.

Hypertensive Hemorrhage

- Severe HTN is a significant risk factor for stroke.
- CT readily permits identification of parenchymal hematoma or petechial hemorrhage.
- MRI is useful for the detection of blood products in various stage of Hb degeneration and reflects the timing of hemorrhage.
- Hypertensive hematoma occur in the elderly are most commonly located in the basal ganglia and internal capsule. The lateral putamen is the most common site of origin, although the caudate nucleus, brainstem and the thalamus are all frequent locations. Larger parenchymal hematoma frequently ruptures into the ventricular system resulting in hydrocephalus, ventricular obstruction and mass effect on the adjacent normal parenchyma.

NCCT

- The acute hypertensive parenchymal hematoma appears as a homogenously dense, well defined lesion with mass effect and initially little surround edema.

MRI

T1WI–Iso to slightly hypointense to gray matter.
T2WI – markedly hypointense.

Age of hemorrhage	T1W – MR	T2W MR
Hyperacute (<24 hrs) Oxy Hb begins changing to deoxy Hb within 3 hrs becomes hypointense within 1-2 days	Isointense	Initially hyperintense
Acute (1-3 days) deoxy Hb	Iso to hypointense	Hypointense
Subacute (early 1-2 weeks) Intracellular met. Hb (later 2-4 weeks) Extracellular met Hb	Hyperintensity begins peripherally, solid hyperintensity at 2-3 weeks	Hypointense until 2 weeks then peripheral hypointensity progress to solid hyperintensity at 2-3 weeks.
Chronic > 1 month	Isointense to mildly hypointense the periphery begins more hypointense with time	Hypointense periphery progresses to complete hypointensity

Chapter 3

Intracranial Infections

1. **Congenital/Neonatal Infections**
   - TORCH.
   - HIV infection.
   - Varicella.
   - Enteroviruses.

2. **Meningitis**
   - Acute pyogenic meningitis.
   - Acute lymphocytic meningitis (Figure 3.1).
   - Chronic meningitis.

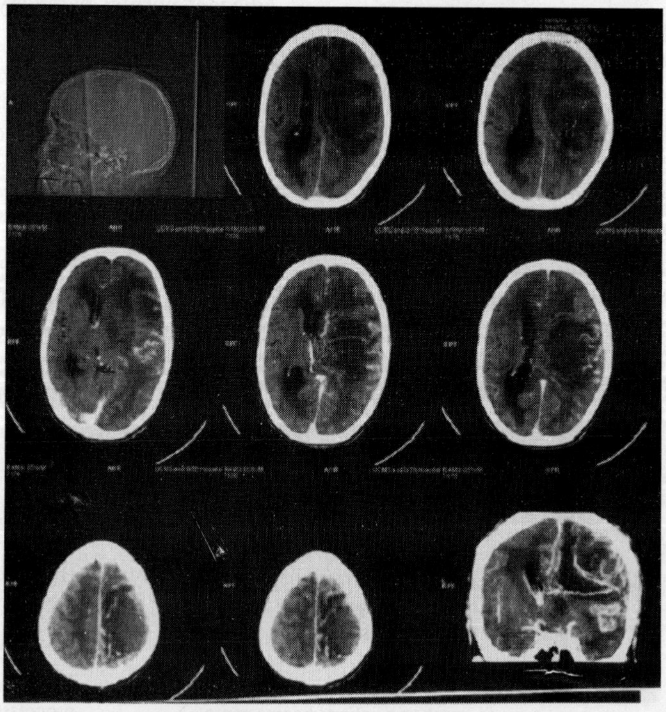

Fig. 3.1: Serial axial non-contrast and contrast-enhanced CT images shows features of meningitis, abscess formation with multiple satellite lesions

3. Pyogenic Parenchymal Infection

- Cerebritis and abscess.
- Complications of cerebral abscess (Figure 3.2).

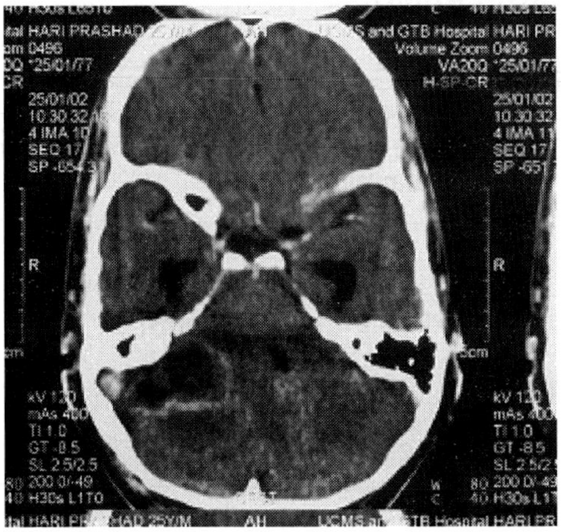

Fig. 3.2: Axial CT image shows cerebellar abscess on right side

4. Encephalitis

- Herpes simplex encephalitis.
- HIV encephalitis and other CNS infections in AIDS.
- Misc. viral encephalitis.
- Post-infection encephalitis.

5. T. B. and Fungal Infections

- CNS T.B.
- Fungal infections.

6. Parasitic Infections

- Neuro cysticercosis (Figure 3.3).
- Misc. parasitic infections.

CONGENITAL CNS INFECTIONS

Agents

- TORCH.
- HIV.

Routes

- Hematogenous-transplacental (toxoplasmosis, most viruses).
- Ascending cervical infection (bacteria).
- At birth (herpes virus).

Results (Vary with Timing of Infection Relative to Fetal Development)

- Malformations (e.g. neuronal migrational abnormalities).
- Brain destruction.
- Dystrophic calcification.

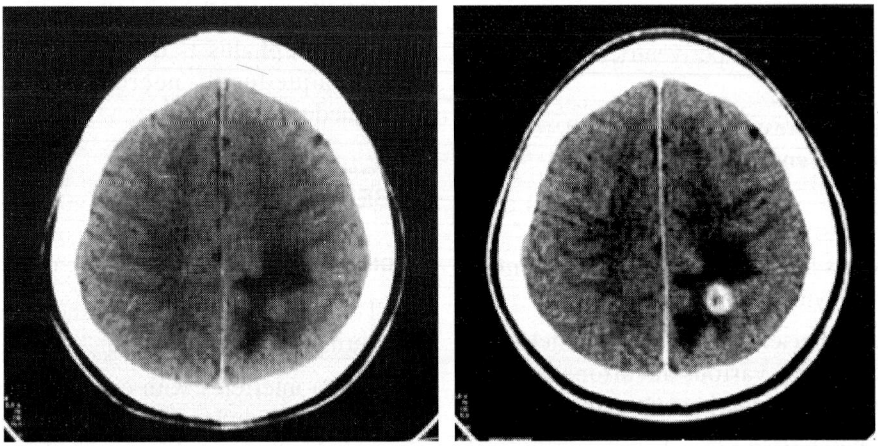

Fig. 3.3: Cranial CT scan without (left) and with (right) contrast medium, showing a rounded lesion with prominent ring enhancement in the left parieto-occipital subcortical region— neuro cysticercosis

CMV

Etiology

- DNA virus that belong to herpes virus group.
- Humans are the only reservoir.

Location

- 60% multiple organ system involvement.
- 70% intracranial abnormalities.
- 1/3rd cardiac anomalies and HSM.

CMV has a particular affinity for the developing germinal matrix. Widespread periventricular tissue necrosis with subsequent calcification occurs. Other frequently effected sites are cerebral white matter and cortex, cerebellum, brain stem and spinal cord.

C/F

- Premature birth.
- Hepato splenomegaly, jaundice, thrombocytopenia and chorio retinitis are common manifestation.
- Seizures, MR, OA, SNH H and hydrocephalus.

Imaging

Plain film radiography: Encephaly with periventricular calcifications.

USG: Bilateral periventricular calcifications preceded by hypo echoic periventricular ring like zones.

CMV can also result in widespread cerebral death with severe encephalomalacia.

CT

- NECT scans atrophy, ventricular enlargement and parenchymal calcifications.
- CMV can cause widespread parenchymal calcification in various locations but the periventricular region is most common.
- Neuronal migration anomalies are common.

MR migrational anomalies, encephalomalacia with non-specific ventricular enlargement and prominent nuclei, delayed myelination and subependymal paraventricular cysts and calcifications.

TOXOPLASMOSIS

Etiology

- Caused by T. gondii which is an obligate intracellular parasite.
- Oocysts in infected meat or cat feces.
- Hematogenous spread to the placenta and fetus occurs during maternal parasites.

Location

- Basal ganglia.
- Periventricular.
- Peripheral location.

C/F

- Mild undiluted cases to seizures with encephaly, very early infectious-abortions.

  Unilateral, bilateral chorioretinitis and intracranial calcifications form the typical triad found in infants.
- Host most common site of calcification – basal ganglia and cortex.
- Hydrocephalus is due to ependymitis with periaqueductal necrosis that results in aqueductal stenosis.

RUBELLA

Etiology

- Transmitted through the plancenta to the fetus during maternal uraemia.

Rubella interferes with cellular multiplication, inhibiting proliferation of immature undifferentiated progenitol cells located in germinal matrix.

C/F

Mild manifestions to spontaneous abortions, stillbirth of devastating abnormalities:

- Cataract, glaucoma, chorioretinitis, enophthalmos, cardiac malformations and microcephaly.
- Severe infections and deafness are later manifestations.
- Meningoencephalitis, thrombocytopenia HS and LAD.

Imaging

USG

- Sub ependymal cysts in nucleus and the striothalamic regions (+).
- Echogenic foci in the basal ganglia represent mineralizing vasculitis with calcification.

CT

- Microcephaly and parenchymal calcification (+) cortex and BG are affected.

MR

- Deep and subcortical white matter lesions caused by vascular injury and ischemic necrosis.

Delayed Myelination

Herpes Simplex

- Type 1.
- Type 2 → genital herpes.
- Most neonatal infections are posturitional acquired through direct contact between the infants skin, eyes or oral cavity and maternal herpatic lesion in the cervix or vagina.
- Associated infection can also occur after membrane rupture during delivery.
- Gross microphaly, AC enopthalmia, and chorioretinitis are seen.

Location

- Acute neonatal HSV infections cause diffuse brain involvement.
- The limbic system localization (temporal, lobes, angulate gyrus) that is so characteristics in older children and adult infections does not occur.
  1. Cerebritis stage.
  2. Early capsule stage.
  3. Late capsule stage.

MR

- Early cerebritis stage.
- Late cerebritis stage.
- Cerebral abscess.

C/F

Neontal herpetic infections are divided into the following 3 clinical categories:

1. Skin, eye and mouth lesions.
2. Disseminated diseases.
3. CNS infections.

Imaging

CT

NECT – Focal or diffuse white matter lucency, the relative hyperdensity of cortical gray matter appears accentuated.

- Hemorrhagic infarction may occur.
- Long-term sequelae-diffuse atrophy and multicystic encephalomalacia.

MR

- The neonatal brain is largely uncomplicated. Diffuse white matter oedema is difficult to detect. Hemorrhage change are occ (+).
- Parenchymal and meningeal enhancement following contrast administration (+).

HIV INFECTION

- Perinatal transmission is the most common route of HIV infection.
- Nearly 80% of all childhood HIV infections are maternally transmitted.

CT

NECT–Diffuse cerebral atrophy in 90% of cases. BL calcification are seen in few cases:

- Hemorrhage can occur in children with thrombocytopenia.

MR

Most common findings is non-specific cerebral atrophy:

- Foci of increased signal on T2W are seen in the peripheral and deep white cerebral matter.
- Hemorrhagic cerebral infarcts.

MENINGITIS

Acute pyogenic meningitis.

Etiology

Neonates – Group B streptococcus, E. coli.

Children under 7 – H. influenzae.

Older children – N. meningitis.

Adults – S. pneumoniae.

Pathology: Purulent exudate in basilar cistern, sulci, perivascular inflammation, vasospasm common.

CT

A normal scan is the most common finding in children with acute bacterial meningitis.

- Mild ventricular dilatation and subarachnoid space enlargement are early abnormalities on NECT scans.
- Effacement of the basilar or convexity cisterns by inflammatory exudate can be seen.
- Less than 1/3rd of all children with clinically documented meningitis have abnormally enhancing meninges on CECT.

MR

- Precontrast T1W1 may show obliterated cisterns that enhance strongly following contrast administration.
- Extension of enhancing subarachnoid exudate deep into the sulci can be seen in severe cases.

Complications of Meningitis

1. Hydrocephalus and ventriculitis.
2. Subdural effusion.
3. Subdural empyema.
4. Parenchymal lesions:
   - Cerebritis.
   - Abscess.
   - Oedema with or without cardiac herniation.
5. Cerebral infarction.

Hydrocephalus and Ventriculitis

- Extensive fibrinos purulent exudate can obstruct the subarachnoid space and result in extra ventricular (communicating) hydrocephalus.
- Aqueductal or outlet obstruction cause intraventricular (non communicating) hydrocephalus.
- Ventriculitis occurs in 30% of all patients and over 90% of neonates with meningitis.
- The ependymal lining of the ventricles enhance intensity.
- Choroid plexities is sometimes present.

Subdural Effusion (SDE)

- SDE are caused by inflammation of subdural veins with fluid and albumin seepage into the subdural space.

- Imaging findings of SDE are concentric extra axial fluid collections that are similar to CSF on both CT and MR.

Empyema

- Nearly half of all cases are caused by sinusitis; the frontal sinus is the most common source.
- Imaging findings in cerebral emphysemas show concentric or lentiform extra axial collections that are low density on CT and mildly hyperintense compared to CSF on T2 weighted MR studies.
- The cerebral convexities and interhemispheric fissures are common site.
- A surrounding membrane that enhance intensely and uniformly following contrast administration is typically identified.

Cerebrovascular Complications

- These include cerebral infarction, vessel wall irregularities, focal dilatations, arterial occlusion, venous infarcts and dural sinus thrombosis.

CHRONIC MENINGITIS

Etiology

- Caused by mycobacterium tuberculosis. Other organisms include coccidiodomycosis imitans and cryptococcus neoformans.

Location

- It has predilection for basal cisterns although more generalized disease can occur.

Imaging

CT

NECT scans chronic meningitis shows 'on plaque' dural thickening. Popecorn like dural calcification are seen around basal cistern.

NECT

It shows abnormal meningeal enhancing sequelae include atrophy and cerebral infarction.

MR

- Contrast enhanced T1W MR scans show characteristic basal meningeal inflammatory pattern.
- Calcific meningeal nodules are markedly hypointense on all pulse sequence.
- Peripheral enhancement often persists.

PYOGENIC PARENCHYMAL INFECTIONS

Etiology

- The most common cause is hematogenous spread from an extra cranial site.
- Mastoid and sinus infections spread directly to the CNS then retrograde thrombophlebitis and may be preceded by emphysema, meningitis or both.
- Congenital or acquired dural dehiscence and dermal sinus are less common cause.
- The organisms most frequently isolated from cerebral abscess are streptococci (both aerobic and anaerobic) and staphylococci, although gram negative organisms are an increasing cause of cerebral abscess.

Neonates

- Citrobasiter.
- Proteins.
- Pseudomonas.
- Serratia.
- Staphylococcus aureus.

Pathology

- Stages of intracranial abscess development.
- Early celebritis 3 to 5 days.

- Late cerebritis 4 to 5 days to 10 to 14 days.
- Early capsule–begins at about 2 weeks.
- Late capsule–may last for weeks/months.

Early Cerebritis

During this stage infection is focal but not yet localized. An unencapsulated mass of congested vessels with perivascular PMNCs infilterates and edema is seen. Scattered necrotic foci and microscopic petechial hemorrhages without frank tissue destruction is seen.

Late Cerebritis

The infection becomes more focal as small necrotic zones coalesce. Vessels proliferate and a central necrotic core is formed that is surrounded by an ill-defined ring of inflammatory cells, macrophages granulation tissue and fibroblast.

Early Capsule

- Collagen and reticulin form a well-delineated capsule around a core consisting of liquefied necrotic and inflammatory debris.

Late Capsule

- During the late capsule stage, the capsule is complete and consists of the following 3 layers:
  a. An inner inflammatory layer of granulation tissue of macrophage.
  b. A middle collagenous layer.
  c. An outer gliotic layer.

Location

- The corticomedullary (gray-white matter) junction is the most common location of the frontal and parietal are the most frequent sites.

Imaging

Nuclear medicine: 99m Tc HMPAO, a new radionuclide imaging label for leukocytes and radio labelled polyclonal immunoglobulin (IgG) antibodies may be helpful.

CT

Early Cerebritis

NECT scans may be normal or show only a poorly marginated subcortical hypodense area. In CECT studies disclose an ill-defined contrast enhancing area within the edematous region.

Section 1—Central Nervous System

Chapter 4

Intraventricular Masses

Intraventricular masses comprise 1/10th of all CNS neoplasm. Are readily seen on cross-sectional images, but myriad possibilities make a focus differential diagnosis elusive.

By using clinical, demographic and imaging findings, one can significantly limit the D/D for many of most common intraventricular neoplasm.

Lateral ventricles are paired C-shaped structure; each is sub-divided into frontal born, body atrium, occipital horn and temporal horn.

50% of intraventricular tumor in adults and 25% in children are found in lateral ventricle.

Frontal Horn

CSP and CV are common developmental anomaly. 80% of normal neonates have CSP M; CV is seen in 30% term infants. Both CSP and CV shrink and eventually disappear after birth. A persistent CSP is seen in 2-4% of normal adults and which is seen as CSF filled collection contained between two septal leaves. CV never occurs without CSP. A CV is seen as finger like CSF collection that lies in midline below corpus collosum and between fornices.

Primary septal neoplasms are uncommon astrocytoma being the most common. A septum pellusidum >3mm is suspicious for infiltrating neoplasm.

Body

PNET (Primitive neuroectodermal tumor) most common (Medulloblastoma) in children and astrocytoma in adults is the most common neoplasm in this location.

Atrium

CPP is most common trigone mass in young children, ependymoma and astrocytoma occur in older children. Meningioma, metastasis and lymphoma are typical lesions in older adults.

Occipital and Temporal Horns

Primary intraventricular masses are very uncommon in occipital horn.

Foramen of Monro (FM) and Anterior Third Ventricle

FM is a Y shaped structure that connects two lateral ventricles with third ventricle. FM masses are uncommon young children. Subependymal Giant Cell Astrocytoma (SGCA) occur in older children and young adults with tuberous sclerosis.

Anterior Third Ventricle

Colloid cysts are most common mass in this location, common in adults 20-40 years) M=F. Smooth gelatinous filled cystic masses on CT 2/3 hypodense, noncalcified, rim enhancement.

On MR variable signal, most common hypointense or T1W, hypointense on T2W, turbulent CSF flow mimics a colloid cyst; however less inferiorly in the third ventricle.

Primary third ventricular neoplasm are rare at any age, most are astrocytomas in adults third ventricular masses are usually secondary to extra ventricular lesions.

Aqueduct

The cerebral aqueduct communicates antero-superiorly with third ventricle and posteroinferiorly with the 4th ventricle. Stenosis is the most common intrinsic aqueduct abnormality.

4th Ventricle

Primary 4th ventricle neoplasms are common in children but none in adults. Cerebellar astrocytoma are most common post fossa tumor followed by PNET-MB. In adults metastases are most common neoplasm. Primary post fossa tumors are rare.

Ependymoma

Arise from differential ependymal cell that line cerebral ventricle and central canal of S.C. 3-9% of neuroepithelial neoplasm 6-12% of paed brain tumor and 1/3 of all brain tumor of patient younger than 3 years. May present at any age and no gender predilection.

Post fossa ependymoma arise in children with mean age of 64 years for supratentorial (T) mean age is higher are extra ventricular.

58% originate in 4th ventricle and rest in lateral and 3rd ventricle.

Children have bad prognosis than adults and supratentorial tumor have better survival rates. They are well-circumscribed, greyish red masses that usually fill ventricular lumen and extent into adjacent brain parenchyma and into CP angle and foramen magnum.

Subependyoma

Prevalence 0.4%, smaller than 2 cm. However, symptomatic (T) are larger. Are well circumscribed, grow in slow fashion, are usually avascular and attached with ventricular wall with marrow pedicle. The prognosis with intraventricular subependyoma is good with gross surgical dissection being curative.

Central Neurocytoma

It is reserved for (T) in lateral and 3rd ventricle. Lesions with similar histological characters but located outside these location should be referred to extraneural central cytoma. Arise from septum pellucidum or ventricular wall and often contain calcification or hemorrhage strikingly similar to oligodendroglioma (the classic Friday appearance). Total surgical resection is treatment of choice and typically curative. But with extraneural extension (T) outcome is poor.

Subependymal Giant Cell Astrocytoma

In most common cerebral neoplasm in tuberous sclerosis (6-16%) but it itself is present in almost all patient of tuberous sclerosis. It is characterized by slow growth and benign biological behaviours. Earlier diagnosis is associated with increased survival. Neurosurgical resection is treatment of choice.

Choroid plexus papilloma and carcinoma neoplasm can arise anywhere this tissue exists. Most of these (approx 80%) occurs as benign, slowly growing with favourable prognosis – The other 20% of cases manifest as more biological aggressive C.P. carcinoma which is more common in children. They have been associated with hydrocephalus and symptoms related to increased intracranial pressure due to increased CSF production by the tumor. These are soft well circumscribed, cauliflower like masses with prominent lobulation periphery. Hemorrhage and cyst formation may be seen. Necrosis and parenchymal lesion are characteristic of CPC.

Transformation of CPP to CPC has been reported in small number of patients.

When these tumors occur in region of trigone engulfment rather than invasion of choroid plexus has been described, extension from one ventricle to other or into CP angle is characteristic feature of choroid plexus (T).

Choroid plexus papilloma (Figure 4.1) appear lobulated uniformly echogenic masses at USG and demonstrate bi-directional flow continuing throughout diastole. Enlargement of choroidal artery is common feature in cross-sectional and angiographic images.

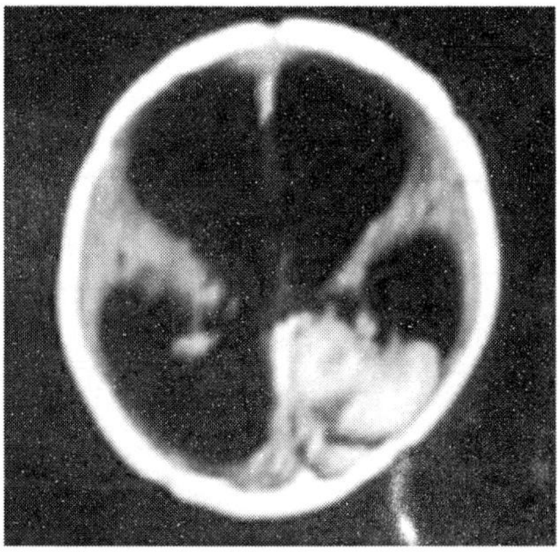

Fig. 4.1: Axial CT image shows choroid plexus papilloma with severe hydrocephalus

Intraventricular Meningioma

Are rare ~ 0.7% of all meningioma. Still it is more common intraventricular (T) (atrial) in adult population. They arise from arachnoid cap cells trapped within choroid plexus tele choroidae or velum interpositum. Correspondingly trigone of lateral. Ventricle is the most common site, left side slightly more common.

Nearly all of these (T) have benign histological characteristics except in children, which has predilection for sarcomatous changes. Metastasis is rare.

MR spectroscopy of intraventricular meningioma have revealed pattern similar to meningioma outside ventricle system with decreased amount of N-acetyl aspartate and creatinine; ↑ed amount of choline. Preoperative embolisation may be efficacious in limiting blood loss and reduction is size of mass before surgery.

Metastasis

To choroid plexus is rare accounting for 0.9% to 4.6% of all cerebral metastasis. The most common source is renal and lung carcinoma. In children neuroblastoma, retinoblastoma and Wilm's tumor is the most common primary tumor. Lateral ventricle is the most common site for metastatic spread followed by 3rd ventricle. RCC is noteworthy for its propensity to produce solitary metastasis upto 50 years after detection of primary lesion and for its imaging appearance that mimics intraventricular meningioma.

PAEDIATRIC TUMOR

Cerebellar Astrocytoma

Most common post fossa tumor in children accounting for 1/4th of all 4th ventricle tumor in this age group. Most of them are pilocytic type with appearance of large cystic mass with a mural nodule. They arise from vermis and extent anteriorly into 4th ventricle.

Medulloblastoma (PNET-MB) is the 2nd most common post fossa tumor in children accounting for 25% of all intracranial tumors. 90% are midline originating in inferior vermis and fill the 4th ventricle. Subarachnoids dissemination is common.

SUMMARY

By using clinical, demographic and imagined findings one can significantly limit the differential diagnosis for many of the most common intraventricular neoplasms. Ependymomas are typically calcified, more common in children are more common in 4th ventricle and shows intense enhancement. Subependymoma and central neurocytomas have affinity for anterior portion of lateral ventricles and both commonly demonstrate heterogeneous cystic appearance. Subependymoma are more common in older adults whereas central neurocytomas are more common before 40 years of age. SEGA always was near foramen of monro, characterized by frequent calcification, intense enhancement on contrast enhanced studies and presence of other stigmata seen in TS when a mass is centred in choroids plexus, a highly vascular tumor either CPP, CPC, meningioma or metastasis should be suspected.

Sellar and Suprasellar Masses

Sella Turcica

Is a cup shaped depression in the central basisphenoid bone that contains pituitary gland and infundibular stalk. Length–11-16 mm, depth 8-12 mm, side to side 11-19 mm.

Loss of definition dorsum sellae–elderly, prolonged hypertension, chronic raised intracranial pressure.

Pituitary Gland–Two Lobes

- Adenohypophysis–pars tuberalis, pars intermedia, pars distalis.
- Neurohypophysis–post pituitary lobe, infundibular stalk, supra optic and para ventricular hypothalamic nuclei.

CT

It appears homogenous and isodense to cavernous sinus. Mildly inhomogeneous– adolescents and menstruating women.

MRI

A well demarcated zone of higher signal on both T1 and T2W images.

Empty Sella

Is a very common anatomic variant in which the sella is partially filled with CSF. The gland itself appears thinned and confined against the bony floor.

- Sella often enlarged due to pulsating CSF.

Secondary Causes

- Hypophysectomy.
- Radiation therapy.
- Pituitary necrosis.

Size and shape of sella occurs as per age and gender.

Infundibulum: 3-3.5 mm near the med. Eminence 2 mm–pituitary gland.

Intrasellar

1. Neoplasms and cysts.
   - Common–adenoma.
     - Non-neoplastic cysts (pars intermedia, colloid RCC).
   - Uncommon–craniopharyngioma-mets, Meningioma, epidermoid or dermoid cyst.

Vascular Lesions

- Aneurysms.
- Para median C-art.

Inflammatory

- Hypophysitis.
- Abscess.

Suprasellar

i. Neoplasms

- Common
  - Macro adenoma.
  - Meningioma.
  - Craniopharyngioma.
  - Glioma.
- Uncommon
  - Lipoma.
  - Dermoid.
  - Metastasis.
  - Germinoma.

ii. Vascular lesions

- Vascular ectasias.
- Supraarachnoid ICA aneurysms.

iii. Cong lesions

- Arachnoid cyst.
- Rathkel's cleft cyst.
- Hypothalamic hematoma.

iv. Inflammatory and infections

- Meningitis.
- Sarcoidosis.
- Cysticercosis.

PITUITARY ADENOMA

- 7-8% of intracranial tumors, peak in 4th and 5th decade.
- Virtually all originate in anterior lobe.
- Majority are now believed to be secretory.
- Macro and micro adenoma (Figure 5.1).

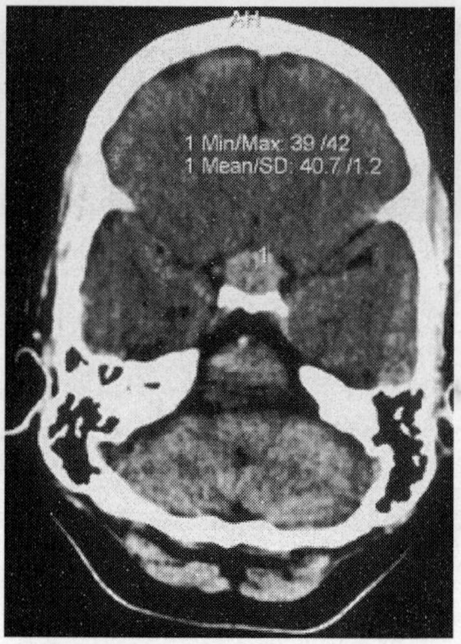

Fig. 5.1: Axial contrast enhanced CT image shows pituitary macroadenoma

Symptoms

- Amenorrhoea.
- Galactorrhea.
- Gigantism.
- Endocrine active – 80%.

IMAGING

Plain X-ray

- Expand and erode the pituitary fosse (Figure 5.2).
- Ballooned sella–classically.
- Local bulging of the sellar floor–double floor.

CT

Microadenoma–Hypodense or isodense on NECT.

- Delayed enhancement compared to the immediate intense enhancement of normal pituitary gland.
- 1/3rd may show early enhancement.

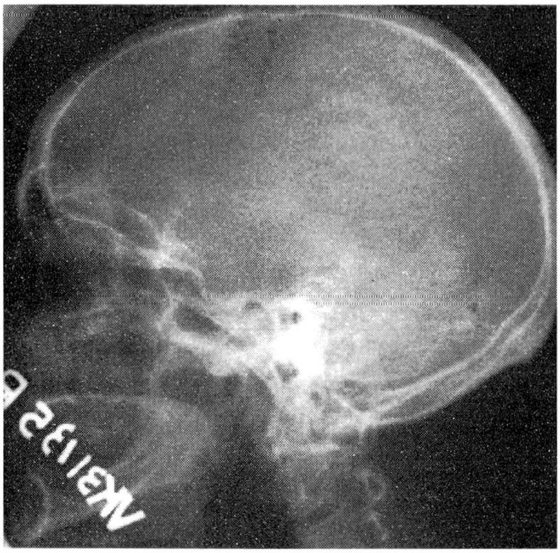

Fig. 5.2: Radiograph of the skull shows enlarged sella due to sellar mass

Macroadenoma

- Variable appearance isodense with artery on NECT and show moderate enhancement.
- Necrosis, cyst formation and hemorrhage may result in mixed density lesions.
- Large adenomas seen producing chiasmal compression extending to suprasellar cistern and then anterior end of 3rd ventricle.
- Invasion is common with prolactin or GH producing adenoma features like – infundibular deviation and upward bulging of the upper surface.

MRI

- Appear hypointense on T1W and hyperintense on T2W. Delayed enhancement on dynamic scanning.

Rathke's Cleft Cyst

- Develops as a nostril out pouching from the primitive stomodeum during the 3rd and 4th gestation week.
- Cystic lesion with mucoid or serous content.
- 4th-6th decade, F: M – 2:1:1.
- 70% both intra-supra, 20-25% - intrasellar.
- Usually a symptomatic.

CT

Well refined low density on NECT -75%, no calcification, capsular enhancement – 50%.

MR

2/3rd – hyperintense to brain on T1WI.

1/3rd low signal like CSF.

More unpredictable on T2W–50% hyperintense typically do not entrance.

Colloid Cysts

Assumed to be neuroectodermal origin. Recent studies suggest endoderm origin.

- Range from a few mm to 3-4 cm in size.
- Grossly, smooth spherical gelatinous filled cystic mass.
- 20-40 cm.

Type anterior 3rd ventricle/foramen of monro attached to roof of 3rd ventricle and choroids plexus.

Symptoms due to typical location–intermittent or prolonged ↑ ICT. Headache, vertigo, memory deficits, coma and death have been reported.

CT

2/3 hyperdense, 1/3rd isodense, non-calcified lesions. Occasional rim enhancement.

MRI

Variable signal.

MC

Hyperintense on T1W1.

Hypointense on T2W.

Craniopharyngioma

- Arise from squamous epithelial rests along the involuted hypophyseal Rathke's duct.
- Typically it is a lobulated, well delineated cystic mass with a mural nodule.
- 50% of paediatric suprasellar tumors.
- Headache most common symptoms.

  70% combined supra/intrasellar.

CT- NECT

Cystic, lobulated, suprasellar mass with a mural nodule.

- Nodular or rim calcification.

Cyst contents – Higher attenuation than CSF.

- Nodular or rim enhancement >90%.

MRI

Very variable. Most common of a cyst.

ASTROCYTOMA OF VISUAL PATHWAY

- Accounts for 25-30% paediatric suprasellar masses.
- NF-1 in 20-25% low-grade artrocytoma.
- On CT – isodense to hypodense and frequently enhance following contrast administration.

MRI

Hypo on T1W and hyperintense on T2W.

- Post chiastmatic enhancement or signal abnormality on T2W is suggestive of but not pathognomonic of glioma because long standing compressive lesions such as adenoma or craniopharyngiomas also occasionally shows enhancement.

Meningiomas

Second most common suprasellar neoplasm – adults 40-60 years.

- Most parasellar meningiomas originate in sphenoid ridge, diaphragm or tuberculum sellae.
- Appear as smooth, slightly hyperdense, well delineated lesions. Homogenous ball like calcification.
- Dural tail sign.
- Contrast enhancement is strong and uniform but not as intense as the adjacent pituitary. Gland and cavernous sinus.

Germinoma

Preference for midline sites.

- Pineal gland >sellar/suprasellar.
- Often both intra and suprasellar.
- 30 years of age, mostly females.

CT

Well-defined, hyperdense masses, significant long contrast enhancement.

MRI

Typically demonstrate an infiltrating mass that is isointense to brain on T1W, moderately hyperintense in T2W, enhances strongly and homogenously.

Epidermoid Tumor

- Occasionally occur in suprasellar region.
- Contain desquamated epidermal debris and cholesterin, which gives characteristic pearly appearance.
- Tend to infiltrate widely around vessels and nerves.

CT homogenously hypodense (0-20HU) with well defined borders that follows contours of the adjacent brain.

No contrast enhancement.

MRI

Hypointense on T1.

- Strongly hyperintense on T2WI. Their signal density is usually greater than CSF.

Metastasis

1% of sellar/parasellar masses.

Overall breast cancer–most common ~50% of secondary.

In man lung, prostrate, bladder, stomach.

Permeative destruction of sphenoid bone with irregular indistinct margins.

Vascular Lesion

Vascular ectasias and supraclinoid ICA aneurysms are the most common non-neoplastic suprasellar masses in adults.

ICA aneurysms eroding into the sella-pose differential diagnostic problem.

On CT–intracavernous and pre cavernous aneurysms may appear as homogenously enhancing rounded or lobulated masses.

May have calcifications, along rim. When an organized thrombus is present, the area appears homogenous on CECT.

Aneurysms present in number of ways as nerve palsy, visual impairment, headache, etc.

Section 1—Central Nervous System

Chapter 6

Posterior Fossa Cysts

DIFFERENTIAL DIAGNOSIS

1. Dandy-Walker malformation and variant.
2. Arachnoid cyst (Figures 6.1 and 6.2).
3. Mega cisterna magna.
4. Enterogenous cyst.
5. Inflammatory cyst.
6. Dermoid.
7. Epidermoid.
8. Cystic neoplasm.

Dandy-Walker Malformation

Etiology

- Theories include–failure of development of roof of 4th ventricle.
- Atresia of 4th ventricle outlet foramen.

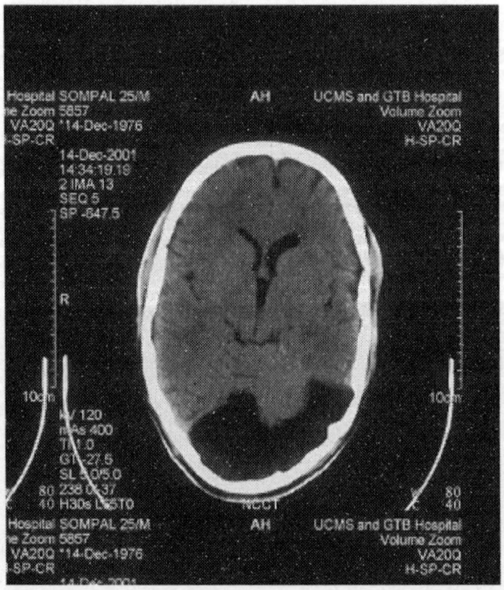

Fig. 6.1: Axial CT image shows a large posterior fossa cyst in a case of Dandy-Walker syndrome

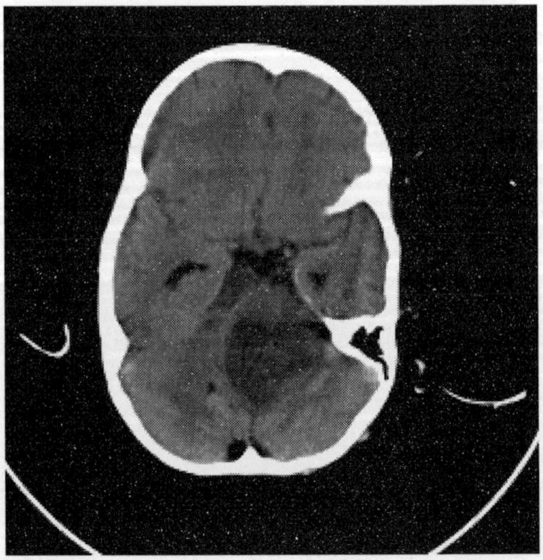

Fig. 6.2: Axial CT image shows arachnoid cyst in the posterior fossa arising from the cerebellopontine angle cistern

- Insult to developing cerebellar hernia and 4th ventricle.

Pathology and Imaging

1. Skull and dura
   - Enlarged posterior fossa
   - High tentorial insertion.
   - High position of transverse and straight sinuses and torcular (lambdoid torcular inversion).
2. Ventricles and posterior fossa cerebrospinal fluid space
   - Cystically dilated 4th ventricle opening dorsally in to a posterior fossa cyst between widely separated cerebellar hemispheres.
   - Generalized obstructive hydrocephalus – in 80% cases.

erebellum, vermis and brain stem
   - Varying degree of cerebellar and vermin hypoplasia.
   - Vermis typically rotated antero superiorly above cyst.
   - In severe cases cerebellar hemispheres appear winged outward and displaced antero laterally against the petrous bone.
   - Brain stem may be hypoplastic or compressed.
4. Associated anomalies
   - Corpus callosum agenesis 20-25%.
   - Heterotopias, gyral anomalies, schizencephaly and cephaloceles.
   - Non-CNS anomalies–polydactyly and cardiac anomalies.

Dandy-Walker Variant

1. Mild vermin hypoplasia with variable sized cystic space due to communication of post inferior fourth ventricle and cistern a magna through enlarged vallecular "Key Hole" appearance.
2. Posterior fossa normal sized.
3. Fourth ventricle normal to moderately enlarged.
4. Brain stem usually normal.
5. Hydrocephalus ± usually mild.

MRI

1. Well defined non-enhancing masses isointense to CSF (low on T1 and high on T2).
2. Displacement of adjacent brain.
3. If hemorrhagic or proteinaceous fluid–high signal on T1.

Mega Cisterna Magna

- Now included in spectrum of Dandy-Walker complex.
- Vermis is intact and cerebellar hemispheres are normally formed.
- Fourth ventricle is normal.
- Large cisterna magna is present and may extend around and above vermis upto the straight sinus.
- Posterior fossa can be enlarged with prominent and scalloping of occipital squame.
- Mega cisterna magna can be asymmetric and may exhibit mass effect.
- A large cisterna magna may be confused with arachnoid cyst.

Intrathecal contrast instillation leads to ready opacification of cisterna magna but not arachnoid cyst.

Epidermoid Tumor

- Occur due to inclusion of ectodermal elements during neural tube closure or due to implantation of epidermis following trauma.

- Contain soft, waxy kerato hyaline material within a cyst.
- Age 20 to 60 years with peak in 4th decade.

Location

- 90% intradural–primarily in basal subarachnoid spaces.
- 40-50% in CP angle cistern.

Imaging

CT

Noncontrast CT. (NCCT) scan shows well defined lucent lobulated masses with attenuation similar to CSF with no post contrast enhancement.

- Calcification in 10-25%.
- Have irregular frond like surface and insinuates along CSF spaces.

MRI

- Attenuation similar to CSF.
- Some epidermoids may show hyperintense rim.
- Some epidermoids have high signal on T1 due to high lipid content known as white epidermoids.

Differentiation of Arachnoid Cyst and Epidermoid

1. Both masses have similar characteristics on T1W and T2W images.
2. Proton density images–epidermoids are slightly hyperintense to CSF.
3. FLAIR sequence–suppress CSF signals, so arachnoid cyst containing CSF shows low signal whereas it is not low in epidermoid.
4. Diffusion weighted MRI–epidermoid are bright whereas arachnoid cysts are dark.
5. Epidermoid encase and engulf arteries and cranial nerves whereas arachnoids cysts displace adjacent structures.

Enterogenous Cysts (Neuroenteric Cysts)

- Only 10-15% are intracranial.
- Can occur at any age.
- They are typically intradural extramedullary posterior fossa masses.

  CP angle and cranio cervical junction. Anterior to brain stem are most frequent sites.
- NCCT scan shows a well-defined, non-calcified non-enhancing lobulated hypodense mass.

MRI

- Isointense or mildly hyperintense on T1.
- Moderately hyperintense on T2.

Inflammatory Cysts and Abscesses

- Usually rounded well defined with enhancing wall surrounding edema and mass effect calcification ±.

Cystic Neoplasms

1. **Cystic Astrocytoma**
   - CT round or oval sharply demarcated hypodense masses with an enhancing mural nodule mass effect with obstructive hydrocephalus may positive.

     On MR–hypointense on T1 and hyperintense on T2 WI with enhancing mural nodule.
2. **Cerebellar Hemangioblastoma**
   - 3rd to 5th decade
   - CT large low-density cystic mass with enhancing mural nodule.
   - MR–hypo on T1 and hyperintense on T2 WI–serpentine flow voids may be seen.
3. **Dermoid Tumors**
   - These are ectodermal inclusion cysts, containing thick viscous only fluid.

- Present during 2nd-3rd decade.
- Occur in or near midline–LS spine, parasellar, frontobasal and posterior fossa regions, midline vermis and 4thntricle are the most common.
- Seizures and headache may occur.

  Imaging – NCCT – Rounded well defined hypodense (-20 to -40 HU) mass.

  Capsular calcification is common.

  Post contrast enhancement is absent.

MRI

- Increased signal on T1W images.
- Variable signal on +T2.
- Dermoids may rupture and cause chemical meningitis and MR shows high signal fat droplets in CSF spaces.

Posterior Fossa Arachnoid Cyst

- Arachnoid cysts are benign, congenital, intra-arachnoidal space occupying lesion that are CSF filled.

Etiology

- Meningeal maldevelopment with focal splitting of developing meninges with formation of cyst in between.

Age and Gender

- 75% occur in children 3:1 male to female ratio.

Location – Mostly Supratentorial

50-60%	Middle cranial fossa.
10%	Quadrigeminal and suprasellar region.
5%	Frontal convexities.
5-10%	Posterior fossa (CP angle and cisterna magna).

Clinical Presentation

Headaches, seizures and focal neurological signs.

Imaging – CT scan

1. Cystic unilocular or septate, sharply marginated non-enhancing extraxial mass.

   Attenuation similar to CSF.
2. Minimal mass effect on subjacent brain may be positive.
3. Pressure erosion of adjacent calvarium can occur.
4. CT cisternography–no filling of contrast or some cyst showing delayed filling.

Section 1—Central Nervous System

Chapter 7

Cerebellopontine Angle Cistern Masses

Normal anatomy: The CPA cisterns lies between the anterolateral surface of the pons and the posterior surface of the petrous temporal bone. Important structure within the CPA cistern includes the Vth, VIIth and VIIIth cranial nerve, the superior and anterior inferior cerebellar arteries and tributaries of the superior petrosal veins.

CPA CISTERNAL MASSES

- Cystic.
- Solid.

Cystic

- Epidermoid tumor.
- Dermoid tumor.
- Arachnoid cyst.
- Cerebellar brainstem astrocytoma.
- Abscess.
- Neurocysticerosis.
- Metastasis.
- Hemangioblastoma (Figure 7.1).
- Neuroenteric cyst.

Solid

- Acoustic schwannoma.

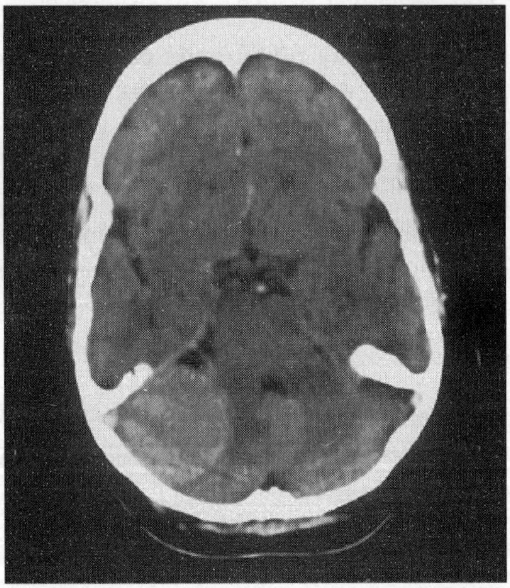

Fig. 7.1: Axial contrast enhanced CT image shows tentorial meningioma in the right cerebellopontine angle cistern

- Meningioma.
- Vascular (vertebrobasilar ectasia/aneurysm).
- Paraganglioma.
- Ependymoma.
- Choroid plexus papilloma.
- Cholesterol granuloma.
- Osteocartilaginous tumors.

EPIDERMOID TUMOR

- 0.2% to 0.1%.

Age

Occur between the age of 20 and 60. The peak incidence is in the 4th decade.

Gender

There is not gender predilation.

Duration

- Intradural→basal subarachnoid space.
- Intra-axial, sellar and suprasellar region IVth ventricle.
- Extra dural→mostly interdiploic.

Imaging

Plain Film Radiography

- Diploic epidermoid cysts have round or lobulated well-defined focal bone erosions with sclerotic margins.

Angiography

- It is usually normal or has avascular mass effect.

CT

- NCCT well defined lucent appearing lobulated mass with attenuation similar to CSF. Calcification is seen in 10% to 25% cases.

MRI

- Does not enhance on contrast administration.
- Depend on the relative proportions of cholesterol (short T1) and keratin (long T1) within the tumor.

T1W – Isointense with CSF.

T2W – Isointense or slightly brighter.

DERMOID TUMOR

Incidence

- 0.04% to 0.6%. Intradural dermoid cyst are 4 to 9 times less common than epidermoid cysts.

Age

- Spinal dermoids present during the 1st two or three decades of life. Intracranial dermoid become symptomatic during the 3rd decade.

Gender predilection–Slight male predilection.

Location

- Occur in or near the midline. The L-S spinal canal is the most common site following by parasellar, frontobasal and post fossa regions. The midline vermis /IVth ventricle, rupture and spreads through SA space.

Angiography–Normal or avascular mass effect.

	Epidermoid cyst	Arachnoid cyst
FLAIR	Slightly higher signal to CSF	Usually isointense with CSF
Diffusion weighted	There is restriction of free diffusion due to the presence of protein molecules, hence they are of ↑ed signal	Free diffusion of water within arachnoid cysts hence they are of low signal
Relation to adjacent	It may be encase and engulf arteries and cranial nerves.	These displace adjacent structure
	Does not erode the skull	Erode the skull
ADL	It is similar to brain parenchyma	It is similar to water

CT

- NCCT–Round well delineated, uniformly hypodense (-20 to -40 MU) mass. Capsular calcification in common. Ruptured dermoids may show low-density fatty drops in SA space. Enhancement is uncommon.

MR T1W–increased signal intensity.

T2W–Variable intensity that ranges from hypointense to inhomogenously hyperintense.

	Epidermoid	Dermoid
Incidence	0.2-0.1%	0.04 to 0.6%
Location	Off midline	Midline
Age	20 to 60 years	30 to 50 years
Gender	M=F	Slight male predilection
Imaging	CT- Low density, periphery occ. Enhances	Very low density (like fat) no enhancement T1W-Hyperintense
	MR T1 and T2W →often like CSF	T2W-Hypointense

ARACHNOID CYST (Figure 7.2)

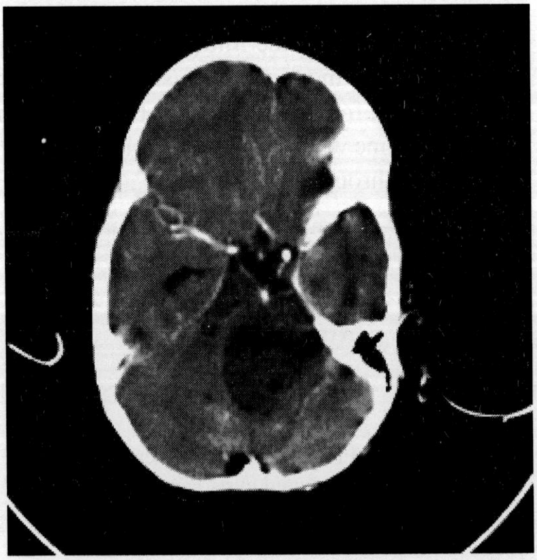

Fig. 7.2: Axial CT image shows arachnoid cyst in the left cerebellopontine angle cistern

Definition

These are benign, congenital, intra arachnoidal SOL that are filled with clear CSF like fluid.

Etiology

Minor aberrations of CSF flow through the loose primitive perimedullary mesenchyma may result in focal splitting of the developing meninges. Formation of pocket in the space thus created between arachnoid and pia results in arachnoid cysts.

Age

- More common in children

  M: F →3:1 ratio.

Location

- Supratentorial → Middle cranial fossa–50% to 65%
  → Suprasellar and quadrigeminal–10%
  → Frontal convexities–5%
- Infratentorial → Post. fossa and cisterna magna

C/F

- Headache.
- Seizures.
- Focal neurologic signs.

Imaging

CT

- Pressure erosion of the adjacent calvarium positive.
- Unilateral pneumosinus dilatans and asymmetric sinus aeration positive.

MRI

Sharply demarcated extra axial mass that may displace or deform adjacent brain.

- They parallel CSF in signal intensity on all pulse sequences–has no internal architecture and does not enhance.

PILOCYTIC ASTROCYTOMA

Etiology

- They arise from a class of astrocytes that is inconspicuous in normal brain but may become prominent in reactive gliosis and neoplasia.
- Incidence: 5% to 10% of all glioma.
- 1/3rd of pediatric gliomas.
- Second overall most common pediatric brain tumor.

Age

Children and young adults:

- First two decades of life and have a peak incidence at the age of 10.

Location

- 3rd and 4th ventricle.
- Optic chiasma and hypothalamous.
- Cerebellar vermis and hemispheres.

Imaging

Angiography

- An avascular mass effect with tethering and draping of otherwise normal vessel.

CT

- NCCT round or oval sharply demarcated and smoothly marginated hypo or isodense masses.
- Calcification —10%.
- Contrast enhancement in strong but variable (mural nodule may enhance intensely but inhomogenously).

MRI

- Cystic.
- T1W → Iso and hypointense.
- T2W → Hypointense.
- Mural nodules enhance strongly but somewhat inhomogenously.

HEMANGIOBLASTOMA

Age Group

- 30 and 65 years.
- VHL–Younger patients, multiple.

Location

- Most common intraaxial tumor of the post fossa in the cerebellum -10%.
- Brain stem.
- Spinal cord.

Angiography

- There is a dense blush of contrast, commencing in the arterial phase and continuing through into the venous phase. The larger modules can be 1-2 cm in diameter and resemble angioma.

CT

- Smooth walled cystic mass within an enhancing mural nodule that abuts the pial surface of the brain.

MRI

- The signal return from the cyst is that of CSF and the mural nodule is normally isointense on T1 and hyperintense on T2 with intense enhancement.

D/D

- Cerebellar astrocytoma.
- Metastases.

BRAIN ABSCESS

Etiology

- Pyogenic.

- Streptococcus.
- Bacteroides.

- Tuberculous.
- Fungal.
- Parasitic.

Location

- Grey, white matter surface.
- Frontal and parietal lobes.

Sequence of Events

- Cerebritis, precedes abscess formation.
- Parenchymal softening with neurosis, oedema, vascular congestion, petechial hemorrhage and an inflammatory exudate.
- Cerebritis is better demonstrated with MRI than CT.

CT

- It will show an area of low density in the large majority of cases and injection of I.V. Contrast medium will demonstrate the abscess capsule as a thin walled regular ring of enhancement.

MRI

T1W → Slightly hyperintense to CSF.

T2W → Central zone of liquefying necrosis is similar to that of CSF and surrounding brain oedema.

T1W → Collagenous capsule is commonly isointense to hyperintense.

T2W → Collagenous capsule is hypo-intense to brain.

D/D

- Tumors.

METASTASIS

- Metastasis to the brain, skull or meninges can occur.
- Primary tumors:
  - Lung (30%).
  - Breast (20%).
  - Melanoma (10%).
  - Kidney (10%).
- GIT (5%).

Extra-Axial Brain Tumors

What is significance of determining origin?

- Location of mass has clinical importance.
- Effects treatment planning.
- Has predictive prognosis.

As extra-axial (extracerebral) masses are most frequently benign in nature.

How to determine origin?

- Intra-axial.
- Extra-axial.

MRI

It is more informative in visualization and complete characterisation of extra-axial masses than CT.

- Provides pathological information regarding.
- Histology and intrinsic tumor vascularity effects of tumor.

Multiplanar Imaging Capability of MRI Provides

- Complete delineation of relationship of extra-axial masses to vital regions of surrounding brain and vascular structures – which can be of great value to neurosurgeon in pre-operative planning.
- Posterior fossa extra-axial masses lie adjacent to dense bone and therefore are not well delineated on CT because of beam hardening artifacts and are well seen on MR.

Extra-Axial Masses

- Meningeal origin
  - a. Meningioma
  - b. Lymphoma
  - c. Sarcoid

	Intra-axial	Extra-axial
Location	• Deep or superficial	• Usually superficial, may invaginate sulcus
Enhancement	• Variable, small nodule or large ring	• Usually dense and uniform when present
Margins	• May be infiltrative, difficult to separate from brain parenchyma	• Smooth margins, often well demarcated
Morphology	• Variable, grey matter only rarely involved	• Dural tail
Most effect cortical buckling	• Intrinsic mass symmetrical/brain expanded	• Extrinsic mass with displaced crumpled sinuses

• Extra-axial metastasis		
• Cerebellospontine angle Cistern masses	a. Acoustic schwannoma	
	b. Meningioma (Figure 8.1)	
	c. Epidermoid	
	d. Metastasis	
	e. Ependymoma	
	f. Arachnoid cyst	
	g. Lipoma	
• Cavernous sinus	a. Metastases	
	b. Meningioma	
• Suprasellar	a. Macro-adenoma	
	b. Meningioma	
	c. Aneurysm	
	d. Craniopharyngioma	
	e. Glioma	
• Intrasellar	a. Microadenoma	
	b. Cyst	
• Pineal gland tumor	a. Germinoma	
	b. Teratoma	
	c. Pinaoblastoma	

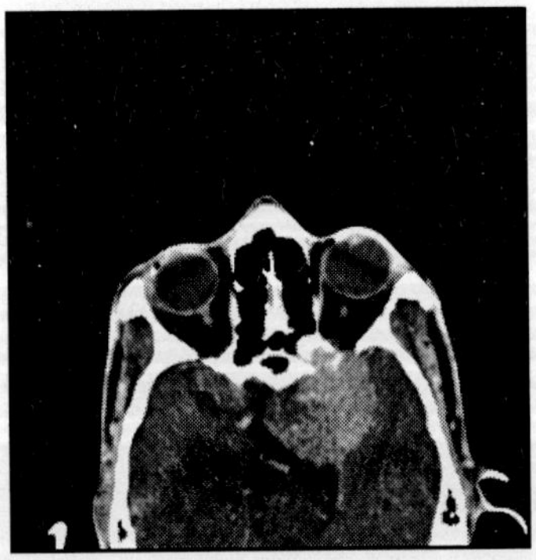

Fig. 8.1: Axial CT image shows a sphenoidal meningioma on left side

Meningiomas

WHO classification Meningioma 88-95%

Atypical meningioma: 5-7%.

Anaplastic (malignant) 1-2%.

Correlates with biological behaviour and hence preferred.

Meningioma: Etiology and Epidemiology

- Arise from specialized meningothelial cells called arachnoid cap. cells.
- Chromosome 22 origin.
- Progesterone, estrogen receptors.

Incidence

- Most common nonglial primary CNS tumor.
- 15-20% of all primary brain tumors.
- Multiple in 1-2%.
- Part of NF-2.

Age, Gender

- Peak incidence 40-60 years.
- Rare in children (often atypical).
- Male: Female 2:1 to 4:1.

Location

Arachnoid granulation, dural sinus, along suture.

- 25% parasagittal — 10% post fossa
- 20% convexity — 2% intraventricular
- 15-20% sphenoid ridge — 1% extra-cranial (nose, sinus, skull)
- 5-10% olfactory
- 5-10% parasellar
- Using WHO criterion, there are significant differences in recurrence rates for different meningiomas (5 years recurrence).

Typical	3% to 7%
Atypical	33%
Anaplastic	75%

- Meningioma metastases are rare (0.1 to 0.2%).

- Location and histopathology do not correlate with metastasis.

Imaging Characteristics

Plain Film Radiography

- Hyperostosis.
- Erosion.
- Enlarged vascular channel.
- Tumor calcification.
- Pneumosinus dilants.

Angiography

- Dual vascular supply (dural to centre, pial to periphery.
- Sunburst of enlarged dural feeders.
- Prolonged vascular stain (mother-in-law sign).

CT

- 70-75% Hyperdense.
- 20-25% Calcified.
- 90% Enhance strongly, uniformly.
- 10-15% Cystic areas.
- 60% Peritumoral oedema.

MR

- Typically isointense with grey matter.
- >95% enhance strongly, heterogenous enhancement common.
- CSF vascular cleft.
- 60% have dural tail (suggestive of but not specific).

Features such as:

- Marked oedema, non-enhancing central low density.
- Absence of visible calcium, poorly defined irregular borders.

All points to invasive characteristics that are more commonly found in malignant meningioma:

- Another important morphologic feature that suggests malignancy is "mushrooming" a lesion whereby intracranial diameter is much larger than its base of dural attachment.
- Mushrooming also seen in hemagniocytomas. lobulation is another important characteristics that increases malignancy.

Cerebellopontine Angle Masses

Schwannomas

- Benign tumors that originate from Schwann cells.
- Well-delineated, encapsulated tumors.
- Arise eccentrically.

  Cystic/fatty degeneration common and hemorrhagic necrosis are common.
- Malignant degeneration not common.
- 6-8% of all primary brown tumors.
- 40-60 years of age.
- When associated with NF 2 appear earlier.
- Slight female predominance 1.5:1.
- CN VIII to most common location for intracranial schwannoma.
- Earliest symptomatic, tinnitus and SNHC though originate from vestibular segment.

Imaging Findings

- Plain radiography
  - Late manifestation.
  - Widening of canal.
  - Anteromedial petrous erosion (5th nerve Schwannoma).
- Angiography
  - Findings vary and no typical pattern.
  - Many are avascular/focal displacement.
  - Stretching and droping of adjacent vessels.
  - ¼ show hypovascularity.

	Incidence	Comments	NECT	TIW	PD	TZW	Post Gd
Vestibular schwannoma	75-80%	C, Ca, Hem	Hypo	Hypo	Hyper	Hyper	++
Meningioma	10%	Durol tail	Iso	Hypo or iso	Usually hyper	Iso or hyper	++
Epidermoid	5%	May have peripheral Ca	Iso-mildly hyper to CSF	Hypo	Hyper to CSF	Iso or ↑ CSF	- (Thin mm)
Arachnoid cyst	1%	Na C, Ca, Hem	Iso to CSF	Iso to CSF	Iso to CSF	Iso to CSF	-
Astrocytoma	1%	Exophytic	Iso	Hypo	Hyper	Hyper	+

CT

- Iso intense to adjacent brain on NECT.
- Calcification, hemorrhages are uncommon.
- Enhance strongly, uniformly.
- Large tumors have heterogenous pattern due to cystic, xanthomatous changes.

MR

- Avascular/CSF cleft.
- Corticomedullary junction of brainstem is displaced.
- Brainstem appears displaced.
- Foraman acute angle.
- Cisternal portion larger than intracanicular part.
- Giving typical icecream on cone.
- Hypo 2/3, iso 1/3.
- Mild/moderate/hyperintense on pD/T2.
- Intense enhancement following contrast.

Extra-Axial Metastases

Leptomeningeal carcinomatosis (arachnoid–subarachnoid):

- Accounts for 8-10% of intracranial metastatic disease.
- Widespread neurological symptoms than can be accounted for by presence of single lesion.
- Signs and symptoms: Cause of widespread dissemination of tumor calls through CSF.
- Tumor spread through meningeal vessels with subsequent spread through CSF.
- Direct leptomeningeal invasion may occur from surrounding/adjacent structures:

Systemic tumors	CNS primary
Lymphoma	Medulloblastoma
Leukemia	Ependymoma
Melanoma	Pineal tumors
Breast	Retinoblastoma

IMAGING FEATURES

- Obliteration of SA space, basal cistern and sulci.
- Sulcal-cestemol enhancement, in sylvian fissure, basal cistern, high convexity cortical sulci.
- Tentorial enhancement (if widespread or is irregular).
- Within ventricle there may be ependymal/subependymal enhancement in diffuse/nodular characteristic of lymphoma D/D infectious/inflammatory/ischemia.
- Communicating hydrocephalous 2nd most common abnormality due to faulty resorption.
- Leptomeningeal carcinomatosis should be strongly suspected in patients with systemic neoplasm who has communicating hydrocephalus (Lumbar puncture for diagnosis).

- CEMR is most useful test for detection of leptomeningeal metastasis. Same findings as above.
- Normal meningeal enhancement is then and discontinuous primarily of dura arachnoid/pia do not enhance.
- Show nodular pattern whereas diffuse linear pattern are positive with inflammatory conditions.

Presence of contrast enhancement not necessarily indicates metastasis→similar meningeal enhancement may occur as in meningitis, sarcoidosis, vasculitis and rest. Surgery, fluid collection, post RT/CT conversely absence of contrast enhancement do not exclude metastasis.

Positive cytology is necessary for diagnosis.

Dural Metastases

- In adult's metastasis from carcinoma of lung, breast and prostrate. In pediatric age esp. medulloblastoma/sarcoma most often.

Unless very aggressive do not transgress dural boundaries, consequently do not involve brain parenchyma. Do not cross the falx to invade contralateral side.

ON CECT/CEMR

- Enhancement of dura not seen (however, should be differentiated from normal enhancement which is more linear and uniform).

Differentiation from meningioma may be difficult.

Hydrocephalus

CSF FLOW DYNAMICS

Capacity of entire cerebral cavity 1600-1700 ml.

↓

150 ml is CSF ± rest is brain and spinal cord. (40 ml in vent).

CSF is produced as an altered filtrate of plasma by:

1. Choroid plexus of ventricles (2/3rd).

   Temporal horns of LV.

   Posterior horn of 3rd ventricle.

   Roof of 4th ventricle.
2. Ependyma of ventricles (1/3rd).
3. Arachnoid membranes.
4. Small amount by brain through perivascular spaces.

FLOW AND ABSORPTION OF CSF

CSF in bilateral ventricle

↓

Both foramen of Monro

↓

3rd ventricle

↓

Aqueduct of Sylvius

↓

4th ventricle

↓

CSF spaces

↓

Cerebral convexities

- Arachoid granulation
- Mirchow robin space.

DEFINITION

"Hydrocephalus is an abnormal increase in the amount of CSF resulting in enlarged CSF spaces within skull, with or without raised intracranial pressure which is not the result of primary atrophy or dysgenesis of the brain."

Pathophysiology

Normal CSF produced at the rate of 0.3-0.4 ml/min or 530-570 ml/day by choroid plexi and extracellular spaces of brain by cerebral vasculature.

↓

Diffuse through ependyma into ventricles.

↓

Sequential flow through lateral 3rd and 4th ventricle

↓

Basal arachoid cisterns

Spinal canal

↓

Passes upward through incision to anach. Vill

Via Sylvian fissure

Lateral convexity cistern

Pen mesencephalic cistern

↓

Primary Gradient (20-50 mmHg) between SSE and CSD leads to primary Gradient resorption.

Etiology

A. Overproduction B. Obstruction

Classification

Hydrocephalus

Causes

A. Non-communicating HC or IVOH

Lateral ventricle

Extrinsic	Intrinsic
Hypothalamic glioma	Post inflammatory
Craniopharyngioma	Post hemorrhagic
Giant cell astrocytoma	Parasitic cyst
Colloid cyst	Congenital membrane
Chorsed plexus papilloma	

Foramen of Monro

Colloid cyst	Lymphoma
Ependymoma	Adenoma
Craniopharyngioma	Fibrosis

Subependymal giant cell astrocytoma

3rd ventricle

Pineal region masses

Aquaductal obstruction

Congenital.

Post meningitis.

Post infective.

Neoplastic.

- Suprasellar tumors.
- Arachnoid cysts.
- CPP.
- Vein of galen aneurysm.
- Peri aqueductal tumors.
- Thalamic and hypothalamic tumors.

4th Ventricle

Congenital	Dandy - Walker cyst
Neoplastic	CPP Cerebellar tumors PNETIS
Post infections	

Non obstructive	Obstructive			Congenital
↓ Overproduction hydrocephalus	↓ Non-communicating or IVOH	↓ Communicating or EVOH		
		Benign external HC	Normal pressure HC	

B. Communicating HR or EVOH (Figures 9.1 and 9.2)
- Subarachnoid hemorrhage.
- Trauma.
- Infection.
- Carcinomatosis.
- Intracranial surgery.
- Hurler's syndrome.
- Achondroplasia.
- Fusing syndrome.

C. Congenital HC
- Dandy-Walker malformation/cx.
- Homi-megaloencephaly.
- Holo prosencephaly.
- Agenesis of corpus callosum.
- Chiari type II malformation.
- Aqueductal stenosis.

D. Benign external hydrocephalus
- Is a form of EVOH – age < 9 months.
- Clinically normal macrocrania.
- Psychomotor retardation.
- Ventricles, cisterns or sulci may be normal or enlarged.
- Etiology–inadequate absorption of CSF by arachnoid granulations.
- DD–subdural collections.
- No shunting reg. and condition resolves by 2 years.

E. Hydrocephalus ex vacuo-dilatation of CSF spaces secondary to atrophy.

Clinical Presentation

Symptoms and treatment - Decreased blood flow
Stretching of fibres.

Depends on age, rapidity, degree of pressure elevation.

8 Months–2 Years

- Enlargement of head or macrocrania.
- Setting sun sign.
- Delayed milestones.
- After sutural closure

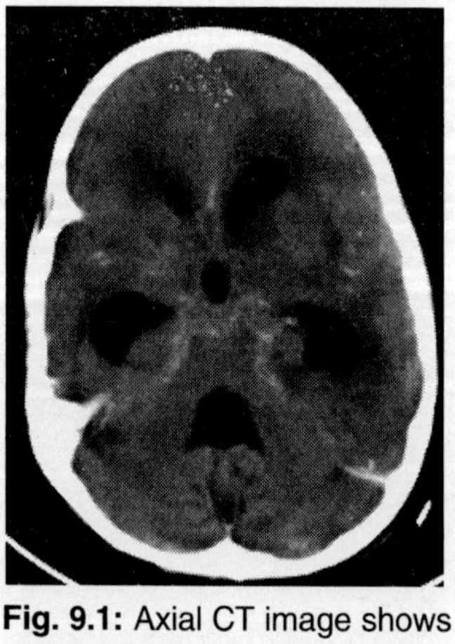

Fig. 9.1: Axial CT image shows communicating, obstructive hydrocephalus in a case of tubercular meningitis

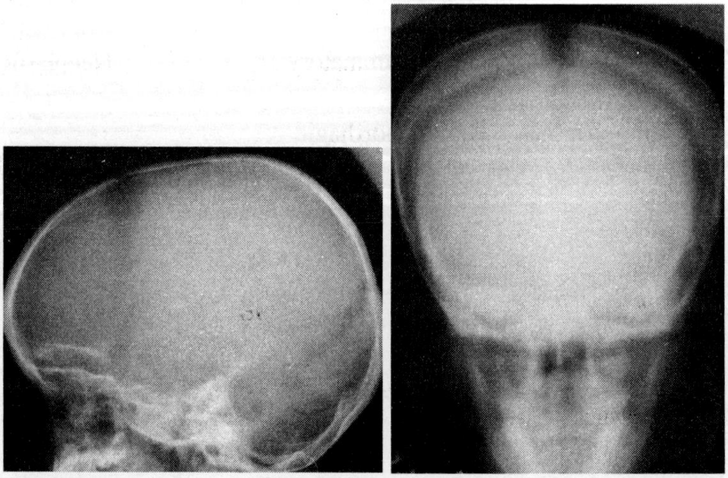

Fig. 9.2: Radiographs of the skull show sutural diastases in a case of hydrocephalus

- Headache.
- Vomiting.
- Papilloedema.

Adults

- Giant disturbances.
- Incontinence of bladder and bowel.
- Mental changes.
- Headache.
- Craze disturbances.
- Sp raised ICT.

Imaging Techniques

A. Plain Radiograph:

Infancy

Thin vault	Posterior fossa–Small, ballooned
Craniolancunac	
Sutural diastasis	Enlarged supratentorial fossa
Loss of lamina dura	

Childhood

Sutural diastasis	Diastasis with deep intro-digitation.
Sular erosions	Deep ant. fossa with enlarged head.
	Orbits laterally placed.
	Prominent convolution marking.
	Sellar erosion.

Adults

No vault changes	Supratentorial vault enlarged
Erosions of lamina dura	Calvarial thinning.
Sellar osteoporosis	Prominent convultional marking.

B. Ultrasound

Causes diagnosed are

Arnold Chiari IV malformation	-	ICH
Dandy-Walker cyst	-	lammation
Holoprosencephaly etc.		

Normal values of lateral ventricle

Lateral dimension	Width
7-11 mm	1-3 mm

Importance of Ultrasound in hydrocephalus:

- Determine the cause of screening at risk.
- Differentiation between enlarged ventricles in HC and HC with brain dysgermin.
- For intra op shunt placement.
- Monitoring the efficacy of therapy.
- Identify post operative ox.

C. Computed Tomography

Site of obstruction is the zone of transition from dilated to non dilated CSF spaces.

Changes in skull and dura.

Sutural diastasis.

Thinned calvarium.

Focal, asymmetric expansion of cahroni in asym. Vent. dilatation.

Head size.

High or low tentorial insertions.

Falcine deviation.

Post Shunting

- Fontanelles–slack–sunken.
- Sutures–narrow.
- Calvarial platio-override/adult.
- Premature sagittal synostosis.

Changes in Brain Parenchyma

- White matter is more severely affect than gray matter.
- White matter rarefaction and gliosis.

Findings on CT are:

1. Ventricular dilatation.
2. Periventricular edema.
3. Atina and occipital hours are more dilated.
4. Thinning of cerebral mantle.
5. Unilator or Bilator pulsion diverticular of vent. wall.

D. MRI

1. Better soft tissue resolution.
2. Localizing exact level of obstruction.
3. Identifying small obstructing pathology.

NORMAL PRESSURE HYDROCEPHALUS (NPH)

It is a form of EVOH; is a disease of elderly.

NPH is characterized by:

- Normal mean intraventricular pressures.
- Raised pulse pressure.
- Water hammer pulse is described.
- Classical clinical diagnosis of – gait apraxia, dementia, urinary incontinence.
- Diagnosis based on S. criteria:
  1. Clinical presentation.
  2. Out of proportion enlargement of ventricles to suture.

On MRI – Aqueduct CSF flow used is seen due to high CSF flow during systole. This magnitude of flow used has been used to predict which patients with clinical VH should undergo shunting.

CSF Flow in NPH

- Using phase contrast CSF velocity imaging with high-resolution axial technique, accurate quantitative measurement of aqueduct CSF stroke volume can be done.
- Aqueduct stroke volume >42μL.

  Hyper dynamic CSF flow.
- All patients with this one finding responded well to shunting.

Thus quantitative CSF flow imaging is an even better technique than routine MRI to determine the shunt responsive NPH and potential shunt malfunctions.

Section 1—Central Nervous System

Chapter 10

Cavernous Angioma

- Accounts for 8-16% of all cerebrovascular malformations.
- 4% of population harbours this lesion.

AGE

Congenital in Origin

Peak incidence of symptoms between 3rd to 5th decade.

SEX INCIDENCE

Intracranial M=F Spinal F>M.

Location

- Superficial location with proximity to either the subarachnoid space or ventricle is particularly common.
- Multiple lesions occur in half of spontaneous cases and 80% of familial cases.
- Change in size, shape and morphology over time.

CLINICAL FEATURES

- Usually a symptomatic.
- Symptoms may be:
  1. **Seizures**
     - Present in 40-60% patients with symptoms.
     - Are due to irritative effect of hemosiderin, gliosis and compression of adjacent cortex.
  2. **Progressive FND**
     - More common with intratentorial lesions.
  3. **Headache.**

Intracranial			Extra-axial	Spinal
Supratentorial (80%)	Infratentorial (20%)			
More common involvement. Of frontal and temporal lobes	Cerebellum	Brain stem ↓ Esp. pons	• Subarachnoid • Intraventricular • Subdural • Dural sinus • Extra dural • Arising from ventricular system or nerves	

COMPLICATION HEMORRHAGE

- Risk of hemorrhage is 0.1% to 1.1% per year for each lesion.
- Highest incidence in 2nd and 3rd decade.
- Clinically significant hemorrhage occurs in 10-13% of patients.
- Hemorrhage may be associated with seizures or acute FNDs with severity depending on location of lesion.
- Hemorrhage may extend to subarachnoid or intraventricular space.
- Intratentorial location and previous gross hemorrhage are associated with increased risk of subsequent neurological disability.

PATHOLOGICAL FINDINGS

- On gross inspection → Dark blue, well defined, lobulated mass lesion with grapelike configuration.
- Site may range from few mm to few cms.
- A rim of gliotic brain is present stained by hemosiderin pigment resulting from prior hemorrhages.
- On microscopic examination → closely approximated endothelial lined sinusoidal spaced without presence of interposed neural tissue and without any muscularis or elastic in vessel wall.
- Venous angioma may coexist with cavernous angioma.

IMAGING FEATURES

Angiography

- Usually angiographically occult except mass effect if acute hematoma is present.
- Occasionally a late minimal contrast stain is seen on late capillary or early venous phase.

CT

- Usually isodense to moderately hyperdense on NECT.
- Enhancement varies from none for minimal to striking.
- Calcification is common.
- Usually no edema or mass effect is associated.

MRI

- More sensitive and is diagnostic in most cases.
- Typical popcorn like lesion is seen on MR with a complex core of mixed signal intensities representing hemorrhage in different stages of evolution.
- Circumferential complete rings of markedly hypointense iron storage produce that bloom on T2W and GRE sequences.
- Usually no associated mass effect/edema.
- No demonstrable feeding artery or draining vein.
- Associated venous angiomas can also be picked upon MR scans as tufts of tubular or stellate vessels of variable signal.
- Extra axial cavernous angioma:
  - May present as classical popcorn like lesion.
  - Hyperintense on T2W with strong homogenous post contrast enhancement.

Differentiating features of benign vs. malignant hemorrhagic lesion.

TUBERCULOMA

Most common radiographic features of CNS TB include:

- Enhancement of basal cisterns.
- Granulomata.
- Calcification.
- Hydrocephalus.
- Meningeal enhancement.
- Infarctions (Usually of basal ganglia).

Malignant	Benign
Hemosiderin rim is usually incomplete	Complete rim
May have few non-enhancing areas	Not so
Evolution of bleed is often delayed/disorders	Orderly evolution
Edema and mass effect are persistent	Resolve with tissue
Usually solitary lesion	May be multiple

Coexistent pulmonary TB is present in 25% to 83% patients with CNS TB.

Location

Most common sites are corticomedullary functions and periventricular location:

Most tuberculomas are supratentorial.

CT

Demonstrates hypo/iso/hypodense lesion on NCCT with rim nodular enhancement:

- One-third patients demonstrate 'target sign' seen as central calcification or punctate enhancement surrounded by hypodensity surrounded by rim enhancement.
- Healed tuberculoma may calcify in 23% cases.

MRI

- Iso to grey matter on T1W segment ± slightly hyperintense rim.
- Iso/hypo to brain on T2W in most cases may be hyperintense if greater degree of necrosis in the lesion.
- Surrounding edema is seen which is more prominent in early stages of granuloma formation.

MR spectroscopy shows prominent lipid peaks with resonance's at 0.9, 1.3, 2.0 and 2.8 ppm for lipids and at 3.7 ppm for phosphoserine.

INTRACRANIAL METASTASES

Causes

Parenchymal		Leptomeningeal	Dural and Calvarial	
Adult	Children		Adult	Children
Lungs	SA	Lymphomas	Prostates	Neuroblastoma
Breast Ca	Germ cell tumor	Leukemia	Breast	SA
Melanoma	Wilm's tumor	Dissemination of primary brain malignancies	Lung	
Genitourinary tract	Neuroblastoma			
Gastrointestinal tract				

PARENCHYMAL METS

Single	Multiple
• Mets from RCC and tumors of abdomen and pelvis are usually single and infra-tentorial	• More common pattern • Lung CA and melanoma mets are usually always multiple

Most common location is corticomedullary function in anatomic watershed areas of main cerebral arteries.

PATHOLOGY

- Grossly rounded solid/partially cystic mass associated with edema disproportionate to the size of lesion.
- Microscopically reasonable tumor of origin.

Clinical Presentation

- Headache–most common symptom (in 50% patients).
- Seizures–In 15% patients more common presenting feature in children.
- Neurological deficits.

CT

NCCT

Hypodense	Hyperdense	Isodense
Lung	GIT	Diagnosed by associated oedema and mass effect
Breast	Small round cell tumors	
Kidney	Hemorrhagic mets: • Melanoma • RCC • Chorio CA	
	• Thyroid CA • Lung CA Calcified mets • Osteo sarcoma Mucinous Aden carcinoma • Treated mets Lymphoma Leukaemia	

Contd.

CECT

- Diffuse/nodular/ring like enhancement Standard contrast dose 40 gm iodine Additional lesions may be identified with delayed scars (1-1.5 hr after contrast) and high dose (80-85 gm iodine).
- Contrast may seep in necrotic areas ® fluid filled level.
- Hemorrhagic fluid levels may be seen in cystic RCC mets.

MRI

- Investigation of choice esp. CEMR.
- Non hemorrhagic mets:
  - Hypo/iso to white matter on T1W.
  - Hyperintense white matter on T2W and PD.
- Hemorrhagic mets → variable signal on both T1W and T2W.
- Surrounding edema–hypo on T1W, hyper on T2W.
- Melanoma mets have variable signal both due to hemorrhage and melanin content which has paramagnetic effect.
- Mucinous adeno CA mets–hypointense on T2W due to high cellularity.
- Contrast enhancement is present (base 0.1 to 0.3 mmol/kg body weight).
- No use of delayed scans.

- Dx of mets is questionable if lesion is non-enhancing. Contrast enhanced magnetization transfer MR imaging is more sensitive.

PRIMARY CNS LYMPHOMA

Pathology

Gross: Vary from well-defined focal masses to poorly defined diffusely infiltrating lesions.

Microscopically: Usually B-cell lymphomas.

Age: Any age but usually 60s in immuno-competent.

Location

- Multiple centrally located lesions are common.
- Common sites are basal ganglia and thalami.
- Periventricular region.
- Corpus callosum.
- Most PCL about ependyma.

Clinical Features

- Seizures, headache, stupor, FND.

IMAGING

CT

Hallmarks are:

- Hyperdensity on NCCT.
- Characteristic periventricular location.
- Fluffy pattern of contrast enhancement.
- A soft tissue mass crossing corpus callosum is also very suggestive esp. if it is hyperdense on NCCT.
- There is absence of significant mass effect or ventricular enlargement.
- Tumor margins are usually poorly defined and irregular (due to perivascular infiltration of tumor cells) seen in 50% of patients.

MRI

Iso/hypointense to grey matter on T1W.

- Iso/hyperintense to grey matter on T2W.
- AIDS related PCL are more heterogeneous.
- Can infiltrate diffusely and mimic white matter disease. Multicentric in 43% cases.
- Induces mild edema and little mass effect.
- Contrast enhancement may be moderate.

Intracranial Metastases

CNS metastatic disease from extra cranial primary tumors has many manifestations.

Common

Skull.

Leptomeninges (Arachnoid/subarachnoid).

Parenchyma.

Less Common

Dura.

Pial/subpial.

Rare

Carcinomatous encephalitis.

Limbic encephalitis.

SKULL METASTASES (Figure 11.1)

- Breast and lung are the most frequent primary tumors.
- Their characteristics are similar to those found in other bones–irregular lysis or sclerosis and multiplicity.
- There may be subtle intradiploic metastases or large mass with extensive areas of bone destruction.

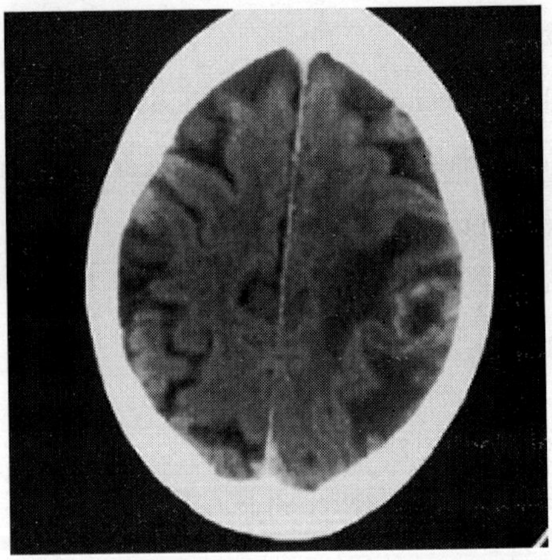

Fig. 11.1: Axial CT image shows intraparenchymal brain metastases on left side

- CT scan with bone algorithm reconstruction best delineates osseous component.
- MRI is superior for detecting subtle.
- Intradiploic lesions for delineating extent and determining involvement of underlying dura or brain.

Dural Metastases (Pachymeningeal Metastases)

- Less common than skull lesions.
- Calvarial metastases commonly involve the adjacent dura.

- They may occur without calvarial lesions.
- Neoplastic cells forming a thickened nodular membrane that covers the brain and spares subarachnoid space, diffusely infiltrate the meningeal fibrous layer of dura.

Leptomeningeal Metastases

- 6-18% of CNS metastases involve the leptomeninges i.e. arachnoid and subarachnoid space, pia or both.

Arachnoid/Subarachnoid Metastases

- Diffuse or widespread multifocal tumor, infiltrates and thickens the leptomeninges.
- Focal tumor nodules are less common.
- Subarachnoid space can be diffusely involved by metastasis–basal cisterns is a common site.
- Thick sheet like homogenous contrast enhancement or nodular enhancement with obliteration of subarachnoid cisterns is diagnostic of this complication.

Pial Metastases

- Typically occur in combination of arachnoid and subarachnoid tumor.
- Diffuse tumor infiltration in sub pial perivascular distribution produces innumerable tiny tumor nodules with a miliary pattern.

  Ependymal or subependymal tumor spread in wall of ventricles appears as sheets, or nodular plaque like intense contrast enhancement.
- This complication occurs occasionally in metastasis particularly seen with melanoma and is more common with glioblastoma, lymphoma, ependymoma and germinomas.

Parenchymal Metastases

- It is the most common CNS manifestation of extracranial primary neoplasms.

Etiology

- Approx 20% of the cardiac output goes to brain and the end artery pattern of distal cerebral arterial branches serves as a trap for circulating tumor cells.
- Most common primary sites are lung, breast, malignant melanoma, and GIT and genitourinary tract.

Pathology

1. Grossly parenchymal metastases are: Well defined circumscribed nodules of varying size that can be:
   - Solid.
   - Partially cystic (fluid with mucinous, necrotic debris or hemorrhagic fluid).
2. Extensive peritumoral edema disproportionate to the size of the metastatic focus.

Age and Incidence

- Uncommon in children.
- In adults 1/4 to 1/3 of all brain tumors.
- 60 to 85% are multiple.

Location

All areas of brain may be affected, but corticomedullary junction is the most common site.

Clinical Presentation

Varies from a symptomatic individuals to patients with severe neurological deficits.

Imaging (A) CT Scan

1. Attenuation of cerebral metastases varies on NCCT scans:
   a. **Most** metastases are **isodense** with adjacent brain and merge imperceptibly with the overlying cortex, being detected only when they distort the inner margin of cortex.

b. **Hyperdense Metastases**
- Small round cell tumors.
- Hemorrhagic metastases like–renal carcinoma, breast carcinoma, melanoma, chorio-carcinoma, thyroid carcinoma and oat cell carcinoma of lung.

c. **Cystic metastases**
- Squamous cell carcinoma of lung.
- Adenocarcinoma of lung.

Some metastases undergo central necrosis and appear as ring like masses with central lucency and peripheral isodense or slightly hyperdense rim of irregular thickness.

d. **Calcified metastases**
- Mucin producing neoplasms.
- Cartilage/bone forming sarcomas.
- Effective radio chemotherapy.

e. **Oedema** of the surrounding white matter is usually extensive and produces considerable mass effect. It may be sometimes the only abnormality on NCCT scans.

Contrast Enhancement

Is usually strong in almost all metastases. Less than 4% of metastases fail to show enhancement.

- Both solid and ring like patterns are seen.
- It enables clear separation of hypodense or isodense masses from peritumoral edema.
- Double dose delayed CT significantly improves detection.

MRI

- The MR appearance of metastatic lesions depends on the cellularity, degree of necrosis, hemorrhage calcification and surrounding edema.
- Most non-hemorrhagic metastasis are slight **hypointense** relative to brain **on T1W** images and **hyperintense on T2.**

Melanoma

Deposits are often hyperintense on T1 due to T1 shortening by melanin content:

- Some metastatic tumors are hypointense on T2W1 e.g. mucin secreting neoplasms such as adenocarcinoma from GIT and densely cellular tumors with N:C ratio.

  If hemorrhage has occurred the signal is determined by the age of hemorrhage.

Contrast Enhanced MR Scans

- Are the most sensitive imaging procedure for evaluating intracranial metaplastic disease.

Most metastases enhance strongly following I.V. gadolinium with solid rim and mixed patterns.

Carcinomatous Encephalitis

- It is a rare form of metastatic disease due to diffuse spread of tumor to cortex and meninges without formation of macroscopic masses.

Limbic Encephalitis

Etiology

Precise etiology is unknown but viral or auto-immune disorders are the proposed cause. It is a type of paraneoplastic syndrome, which are the clinical manifestations with cancer that are not due to the tumor in affected organ.

- Small cell lung cancer is the most common malignancy associated with paraneoplastic syndromes.
- Female genital tract tumors–cerebellar degeneration.
- Neuroblastoma–opsoclonus.
- Hodgkin's disease–demyelineating neuropathy.
- Limbic encephalitis involves the limbic system and is frequently associated with oat cell carcinoma.

Pathology

Mononuclear perivascular and parenchymal infiltrates with reactive gliosis, neuronal loss and microglial proliferation. No tumor cells are positive.

Location

- Hippocampal formations.
- Amygdalate.
- Medial temporal lobe.

Clinically

- Changing mental status with effective symptoms.
- Memory loss.

Imaging

- CT scan is usually normal.

MRI

↑ signal in medial temporal lobes on T2W weighted scans.

Variable Contrast Enhancements.

Complications

1. **Edema**

   Vasogenic type due to breakdown of blood brain barrier and seepage of plasma infiltrate through it.

   - Mainly accumulates in white matter spreading along white matter tracts with finger like extensions into each gyrus.

2. **Herniations**

   May be due to tumor, edema or both may cause mechanical development of brain, CSF or blood vessels from one compartment to another under the rigid falx or territorial incisura.

a. Subfalcine herniation
   - Cingulated gyrus displaced across midline under the free margin of falx.
   - Ipsilateral lateral ventricle is compressed and contralateral lateral ventricle enlarges due to obstruction of foramen of Monroe.
   - Septum pellucidum, 3rd ventricle, and corpus callosum are also displaced.
   - Ipsilateral ACA and subendymal veins are also shifted across the midline.

b. Descending transtentorial herniation
   - Most common.
   - Uncus and parahippocampal gyrus of temporal lobe are displaced medially and protrude over the free edge of tentorium.
   - Initially ipsilateral suprasellar cistern is effaced and then subsequently obliterated.
   - Ipsilateral mid brain is compressed and rotated by impinging temporal lobe.
   - Narrowing of contralateral perimesencephalic cisterns and ipsilateral widening.
   - Inferomedial displacement of PCF, posterior-communicating artery.
   - Midbrain hemorrhage (Duret Hemorrhage).
   - Unilateral or bilateral medial occipital infarction due to occlusion of PCA.

c. Ascending transtentorial
   - Superior cerebellar vermis is displaced upwards through tenotrial incisura.
   - Obliteration of quadrigeminal and superior cerebellar cistern with

flattening of posterior margin of 3rd ventricle.

d. Transalar (trans sphenoidal) herniation
   - In descending type – frontal lobe forced posteriorly with backward displacement of sylvian fissure and MCA.
   - Ascending –sylvian fissure MCA and temporal lobe displaced anteriorly over sphenoid ridge.

f. Tonsillar herniation
   - Downward displacement of cerebellar tonsils.

3. Hemorrhage

- Metastases from chorio carcinoma, melanoma, renal cell carcinoma, carcinoma lung.

Cyst with a Mural Nodule

CAUSES

A. Pilocytic astrocytoma.
B. Ganglioglioma.
C. Pleomorphic xanthoastrocytoma.
D. Glioblastoma multiforme.
E. Hemangioblastoma.

Pilocytic Astrocytoma

- 5-10% of all cerebral glioma, second most common paediatric lesion and is most commonly seen in children and young adults.
- May be associated with neurofibromatosis.
- Most commonly seen in cerebellum, hypothalamus (around 3rd ventricle), optic nerve/ chiasm.
- Presents as a cystic mass with mural tumor nodule.
- CT shows a round or oval sharply demarcated and smoothly marginated hypodense mass. Contrast enhancement is variable and is usually seen of the solid mural nodule. As the wall of the cyst is made of compressed brain tissue, it usually does not enhance.
- There may be extensive perilesional oedema.

Ganglioglioma

- These are hamartomatous malformation and are rare tumors usually seen in children and young adults.
- They usually arise in the floor of the third ventricle and here they are usually referred to as hamartoma of the tuber cinerium. Even more rarely they may be seen in temporal lobe or elsewhere.
- CT shows a small mass in the floor of the third ventricle, which protrudes down into the suprasellar cistern. The mass is isodense or slightly hyperdense and may show as large cystic component and enhances little with contrast media.

Hemangioblastoma

- Benign autosomal dominant tumor of vascular origin, less than 20% occur in childhood especially in patients suffering with von Hippel-Lindau disease.
- Usually infratentorial and if supratentorial it is usually seen in association with von Hippel-Lindau syndrome.
- CT shows a sharply demarcated cystic mass of CSF attenuation with a densely and homogenously enhancing peripheral nodule.

Cerebral Abscess

- Most common cause is hematogenous spread from a distant source or direct spread as in cases of mastoid, middle ear and sinus infections.

- It has for stages:

  a. Early cerebritis (3-5 days).

  b. Late cerebritis (5-15 days).

  c. Early capsule (> 2 weeks).

  d. Late capsule (weeks to months).

In early capsule stage the capsule, is initially thin but becomes thicker as more collagen is produced. During late capsule stage the capsule is complete.

- The corticomedullary junction is the most common location and frontal and parietal lobes are most frequent sites.

CT

- *Early cerebritis:* NCCT may be normal or may show only a poorly marginated hypodense area suggesting oedema. In CECT there is focal gyral enhancement.
- *Late cerebritis:* There is an irregular enhancing rim that surrounds a central low density area and the perilesional oedema is usually marked.
- *Early capsule:* Thin well demarcated capsule is seen that enhances strongly, uniformly and continuously is typical. In contrast to other cystic tumor the abscess wall is thicker on the cortical side and thinner at the epindymomal side.
- *Late capsule:* Abscess shrinks, the peripheral oedema diminishes but the rim enhancement may persist.

Section 1—Central Nervous System

Chapter 13

Radiological Anatomy of Ventricular System and Cisterns

VENTRICULAR SYSTEM

- The interior of brain contains a series of cavities. The cerebrum contains a median cavity. The third ventricle; and two lateral ventricles, one in each hemisphere.
- Each lateral ventricle open into third ventricle through an interventricular foramen.

  The third ventricle is continuous caudally with the cerebral aqueduct, which traverses the midbrain and opens into fourth ventricle. The fourth ventricle is situated dorsal to pons and medulla and ventral to cerebellum. It communicates inferiorly with the central canal, which traverses the lower part of medulla and spinal card.
- An epithelial layer called as ependymal lines the entire ventricular system:
  1. *Lateral ventricles:* Conventionally, the (L) lateral ventricle is labelled as the first followed next by the (R) lateral ventricle.
     - The two lateral ventricles join to the third ventricle via the midline foramen of Monro.
     - The anterior extension into frontal horn is called frontal horn. The frontal horns are separated from each other by septum pellucidum. The head of caudate nuclei outlines the frontal horns laterally.
  2. Anteriorly, the frontal horns are bounded by the genu of carpus callousm. The body of lateral ventricles extends posteriorly over the corpus callosum and is outlined by the body of caudate nuclei. The posterior extension of body of lateral ventricles form occipital horn.
  3. Medially the occipital horns are bounded by the splenium of corpus callosum. The temporal horns are extensions of the lateral ventricles into the temporal lobes. The place where the temporal and occipital horns and the body of lateral ventricles meet is called the atrium. The main portion of choroid plexus is located in the atrium.

THIRD VENTRICLE

- Third ventricle is a midline structure located between two thalami. Anteriorly the floor of third ventricle is formed by tubercinereium. Posteriorly it is bounded by cerebral peduncles. The root of third ventricle is formed by velum interposition.

FOURTH VENTRICLE

- Fourth ventricle is located in the posterior fossa

between pons and cerebellum. The fourth ventricle is connected to the third ventricle via cerebral aqueduct.

CSF FLOW THROUGH VENTRICLES

CHOROID PLEXUS

↓

CSF

Lateral ventricle — Lateral ventricle

Foramen of Monro

↓

Third ventricle

↓

Cerebral aqueduct

↓

Fourth ventricle

↓

Foramen of magendie

Foramen of Luschka — Foramen of Luschka

Cisterna magna

↓

Other parts of subarachnoid space

↓

Arachnoid granulations

↓

Dural venous sinuses

At places, the subarachnoid space far expensive spaces called cisterns.

CISTERNS

1. Cisterna Magna:

- The largest cistern is formed where the arachnoid bridges the interval between the medulla and the inferior surface of cerebellum.
- This cistern is continuous with the lumen of 4th ventricle through median aperture the foramen of magendie and below by the subarachnoid space of spinal cord.
- Ventral to pons, continuous below with spinal subarachnoid space, behind with cisterna magna and rostal to the pons with interpeduncular cistern. The basilar artery runs through pontine cistern into interpeduncular cistern.

2. Interpeduncular Cistern:

- Contain circulus arteriosus (the circle of Willis). Anteriorly the interpeduncular cistern extends into optic chiasma.

3. Cistern of Lateral Fossa:

- Formed by arachnoid as it traverses the lateral sulcus and contain MCA.

4. Cistern of Great Cerebral:

- Lies posterior to the brainstem and the third ventricle and occupies the internal between the splenium of corpus callosum and the superior cerebellar surface. The greater cerebral vein traverse it and pineal gland protrudes into it.

Other minor cisterns include:

- Prechiasmatic.
- Post chiasmatic.
- The cistern of laminar terminalis.
- Supracallosal cistern.

These are extensions of interpeduncular cistern and contain anterior cerebral arteries.

SECTIONAL ANATOMY

Normal Axial CT and MRI Anatomy

- CT scan is reviewed from caudal to cranial levels. The scans are obtained at 15-20° angulation to canthometal line. MRI scans are generally obtained parallel to this line. These scans are divided into posterior fossa cuts of 5 mm increment and supratentorial cuts of 8 mm increments.

POSTERIOR FOSSA CUTS

1. *Above foramen magnum level:* The cerebellar towers can be seen lateral to medulla. Most of the structures in anterior and middle cranial fossa are component of base of skull and the orbits. In the middle fossa foramen evale and spinosum can be visualized if a wide window setting is usual. The inferior portion of cisterna magna outlines the posterior aspect of the cerebellar hemispheres.
2. *Level of fourth ventricle:* The lower pons is seen in front of fourth ventricle, connecting to the cerebellar hemispheres by middle cerebellar peduncles. The anterior and lateral misencephalic cisterns containing CSF on MRI outline the pons. Seventh and eighth cranial nerves can be seen at this level. Posteriorly the 4th ventricle is outlined by nodules in the middle and cerebelllar hemispheres laterally.

ABOVE THE FOURTH VENTRICULAR LEVEL

- The superior cerebellar surface is seen with separation of two hemispheres by the vermis. In the middle fossa, the temporal lobes are separated from frontal lobe by the sylvian fissure. The temporal horn seem as a coma shaped structure in the middle of temporal lobe, is easily visualized in patients older than 50 years of ages. The medial aspect of temporal lobes bounds the suprasellar cistern and contains ICA, the optic chaisma, the infundibulum, the mamillary bodies and the top of basilar artery anteriorly the most inferior part of frontal lobe can be seen separated by the interhemispheric fissure.

1. Tentorial Level

- The V shaped enhancement of the tentorial notch outlines the superior vermis and junction of pones to the midbrain. In axial scan it is sometimes difficult to separate an intratentorial lesion from supratentotrial lesion. If the lesion is lateral to the tentorial notch, it is probably supratentorial.

2. Supratentorial Cuts

a. **Third ventricular level:** The most inferior part of frontal horns can be seen with interhemispheric fissure medial to them. The third ventricles are seen like a slit like cavity. Generally its transverse diameter should not exceed 5 mm. Superficially, the sylvian fissure can be seen extending medially to separate frontal from temporal lobe. Medial to medial aspects of sylvian fissure. The insular cortex, the external capsule, putamin and globus pellidus are visualized. Behind the third ventricle quadrigeminal plates and cistern can be seen.

b. **Low ventricular level:** The superior portion of frontal horns is seen outlines by the head of the caudate nuclei. Anteriorly the frontal horns are shaped by the indentation of the genu of corpus callosum. Pineal gland calcification is located behind the third ventricle. Behind the pineal gland, the great vein of Galen may show slightly - attenuation value in precontrast studies as a result of circulating blood. Within the lateral ventricle, the most commonly calcified choroid plexus can be identified. Posterior horns of lateral ventricles are seen at this level.

c. **Mid ventricular level:** The superior extension of sylvian fissure and superior temporal gyrus is seen. The central sulcus separates the temporal from the parietal lobes. The most superior aspect of the frontal horns is outlines inferiorly by the anterior portion of corpus callosum and the most superior aspect of caudate nuclei binds them laterally. The posterior portion of the singulate sulcus, separating the cingulated gyrus from occipital lobe can be seen connecting to posterior inter-hemispheric fissure.

d. **Above the ventricular level:** Include frontal, parietal and a small portion of occipital lobes. Central sulcus can be identified in midportion. The intra-hemispheric fissure can be seen in its entire length with the falx between.

In post contrast studies, the following structure enhances. Physiologically without any break in blood brain barrier.

1. The pituitary gland and its stalk, which enhance homogeneously.
2. Rural structures, including inter-hemispheric falx, falx cerebelli, tentorium along cavernous sinus and the tentorial notch.
3. Arterial structures in suprasellar region including circle of willis and proximal portion of anterior, middle and posterior cerebral arteries, the deep venous structures such as internal cerebral vein, vein of Galen, dural sinuses do show enhancement.
4. The choroid plexus within the lateral, third and fourth ventricle.

MRI APPEARANCES

CSF–Low signal intensity on T1W.

- High signal intensity on T2W.
- The basal ganglia, dentate nuclei of cerebellum and red nuclei of midbrain show low signal intensity on T2 weighted images due to mineral content.
- The grey matter has slightly higher signal intensity in relation to white matter in almost all spin echo images.
- The very high intensity of fat in T1W images can be appreciated within the diploic space and is outlined by low signal intensity of cortical bone.
- The vascular structures show signal void in all regular T1, T2 and proton density images.

1. USG Skull

- Window
  a. Anterior fontanelle–upto 27 years.
  b. Posterior fontanelle–upto 3 months.
  c. Mastoid fontanelle–upto 3 months.

CORONAL BRAIN SCAN

- Coronal images are obtained by placing the probe transversely across anterior fontanelle. The plane of USG beam is then made to sweep in an anterior to posterior direction.
- The frontal horns of lateral ventricles appear as symmetrical anechoic coma shaped structures with the hypoechoic caudate heads within the concave lateral borders. Structures visualized in midline from superior to inferior include the interhemispheric fissure, the cingulated sulcus, the genu and anterior body of corpus callcum and the septum pellucidum between the ventricles. Echogenic material in floor of the lateral ventricles is choroid plexus.
- In the posterior fossa, the vermis is the echogenic structure in the midline surrounded by the more hypoechoic cerebellar hemi-spheres.

SAGITTAL BRAIN SCAN

- Placing the transducer longitudinally across the anterior fontanels and angling it in each side obtain the sagittal images.

POSTERIOR FONTANELLE SCAN

- Useful view to evaluate the occipital horn for the diagnosis of intraventricular hemorrhage.

MASTOID FONTANELLE SCAN

- Allow assessment of brainstem and posterior fossa that are not well demonstrated in standard planes through anterior fontanelle.

NORMAL CALCIFICATIONS

The following calcifications seen on CT/MRI are considered to be normal:

1. Pineal gland.
2. Choroid plexus.
3. Dura.
4. Basal ganglia.
5. Habenular commissural.
6. Dentate nuclei.
7. Parasellar ligaments.
8. Arachnoid granulations.

MEASUREMENT OF VENTRICLE SIZE

1. Atrium

Normal	-	<10 mm
Borderline ventriculomegaly	-	10-15 mm
Marked ventriculomegaly	-	15-20 mm
Mean arterial diameter	-	5.8±1.3 mm
	-	6.4±1.3 mm

2. Ventricle to Choroid Separation

Normal < 3 mm.

3. Ventricle to Hemispheric Ratio

16 weeks	-	74%
25 weeks	-	<35%

4. Combined Anterior Frontal Horn Measurement

Should not exceed 20 mm at <24 weeks gestation.

Subarachnoid Hemorrhage

Subarachnoid hemorrhage (SAH) is bleeding into the subarachnoid space around the brain and spinal cord. The most common causes of SAH are head trauma and rupture of an intracranial aneurysm. Radiological evaluation is essential in determining the prognosis and treatment of SAH.

Causes of SAH

Common causes of SAH include the following:

- Head trauma.
- Intracranial aneurysms.
- Benign perimesencephalic hemorrhage.

Less frequent causes of SAH include the following:

- Arteriovenous malformation (AVM).
- Arterial dissection.
- Extension from intracerebral hemorrhage.
- Iatrogenic during surgery or intervention.
- Arteriovenous fistulae.
- Meningitis.
- Neoplasm.

Rupture of a saccular intracranial aneurysm causes approximately 80% of nontraumatic SAH. Most intracranial aneurysms occur at typical locations within or near the circle of Willis. The most common specific locations of intracranial aneurysms are at the middle cerebral artery bifurcation and along the anterior communicating artery.

Saccular aneurysms are acquired lesions that rarely, present before the third decade of life. Theories of pathogenesis include underlying congenital weakness in the arterial wall, degenerative weakening in the arterial wall from atherosclerosis, and stress of arterial pulsations on the arterial wall at turning or branching points.

Traumatic SAH must be distinguished from spontaneous SAH. Cerebral angiography may sometimes be avoided if it can be confidently established that the hemorrhage is caused by trauma. When in doubt, it is usually best to obtain a cerebral angiogram to exclude an underlying aneurysm or vascular malformation.

Clinical Details

Headache is the most common complaint in patients presenting with non-traumatic SAH. Severe headache with abrupt onset that reaches maximal intensity within seconds is particularly suggestive of SAH.

Radiological Evaluation

CT

Scanning without intravenous contrast enhancement is the preferred first diagnostic study.

CT Scans

On CT scans, SAH appears as a high-attenuating amorphous substance that fills the normally dark CSF-filled subarachnoid spaces around the brain (Figure 14.1). These findings are most evident in the largest subarachnoid spaces, such as the suprasellar cistern and Sylvian fissures. When CT scanning is performed several days to weeks after the initial bleed, the findings are more subtle. The initial high-attenuation of blood and clot tend to decrease, and these appear as intermediate gray. The sensitivity is 93-100% in patients presenting with SAH within 24 hours of symptom onset. As the time from the onset or the bleeding episode increases, the sensitivity of CT decreases. At 5 days, the sensitivity is approximately 85%, and at 1 week, it is approximately 50%.

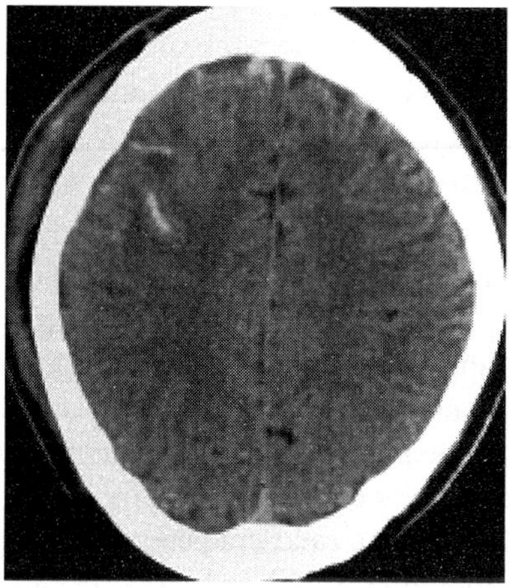

Fig. 14.1: Axial CT image shows acute sulcal bleed in right frontal lobe representing SAH

Fischer scale (CT scan appearance):

- Group 1 – No blood detected.
- Group 2 – Diffuse deposition of subarachnoid blood, no clots, and no layers of blood greater than 1 mm.
- Group 3 – Localized clots and/or vertical layers of blood 1mm or greater in thickness.
- Group 4 – Diffuse or no subarachnoid blood, but, intracerebral or intraventricular clots are present.

Group 3 appears to carry the greatest risk of subsequent vasospasm.

CT helps localize the site of the aneurysm.

- An anterior communicating aneurysm is suggested by blood in the cisterna lamina terminalis, anterior pericallosal cistern, and interhemispheric fissure. Identification of clot within a cistern makes this sign more specific. There may be extension of blood into the septum pellucidum and lateral ventricle, and hematoma in the inter medial frontal lobe.
- Localizing posterior communicating artery aneurysms is more difficult because the blood is usually diffuse within the cisterns. Intracerebral hematoma or ventricular rupture is unusual with posterior communicating aneurysms.
- Rupture of a middle cerebral aneurysm is characterized by blood in the sylvian fissure and a hematoma in the temporal lobe, which may also rupture into the adjacent temporal horn.
- Posterior fosse aneurysms often do not have good localizing findings on the CT scan.

The CT is important to evaluate complicating factors such as cerebral hematoma, ventricular rupture, hydrocephalus, cerebral infarction, and re-bleed.

It is not uncommon to find a small amount of blood in the ventricles in patients with subarachnoid hemorrhage. That does not necessarily mean that direct ventricular rupture has occurred because subarachnoid blood can enter the ventricular system in a retrograde manner. Ventricular rupture from a bleeding aneurysm is usually more dramatic, often showing a cast of blood or clot in a lateral ventricle. A subarachnoid hemorrhage with blood in the lateral ventricle is usually due to an anterior communicating aneurysm. Middle cerebral aneurysms is another possibility, but that should be associated with a temporal hematoma.

Similarly, pericallosal aneurysms can rupture into the ventricle but then there should be hematoma in the corpus callosum as well.

- False Positives/Negatives: Various normally attenuating extra-axial structures may be misinterpreted as SAH, and these can lead to false positive results.
- The falx ceribri, tentorium cerebelli and intracranial blood can be confused for small amounts of SAH.
- Streak artefact from bone at the skull base and partial volume-averaging artefact also may lead to the false diagnosis of SAH.
- False-negative studies may occur from errors in interpretation or from failure of the technology itself.
- An interval of days to weeks between the bleeding episode, and the CT allows for the breakdown and resorption of some or all of the hemoglobin from the subarachnoid space, decreasing the contrast between the SAH and CSF.
- Similarly, small amounts of SAH may be masked by dilution by CSF and/or CT volume averaging with CSF.
- Motion artefact occurring in scans of agitated or confused patients can lead to either false-positive or false-negative SAH diagnosis.

MAGNETIC RESONANCE IMAGING

Fluid-attenuated inversion recovery (FLAIR) is the most sensitive MRI pulse sequence, for the detection of SAH. On FLAIR images, SAH appears as high-intensity signal in normally low signal CSF spaces. FLAIR is similar to CT in its findings in SAH. T2- and T2*-weighted images can potentially demonstrate, SAH as low signal intensity in normally high-signal subarachnoid spaces. On T1-weighted images, subacute SAH may appear as intermediate or high intensity signal in the subarachnoid space.

Aneurysm appearance on MR scans is highly variable and may be quite complex. Signal on routine spin-echo sequences depends on the presence, direction and rate of flow, as well as presence of clot, fibrosis and calcification within the aneurysm itself. In patent aneurysm, flowing spins can produce hyper or hypo intense signals in routine spin-echo MR studies, depending on specific flow, characteristics and pulse sequences used.

Intravenous contrast typically does not enhance patent aneurysms with high flow rates, but wall enhancement may occur.

MAGNETIC RESONANCE ANGIOGRAPHY

The macroscopic motion of moving spins of in-flowing blood together with background suppression of stationary tissue can be used to create images of the cerebral vasculature. The images can be viewed as individual thin sections or reprojected in the form of flow maps or MR angiograms (MRA).

Two standard techniques currently used for MRA are phase-contrast (PC) and time of flight (TOF) acquisitions. PC creates projection angiographic images by using time of flight (TOF) acquisitions. PC creates projection angiographic images by using bipolar pulse sequences to detect the phase shifts that are caused by blood flowing through magnetic field gradients. PC imaging has excellent background suppression, allows for variable velocity encoding and can provide directional flow information.

TOF uses the inflow of fully magnetized spins into saturated stationary tissue to create angiographic images. TOF methods use two dimensional projection and direct 3D acquisitions. 3D TOF images are useful in depicting small and medium sized aneurysms.

3D time-of-flight or phase-contrast is recommended for screening for aneurysms around the circle of Willis. Relatively small imaging volumes can be used to keep imaging times short. Aneurysms 5 mm and larger are detected reliably on good quality studies.

Depending on the size of the aneurysm neck and local homodynamic, the entire aneurysm lumen may be rendered hyper intense, or an internal flow jet may be observed–similar to the first film of a conventional angiographic sequence. The flow jets can be seen as high or low signal intensity, depending on the flow dynamics and the MRA parameters used.

Potentially slow flow areas, such as the anterior and posterior communicating arteries, may not be visualized. The resolution of MRA is insufficient to accurately define the aneurysm neck or adjacent perforating arteries for presurgical planning.

To avoid errors in diagnosis, all images should be reviewed, including the individual 20 sections or partitions, and the projection images of the MRA, as well as any available spin echo scans. Using this approach to screen for aneurysms about the circle of Willis, a sensitivity of 86-95% can be achieved for aneurysms 5 mm or larger, but the sensitivity decreases to 56% for smaller aneurysms.

Patient must be informed that a normal MRA does not absolutely exclude all aneurysm. Conventional angiography remains the definitive procedure. For the same reason, MRA is not recommended in patients with documented subarachnoid hemorrhage.

ANGIOGRAPHY

Conventional catheter arteriography still has a vital role in the evaluation of aneurysm and subarachnoid hemorrhage.

The arteriogram is essential, first of all, to determine the site of aneurysm. CT and clinical, findings can suggest the location of the aneurysm, but the arteriogram is still needed to confirm the specific location of the aneurysm. The information from the clinical and CT findings should be used to guide the sequence of vessels catheterised during the angiogram.

- Secondly, the angiogram must define the neck of the aneurysm so the surgeon can plan his approach for surgical clipping.
- Thirdly, it is important to identify arteries adjacent to or arising from the aneurysm. This information will also help the surgeon in positioning his clip, thus avoiding inadvertent clipping of a branch vessel.
- Fourthly, assessment of vasospasm is essential for planning the timing of the operation.
- Finally, in any patient with an aneurysm, there is a 15-20% chance of finding multiple aneurysms. For that reason, a three- or four-vessel angiogram should always be performed in patients with subarachnoid hemorrhage, even though an aneurysm might be found on the first vessel studied.
- In cases of multiple aneurysms, the angiogram may help determine which one bled. The angiographic evidence for the ruptured aneurysm includes the larger aneurysm, multi lobulation, tits and adjacent vasospasm and mass effect. Again, the CT pattern of subarachnoid blood may also suggest thc site of bleeding.

CT Angiography

There has been increasing interest in computed topography as a non-invasive imaging modality for detection of intracranial aneurysms.

CT angiography and MR angiography are equally accurate in the detection of intracranial aneurysms, and aneurysms 5 mm or smaller are detected substantially less well than are those larger than 5 mm.

Multi-detector row CT scanners provide increased spatial resolution with decreased scanning time, leading to increase in the sensitivity of the technique in depicting aneurysms of less than 5 mm in diameter.

Advantages of multi-detector row CT angiography over DSA and MR angiography include the ability to depict bone landmarks and the proximity or aneurysms to vascular structures, which may play an important role in treatment planning. Given the improved spatial resolution obtainable with multi-detector row scanners compared with single-detector row scanners, bone subtraction is unnecessary if appropriate window and level settings are used.

Arterial and venous structures have nearly equivalent attenuation on multi- detector row CT angiographic images, with resultant benefits and drawbacks. The major benefit is in the delineation of venous anatomy (more variable than arterial anatomy), which has been cited as an advantage of multi-detector row CT angiography in patients for whom surgery is being considered. However, the overlap of arterial structure with venous structures on CT angiographic images can make their interpretation more challenging than that of MR angiographic images or DSA images.

With increasing experience, multi-detector row CT angiography may become the method of choice for aneurysm screening in patients with acute subarachnoid hemorrhage.

Sturge - Weber Syndrome

- Also known as encephalogenital angiomatosis.
- Inheritance — None (sporadic occurrence).
- Clinically — Presents as vascular malformation (portwine stain) in trigeminal nerve distribution (1st division is most frequently affected).
- Etiology — It's unknown, but it is probably due to faulty development of arterial venous drainage.
- Pathology — The paucity of the normal venous drainage results in venous stasis and vascular congestion with hypoxia of the affected cortex. Slowly progressive atrophy of the brain underlying the angioma occurs, with dystrophic calcification in the middle layer of cortical grey matter. Angioma itself is not calcified.
- Patient may present with seizures, dementia, hemiplegia, buphthalmos and glaucoma.

Imaging

Intracranial calcification is the common radiological manifestation of SWS.

- Calcification <2 years of age is uncommon.

Skull X-ray

Shows TRAM-TRACK pattern of calcification which is caused by calcification in the opposing gyri on either side of an intervening sulcus.

CT Scans

Curvilinear calcification in a gyral pattern are observed:

- More common in the occipital and post parietal lobes ipsilateral to the facial angioma.
- Progressive cortical atrophy is commonly seen with secondary manifestation such as:
  - Ipsilateral calvarial thickening.
  - Enlargement of PNS and mastoid.
- Enhancement following contrast administration can be observed on both CT and MR.
- Pial angioma often enhances.
- But gyral enhancement, possibly due to cortical ischemia and striking ipsilateral choroid plexus enhancement from collateral venous drainage may be observed as well.

MR angio in combination with MR imaging can give detailed information regarding the vascular anomalies in SWS.

Associated Abnormalities

- 1/3rd of the patients have ocular vasculitis, congenital glaucoma with buphthalmos is seen in 10-30% of cases, and scleral and choroidal angiomata have also been reported.
- Also associated with angio-osteo-hypertrophy of Kippel-Trenaunay syndrome.

DIFFERENTIAL DIAGNOSIS

Oligodendroglioma

- Arise from oligodendrocytes.
- Arise in the white matter and gyri towards the cortex.
- Adults >> children (8:1, peak 35-45 years).
- Frontal lobes are commonly involved.

Imaging

- Heterogeneous hemispheric mass involving the cortex.
- Mild to moderate in homogenous enhancement is common.
- Dystrophic calcification occurs in 90% of tumors, which may be central, peripheral or even gyriform or ribbon like.
- Overlying skull may show pressure erosion.

POST TREATMENT LYMPHOMA

History of Lymphoma and Treatment

Meningioangiomatosis.

Pathological Intracranial Calcification

- Variable leptomeningeal enhancement.
- Atrophy usually absent.
- May invade brain through Virchow- Robin perivascular spaces.

1. ***Neoplasm***
   - Craniopharyngioma.
   - Glioma.
   - Meningioma.
   - Ependymoma.
   - Papilloma of choroid plexus.
   - Pinealoma.
   - Chordoma.
   - Dermoid, epidermoid and teratoma.
   - Hematoma.
   - Lipoma.
   - Pituitary adenoma (rarely).
   - Metastasis.
2. ***Vascular***
   - Atheroma.
   - Aneurysm.
   - Angioma (Figure 15.1).

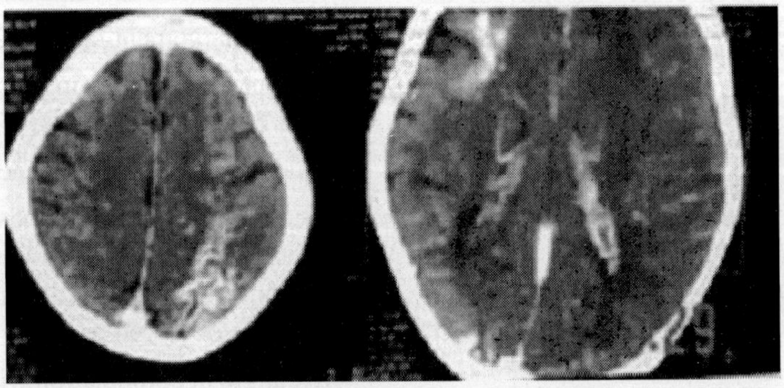

Fig. 15.1: Axial CT images show angiomatosis in the left parietal and right frontal lobe with enlarged bilateral choroid plexus

- Subdural hematoma.
- Intracranial hematoma.

3. ***Infection and Infestations***
- Toxoplasmosis.
- Cytomegalic inclusion body disease.
- Herpes.
- Rubella.
- TB.
- Pyogenic abscess.
- Cysticercoids.
- Hydatid cyst.
- Paragonimus abscess.
- Trichinosis.
- Torulosis.
- Cocidioides.

4. ***Metabolic and Miscellaneous***
- Idiopathic basal ganglia calcification.
- Hyoparathyroidism and pseudo hypoparathyroid.
- Tuberous sclerosis.
- Sturge-Weber syndrome.
- NF.
- Lissencephaly.
- Fahr syndrome.
- Cockayne syndrome.
- X-irradiation.
- Hemodialysis.
- Pb poisoning.
- CO poisoning.

GYRAL CALCIFICATION

1. Sturge-Weber syndrome (Figure 15.2).
2. Post meningoencephalitis.
3. Post treatment lymphoma.
4. Oligodendroglioma.

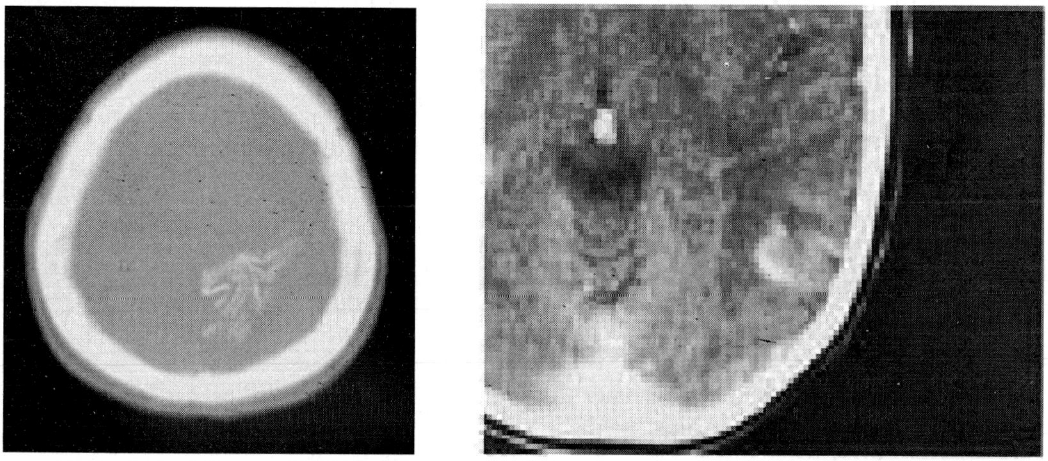

Fig. 15.2: Axial CT sections of brain showing gyral calcification in a patient with Sturge-Weber Syndrome

Arteriovenous Malformations

Intracranial AV malformations (AVM) are subdivided in 3 types:

1. Brian parenchymal (pial malformation).
2. Dual parenchymal (pial malformation).
3. Mixed pial-dual AVM.

PARENCHYMAL (PIAL) AVM'S

Pathology

AVM are complex network of abnormal vascular channels consisting of arterial feeders, arterial collaterals, the AVM nidus and enlarged venous outflow channels.

- Residue of previous hemorrhagic episodes such as dystrophic calcification and blood in different stages of degradation is common.
- Secondary changes occur within and around AVM's:
  - Overlying leptomeninges becomes thick and sometimes hemosidrin stained.
  - Flow related aneurysms on feeding vessels or within AV nidus are in 8-12% cases.
  - Thrombosis or stenosis of feeding artery and draining veins are common.

Microscopic–No intervening capillary beds in AVM.

- There is abrupt transition from thick walled feeding arteries to thin venous type channels.

Location

- 85% is cerebral hemispheres.
- 15% in post fossa.
- Located typically and extends from subpial surface and brain through the cortex and underlying white matter.
- Often cone shaped with base on the cortex and opening pointing towards the ventricle.

Incidence

- Both sexes equally effective.
- Almost always solitary, approximately 2% are multiple.
- Usually associated with extracerebral cutaneous or vascular anomalies.

Age

- These are congenital lesions.
- Peak between 20-40 years of age.

Symptoms

- Hemorrhage ½ of all AVM's present.
- 25% have seizures.
- Neurological deficit, treatment in next 20-25% cases.

IMAGING

Angiography

- Pials AVM's appear tightly packed masses and enlarged feeding arteries and dilated, tortuous draining veins with little or no internal parenchyma within the AVM nidus itself.
- Uncomplicated AVM's has no mass affect unless a hematoma or a lumen varix is present.
- AV shunting with abnormally early filling of veins that drain the lesion is characteristic, no pathognomonic of AVM.
- Flow related aneurysm is seen in 10-12% cases and in some cases stenosis/occlusion of feeding ateries or draining veins may be present representing flow induced angiopathic vascular disease.
- Completely thrombosed AVM's may have normal angiogram, show only a minimal avascular mass effect or show a very subtle AV shunting seen as an early draining vein.
- Occasionally arteries with slow blood flow visible in late arterial or capillary phase can be seen. Such as abnormal vessels have been termed as STAGNATING ARTERIES.

CT Scan

- Finding of patient AVM's include serpiginous isodense or slightly hyperdense vessels that enhance strongly following contrast administration.
- Calcification is identified in 25-30% cases.
- CT is useful for demonstrating acute hemorrhage from AVM's.
- CT also shows all other changes that one will see in angiography. These include local and distant mass effects, the presence of surrounding edema and focal compression, distortion and displacement of normal anatomic structures.
- MR is superior for delineating subacute or chronic hemorrhage as well as secondary changes such as mass affected and edema.

MRI

- Firstly depend upon the flow rate (direction in feeding and draining vessels, presence of hemorrhage and secondary changes).
- On standard spin echo images, the tropical unruptured AVM appears as a tightly packed "HONEY COMB" of "flow void" caused by high velocity signal loss. Among of -ed signal may be seen in thrombosed vessels or vessels with slow or turbulent flow.
- Hemorrhage in different stages is commonly associated with AVM's.

Hyperacute Clot

- Isointense to brain in T1WI and hyperintense on T2WI.

Subacute Clot

- Mixed signal intensities both in T1 and T2 WI.

Chronic Hemorrhage

- Chronic hemorrhage with area of hemosiderin or ferritin appears as areas of hypodense signal within and around the AVM on T2WI gradient echo scan.

Treatment

- Because the risk of hemorrhage is high, complete obliteration of an AVM nidus is the the goal regardless of treatment modality.
- Elective resection is recommended for unruptured AVM's particularly in young patients with lesions that have a favourable location, size and venous drainage.
- Other modalities of treatment include endovascular occlusion, stereo tactic radiation.

- Extravascular techniques are also used to reduce the size of AVM's for the treatment. Pre op embolization with nidus occluding agents such N-butyl cyanoacrylate make larger higher grade AVM's, the surgical equivalent of smaller, lower grade lesion by reducing the operative time and intraoperative blood loss.

DORSAL AVM'S

Pathology

- Thickened arteries and dilated veins form an abnormal vascular network within the wall of venous sinus.

Etiology

- This is an acquired abnormality.
- Dual AVM's arise following sinus thrombosis or occlusion with subsequent recanalization; numerous small direct artery or sinus communications or micro fistulae are formed.
- Other theories that a single AV fistula firmly form in along near a venous sinus and as blood flow increases adjacent dural arteries are recanalized and form dual AVM's.

Location

- Most dual AVM's involve the venous sinuses along the base of the brain. The transverse and sigmoid sinus is most frequently affected. Cavernous sinus is also a common site.

  Superior sagittal sinus and straight sinus are uncommon site.
- Dual AVM's are usually solitary except bilateral cavernous sinus AVM's.
- Multiple are uncommon and account for only 7% of all dual AVM's no known predisposing conditions for multiplication are known, although hypercoagulable status could conceivable lead to thrombosis and subsequent fistulization at several sites.

Incidence

- Dual AVM's account for 10-15% of all intracranial AV malformation.

Age and Presentation

- *Bruit and headache:* Most common symptoms of DAVM involving transverse and sigmoid sinus.
- Proptosis, chemosis, bruit, retro orbital pain – cavernous sinus lesion (ophthalmoplegia).
- *Cranial nerve palsies:* Straight cavernous sinus lesion and DAVM's with intracranial venous varices.

Risk and Complications

- Rarely cause IC hemorrhage, however, intracranial venous varices carries increased risk of hemorrhage and mass affect with subsequent cranial nerve palsies.

Obstructive Hydrocephalus

- Due to mechanical compression.
- Communicating hydrocephalus—increased CSF absorption due to chronic passive congestion.

IMAGING

Angiography

- Any dural vessel is potential source to dural vascular malformation.
- Most DAVM's have multiple feeders.
- As most DAVM's seen in post fossa, communicating vessels that supply are occipital artery and meningeal branches of ECA.
- Particular type of DAVM's, traumatic cortico-cavernous fistula (CCF), often has single direct communication.
- Less common type of CCF may primarily in

middle-aged women with proptosis, bruit and chemosis. These lesions are spontaneous and unrelated to trauma – multiple dural feeders are a rule.

CT Scans

- Often normal.
- Sometimes enlarged dural sinus or draining vein can be identified.
- In CCF's enlarged cavernous sinus is seen in half of the cases and a dilated sup. Ophthalmic vein can be identified in most CECT scans.

MRI

- On MR the finding of dilated cortical vein without an identifiable parenchymal nidus suggests the presence of DAVM's with associated venoocclusive disease.
- Routine spin echo MR is procedure of choice for demonstrating complication of DAVM's including infarction and hemorrhage.
- These contrasts MRA can demonstrate flow direction in draining vein of dural sinus.

Miscellaneous Techniques

Colour flow Doppler USG studies have been used recently to demonstrate flow in the superior ophthalmic vein.

MIXED PIAL-DURAL AVM'S

If a parenchymal (pial) AVM attains sufficient size, it can reconnect vascular supply from dural arterial branches. In such cases the malformation has the imaging characteristics of both pial and dural AVM's.

Section 1—Central Nervous System

Chapter 17

Spinal Cord Malformations

Normal Anatomy

The spinal cord (SC) is:

- Greyish white structure.
- Begins above at foramen magnum.
- Continues with medulla oblongata of brain.
- Inferiorly it terminates as conus medullaris at L1(lower border) in adults and L3 (upper border) in children.
- Prolongation of pia mater from conus is filum terminale, which is attached to back of coccyx.
- Cord has 2 fissures:
  - Ant is anterior median fissure; and
  - Post is posterior median sulcus.

  On cross-section:
- Central is gray matter with H shape configuration formed by dorsal and ventral horn, surrounding is white matter.

Meninges

From outside in:

1. Dura extends till S_2 spindle subdural space small.
2. Arachnoid–loosely attached to inner aspects of dura. Subarachnoid space lies under lepto meninges and contains CSF. SC and nerve roots cervical subarachnoid space is wider, CV junction tapering from Foramen Magnum. To C_2 C_3 C_7 10-15 mm in A.P. diameter. Thoracic subarachnoid 12-13 mm in sagittal diameter and lumbar subarachnoid space is larger 15-20 mm in sagittal diameter.

Congenital Malformations

Types

1. Open spinal dysraphism
   - E.g. Myelocoele.
   - Myelo meningocele (Figure 17.1).
2. Occult spinal dysraphisms

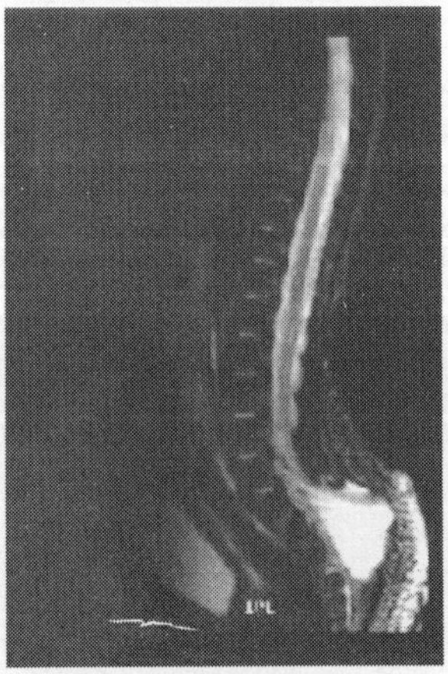

Fig. 17.1: Myelomeningocele of lumbar spine, with neural placode present posterior to enlarged thecal sac. Ventral nerve roots course through CSF-filled sac to exit neural foramina. Tethered spinal cord

- Meningocoele.
- Dorsal dermal sinus.
- Spinal lipomas.

3. Abnormalities of abnormal canalization and retrogressive differentiation
   - Fethered spinal cord.
   - Tight filum terminale syndrome.
   - Caudal spinal anomalies.
4. Split Notochord syndrome
   - Dorsal enteric fistula (most severe) and rarest.
   - Dorsal enteric sinus.
   - Diastematomyelia.
   - Spinal enterogenous cyst.

Tethered SC and Tight Filum Terminale Syndrome

- Etiology – Failure of terminal cord involution or normal nerve fibre lengthening.
- Syndrome is complex of neurological and orthopaedic deformity associated with short thick filum terminale and low lying conus medullaris.
- Tethered cord is common feature of much spherical malformation and thick filum terminale is usually associated with clinical tethered S.C. syndrome.

Incidence

- Seen at any age.

Symptoms

- Begins between 3-35 years.

Gender Predilection

- Nil.

Clinical Presentation

- Pain, dyesthesias, neurogenic bladder and spasticity, congenital/developmental kyphoscoliosis.

Imaging

- Plain film – dysraphic spine.

Myelography

- Low lying conus, with or without lipoma. Existing nerve roots have lateral/uphill course in severe cases.

CT Myelography

- Low-lying conus below L2 thickened filum terminale > 1.5 mm in diameter and sometimes, fibrous adhesion band. Tethered cord may terminate in lipoma.

MRI and MR Myelogram

- Axial T2W are diagnostic, sagittal view can be misleading (lumbar nerve root usually larger dorsally and can mimic tethered cord).

CAUDAL SPINAL ANOMALIES

- In which malformation of distal spine, SC and meninges are associated with hindgut, kidney, urinary bladder and genital anomalies.
  a. *Caudal regression syndrome (VACTER L)* – Varying degree of lumbosacral agenesis with associated anomalies as imperforate anus, malformed genitals, and renal dysplasia. On investigation – absent coccyx, sacral or lumbosacral agenesis may be present.
  b. *Terminal myelocystocel (syringocele)*– Localized cystic dilatation of distal S.C. consists of post spinal bifida or partial sacral agenesis, tethered spinal cord with hydromelia. Cord, meninges and subarachnoid space protrude into dorsal subcutaneous plane. MRI is diagnostic.
  c. *Anterior sacral meningocele*–Herniation of meninges through defect in sacrum, coccyx or adjacent disc spaces to form a CSF filled hernial sac within pelvis. It may be isolated defect or part of caudal regression syndrome.

On Investigation

- Widen sacral foramina with smoothly scalloped margin and protruding CSF sac is present.

d. *Occult intrasacral meningocoele*

The arachnoid herniates through dural defect expanding and scalloping the bony sacrum.

On imaging studies – It is seen as expansile smoothly marginated, well delineated cyst that are often slightly higher in signal intensity than CSF.

- Symptoms are unrelated to cyst size.
- Communicating cysts are asymptomatic.
  Non-communicating cysts are symptomatic.
- Occurs in isolation but are commonly associated with lipoma, hyperkeratosis, sacral pigmentation, sacrococcygeal dimple and neurofibromatosis.

e. *Sacrococcygeal teratoma*

Developmental in origin, commonly encountered presacral masses in children classified into four types:

Type I (47%) - Ext mass predominant.
Type II (34%) - Ext mass with significant internal component.
Type III (9%) - Int masses with small external compression.
Type IV (10%) - Presacral mass only.

- On prenatal USG, most teratomas are solid or mixed, 15% are cystic, calcification present, large masses may displace and distort neighbouring structures as rectum or urinary bladder. Large (-) may develop AV shunting causing fetal cardiac failure, hydrops (Carries poor prognosis).

D/D of Presacral Fetal Masses

- Most frequent
  – Sacrocoxygeal teratoma - a fetal part and acetyl elionesterase in amniotic fluid.
  – Cordomas.
  – Ant. Myelomeningocoele.
  – Sarcoma.
  – Lipoma.
  – Neuroenteric cyst.
  – Lymphoma.
  – For masses <4.5 cm in dia without associated abnormality, elective vaginal delivery is recommended.
  – For masses >4.5 cm elective c.s. is recommended.

Spinal Notochord Syndrome

Results from splitting of notochord with a persistent connection between gut and dorsal ectoderm.

Diastematomyelia

- *Etiology and pathology:* Characterized by sagittal clefting of spinal cord. Or filum terminale. Recent theory postulate arises from adhesion between embryonic ectoderm and endoderm, which leads to accessory neuro enteric canal. Endomesenchymal tract condenses around accessory canal bisecting developing notochord and causing two hemi neural plates to form S.C. split into 2 I/V halves by fibrous, bony or osteocartilagenous septum. Cleft extends completely though out cord although partial clefting occasionally occurs two hemichord contains a central canal and one set of dorsal and ventral horn.
  – Split spinal cord (not duplicated cord).
  – Hemicords in separate (50%) or common (50%) dural lobe.
  – Usually between T_9-S_1 (85%).
  – Spine nearly always abnormal.
  – Osseous spur in only 50%.
  – Associated with Chiari syndrome II malformation, tethered spinal cord, hydromelia of one or both hemicords.
  – Distinct female predominance.

– Age at symptom onset varies.

Imaging Findings

- If there is associated fibrous or bony septum prenatal sonography will not detect abnormality. Post natal USG, CT and MRI can demonstrate the lesions. Plain films and NCT shows grossly abnormal osseus spine (hemivetebrae block), butterfly vertebrae, narrow I/V disc space intersegmental laminar fusion with spina bifida, increased interpediculate distance. The hemicords and subarachnoid space well delineated at CT, myelography and MRI.

Enterogenous Cyst

- *Etiology and pathology:* Results from failure of notochord and foregut. Separation during formation of elementary canal. The elementary canal is well-delineated, fluid containing masses incidence, age and gender. Mostly less than 40 years of age with peak incidence in 1st and 2nd decade.

Male Predominance

Clinical Sudden and Severe Pain and Myelopathic Symptoms

Imaging – myelopathy typically discloses intradural extramedullary mass interior to SC, CT or CT myelography shows a low density mass – MRI shows T1W, iso to slightly hyperintense compare to CSF and slightly hyperintense on PD and T2W. Associated anaomaly – vertebral anomaly.

D/D Arachnoid Cyst (Dorsal to Cord/Intensity < CSF)

Epidermoid cyst (DW and FLAIR sequences).

Miscellaneous Malformations

- Chiari malformations.
- Hydromelia.
- Syringomelia.

Chiari I Malformation

- Peg like, pointed tonsils displaced into upper cervical canal.
- At least 6 mm in first decade of life 10-30 years: 5 mm.
  30-80 years: 4 mm.
  Associated anomalies.
  Brain – usually none.
  Ventricles – mild, moderate hydrocephalus (20-25%).
  Spinal cord – syringomyelia in 30-60% in all patients; 60-90% in symptomatic patients.
  Skeletal anomalies in 25%.
  Basilar invagination (25-50%).
  Klippel-Feil (5-10%).
  Atlanto-occipital assimilation (1-5%).

Chiari II Malformation (Figure 17.2)

- Internal herniation of medulla with elongaged 4th ventricle and vermis displaced inferiorly into cervical canal.
- Myelomeningocele in 100% patients.
- Syringohydromyelia 50-90%.
- Diastometamyelia.
- Segmentation anomaly <10% in complete C arc.

Hydromelia and Syringomyelia

- Congenital.
- Acquired post traumatic.

Pathogenesis

a. Dysraphic theory suggest neural tube defect of closure.

b. Hydrodynamic theory disturb CSF outflow from 4th ventricle is responsible.

Patho: It is ependymal line distention of central canal whereas syringomyelia is CSF dissection through ependymal lining to form paracentral cavity.

Because histological and imaging studies are indistinguishable, they are often grouped under terms hydrosyringomelia.

- Communicating (15% - 20%).
- Non-communicating (80%).

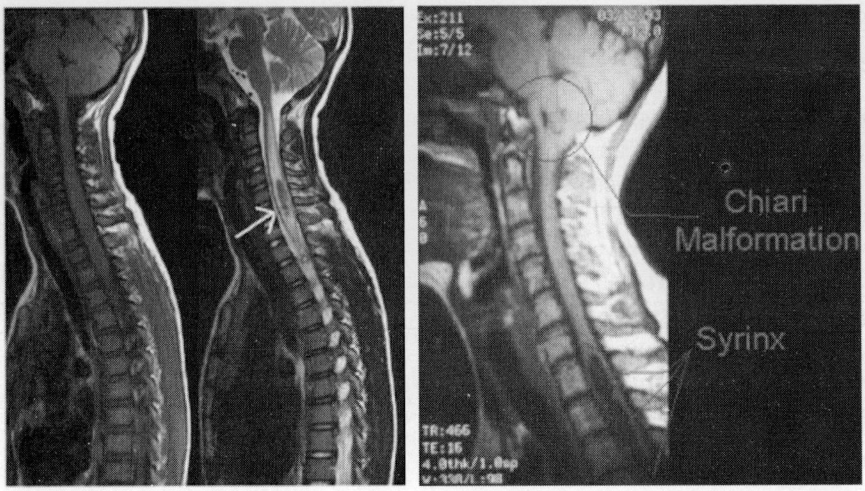

Fig. 17.2: Sagittal MRI sections showing Arnold Chiari malformation with syrinx formation in upper cervical canal

Communicating

- Continues with 4th ventricle via obe.
- Typically associated with hydrocephalus, SAH, meningitis.

Non-communicating

- Separated from 4th ventricle by syrinx free segmentospinal cord associated with Chiari I and Chiari II malformation, S.C. Trauma, intramedullary (T), those associated with Chiari II malformation is asscoaited with hydrocephalus. Those with Chiari I typically are not.

  Location: Any location but cervical cord is most common. Chiari I and neoplastic syringes occur in cervical spinal cord.

  Sudden and Severe - Sensory disturbances
  - Muscular atrophy.
  - Diminished deep tendon reflexes.

Imaging Finding

- MR is diagnostic. Enlarged cord with central or slightly fluid filled cavity that parallels CSF and signal intensity. Beaded shapes are typical of Chiari-associated hydromelia.
- Increased signal around syrinx in T2W images represent cord gliosis, edema or myelomalasia.
- Benign syrinx does not enhance following contrast administration.

Neurocutaneous Syndrome

- Neurofibromatous type I- scoliosis, wide spinal canal with dural sac and meningocele are characteristic. Neurofibroma of existing nerve roots are common. S.C. lesions are less frequent in NSI as compared to NF-2.

  Intramedullary hyperintensity on T2W images represent glial hematomatous proliferation; SC neoplasms are rare when they occur, they arre low-grade astrocytomas.

  NF-II characterized by multiple Schawan-nomas and meningiomas. Are equally divided into cervical thoracic and lumbar routes.
- 70% are intradural extramedullary lesions.
- SC neoplasms are also common.
- Ependymomas are most frequent (T).

  Von-Hippel-Lindau syndrome – autosomal dominant, multisystem disorder with RCC, pheochromocytoma, cysts.
- Hemangioblastomas of cerebellum, brain and spinal cord as well as retinal angiomatoses are typical 10-30% of S.C. hemiangioblastomas occur in VHL.

Paraplegia

Disc and vertebral	Plain film	Myelography	CT	MRI
Trauma	• Widening of inter pedicular distance/ disc space • Paravertebral swelling • Burst fracture, Wedge fracture • Crunch fracture	Extradural compression (Figures 18.1 and 18.2)	Post displacements of fragments and impingement upon the spinal cord	Cord hematoma Variable signal Intensity Cord oedema T2W hyper intense Epidural hematoma may be seen
Chronic degenerative changes	• Apophyseal joint ↓ed space Sclerosis Osteophyte Subluxation (instability) IVD ↓ed height Vacuum Osteophyte Canal stenos is Body sclerosis	Extradural compression by osteophytes	Interdiskal gas (vacuum phenomenon) osteophyte compression of cord ↓ed height	Modic 1-T1w-↓ed T2W–↑ed Modic 2-T1W–↑ed T2W Isointense or hyperintense Modic 3-T1W-↓ed T2W-↓ed
Inflammatory epidural abscess	(-)	Extradural compression		Fluid collection of slightly higher density than CSF and the involved duration is markedly thickened and enhances
TB	• Lytic destruction at the ant subchondral plate • Loss of disc ht.	Extradural compression		Lytic destruction at the anterior subchondral plate

Contd.

Contd.

	• Vertebral collapse • Obliteration of disc space • Abscess formation Para vertebral psoas • Multiple segments involved • Ant. vertebral scalloping			• Loss of disc ht • Vertebral collapse • Obliteration of disc space • Abscess formation with calcification Para vertebral psoas • Multiple segments involved • Ant. vertebral scalloping (gouge defect)
Metastasis	• Pedicle destruction • Osteolytic (80%) • Loss of bone density after 50% has since lost • Pathologic compression fracture • Paraspinous soft tissue mass	Extradural compression	Earlier than plain film osteolytic/osteoblastic lesions intrathecal contrast is required to delineate the precise extent	– Most sensitive – Marrow adjacent to post cortical margin is effective first – Replacement of normal fatty marrow within the V. body – Four patterns – Focal lytic – Focal ulceration – Diffuse inhomogenous – Diffuse homogenous – T1W low signal –T2W high signal

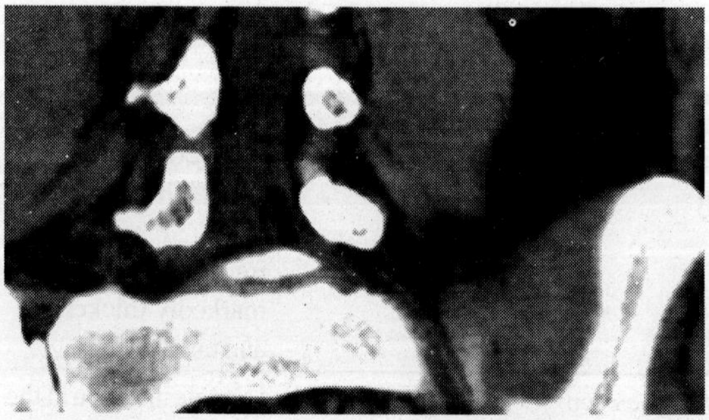

Fig. 18.1: Sagittal and coronal MPR CT images showing a hypodense extradural mass on the right side of midline

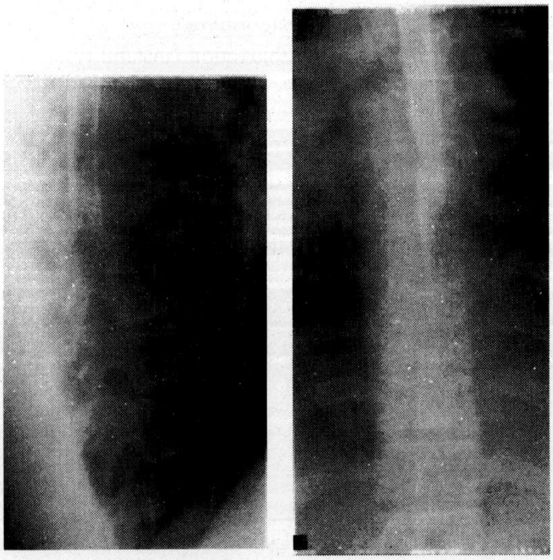

Fig. 18.2: Myelography shows extradural block secondary to spinal tumor

PARAPELGIA

Definition

It means weakness of both lower limbs.

Causes of Paraplegia

I. Spinal Lesions

i. Spinal cord compression

a. Disc and vertebral lesions
- Trauma.
- Chronic degeneration.

b. Inflammatory
- Epidural abscess.
- T.B.
- Granuloma.

c. Vertebral neoplasms
- Metastases.
- Myeloma.

d. Epidural hemorrhage

e. Rarities
- Paget's disease.
- Epithelial, endothelial and parasitic cysts.
- Aneurysmal bone cyst.
- Vertebral angioma.
- Hematomyelia, arachnoiditis.
- Osteoporosis.

ii. Multiple sclerosis.

iii. Myelitis (e.g. VZU).

iv. Motor neuron disease.

v. Subacute combined degeneration of the cord (Figures 18.3 and 18.4).

vi. Syringomyelia.

vii. Syphilis.

viii. Familial or sporadic para paresis.

ix. Vascular disease of the cord.

x. Non-metastatic manifestation of malignancy.

xi. Tropical spastic para paresis (HTLV-1).

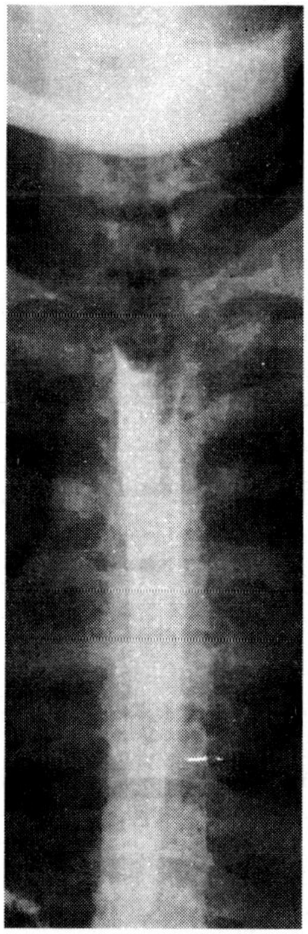

Fig. 18.3: Myelogram shows extramedullary intradural lesion in the cervical region

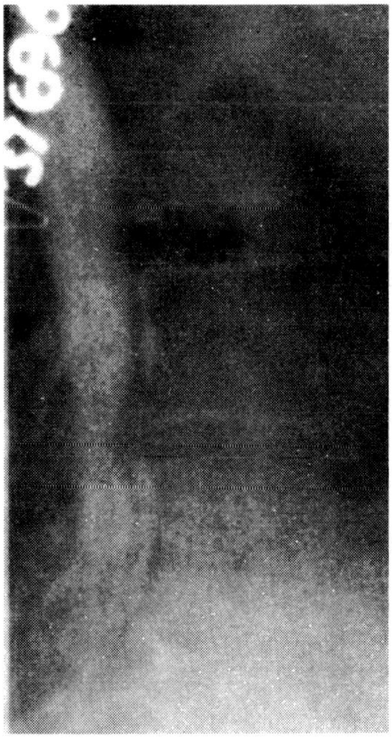

Fig. 18.4: Myelogram shows partial extradural block due to intervertebral disk prolapse

Chronic Degenerative Changes

Aetiology and Pathology

- Osteophytosis is a primary pathologic finding. Osteophytes are bony expressions that originate near the margin of vertebral bodies or facet joints.
- Vertebral body osteophytes results from weakening of annular fibres with disk bulging and traction on sharply fibres.
- Osteophytes typically develop where these fibres attack to the V. body, usually several mm from the disk vertebral joint muscles.
- Schmorls nodes, herniation of disk material then the plates into V. body are common manifestation.

Incidence Age and Gender

- The prevalence of osteophytes in patient 50 years of age or older is estimated to be 60% to 80%.
- Men are more frequently affected than women.
- Individuals engaged in occupations that require heavy physical labour are more often affected.

Location

- Lumbar and cervical areas are the most common sites.
- In the cervical spine the levels most frequently affected for both disk herniation and chronic spondylosis are C6-C7 and C5-C6. In the lumbar spine L4-5 and L5-S1 are the MC and most severely affected.

Epidural Abscess

Etiology and Pathology

Spinal epidural abscess results from direct hematogenous seeding of epidural spaced from a cutaneous, pulmonary urinary tract source.

- S. aureus is the most common organism.
- *Two basic stages are seen SEA:* Initially there is thickened inflamed tissue with granulomatous material. This represents a phlegmonous.

II. Cerebral Lesions

- Parasagittal cortical lesions.
  - Meningioma.
  - Venous sinuses thrombosis.
- Hydrocephalus.
- Multiple cerebral infarctions

Stage: In the 2nd stage a collection of liquid pus forms a frank abscess.

Incidence, Age and Gender

- One case per 10,000 hospital admissions in tertiary institutions.
- The mean age affected in 50 to 55 years.
- There is moderate male predominance.

Location

- All area of the spine are affected.
- SEA are often extensive in 1/3rd cases the infection extends over more than 6 vertebral segments.
- Concomitant diskitis or osteomyelitis is seen in 80%.

Granulomatous Spondylitis

Etiology and Pathology

Granulomatous lesions are treated with a spectrum of bacterial, viral, parasitic and fungal infection as well as bone tumors, autoimmune disease and idiopathic disorders. Granulomatous spondylitis is most commonly caused by mycobacterium tuberculosis. Other organisms include B. malenosis some fungal infection such as blasto mycosis and aspergillus's can cause it.

Parasitic infections: Echinococcus.

Incidence Age and Gender

In developing countries, TB spondylitis is a disease

of children whereas in North America and Europe it is most prevalent in middle-aged adults.

- The mean age at diagnosis in 40 and 45 years.
- Debilitation, immunosuppression, alcoholism and drug addiction are predisposing conditions.

Location

The lower dorsal and lumbar spine is affected in nearly 3/4th of all T.B. spondylitis.

- Nearly 90 of cases have at least 2 affected V. bodies, 50% have 3 or more levels affected "skip" lesion are common.

Multiple Sclerosis (MS)

Etiology and Pathology

- Spinal cord plaques are an almost universal autopsy finding in patients with multiple sclerosis.
- Plaques occur preferentially in the dorsolateral cord and do not respect boundaries between specific tracts or between grey and white matter.

Incidence, Age and Gender

- The greatest prevalence is in temperate zone

Disc and vertebral	Plain film	Myelography	CT	MRI
Multiple myeloma	Focal or diffuse lytic defects in	Extradural compression V.body	Focal/diffuse lytic defects in V. body	T1W hypointense to a adjacent marrow and iso or slight hyperintense compared to adjacent muscle T2W hyperintense fat suppressed and T2W helps in delineating lesion extent.
Multiple sclerosis	(-)	(-)	Location-callo septal interface NCCT iso or hypo-intense CECT-variable contrast enhancement both solid and ring pattern	T2W–ovoid high signal intensity foci Periventrcular extension (1 to ventricles) bevelled or "targets) (lesion within a lesion) appearance, common on T1W PD weighted e.g. variable enhancement (solid, ring).
Subacute combined degeneration of cord	-	-	-	Not always visible on MRI. Swelling and enhancement after Gd administration striking column change confined to dorsal column.

such as United States, Canada and Great Britain and Northern Europe.

- Disease onset is between 15 and 30 years with a peak in the 3rd and 4th decade.
- There is a distinct female predominance, particularly in children and adolescents with MS.

Location

Spinal cord plaques are found at any segment:

- In later stages, plaques are evenly distributed in early disease there is distinct predilatation for the cervical spinal cord.
- An MS called variant neuromyelitis optica is a rapidly progressive fulminant demyelination that is restricted to the optic nerves and spinal cord.

Syringomyelia

Etiology and Pathology

- Syringomyelia may be congenital or acquired (e.g. post traumatic syringomyelia).
- The dystrophic theory suggests that a neural tube closure defect is responsible, whereas the hydrodynamic theory maintains that disturbed CSF outflow from the 4th ventricle is responsible.
- Syringomyelia supervenes as the dilated ependymal canal rupture into the spinal cord parenchyma.
- Syringomyelia is defined as CSF dissection through the ependymal lining to form a parenteral cavity.
- Syringomyelia may be communicating or non-communicating. Between 15% and 20% of syringes are anatomically communicating with the 4th ventricles. These so called communicating syringes are typically associated with hydrocephalus and occur with SAH, meningitis and leptomeningeal carcinomatosis.
- Nearly 80% of syringes are non-communicating i.e. they are separated from the 4th ventricle by syringe free segment of spinal cord.
- Non-communicating segments occurs with Chiari I and Chiari II malformations, as well as acquired disorders such as spinal cord trauma, intramedullary tumors and extra medullary compressive lesions.

Locations

- Cervical cord is the most common site.
- Syringes associated with Chiari I malformation are most often cervical or cervicothoracic neoplastic syringes occur mostly in the cervical spinal cord.

NEUROGENIC BLADDER

- It may be caused by spinal dysraphism, cord compression or cord injury.
- Cystography is very helpful in diagnosis of neurogenic bladder.
- US is also useful to assess bladder size, shape, volume post cord residue, renal parenchyma change and secondary calculi.
- In the condition called as detrusor – external sphincter dysnergia (DESD), contraction of the external sphincter occurs involuntarily at the same time as detrusor contraction thus impeding urinary flow and resulting in bladder outlet obstruction.
- In this condition bladder is often vertically oriented within irregular contour with trabeculation, frequently with multiple diverticular and is referred to as X-mas tree or "pine tree" bladder.
- On voiding cysto urethrography there may or may not be VUR.
- In detrusor are flexia voiding cystourethrography often reveals a smooth, thin walled bladder with increased capacity occur upto several litre and extending high into the abdomen.
  - Significant post void residue is seen in both these conditions.

Disc and vertebral	Plain film	Myelography	CT	MRI
Syringomyelia	• Symmetric tapering of the contrast column	Cavities are well shown gen. CT myelography is required with imaging early and late (6 to 10) after contrast. Administration	On T1W image axial and sagittal images, syringes area best demonstrated, where the low signal intensity CSF creates a black column relative to the surrounding high signal intensity spinal cord parenchyma	
Syphilis	• Lumbar spine • Prominent loss of the disk height • Sclerosis • Osteophyte • Vacuum phenomenon • Fragmentation of V. body (jigsaw vertebrae) • V. malalignment with ant, post and lat. displacements (tumbling building block spine)	-		
Angiomatous malformation and fistula	• To localise the AV shunt prior to surgery	Abnormal vessel sometimes minor cord swelling is also positive	-	T2W done signal linear strand. High signal intensity within the spinal cord usually through its lower half or so down to the conus medullaris due to oedema and/or infarction.
Epidural hematoma	• May reveal signs of trauma	Extradural compression from post aspect of spinal cord	Extradural mass (Fig. 18.5)	Intensity patterns will suggest with axis and the degree of narrowing of the these and compression will be shown.
Meningioma	• Hyperostosis erosion enlarged	-	Hyper dense, enhances strongly	Typically isointense with grey matter

Contd.

Contd.

	vascular channels tumor calcification pneumosinus dilatation Angiography • Dual vascular supply –"sunburst" of enlarged dural feeder prolonged vascular stain		and uniformly 20% to 25% calcified 8% peritumoral oedema	>95% enhance strongly; heterogeneous enhancement common CSF/vascular cleft 60% has duration "tail".
Venous sinus thrombosis	• –	Thrombosed sinus appears as an empty channel devised of contrast and surrounded by dilated collateral venous channels in the dural leave	NCCT hyperdense thrombus in the thrombosed dural sinus or veins CECT – engorged dural cavernous spaces, meningeal venous, tributaries and collateral venous channels that surround a relatively hypodense occluded sinus may enhance around the thrombus in empty delta sign	T1W acute infarct ↓ isointense Late acute infarct T1W1 hyperintense T2W hypointense Sub acute thrombin ↓ Hyperintense on all tube sequences

EPIDURAL HEMATOMA

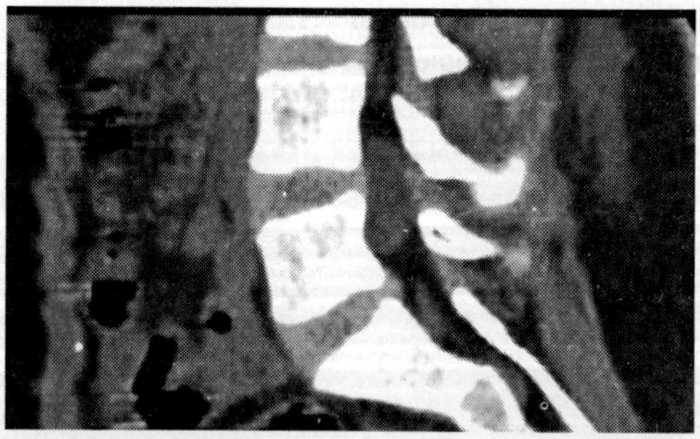

Fig. 18.5: Sagittal CT images showing hyponense extra dural mass–epidural hematoma

Interventional Neuroradiology

ENDOVASCULAR PROCEDURE

- The femoral approach is almost exclusively used. A shear of appropriate size is always used.
- A guiding catheter is used to ensure stable access and provide a route for injection of contrast for road mapping.
- Micro catheter, either flows guided or over the wire, are usually used to reach the catheter.
- The anatomy of the vessels used for access to the target and the target itself must be carefully defined by high quality angiography.
- The possibility that flow patterns will change in the course of the procedure must always be kept in mind and close attention must be given to the appearance of previously non-visualized collateral pathways.
- Heparin is often administered to decrease the risk of thrombosis during the procedure.
- Endovascular procedures can be broadly divided into two categories:
  1. Those that aim to restore a narrowed or obliterated vascular lumen supplying normal tissues.
  2. Those that aim to exclude abnormal blood vessels from circulations.

ENDOVASCULAR TECHNIQUES FOR LUMEN RESTORATION

Intra-Arterial Thrombolysis

- Intravenous thrombolysis with recombinant tissue plasminogen activator (rTPA) is used for the diagnosis of acute ischemic stroke within 3 hours of onset. It is more successful in distal middle cerebral artery occlusions, in recanalization of larger vessels such as the internal carotid artery (ICA) or proximal (MI) segment of the middle cerebral artery.
- Inter arterial thrombolysis achieves a higher local core of the thrombolytic agent in the vicinity of the clot but it is more complex to achieve and therefore takes longer, increasing the delay between onset and treatment.
- The randomized trial has shown all overall benefit from intra-arterial thrombolysis in MCA occlusion within 6 hours. After the onset of stroke, despite a greater risk of hemorrhagic complication.
- In this trial 9 mg of recombinant urokinase has been infused through a single end hole microcatheter placed in the proximal third of the MCA thrombus over a period of 2 hours.

- The trial provided a proof of principle that intra-arterial thrombolysis work and alternative pharmaceutical agents such as streptokinase and rTPA remain available for intra-arterial thrombolysis.
- Intra-arterial thrombolysis is also successful in ICA and vertebro basilar occlusions.
- Success of recanalization is decreased in distal ICA or T-junction occlusion.
- Young patients with short segment basilar occlusions benefited from thrombolytic treatment and had better chances of recovery.
- New developments in the endovascular treatment of acute stroke include the use of mechanical devices for extraction of acute thrombus.
- These have the advantage of reducing the treatment time (with a corresponding prolongation of the therapeutic window) and of a theoretical reduction in hemorrhage complications associated with thrombolytic agents.

TREATMENT OF CEREBRAL VASOSPASM

- Cerebral vasospasm represents a significant cause of morbidity and mortality in patients with SAH.
- Early treatment of ruptured aneurysm together with refinement of endovascular and surgical techniques have led to a reduction of morbidity and mortality from aneurysm re-rupture, but management of cerebral vasospasm remains still a challenge.
- Approximately 1/3rd of patient with SAH develop symptomatic vasospasm with delayed ischemic deficit of which 30% will die and a further 30% will have a permanent deficit.
- Medical treatment consists of hypertension, hypervolemia and hemodilution (triple H therapy).
- Patients who fail to respond to medical therapy may benefit from endovascular treatment, which falls in two categories, mechanical dilatation of stenotic segments (balloon dilatation) and pharmacological relaxation of the contracted vessels with intra-arterial papaverine infusion.
- Intracranial balloon angioplasty is performed with a small, compliant balloon attached to a micro catheter. It is only suitable for treatment of the proximal segments of intracranial vessels, as dilatation of smaller branches carries a high risk of vessel rupture.
- Balloon dilatation has a more permanent effect than the infusion of papavarine through a catheter which often leads only to a transient increase of the vessel lumen.
- Papaverine may be useful to facilitate access for endovascular diagnosis of a ruptured aneurysm if this is impeded by vasospasm. It can also be used to treat vasospasm in distal branches of cerebral arteries that are not suitable for balloon dilatation.
- The complications of both technique include vessel dissection and rupture, vessel thrombosis or at embolus and rupture of an unsecured aneurysm.

ANGIOPLASTY AND STENTING OF EXTRACRANIAL VESSELS

- The ECST and NASCET demonstrated that carotid endo stenectomy significantly reduced the risk of recurrent stroke in patients with over 70% carotid artery stenosis.
- Subsequently PTA and stenting have emerged as alternatives to surgery in these patients.
- The CAVATAS have revealed that endovascular treatment was safer in terms of minor morbidity such as cranial nerve palsies and hematoma.
- Three-year follow up data suggested no difference in outcome between the two treatments, suggesting both are equally effective in preventing stroke.

- The majority of the patients in the endovascular arms of CAVATAS was treated with balloon angioplasty alone and only 22% were treated with stents. In the meantime primary stenting has become the endovascular technique of choice for carotid artery stenosis, replacing PTA.
- In majority of major strokes after carotid PTA is the result of dissection of the carotid artery at the time of balloon inflation with subsequent thrombosis.
- Dissection and occlusion of the carotid artery are lesss likely to occur with stenting because the stent maintain laminar flow across the stenosis and scale the site of dissection, preventing a free intimal flap.
- Carotid stenting is generally performed under local anaesthesia.
- The patient should receive antiplatelet therapy to minimize the risk of thromboembolic complications.
- Following preliminary angiography, a guiding catheter is placed in the common carotid artery, the stenosis is crossed with a soft tip guide wire and a self-expandable stent is placed across the stenosis, normally bridging the carotid bifurcation.
- The self-expandable stent allows differential expansion of its distal and proximal portion adapting to the different diameters of the common and internal carotid arteries.
- Additional dilatation of the stenosis with a balloon catheter placed within the stent is usually performed.
- Recent developments in carotid stenting include protection devices such as filters and occlusion balloon.

ANGIOPLASTY AND STENTING FOR INTRACRNIAL ARTERIOSCLEROTIC DISEASE

- Intracranial arteriosclerotic disease is a significant cause of ischemic strokes.
- The surgical diagnosis option consists of an extracranial intracranial bypass operation, which has not been shown to confer any additional benefit over aspirin therapy.
- The possibility of treating these patients with endovascular techniques such as balloon angioplasty and stenting represents an important development.
- This is a technique in evolution and delineated intracranial stents have recently become available.
- Recent devices suggest that intracranial balloon dilatation and stenting have reached an acceptable safety level.

ENDOVASCULAR TECHNIQUE FOR LUMEN OBLITERATION

- Various techniques such as mechanical devices (coils and balloons), particles and liquid embolic agents are available.
- Detachable balloons made of either silicone or latex is used to occlude large vessels or large fistulas such as cortico cavernous fistulas. One of the risks of this technique is accidental detachment of balloon in an unwanted position, which can lead to obstruction of normal cerebral vessels. Systems with non-detachable balloons are available for temporary test occlusions.
- Guglialmi detachable coils (GDC) are the standard devices for embolization of cerebral aneurysms. They are made up of platinum and attached to a stainless steel delivery wire. The coils have a circular memory and are available in many different diameters and lengths. Detachment of the platinum coiled from the delivery is achieved by electrolysis following application of an electrical current once the coiled is deemed to be in a safe position. The advantage of such a system is that the coil remains firmly attached to the delivery wire until the current applies which allows the retrieval of a coil in an inappropriate position or of inappropriate size.

- Embolisation with particles leads to a less permanent occlusion than embolization with liquid agents. Particles are therefore used for preoperative embolisation. PVA particles are the most frequently used particulate embolic agent and are supplied in sizes ranging from 50 to 1000 μm small particles (50-150 μm) are more effective in inducing tumor necrosis but carry a higher risk of cranial nerve or skin damage.
- Gelfoam sponge is prepared from pork skin gelatine and is pliable material that can be cut to appropriately sized particles. It is used for occlusion of more proximal vessels following embolization of distal vessel with PVA. It has no significant sclerosing effect and recanalizes within approx. 6 weeks.
- Tris acryl gelatine micro spares (embospheres) area a new non-absorbably embolic agent. They tend not to aggregate, area deformable and appear to penetrate cheaper into the vascular system than PVA particles.
- Dehydrated (98%) alcohol is a potent liquid embolic agent. It has sclerosing effect on cells by causing dehydration and dematuration of peptides. It is used in the percutaneous treatment of hemangiomatous malformations in the head and neck. It should be used with extreme care.
- Acrylate glues such as N-butyl cyanomerylate (NBCAs) are liquid embolic agents, mainly used for embolisation of cerebral AVMs and dural fistulas. Prior to injection they are diluted in a lipophylic contract agents (liphodols) or made radiopque with tantalum power. On contact with an ionic solution, such as blood, NBCA solidies rapidly, causing permanent vascular occlusion. The micro catheter through which it has been delivered has to be swiftly withdrawn to avoid the risk of gluing the catheter in situ.
- Onyx is a new non-adhesive liquid embolic agent and consists of a mixture of ethyl vinyl alcohol polymer (EVOH), dimethyl sulfoxide (DMSO) as a solvent and tantalum to render it radiopaque.In contrast to NBCA, it solidifies slowly, minimizes the changes of in situ gluing of a uretherter. Onyx has been used for cerebral AVMs and giant cerebral aneurysms.

CAROTID AND VERTEBRAL ARTERY TEST OCCLUSION

- It is performed to assess the ability of the cerebral circulation to tolerate permanent sacrifice of vessel. Sacrifice of the ICA or VA may be contemplated in the context of surgery for skull base and cervical neoplasms encasing these vessels or for the treatment of giant aneurysms, where surgical or endovascular diagnosis with preservation of the parent artery is not possible.
- Testing the clinical tolerance of an occlusion is the most important part of the procedure, which has therefore to be performed under LA. A temporary (non detachable occlusion balloon, fixed at the tip of a micro catheter is advanced to the point of the anticipated/ permanent occlusion and then inflated for approx. 30 min. with careful monitoring of the patients neurological status which is best undertaken by a separate operator.
- In the event of neurological deterioration, the balloon has to be deflated immediately to prevent a permanent deficit.
- In addition to clinical criteria, an injection of the contralateral ICA during inflation of the test occlusion circle of Willis and to detect any delay in the transit best done by comparing the appearance of cerebral veins in the cerebral hemispheres.
- A delay in venous opacification of 2 seconds or more indicates that the occlusion is unlikely to be tolerated.
- Complications of test occlusion include arterial

dissection (symptomatic and asymptomatic) and transient or permanent neurological deficit).

TRAUMATIC CAROTICO-CAVERNOUS FISTULAS

- Trauma can result in a tear in the cavernous segment of the ICA, leading to a defect in the arterial wall with blood shunting directly into the cavernous sinus surrounding this arterial segment (direct carotio cavernous fistula).
- From the cavernous sinus arterilised blood drains to reverse the flow in the ophthalmic veins, cerebral veins or the petrosal venous sinuses.
- Patient present with symptoms of venous HTN, sometimes month after trauma.
- Increased pressure in the ophthalmic veins typically cause proptosis, scleral injection and conjunctival hemorrhages.
- Increased cerebral venous pressure can cause headaches, seizures and venous hemorrhages.
- The goal of treatment is the occlusion of the AV fistula with preservation of the lumen of the ICA. This is best achieved from an intra-arterial approach using detachable balloons.
- A microcatheter with a deflated attached balloon is passed from the carotid artery through the defect in its wall into the cavernous sinus. The balloon is then gradually inflated until the fistula is occluded from the venous side, preserving patency of the ICA and flow to the epilateral intracranial vessel.
- If this is achieved the balloon is detached by a gentle pulling action. Insertion of more than one balloon may be necessary in large fistulas.
- Alternative treatment options include coil embolisation either transarterially or using a transvenous approach via the inferior petrosal or ophthalmic veins.
- Risks of this procedure include stroke following arterial occlusion after unintentional balloon detachment and cranial nerve palsies due to pressure from balloon or coil.

TREATMENT OF EPISTAXES

- The most common cause of epistaxis is the spontaneous or idiopathic form, frequently related to smoking and HTN. Other causes of epistaxis include tumors (juvenile angiofibroma in male adolescents and malignant tumors in adults) trauma (Carotico cavernous fistulas, traumatic false aneurysm or iatrogenic following endoscopic sinus surgery) and Osler Weber Render disease.
- Most cases of spontaneous epistaxis occur in the ant. septal areas of the nose (Kiesselbach's plexus) a location that is easily accessible for cautery and packing.
- Post epistaxis is often more difficult to treat, requiring post nasal packing and endoscopic cauterization. Endovascular embolization is indicated if the bleeding is refractory to this diagnosis.
- Blood supply to the nasal fossa derives from the ICA (ethmoidal branches of the ophthalmic artery) and ECA (maxillary artery and facial artery). The main blood supply from the sphenopalatine artery, a branch of the maxillary artery can be super selectively catheterised and catheters.
- Refractory idiopathic epistaxis is typically embolised with polyvinyl alcohol particles. This has an 87% success rate after embolisation of internal maxillary branches alone and a 97% success rate with additional fascial artery embolisation.
- Potential complications include stroke and blindness as a result of inadvertent embolisation of ICA breaches.

ENDOVASCULAR THERAPY OF INTRACRANIAL ANEURYSMS INDICATIONS

1. Aneurysms is the post fossa where surgical access is often difficult.

2. Patients in poor medical condition.
3. Following diagnostic angiography.
4. Following acute SAH where two aneurysms are found and it remains unclear which one has ruptured.

DRAWBACK

- Recurrence of aneurysms, especially at the basilar and carotid terminations.
- The most widely used technique is coil embolisation. This is achieved by careful placement of a micro catheter within the aneurysm lumen, through which detachable coils are deployed. If a satisfactory position cannot be obtained, the coils are retrievable before detachment.
- The aim is total exclusion of the aneurysm lumen with preservation of the parent artery and its branches. This is achieved in narrow neck saccular aneurysms.
- Aneurysms with wide neck are increasingly amenable to endovascular treatment since the development of techniques preventing the prolapse of coils through the aneurysm neck, such as balloon remodelling, stenting devices, to bridge the aneurysm neck.
- Potential complications of endovascular diagnostic aneurysm perforation or rupture, inadvertent occlusion of the parent or branch arteries by coils and thromboembolic events.
- Where preservation of patency of the parent vessel cannot be assured, sacrifice of the parent vessel can be considered usually preceded by test occlusion. This is achieved with either coils or detachable balloons, depending on the vessel configuration and indication for diagnosis.

ENDOVASCULAR DIAGNOSIS OF INTRACRANIAL A-V SHUNTS

Endovascular Diagnosis for Cerebral AVMs

- Most patients with cerebral AVMs develop symptoms before the age of 40 years which is in contrast to cerebral aneurysm where only a quarter of patients present by the age of 40.
- Cerebral AVMs are an important cause of cerebral hemorrhage in young adults.
- 60% of patient with cerebral AVMs present with hemorrhage, epilepsy followed by non-hemorrhagic neurological deficit and headache.
- AVMs can be treated by endovascular embolisation, microsurgery, radio surgery or a combination of these methods.
- The choice of diagnosis is often governed by local expertise and the goal of diagnosis may vary in individual patients depending on the clinical presentation, AVM location and size and age of the patient.
- Main aim is the prevention of cerebral hemorrhage or rehemorrhages. The mean risk of hemorrhage is increased in patients within the presence of certain factors and angiographic features. The former include older age and the initial presentation with hemorrhage and the latter include false aneurysms, venous ecstasies or stenoses, a single draining vein, deep venous drainage and venous congestion.
- The MC used endovascular approach is arterial embolisation using a permanent fluid such as NBCA, which is diluted and rendered radio opaque with lipiodol or tantalum. Onxy can also be used.
- Small AVM's can be treated by endovascular means, radio surgery or if in superficial location by microsurgery. Radial obliteration of medium sized or large AVMs represents a challenge for endovascular diagnosis as well as other diagnostic modalities. It requires several staged embolization procedure and complete AVM obliteration is often not possible. Endovascular diagnosis can be combined with others form of diagnosis. It is performed to reduce the size of AVMs prior to radio surgery.
- Partial AVM embolisation is effective in improving the control of epileptic seizures and

in reducing the risk of hemorrhage by target embolization of specific components such as false aneurysms. Partial embolisation can bring relief of symptoms related to venous HTN and the elimination of ECA supply is effective in alleviating headaches.

ENDOVASCULAR DIAGNOSIS OF VEIN OF GALEN ANEURYSMAL MALIGNANCY (VGAM)

- VGAM is characterized by AV shunts at the choroidal level, within the subarachnoid space in the region of the vein of Galen. They must be distinguished from cerebral AV shunts draining into the vein of Galen and producing dilatation of it as these lesions have entirely different natural histories and prognosis.
- In VGAM there is associated aneurysmal dilatation and abnormal persistence of the median vein of prosencephalon and embryological midline venous structure and precursor of the vein of Galen.
- The malformation often drains into a persistent falcina sinus and there may be agencies of the straight sinus and anomalies of other dural venous sinuses.
- VGAM and dural sinus malformations are the only intracranial AVMs, present in the fetal period. They are more common in males. Most present in either the neonatal period or in infancy. In general the high flow AV shunt of VGAM is initially well tolerated from a neurological point of view and early presentation is with cardiac failure or altered CSF dynamics and macrocephaly.
- If possible, treatment of the shunt in VGAM is deferred to allow for growth of the child, as intervention in neonates is technically difficult and hazardous.
- Criteria for intervention in infancy include progressive, macrocephaly, developmental delay, and seizure and reversible neurological deficit.
- Cardiac failure unresponsive to medical management is an indication for urgent embolisation in the neonatals period.
- An arterial approach using a permanent embolic agent (NBCA) is most often used.
- The initial aim to reduce the level of AV shunting to a degree that the cardiac failure can be managed.

ENDOVASCULAR TREATMENT OF DURAL AV SHUNTS

- Dural AV shunts occur in the walls of dural venous sinuses or their tributaries. They may be related to previous episodes of sinus thrombosis.
- Depending on their location and severity of shunting, they may present with pulsatile tinnitus, bruit, ophthalmic symptoms (cavernous sinus DAVS), seizures, intracranial hemorrhage or decreased mental function or neuropsychiatric symptoms.
- Impediments to venous outflow result in venous reflux and congestion, which predispose to hemorrhage and cerebral parenchymal damage.
- Cerebral venous congestion is an indication for treatment.
- Endovascular technique is the first line intervention in DAVS.
- An arterial approach utilizing a permanent embolic agent is often used.
- The goal should be occlusion of the site of AV shunting with preservation of patency of the dural venous sinuses.
- Venous approach may also be used, though this necessitates sacrifice of a segment of dural venous sinuses at the zone of AV shunting.
- Venous approaches are particularly useful in the diagnosis of cavernous sinus dural fistulas.

HEAD, NECK AND BRAIN TUMOR EMBOLISATION INCLUDING CHEMOTHERAPY

- Embolisation of vascular tumor of the head, neck and CNS prior to surgery can significantly reduce intra operative blood loss, shorten the operative procedure time and facilitate the removal of these tumors.
- Hyper vascular tumors, which may benefit from pre operative embolisation, include meningiomas, metastases, glomus jugular tumors, benign and malignant bone tumors and juvenile nasopharyngeal angio fibromas.
- Embolisation is usually performed via the endovascular route but can also be achieved by direct ingestion of embolic agent into the tumor.
- The aim is a reduction of blood supply to the tumor and this is most efficient if the embolic agent can penetrate into the small vessels within the tumor, which is best achieved using particles (PVA or embospheres) of a small size.
- The choice of particle size is a balance between safety and efficiency and depends on whether a highly selective catheter position could be achieved.
- Smaller particles penetrate deeper into the tumor but carry a higher risk of skin necrosis and cranial nerve palsies, risks they share with liquid agent such as glue or concentrate alcohol which are occasionally used.
- Endovascular tumor embolisation may also be indicated as palliative procedures, to reduce tumor size or associated symptoms in patient with lesions not amenable to surgery.
- Intra-arterial chemotherapy is an established form of diagnosis in head and neck tumors that fail to respond to conventional chemotherapy.
- Chemotherapeutic agents can be infused following:
  - Catheterisation of ECA branches via the femoral route or through an inferior pump, implanted via surgical cutdown of the superficial temporal artery.
  - Local toxicity of this treatment includes alopecia, mucositis, skin necrosis and cranial nerve palsies.

SPINE

Endovascular Treatment of Spinal Cord Arteriovenous Shunts

- Spinal cord AVMs are seen in young patients, spinal dorsal fistulas most commonly present in elderly male patients and are thought to be associated with venous thrombosis, like cranial dural fistulas.
- Clinical symptoms may have an insidious onset with a gradual or of stepwise loss of power in the legs, walking difficulties and sphincter disturbances.
- The symptoms are due to increased (arterial) pressure in the veins draining the spinal cord leading to venous congestion and cord oedema, evident as increased T2 signal intensity within the coral on MR images.
- Definitive diagnosis of spinal dural fistulas requires high quality spinal angiography, which should be performed under general anaesthesia.
- Spinal dural fistula may be treated by embolisation or surgery.
- Embolisation is an option if the fistula arises from purely radicular artery, which does not provide any arterial supply to the cord. It involves the ingestion of permanent occlusive agent such as NBCA glue, which must reach and occlude the fistulous point.
- Surgery of these lesions is usually straightforward and consists of exposure and electrocoagulation of the fistula is located on the dura.
- The chief aim of treatment is to prevent further progression of symptoms.

- Recovery from existing symptoms is possible but is now and depends on the degree of established cord damage, which is related to the length of the clinical history.
- The definitive diagnosis of spinal dural fistulas requires high quality spinal angiography.

ENDOVASCULAR TREATMENT OF VERTEBRAL TUMORS

- Embolisation for vertebral tumors is usually performed preoperatively, aiming to reduce intra operative bleeding.
- Both benign (ESP hemangioma) and malignant (usually metastatic hyper vascular lesions may benefit from endovascular diagnosis.
- High quality diagnostic spinal angiography must be performed first. This should demonstrate the blood supply to and degree of granularity of the lesion.
- The arterial supply to vertebral bodies is from the two adjacent metameric levels and these should be examined bilaterally.
- The blood supply to the spinal cord must be carefully examined as inadvertent embolisation of radiculopial or radiculo medullary artery may have terrible consequences.
- If the lesion is hyper vascular and there is no radials medullary or radiological artery arising from the same level, embolisation can be performed safely.
- The possibility of a previously unopacified vessel contributing to the supply of the spinal cord should be excluded.
- Embolisation may be performed either through a catheter position in the segmental artery supplying the tumor or more selectively than a catheter in the feeding pedicles of the tumor itself.
- Occlusion of the segmental artery distal to the origin of supply to the tumor may be useful to reduce passage of embolic material to vessels supplying the skin and body wall.

DIRECT PERCUTANEOUS EMBOLISATION

- How flow vascular malformations of the head and neck such as hemangio-lymphangiomas and venous malformations can be treated with direct injections of concentrated alcohol under fluoroscopic guidance.
- This procedure has to be preceded by an angiographic sum during the injection of a contrast medium through the percutaneously placed needle to delineate the vascular compartment and venous drainage route.
- Inj of concentrated alcohol should not be undertaken in the presence of intracranial venous drainage.
- Spinal tumors or intracranial extra dural tumors can be directly punctured using imaging guidance and embolised with particles or glue through a percutaneous needle, preoperatively or for palliation. Direct P.C. tumor embolisation can be most efficient transembolisation of several feeding radicle via endovascular route.

Section 2—Face, Neck, Orbit and Ear

Chapter 20

Laryngeal Mass in Paediatric Age Group

ANATOMY

It is a cylindrical system of mucosal folds separated from an outer cartilaginous skeleton by intervening spaces filled with fat and muscle. The skeleton of larynx comprises (Figure 20.1):

3 Paired cartilages	3 Unpaired cartilages
a. Arytenoids	a. Thyroid
b. Corniculate	b. Cricoid
c. Cuneiform	c. Epiglottis

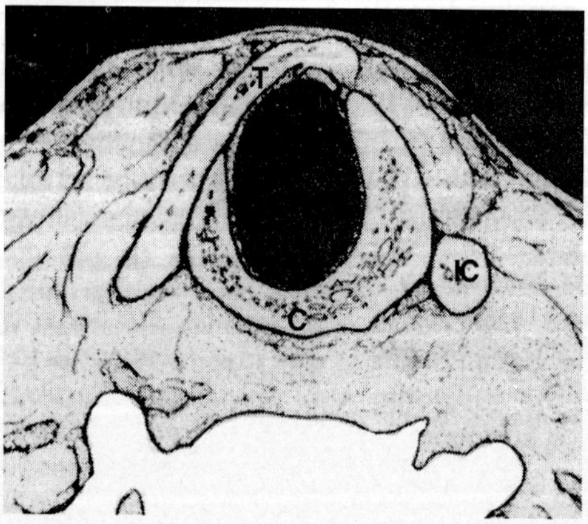

Fig. 20.1: Level: cricoid cartilage (C). Central medullary space of cricoid is of low density. T= thyroid cartilage; IC = interior cornu of thyroid cartilage

Axial Anatomy of Larynx

Compared with the larynx of an adult, paediatric larynx is smaller in relation to overall body size.

- The superior free edge of epiglottis is at the level of C1.
- Caudal portion of cricoid cartilage is at the level of C4/C5.

Imaging of Larynx in Paediatric Age Group:

A. *Plain Radiograph*

This shows an air soft tissue interface with the surrounding bony structures.

- High kV technique is used to optimise soft tissue details. Anteroposterior (AP) and lateral views should be taken.
- Lateral film shows a normal air filled structure comprising nasopharynx/oropharynx/hypopharynx, supraglottic airway, vallecula, laryngeal ventricle, infraglottic airway and trachea. Soft tissue structures are also visualized.
- *AP film:* Shows tracheal and laryngeal airway, specifically false and true vocal cord and subglottic region.

B. *Computed Tomography* (Figure 20.2)

It adds important information about the soft tissue

surrounding the airways. Current spiral and multidetector CT allow volume scanning of neck during a single breath hold and obviates the need for sedation and also sections that are 1 mm thin can be obtained with special technique when evaluating a newborn/infant with a suspected hemangioma/papilloma.

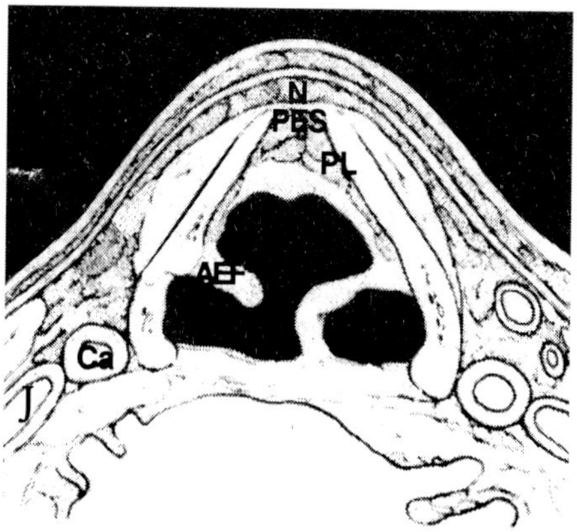

Fig. 20.2: Level: aryepiglottic folds (AEF). N = thyroid notch; PES = pre-epiglottic space; PL = paralaryngeal space; Ca = carotid artery; J = jugular vein

C. *M.R.I.*

Most children between 3-5 years of age require sedation in order for undergoing MRI. The choice of coil and pulse sequence for MR imaging of pediatric neck and airway will depend upon the clinical indication for examination. Multiplanar imaging should be acquired with TIW, T2W and fat suppressed T2W or fast spin echo inversion recovery (FSEIR) sequences.

Laryngeal masses can be divided into:

A. SUPRAGLOTTIC (includes lesion above the level of vocal cords).

B. GLOTTIC (includes vocal cords, anterior and posterior commissure).

C. SUBGLOTTIC (includes area of larynx between vocal cords and lower border of cricoid).

SUPRAGLOTTIC MASSES

Congenital: Aryepiglottic fold cyst.
Inflammatory: Epiglottitis, angioneurotic edema.
Neoplastic: Retention cyst, cystic hygroma.
Traumatic: Foreign body, hematoma.

GLOTTIC MASSES

Neoplastic: Laryngeal papillomatosis (Fig 20.3).
Miscellaneous: Foreign body, laryngocele.

SUBGLOTTIC MASSES

Traumatic: Granuloma.
Neoplastic: Hemangioma, papillomatosis.
Idiopathic: Mucocele.

LARYNGEAL CYST

These may be located anywhere in the larynx. These are fluid filled lesions and are most frequently found in vallecula and true vocal cords.

- Plain film might show smooth mass projecting into airways.
- CT will demonstrate a well circumscribed submucosal, low density, non enhancing masses.
- *MRI:* On TIWI, SI is usually low but may be high in infection and hemorrhage; on T2WI, SI is high.

LARYNGOCELE

It is an air or fluid filled dilatation of laryngeal saccule that communicate with laryngeal ventricle and is a rare cause of laryngeal obstruction in infants. Usually it is unilateral, may be internal or external depending upon whether it lays inside/ outside the thyrohyoid membrane.

- *Plain Films:* Air collection in lateral neck projected over supraglottic larynx is highly suggestive findings.

- *CT Scan:* Cross-sectional imaging demonstrates a small internal laryngocele and combined laryngocele which extends through the thyrohyoid membrane into the lateral neck.
- CT density or the MR intensity of laryngocele is variable depending on whether the cyst is filled with air/fluid or proteinaceous debris.

HEMANGIOMA

It is the most common subglottic soft tissue mass causing upper respiratory tract obstruction in neonates. Associated hemangiomas elsewhere in the body may be present in about 50% cases.

Plain Film

- *AP view:* Eccentric thickening of subglottic portion of larynx.
- *Lateral view:* Shows a subglottic mass arising from posterior wall below the cords.

CT Scan

Hemangioma appears as lobulated, solid, soft tissue tumor that is isodense with muscle and enhances rapidly following contrast administration.

- Areas of calcification may be seen in the mass.

MRI

It reveals a lobulated, moderately hyperintense mass on T2W images with intense enhancement on contrast enhanced TIW images.

Prominent vascularity within tumor appears as flow voids on spin echo pulse sequences.

LYMPHATIC MALFORMATION (LM)

- These are cystic masses composed of lymphatic channels filled with protein rich fluid.
- These may be detected antenatally but usually present at birth.
- These anomalies may remain clinically silent until sudden enlargement occurs due to infection or hemorrhage.

Plain Film

This does not give enough information except for a soft tissue mass which may be distorting the laryngeal air passage which further depend upon size, location and extent of the lesion.

USG

- It may show multilocular, cystic mass with thin/thick walls components and sometimes solid components within due to infection and hemorrhage.

CT

- It adequately delineates the extent of lesion in most cases.
- Lesion generally appears cystic and septate. A very characteristic feature is multiple fluid levels. They are usually hypodense on NCCT and do not enhance on contrast enhanced images except for the septae.

MRI

- It is the modality of choice for diagnosing and demonstrating the extent of the lymphatic malformation. The SI on MRI depends upon the protein contents and blood products.

PAPILLOMA

- It is the most common tumor (benign) of larynx in children.
- It is caused by HPV.
- It is usually small and asymptomatic. When symptomatic it presents with progressive hoarseness, with increasing stridor and respiratory distress.
- Often these are multiple and occur most commonly in glottic region.

Plain Film

- It shows small, pedunculated, nodular masses within the airway.

CT/MRI

- These may show small nodules adherent to the airway wall projecting into the lumen.

ACUTE EPIGLOTTITIS

- It is an acute fulminating infection that occurs in children between 2-6 years of age with edema of epiglottis and aryepiglottic folds.
- It presents with respiratory distress and inspiratory stridor.
- *Site:* Purely supraglottic lesions.

  Diagnosis is based on clinical findings and endoscopic examination. However, plain X- ray lateral view may help in confirming the diagnosis. Findings may be:
- Enlargement of epiglottis and thickening of aryepiglottic fold.
- Circumferential narrowing of subglottic portion of trachea.
- Ballooning of hypopharynx.

FOREIGN BODY

- Laryngotracheal inhaled foreign bodies are less common but more hazardous than those lodged in bronchus. It usually presents with stridor.

Plain Film

- Detect foreign bodies that are radio opaque. E.g.: Pine, coins, screw, and fish bone. However a significant proportion of foreign bodies like food particles, peanuts may not be seen even with magnification views.
- Both AP and lateral views should be taken to localise the object and also to know about the contour of object.

CECT Scan

- It should be done if local complications such as abscess formation occur at the time of presentation or following removal of foreign body.

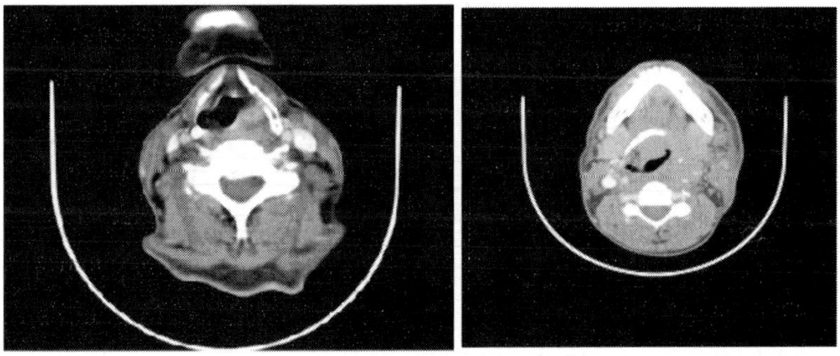

Fig. 20.3: Axial CT scan of neck in two patients showing carcinoma left pyriform fossa and carcinoma glottis with transglottic spread

Section 2—Face, Neck, Orbit and Ear

Chapter 21

Anomalies of the Inner Ear

Imaging Technique

HRCT of the temporal bone:

- Readily identifies the bony anomalies and also give information regarding concomitant external and middle ear anomalies.

MR IMAGING

- Thin section, high resolution MR imaging using GRE and FSE T2W techniques gives exquisite details of membranous labyrinth.
- Thin section, SE TIW images both pre and postcontrast are required to give adequate results.

Membranous and Bony Labyrinthine Anomalies

1. Semicircular canals (S.C.C.)

   Malformation of LSCC is one of the most common inner ear anomalies.

   Abnormal Narrow or Wide/short

   ↓

   When extensive

   ↓

   Vestibule merges with LSCC

   ↓

   Lateral semi circular duct – vestibular dysplasia are common, utriculosaccular – lateral semicircular duct cavity.

2. Semicircular duct aplasia
   - Far less common than dysplasia.
   - May be bilateral.
   - May occur in combination with a normal or near normal cochlea.
   - Common in patients with CHARGE syndrome:

     C – Coloboma

     H – Heart anomaly

     A – Choanal atresia

     R – Retardation

     G – Genital and

     E – Ear anomalies

     - Mondini's dysplasia of pars inferior.
     - Absent pars superior.
     - Short cochlea.
     - Hypoplastic vestibular sense organs/nerve.
     - Waardenberg/Alagille's syndromes – PSCC affected.

3. Dehiscence of the roof of the superior SCC.

- Best seen on coronal images of temporal bone.
- Always with Tullio's phenomenon which consists of sound induced vertigo/ nystagmus/or both.

Mechanism

Sound → stapes → oval window → cochlea → hair cells activated → nerve stimulating → round window dissipitatcs sound waves → middle ear.

When dehiscence is present

↓

Superior SCC acts as mobile window

↓

Sound pressure goes to vestibular apparatus

↓

Stimulates hair cells

↓ Results in

Vertigo

Vestibular and Utriculosaccular Anomalies

- Isolated anomalies are rare.
- Spectrum include:
  - Complete or partial assimilation of SCC into the vestibule.
  - Subtle enlargement or malformation of the vestibule.
- Semicircular ducts can be detected on MR imaging.
- Enlarged globular vestibule is seen in thalidomide - induced deafness.

Cochlea

These anomalies occur because of arrest of development of cochlea at different stages of organogenesis.

Jackler's *et al.* Classification of cochlear anomalies:

- Complete labyrinthine aplasia (Michel's deformity).
  - It is very rare and is due to arrest of development at 3rd to 4th week of IUL.
  - No inner ear development.
  - There is a single, small, common cystic cavity representing vestibule and cochlea with no internal architecture.
  - Semicircular canals may be normal or malformed.
  - Cochlear aplasia.
  - Cochlea fails to form at 5th week of IUL.
  - The other elements of inner ear may be normal or malformed.
- Cochlear hypoplasia:
  - Small rudimentary cochlear band is present due to arrest at 6th week of IUL with normal or abnormal vestibular and SCC.
  - Incomplete partition with dilatational defects (including classic Mondini's dysplasia) due to arrest at 7th week of IUL.
  - Small cochlea with incomplete partitioning of or absent intrascalar septum.
  - Only basal cochlear turn present with common cavity in the region of middle and apical turns resulting in scalar communis cochlea:
    i. Vestibule and SCC may be normal or malformed.
    ii. Mondini's documented flat cochlea having 1½ times with large vestibules (Figure 21.1).
- Dwarf cochlea:
  - On CT cochlea appears to be normal but smaller.
  - Quite rare.
  - Functionally may be abnormal.
  - Labyrinthine segment can be anteriorly positioned.

IAC and Vestibulocochlear and Facial Nerve Anomalies

- Normal range of IAC diameter – 2-8 mm (average – 4 mm).

  < 2 mm - stenotic.

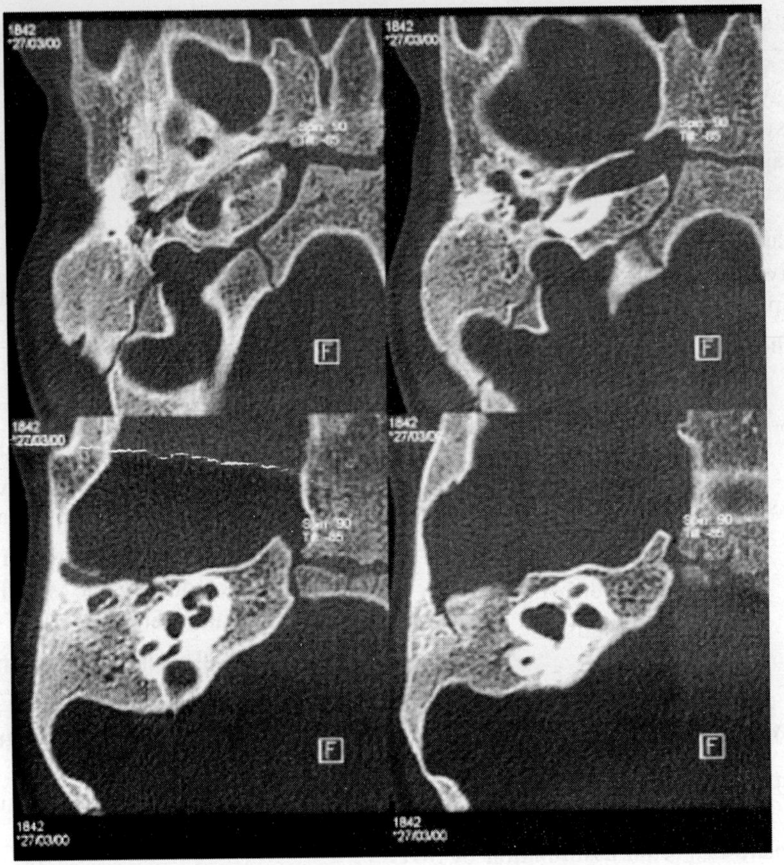

Fig. 21.1: Serial HRCT images of the right petrous bone in a case of Mondini's malformation of the inner ear

IAC may also be atretic on MRI. Decrease of CSF between CP angle and intra-labyrinthine fluid is a reliable sign of atresia.

- Sagittal MR images required for Vestibulocochlear nerve (VCN) lesions:
  - Type-I – IAC stenotic and VCN is absent.
  - Type - II A – Common VCN with aplasia or hypoplasia of its cochlear branch in the presence of labyrinthine malformation.
  - Type II-B–Labyrinthine structures are normal.
- Facial nerve may also be hypoplastic/aplastic. This anomaly may occur in isolation or as part of Mobius syndrome/congenital facial diplegia congenital oculofacial paralysis/ congenital abducens–facial paralysis.
- Duplication of facial nerve or bifid facial nerve-commonly bifurcate along the proximal aspect of tympanic segment inferior to lower semicircular canal into larger lateral and small medial branch.

Vestibular Aqueduct Anomalies

Large vestibular aqueduct syndrome, on CT >1.5 mm.

On T2W GRE images–fluid filled endolymphatic duct and the sac within the bony vestibular aqueduct are hyperintense and are surrounded by hypointense bony structures. This sac extends in the posterior fossa.

It is associated with cochlear anomalies including motility deficiency, gross dysmorphism and scalar asymmetry.

Various syndromes associated with inner ear abnormalities are:

Other Anomalies

Achondroplasia	Pendred's syndrome
Alagille syndrome	Pierre Robin syndrome
Apert's syndrome	Refsum syndrome
Melwik Fraser syndrome	Thalidomide embryopathy
CHARGE syndrome	Tracher Collin's syndrome
Cleidocranial dysplasia	Paten syndrome
Craniometaphyseal dysplasia (Pyle's)	Edwards syndrome
Di George syndrome	Down's syndrome
Gorlin Holt syndrome	Usher syndrome
Goldenhar's syndrome	VATER
Klippel Feil syndrome	Waardenberg syndrome
Mobius syndrome	Weldervanek syndrome
Osteogenesis imperfecta	
Osteopetrosis	

1. X-linked progressive mixed hearing loss or X-linked congenital mixed deafness.

↓

Olson and Lehman

↓

Dilatation of lateral part of IAC + absence or severe hypoplasia of the bony modiolus with normal number of cochlear turns and hypoplasia of the cochlear base, with or without widening of the labyrinthine segment of the FNC and dilatation of vestibular aqueduct and fixed foot plate of stapes

↓

Abnormal fistulous communication between CSF within IAC and perilymphatic fluid in scalar vestibula

↓

Increased pressure within cochlea and at oval window

↓

SNHL and CHL

↓

Stapes gusher at surgery

2. Scalar asymmetry within cochlea

   Normal anterior scalar chamber (S. vest. + S. media) = post scalar chamber (S. tympani) abnormal – anterior: posterior = 1.45:1.

Chapter 22

Chronic Otitis Media (OM) and Mastoiditis

Ac OM with effusion → is an infection of the middle ear, associated with pain and an effusion behind an intact Tympanic Membrane.

If fluid persists for 3 months, the disease is considered chronic.

CSOM – indicates that otorrhea has existed for at least 6 weeks.

Otorrhea

Ch. Mastoiditis → There is progressive obliteration of the mastoid air cell system with reactive sclerosis.

Pathogenesis → Middle ear effusion results from ↓ed intratympanic pressure.

↓

Resorption of O_2

↓

Negative pressure in the middle ear

↓

Collapse of ET wall

↓

Extravasation of fluid

Etiology

1. Malfunction or obstruction of ET:
   - Abnormal development of temporal bone.
   - Bony dysplasia.
   - Trauma.
   - Adenoid hyperplasia.
   - Tumor, and
   - Surgery.
2. Mucosal oedema secondary to rhinopharyngitis, allergy or neoplasm–Nasopharyngeal.
3. Trigeminal motor dysfunction:
   - Tumor in the cavernous sinus region.
   - Perineural spread of malignancy.
   - Persistance eustachian tube dysfunctions.
   - Atrophy of the drum with or without attic retraction pockets.

SEQUELE OF CHRONIC OTITIS

Granulation Tissue

- Most common cause of debris in the middle ear.
- CT–Soft tissue density mass with no ossicular displacement or bone erosion (Figure 22.1).
- MRI–Because of vascularity they enhances on GD DTPA T1 W images.

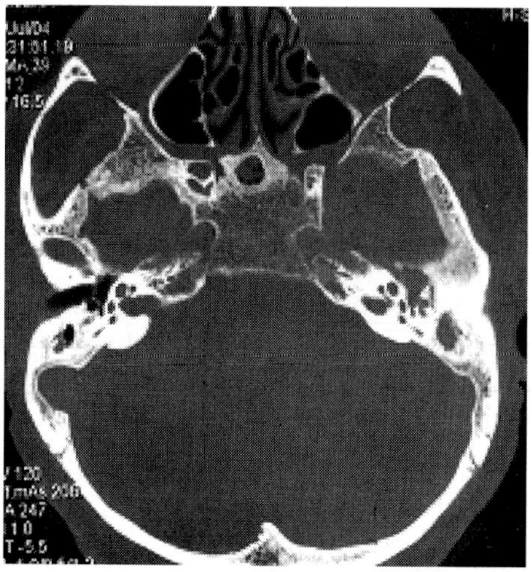

Fig. 22.1: Axial CT image show chronic otitis media and mastoiditis on left side

CHOLESTEATOMA

Consists of a sac lined by sratified squamous epithelium filled with exfoliated keratin debris:

1. Congenital.
2. Acquired
   a. Primary.
   b. Secondary.

Etiology

1. Retraction Pocket or Negitive pressure theory.
2. Epithelial invasion through the T.M. perforation.
3. Metaplasia theory.

Imaging Findings

Pars flaccida cholesteatoma known as primary acquired → Non-enhancing soft tissue mass:

- Erosion of anterior portion of lateral epityme wall.
- Erosion of ant tymp. spine, scutum.
- Soft tissue mass in epitympanic lateral to the ossicle.
- Increased distance between lateral epitympanic wall and the ossicles.
- When cholesteatoma is limited to the anterior portion of epitympanicum, malleus head is eroded, has concave outline.

Posterior portion → body of incus.

Long process of incus is usually spared.

Pars tensa cholesteatoma → secondary acquired.

- Now enhancing soft tissue mass in the middle ear.
- Long process of incus is eroded – non-specific.
- Soft tissue mass of the middle ear extended into the epitympanus medial to the ossicles.
- The malleus head and incus body are displaced.

Laterally by the soft tissue mass. Displaced incus body is often eroded.

- Most common pars tensa cholesteatoma arise from the postero superior margin of the membrane – blunting of post portion of lateral epitympanic wall and erosion of posterior superior bony canal wall.

Combined P. flaccida and P. tensa cholesteatoma.

EVALUATION OF EXTENT OF CHOLESTEATOMA

- Aditus → enlargement of aditus indicates extension of cholesteatoma postero superiorly.
- Short process of incus is usually eroded.

Antrum

- Mass without partially or completely fills the lumen.
- Enlargement of antral cavity.
- Superior extension of the cholesteatoma causes progressive erosion of Koerner's septum.
- Complete amputation of septum indicates extension to the tagmen of antrum.

Mastoid

- Progressive destruction of the trabecular pattern and formation of a large, smooth walled cloudy cavity.

Complications

1. Erosion of tagmen or sinus plate:
   - Meningeal or intracranial complications.
   - CT and MR after injection of contrast.

   Erosion of posterior wall of mastoid and sinus plate–septic thrombophelebitis of the lateral sinus and cerebellar abscess formation (Figures 22.2 and 22.3).
2. Labyrinthine fistula

   Incidence of 5-10%.

   Most common lateral portion of lateral semicircular canal, which bulges into the antrum.

   Pars tensa–more prone to fistula formation.
3. Facial nerve
   - VII nerve dysfunction occurs in 1% of patients with cholesteatoma.
   - Even if there is facial nerve canal erosion, facial nerve function may be normal.
   - Most common site of facial nerve compression is tympanic segment.
4. Tympanosclerosis is caused by ch. osteomyelitis followed by healing.

- Involvement of tympanic membrane is common, but often asymptomatic.
- CHD results when the process involves ossicles on their suspensory ligaments and tendons.

Congenital Cholesteatoma

Histologically is epidermoid tumor, originating from embryonic epidermoid rests located anywhere in the temporal bone or in the adjacent, extradural or epidural spaces.

- Whitish globular masses lying medial to an intact TM.
- No history of antecedent inflammatory ear disease.
- CT – well defined soft tissue mass.
- TM often bulges laterally D/D serous OM.
- Inf margin of lateral. Epitympanic wall – intact.
- Congenital cholesteatoma arisng within the mastoid – very rare but the middle ear cavity appears normal in congenital variety.

D/D of a destructive middle ear masses.

Cholesterol granuloma–is a nonspecific chronic inflammation of middle ear and mastoid.

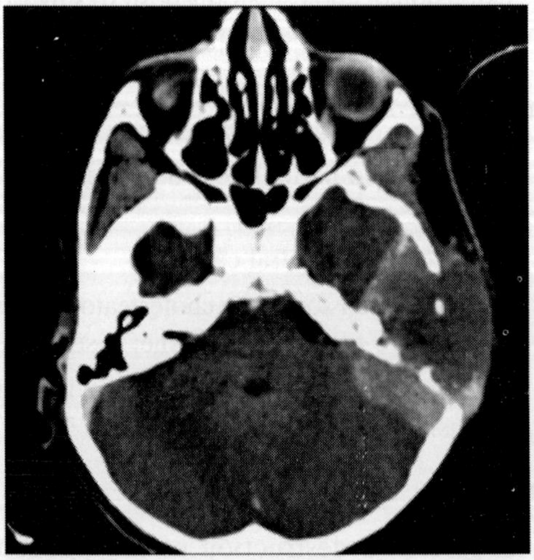

Fig. 22.2: Axial CT image showing a large intra and extracranial abscess in a case of left sided CSOM

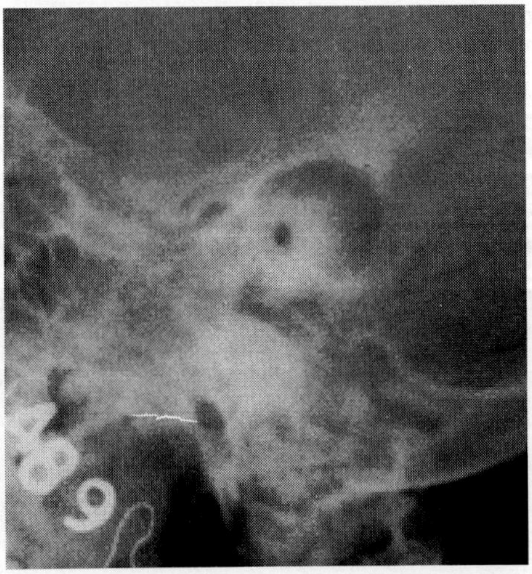

Fig. 22.3: Schuller's view of the mastoid shows mastoid abscess

Consists of a mass of chronic inflammatory tissue-containing clefts of cholesterol crystals surrounded by giant cells.

- Intact TM.
- Well-defined ST mass.
- Ossicles often eroded by the granulomatous process.
- Rhabdomyosarcomas.
- Usually seen in children.
- Arise from middle ear/petrous pyramid.
- CT—Soft tissue mass which causes lateral bulging of TM mastoid air space – appear cloudy in early lesion, but with growth of fat they are destroyed.

3. **Neoplasm** – sq. cell carcinoma.
   - Excessive bone destruction.
   - Accompanied by sclerosis and bloody discharge.

   Metastasis – Rare

   Ca breast, lung, prostate, kidney etc.
4. **Eosinophic granuloma** of temporal bone, usually improves the mastoid bone.

   As the disease progresses, EAC and middle ear cavity become involved with the destruction of their walls.

Section 2—Face, Neck, Orbit and Ear

Chapter 23

Parotid Masses

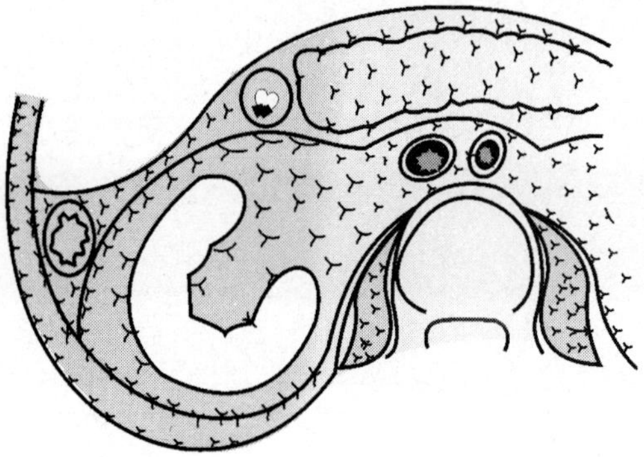

Fig. 23.1: Anatomy of masticator space

Masticator Space

Masticator space consists of vessels of mastication.

- SL of DCF splits to enclose the MS/s of mastication and forms the borders of this space.

Contents

- Masticator muscles.
- Ramus of mandible.
- 3rd division of 5th nerve, fat.

Clinical Presentation

Pain and Trismus

Boundaries

Medial boundary–interpterygoid fascia extends from the mandible to the skull base (sphenoid spine).

- Lateral boundary – lateral fascia extends from bottom of mandible to temporal ridge of calvaris.
- Both fascia join anterior and posterior around the mandibular ramus, closing this space.

Mastication Space Masses

I. Arising Within Vessels

- Hemangioma–usually within masseter muscle.
- Lymphangioma.
- Benign mastication muscle hypertrophy.
- Divarication of masticator muscle.
- Rhabdomyosarcoma.
- Rhabdomyoma.
- Leiomyoma.
- NHP.
- Metastases.

II. Arising Within Mandible

- OM.
- Radiation necrosis.
- Osteoblastoma, sarcoma, chondrosarcoma.
- Odontogenic
  - Dentigerous cyst.

- Keratocyst.
- Ameloblastoma.
- Metastases.

III. Arising Within Nerve

- Schwannoma.
- Neurofibroma.
- Neurosarcoma.

IV. Spread From

- Acute sialadenitis – either parotid gland on accessory parotid tissue.
- Salivary gland malignancy.
- Retromolar trigone squamous cell carcinoma.
- Oropharyngeal squamous cell carcinoma.

CAVERNOUS HEMANGIOMA

- Venous malforamtion, do not involute and involves bones.
- Most commonly affects the oral cavity.
- Soft tissue mass, may infiltrate deeply along fascial planes and may be entirely within the mass.
- Of all the skeletal muscle hemangioma, 14% occur in the head and neck region – masseter, trapezius and sternocleidomastoid.

CTIsoattenuation on NECT.

CECT–Slow flow lesion–supplied by small arteries – may not demonstrate sufficient enhancement.

MRI – Iso to hyperintense on T1 hyper to iso intense on T2.

Venous lakes with phleboliths is specific for hemangioma.

Lymphangioma

Congenital lymphatic malformation, 5.6% of all benign lesions of infancy and childhood.

No predilection for either sex.

On imaging – multiloculated cystic mass.

If infection occurs within the lesion, the cyst wall thickens and enhances along with inflammatory infiltration of adjacent fat planes.

CT – Cyst content is typically of mucoid attenuation (10-25 HU).

Fluid – fluid level – after hemorrhage.

MR – Low T1 (can vary), T2 always high.

Benign Muscle Hypertrophy

- It can affect all the muscles of mastication.
- Either unilateral or bilateral.
- Most common–Masseter alone affected.
- Muscle enlarged upto many times, however normal on all imaging studies.
- Usually starts in adolescence or early adulthood.
- Facial fullness is located anterior to the usual location of parotid gland.
- Not tender/not painful.
- Plain film–an exostosis of the lateral aspect of the angle of mandible at the site of attachment of the masseter muscle.
- Sialogram–show lateral bowing of Stensen's duct around an enlarged vessel.
- CT/MR–an enlarged, otherwise normal vessel.
- Maximum cross sectional area (MCSA) of its location relative to mandibular foramen.
- MCSA of masseter is centered 8 mm above the foramen.

Denervation Atrophy

Patient usually has prior history of trauma or surgery involving the mandibular nerve.

- While weakness and flattening of the side of the face, pain is rarely that within the 1st 4 weeks – mild muscle enlargement with mild enhancement and - T2 signal.

During next 20 months – muscle volume starts

to ↓ as vessel fibers progressively undergo fatty replacement–low on CT and high T1 signal intensity.

Long-standing denervation →↓ in vessel size, and loss of high SI on T2 WI.

Rhabdomyosarcoma/Rhabdomyoma

Malignant tumor of striated muscles accounts for 8-19% of all ST sarcomas and 35-45% of such sarcoma occur in the head and neck.

RMS–tumors of children and young adults.

Most cases less than 12 years

Most common sarcoma in children, 7th most common malignancy in child.

Regional nodal mets occurs in 10-38% of cases.

- Clinically usually a solitary, rapidly enlarging firm mass.

CT/MR–Homogeneous mass with adjacent bone destruction (mandible) with poorly defined margin.

Necrosis can be seen, hemorrhage–very rare, isointense on T1 and hyperintense on T2.

Enhances homogeneously.

Metastases

Hematogenous spread is rare:

Decreased incidence may be due to vessel enzyme inhibited acidic environmental of vessel, or vessel squeezing effect of vessel contractions.

Most frequent primary sites are lung, colon, pancreas, breast and kidney.

Myositis

It can be secondary to an adjacent cellulitis on abscess.

NCCT low attenuation of the affected muscle.

The muscle typically is swollen and enhances on both CT and MR images.

MR – Higher than normal SI on T2.

With associated inflammation in adjacent structures.

Clinically, the patient has an acute history with pain, swelling and redness over the masticator space.

Differential Diagnosis of Opacified Sinus with Bone Destruction

INFLAMMATORY

A. Fungal Infections

Mucormycosis.
Aspergillosis.

B. Granulomatous Diseases

Wegener's granulomatosis.
Midline destructive granuloma.

NEOPLASTIC

A. Benign

Inverting papilloma.
Juvenile angiofibroma.

B. Malignant

Squamous cell carcinoma.
Adenocarcinoma.
Adenoid cystic carcinoma.
Lymphoma.

INFLAMMATORY

A. Fungal Sinusitis

1. *Non Invasive*

a. Allergic fungal sinusitis – Results in recurrent sinonasal polyps seen on imaging as mucoid attenuation masses.

b. Mycetoma – Soft tissue mass in sinus with hyperattenuating strands. Due to magnesium, manganese and iron in fungal mucin.

2. *Invasive*

a. Acute fulminant type.

b. Chronic invasive type.

- Invasive fungal sinusitis occurs commonly in mucormycosis and aspergillosis and causes sinus opacification with bony thickening, erosions and remodelling of bone.
- There is vascular invasion with intracranial and extracranial thrombosis and infarction. Cavernous sinus thrombosis is commonly seen.
- It commonly invades orbits, base of skull and brain.

IMAGING FEATURES TYPICAL OF FUNGAL INFECTION

1. Soft tissue changes in sinus with thick reactive bone, erosions and localised areas of osteomyelitis (Figures 24.1 and 24.2).

2. Association of inflammatory sinus disease-with disease in nasal-fossae and extension into soft tissues of cheek.
3. Lack of air fluid levels (differentiation from bacterial infections).

GRANULOMATOUS DISEASES

E.g.: Nocardia, syphilis, tuberculosis.

Wegener's granulomatosis, midline granuloma and sarcoidosis.

Imaging:

1. Non-specific inflammatory mucosal thickening and increased secretions.
2. Nasal septum may exhibit focal thickening or septal erosions may be seen in later stage.
3. Bony changes of nasal cavity and PNS may include sclerotic walls, bone erosion, as well as destruction.

Wegener's Granulomatosis:

- Progressive thinning and disappearance of part of nasal septum is characteristic.
- Degree of bone destruction is less because systemic nature of disease allows less time of progression.

Midline Granuloma:

Is a localized mid facial destruction with severe mutilation and bone necrosis involving nasal septum and sinuses.

There is relatively smaller soft tissue mass as compared to fungal infections.

NEOPLASTIC LESIONS

1. *Inverting Papilloma*

CT characteristically shows a mass extending from middle meatus of nose to maxillary sinus. Tumor

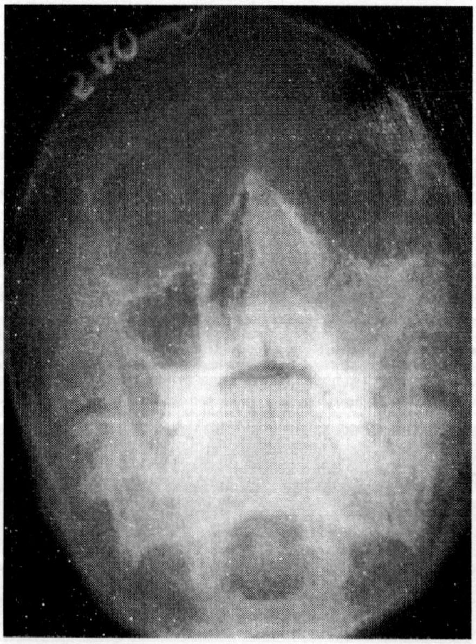

Fig. 24.1: Radiograph of PNS shows opaque maxillary sinus and nasal cavity on left side

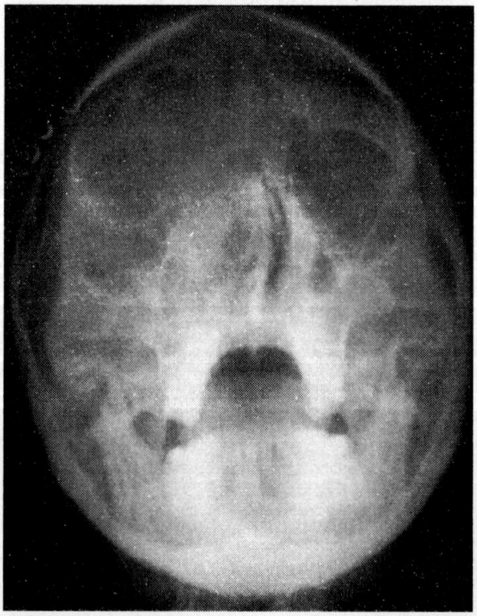

Fig. 24.2: Radiograph of the PNS shows a large expansile, destructive mass of the right maxillary sinus extending in to the nasal cavity

may show areas of calcification and produces sclerotic changes in walls of sinus.

There is remodelling of bone due to pressure erosion rather than destruction.

2. Malignancies

Most common sinonasal malignancy is squamous cell carcinoma.

Imaging:

- Heterogeneous soft tissue mass in sinonasal cavity with surrounding bone destruction. Orbital invasion, intracranial extension may be present.
- Associated lymphadenopathy and distant metastasis may be present.
- Fungal infections and malignancies cannot always be differentiated on imaging, however certain features might help in differentiation.

1. On CT scan fungal infections show serpiginous areas of increased density mixed with mucoid and soft tissue attenuation due to higher levels of magnesium, manganese and iron in fungal mucin. This is known as double density sign. No such hyperdense areas are seen in malignancies.
2. MRI in fungal sinusitis shows on T1 weighted images show isointense or slightly hypointense areas surrounded by mucosal inflammation. And T2 weighted image shows signal void areas due to paramagnetic effect of iron in fungal mucin.

   In malignancy and also in bacterial infections T2 weighted images show hyperintense mass rather than signal void areas.

Extraconal Masses of the Orbit

1. Orbital cellulitis and abscess.
2. Lymphoma and metastases.
3. Dermoid and teratoma.
4. Lymphangioma (Figure 25.1), lymphohemangioma.
5. Spread from lacrimal gland tumors.

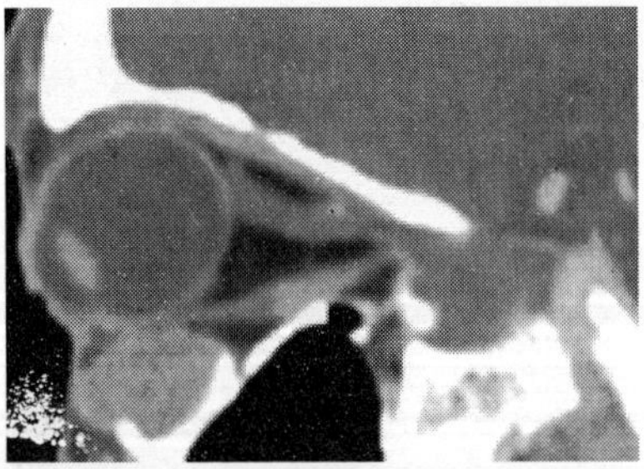

Fig. 25.1: Sagittal CT scan showing extraconal nonenhancing mass lesion in an old patient

MASSES ARISING FROM MUSCLE CONE

1. Inflammatory orbital pseudotumor.
2. Dysthyroid ophthalmopathy.
3. Rhabdomyosarcoma.

ORBITAL CELLULITIS AND ABSCESS

- Most common orbital pathology in children.
- Usually secondary to direct injury or spread from adjacent focus.
- Most – bacterial.
- Usually pre septal. Orbital septum is a strong barrier to posterior extension.
- Most post septal cases are extraconal.
- Cellulitis – poorly defined area of increased CT density or T2 signal intensity within the fat.
- Abscesses – more discrete mass like may contain low CT density or higher T2 signal with peripheral enhancement.
- Fungal infection → bony destruction.

Inflammatory Orbital Pseudotumor

- Most common cause of orbital mass in adults.
- Auto immune etiology is suspected.
- Can be Unilateral → more common
  Bilateral
- All compartments may be affected.
- Imaging.
  - Heterogeneous poorly marginated increased CT density and decreased T1 and T2 intensity within intraconal fat with adjacent scleral/uveal thickening.
  - Diffuse changes.
  - Discrete mass lesion.
  - Lacrimal gland may be enlarged.
  - Enhances follow contrast administration.

- Rapid response to steroids.

  D/D lymphoma
  - Atypical features.
  - No response to medication.
- Muscle cone invovement
  - Tendinous insertions involved.
  - Isolated LR thickening favour diagnosis especially with enlarged lacrimal gland.

Lymphoma

- Most common orbital neoplasm.
- Usually B-cell NHL, usually primary, occasionally secondary.
- Lacrimal gland most frequent involved.
- Imaging
  - Usually homogeneous lesions with well-defined margins, which may enhance on contrast administration.
  - May mimic pseudotumor.
  - Less commonly extraconal masses or diffuse infiltration of orbital fat can be seen.
- Respond well to radiotherapy.

Metastases

- Represent 3-10% of all orbital masses.
- In children – from embryonal tumors, neuroblastoma, Ewing's sarcoma and Wilms tumors–In adults – breast in female, lung in male, colon, prostate.
- In child – Orbit more freq. involved than globe.
- In adults–70% are ocular and 30% orbital.

Imaging

- Non-specific and variable.
- Usually ill-defined, diffusely infiltrating with in distinct boundaries.
- Metastasis to muscle, optic nerve and lacrimal gland may cause enlargement.
- Irregular borders, may be multifocal.

DERMOID/EPIDERMOID

- Usually located near lacrimal fossa or nasal bone and are homogenous.
- Fat clearly seen on CT or MRI.

Neurofibroma/Neurinoma

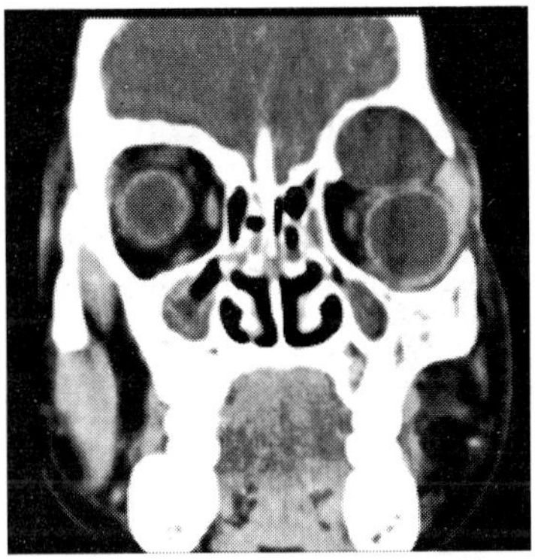

Fig. 25.2: Coronal CT image shows a cystic lymphangioma in the extraconal compartment of the right orbit. Incidentally noted is bilateral maxillary and ethmoid sinusitis

Section 2—Face, Neck, Orbit and Ear

Chapter 26

Embryological Development of Thyroid and Parathyroid Gland

- Thyroid gland develops from median bud of pharynx thyroglossal duct, which passes from foramen caecum from base of tongue to the isthmus of thyroid.
- The ultimobranchial body, which arises from diverticulum of 4th pharyngeal pouch of each side, amalgamates with corresponding lateral lobe.
- Parafollicular C cells are derived from neural crest reach thyroid via ultimobranchial body.

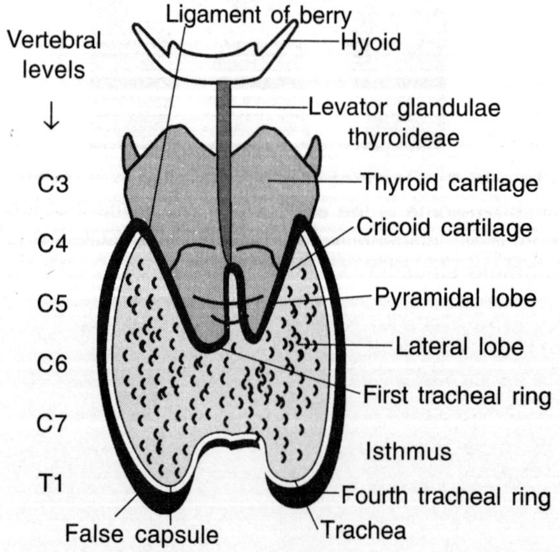

Fig. 26.1: Scheme to show the location and subdivisions of the thyroid gland including the false capsule

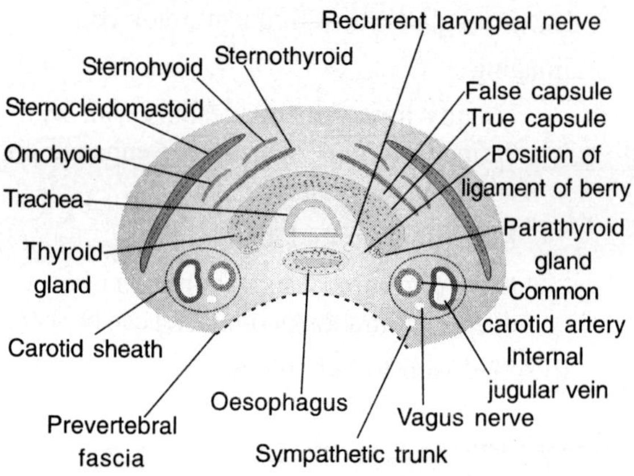

Fig. 26.2: Transverse section through the anterior part of the neck at the level of the isthmus of the thyroid gland

APPLIED

1. Ectopic/Aberrant Thyroid

A/B → Ectopic thyroid
- Lingual
- Cervical

C → Intrathoracic aberrant thyroid

D → Lateral aberrant thyroid

↓

Usually papillary carcinoma thyroid

2. Thyroglossal Cyst

May present in any part of thyroglossal tract. The common situations in order of frequency are:

- Beneath the hyoid.
- Region of thyroid cartilage.
- Above hyoid.

ANATOMY

- The thyroid gland is located in anteroinferior part of neck (intrahyoid compartment). It consists of two lobes that are joined along midline by isthmus opposite 3rd/4th tracheal ring. A pyramidal lobe arising superiorly from isthmus and lying in front of thyroid cartilage is present in 10-40% of normal individuals especially younger one and disappears gradually with age. The size/shape of thyroid varies in normal individuals.

Age group	Mean length	AP diameter
Newborn	18-20 mm	09-09 mm
1 year	25 mm	12-15 mm
Adults	40-60 mm	13-18 mm

The thyroid glands overlie vertebrae C5→T1. The thyroid gland is surrounded by:

→ True capsule – connective tissue condensation.

→ False capsule – formed by pretracheal fascia.

ARTERIAL SUPPLY

1. Superior thyroid artery – external carotid upper pole of each lobe.
2. Inferior thyroid artery–thyrocervical trunk.
3. Thyroid in an artery– brachiocephalic trunk.
4. Accessary thyroid arteries.

VENOUS DRAINAGE

- Superior/ middle/inferior thyroid vein which term plexus deep to capsule of gland.

RELATIONS

- On cut section each lobe of thyroid seem to have 3 surfaces.

LATERAL SURFACE

- Directed anterolaterally.

Covered by

- Skin/fascia.

  Sternohyoid and sternothyroid.

  Superior belly of omohyoid.

  Anterior part of sternomastoid.

Medial surface related to

- The thyroid and cricoid cartilages.
- Upper most part of trachea/oesophagus.
- Parts of two muscles: inferior constrictor and cricothyroid.
- Longus coli muscle.
- Nerves
  - Recurrent laryngeal nerve.
  - External laryngeal nerve.

Posterior surface

- Related to carotid sheath and its contents.

Anterior border

- Related to branch of superior thyroid artery.

Posterior border related to

- Inferior thyroid artery.
- Parathyroid glands.
- Thoracic duct on left side.

Radiological Anatomy

1. X-ray

Thyroid gland is normally not visualized on X-ray STN. However, it can be visualized if calcified increased pretracheal space thickness can be the only clue to thyroid enlargement on X-ray STN.

Vertebral level	Normal pretracheal space thickness
C2 → 7 mm	
C4 →14 mm	
C6 →21 mm	

2. USG/USG Doppler

- Normal thyroid parenchyma has a homogenous medium to high level echogenicity which makes detection of focal cystic or hypoechoic lesions relatively easy.
- Capsule appears as a thin hyperechoic line.
- The high vascularity of gland can be seen with high sensitivity Doppler instruments and is most pronounced at superior/inferior poles.

Mean diameter of arteries	-	1-2 mm
Mean diameter of veins	-	Upto 8 mm
Peak systolic velocities		
1. Major arteries	-	20-40 cm/sec
2. Intraparenchymal arteries	-	15-30 cm/sec

- Sternohyoid/sternothyroid – thin hypoechoic band.
- Sternoleidomastoid – large oval band.

  An important landmark is longus colli muscle located posterior to each thyroid lobe, in close contact with the prevertebral space.
- On longitudinal scan, the recurrent laryngeal nerve and inferior thyroid artery may be seen as thin hypoechoic band located between thyroid lobe and esophagus on left and thyroid gland and longus colli muscle on right.

Thyroid Volume

- Sonography is an accurate method for calculating thyroid volume assessment of which may be useful for goitre size determination thyroid volume can be calculated by linear parameter like AP diameter.

  AP diameter >20 mm in decisive thyroid enlargement.
- In neonate thyroid volume ranges from 0.40 to 1.40 ml increasing by approximately 1.0 to 1.3 ml for each 10 kg weight for upto a normal adult volume of 10 to 11± 3 ml.

Larger thyroid volume	Smaller volume
1. Regions with iodine deficiency	1. Chronic hepatitis
2. Acute hepatitis thyrocine or chronic renal failure	2. Treated with radioactive iodine

3. CT/MRI

- Well visualized due to its higher than average soft tissue attenuation caused by physiological high iodine content of gland.

4. Radionuclide Imaging

Agents used:

- $99mT_cO_4$ (sodium pertechnate).
- ^{123}I.

On radionucleide imaging, left/right lobe appear equal in size, however, minor degree of asymmetry is acceptable.

Uptake of tracer is unifom or at least equal or slightly more than uptake in parotid and submandibular gland.

99 mTc petechnate	^{123}I
- Used for routine thyroid Imaging	- Far functional assessment
	- Retrosternal/ectopic thyroid
	- Neonatal hypothyroidism
	- Follow up after surgery
- HOT AREAS	- COLD AREAS
- Area of ↑ activity e.g.	- Areas of ↓ activity e.g.

1. Functioning thyroid adenoma	1. Colloid cyst
	2. Nonfunctioning adenoma
	3. Carcinoma
	4. Thyroides
	5. Hemorrhage/infarct
	6. Abscesses
	7. Artifacts

EMBRYOLOGICAL DEVELOPMENT OF PARATHYROID GLAND

Superior Parathyroid Glands

- Fourth pharyngeal pouch along with more thyroid gland.
- More constant in position

  80% Posterolateral aspect of thyroid immediately above crossing of inferior thyroid artery and recurrent laryngeal nerve close to cricothyroid articulation.

  20% Posterolateral to upper pole of thyroid.

Inferior Parathyroid Glands

- Third pharyngeal pouch along with thymus.

  During fetal development these migrate caudally along with thymus in a more anterior track. The inferior parathyroid more variable in position.

  60% At or just inferior to posterior aspect of thyroid lower pole

  25% Fail to dissociate from thymus and continue to migrate lower in neck tissues or into mediastinum usually within thyrothmic ligament.

Ectopic Parathyroid Glands

- A significant percentage of parathyroid glands lie in relatively or frankly ectopic locations in week or mediastinum.
- Ectopic superior parathyroid lies far posteriorly in tracheoesophageal groove/posterosuperior mediastinum.
- Ectopic inferior parathyroid → lower neck/ anterosuperior mediastinum associated with thymus/carotid sheath/carotid bifurcation.

ANATOMY

- Most adults have four parathyroid glands each measuring 5 mm × 3 mm × 1 mm and weighing an average 35-40 m supernumerary fifth glands are present in upto 13% of the population.

  Each gland has a delicate capsule supplied by a single lesh of blood vessels running in subcapsular space. Very often parathyroid are embedded within a pad of fat which gives a useful clue for identification.

Radiological Anatomy

1. **X-ray:** Not visualized unless calcified.
2. **USG:** Generally the abnormal parathyroid gland is of lower reflectivity than normal thyroid and echogenic capsule separates one from other.
3. **CT/MRI** can identify ectopic parathyroid adenoma in neck/upper mediastinum.

   Density lower than nearby thyroid tissue.
4. **Radionuclide Imaging**

   Used to localise parathyroid adenoma.

   Hyperplastic glands are ectopic source of parathyroid hormone secretion.

   Radiopharmaceuticals used:

   1. 99 m Tc – methoxyisobutyl ionitrite (MIBI).
   2. 99 m Tc – tetraformin.
   3. Thallium 201.

   Appearance

   1. Normal parathyroid not visualized smallest adenoma currently detected by imaging are in region of 150-200 mg.
   2. Adenomas usually demonstrated as areas of activity adjacent to or overlapping thyroid.

Section 2—Face, Neck, Orbit and Ear

Chapter 27

Role of Imaging in Thyroid and Parathyroid Gland

ANATOMY

- The gland lies in front of thyroid cartilage. Normal gland consists of 2 lobes joined by isthmus.
- Lobes are on either side of trachea and has a
  - Superior pole.
  - Inferior pole.
- Average thyroid lobe measures 3 cm × 2 cm.
- Entire thyroid gland lies in the neck above clavicles. However substernal extension into superior mediastinum may occur.
- An accessory (pyramidal) lobe may be present in 50-70% of people.
- Thyroid gland has a rich vascular supply.
- *Superior:* Thyroid vessels are found at upper lobe of each pole.

  Inferior: Thyroid artery is present post to the lower 1/3rd of lobe.

  In color Doppler normal PSV is 20-40 cm/sec.

THYROID IMAGING

- Nuclear scintigraphy and USG are frequently the first imaging modalities used to assess patients with suspected thyroid disorders.
- CT and MR imaging is useful in assessing the morphological and anatomical features of thyroid along with extent of thyroid goitre, extension of neoplasm outside the thyroid capsule and into the adjacent structures in the neck. They are also useful in assessing regional modal metastasis and in the evaluation of recurrent disease following treatment of thyroid cancer.

Nuclear Scintigraphy

- Provides excellent functional information about thyroid.
- In the evaluation of local thyroid mass to determine whether a lesion is 'hot' or 'cold'.
- Currently morphological details of thyroid gland are obtained using Tc-99 m pertechnetate, I-123, I-131.
- Normal thyroid gland shows homogenous radionucleotide uptake and distribution.
- The isthmus may demostrate slightly less activity than right and left lobe.
- I-131 is used in both the evaluation and treatment of patients with thyroid cancer that concentrate iodine and particularly useful in follow up of patients after thyroidectomy to evaluate for residual thyroid tissue.

Ultrasonography

- It is an accessible, inexpensive and non-invasive technique (Figure 27.1).
- It is performed with high-resolution linear array transducers ranging from 7.5-10 MHz.
- Thyroid gland normally is uniformly hyperechoic. It can easily distinguish cystic from solid lesions.
- USG may also be used to guide FNAC of nodular diseases.

Limitations

- Its interpretation is dependent on the operator.
- It is not as good as cross sectional imaging in identifying lymphadenopathy or in evaluating the extent of thyroid mass into the adjacent soft tissue.

CROSS SECTION IMAGING

- CT and MRI provide better delineation of the lesion within thyroid gland and play a critical role in detection of lymph node meets and extension of thyroid disease to adjacent tissue of neck.
- Normal thyroid has a density of approx 80-100 HU on CT.
- MR imaging is performed with ant. neck coil centres over the thyroid gland.
- Nodules as small as 4 mm may be detected. Pulse sequence used is:
  1. Non contrast sagittal and axial T1W.
  2. Axial FSE T2W with fat saturation; and
  3. Post contrast axial T1W image with fat saturation.
- On T2W image, the thyroid gland is hyperintense related to neck musculature.
- Following contrast administration, the normal gland enhances diffusely and homogenously on both CT and MRI.

PATHOLOGY OF THYROID GLAND

Congenital Anomalies

- During foetal develoement. Thyroid gland must descend from its origin is foramen caecum located at the ant midline base of tongue to its final adult position in the lower neck both anterior and lateral to trachea.

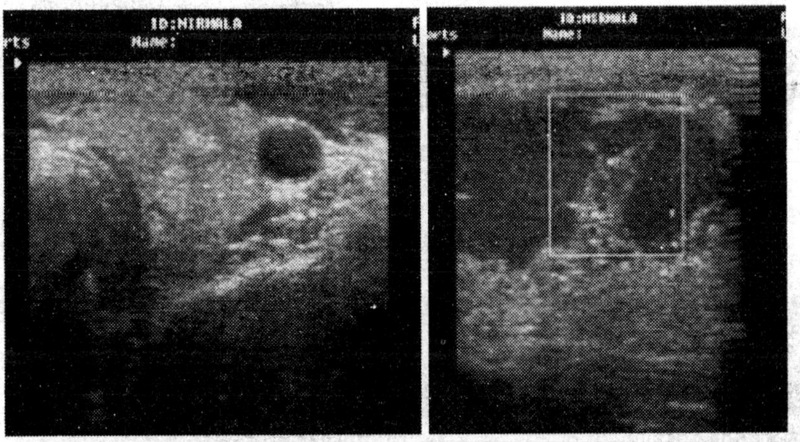

Fig. 27.1: US scans shows a large, cystic mass in the right lobe with color flow in the solid part and a calcified lesion in the left lobe of thyroid

- Arrest of descent can occur anywhere from tongue to lower neck.
- Thyroid tissue may be present elsewhere ectopically.
  - Lingual thyroid.
  - Ectopic thyroid.
  - Thyroglossal cyst.

A. *Lingual Thyroid*

- Results due to failures of descent of thyroid gland.
- Upto 70% of patients may have no functioning thyroid tissue in neck.

Nuclear Imaging

- Has major role in diagnosing lingual thyroid. Also it determines whether there is normal thyroid tissue in neck.

  NCCT: Hyperdense due to iodine content.

  MRI: High SI on T1W and T2W images compared to tongue musculature. Marked enhancement seen after IV contrast.

B. *Ectopic Thyroid*

- Overdescent of thyroid may result in ectopic normal thyroid in lower neck of mediastinum.
- Rarely thyroid tissue may be found in heart and within ovarian teratomas.

  NI: Using Tc-99 and I-131, it should be done when ectopic is suspected.

C. *Thyroglossal Cyst*

Due to incomplete degeneration of thyroglossal duct, these are often medline ant. neck masses and mostly infrahyoid.

NI: Usually not necessary.

USG: Shows typical features of cyst. May demonstrate internal echoes when proteinaceous/infected large cyst may show multiple septations.

CT: Isodense to water.

- May be hyperdense when protein content.

MRI: SI low on T1W and high on T2W.

No contrast enhancement seen.

AUTOIMMUNE DISEASE AND THYROIDITIS

Thyroiditis may be

- Acute and self-limiting.
- Chronic and progressive.

Thyroiditis can be divided into:

1. Auto immune
   - Grave.
   - Hashimotos.
   - Post partum.
2. Inflammatory.
3. Infective.

Autoimmune: Grave's Disease

- Most common autoimmune disorder.
- Occur in 3rd/4th decade: Female >> male.
- Associated with hyperthyroidism.
  - *NI:* Diffusely enlarged with intense radiotracer uptake.

    D/D thyroidits: ↓ Uptake of radionucleotide often inhomogenous.
- *Toxic multinodular goitres:* ↑ and ↓ uptake within enlarged gland.
- *Thyroadenoma:* Focal uptake in single nodule.

  USG: Thyroid is enlarged and diffusely hyperechoic without discreet nodule.

  Colour Doppler: ↑ in thyroid vascularity both in systolic and diastolic. The appearance. Has been referred as "Thyroid inferno". PSV may exceed 70 cm/sec.
- *CT/MRI:* Enlarged thyroid may demonstrate clear enhancement.
- *On NCCT:* Density is ↓ due to ↓ in iodine concentration.

HASHIMOTO'S THYROIDITIS HASHIMOTO'S THYROIDITIS (CH. LYMPHOCYTIC THYROIDITIS)

- More common in females (4th/5th decade).
- Associated with of hypothyroidism.

  NI: No typical pattern. Uptake of radioiodine is usually heterogenous and patchy.

  USG: Thyroid may be normal or enlarged with diffusely heterogenous echogenicity. There may be numerous poorly defined hypoechoic regions separated by fibrous strands.

  USG may be used to follow patient of Hachomotor disease to detect occult malignancy.

Color Doppler

- Marked hyperemia seen.

CT

- Intromogenous distribution of contrast seen.

MRI

- T2W images may show areas of -SI. Linear septate low-density bands represent fibrosis.

CEMR

- Shows patchy inhomogeneous enhancement.

DE QUERVAIN'S THYROIDIS

- Self-limiting inflammatory process following post-viral URTI.
- Occur in 5th/6th decade Female > Male.
- *C/F:* Painful enlargement of gland, fever, thyrotoxicosis.

  NI: ↓ radioactive iodine uptake. May revert to normal when patient returns to euthyroid state.

  NCCT: Gland is slightly enlarged and has lower than normal attenuation.

ACUTE SUPPURATIVE THYROIDITIS

- Etiology is mainly fungal and bacterial.

  USG – Focal/diffuse enlargement of gland with decrease echogenicity.

  Sometimes abscess may be seen within gland.

CT

- Affected portion of gland is enlarged and heterogenous in CT density and MR signal intensity and shows variable enhancement after IV contrast.
- Rim enhancement is seen if focal abscesses develop.

REIDEL'S THYROIDITIS

Rare form of thyroiditis characterized by fibrous reaction and extends to the adjacent soft tissue of neck.

USG

- Thyroid may be hypoechoic.

CT

- Involved thyroid may be hypodense compared to normal thyroid.

MRI

- Give characteristic appearance of ST on T1W and T2W images which correspond to fibrosis. It also demonstrates infiltration of adjacent soft tissue of neck.

Goitre

- Diffuse non-toxic goitre is a diffuse non-nodular enlargement of thyroid associated with an euthyroid state.
- *Endemic goitre:* Prevalent in iodine deficient areas.
- *Sporadic goitre:* Female > male; peak incidence of puertal age group.

- Most simple goitre in due course of time progress to multinodular goitre and may remain non-toxic.
- Multi nodular goitre is characterized by nodularity, focal hemorrhage, calcification, and cyst formation and scarring.

Diffuse Goitre

USG

- ↑ in glandular size RT lobe > left.
- No focal textural change. Homogenous echogenicity.
- May extend substernally into mediastinum.
- Multinodular goitre.
  - *NT:* Radioactive I may accumulate in multiple foci throughout the gland.
  - *USG:* Often irregular with diffuse inhomogenous or multiple focal hypoechoic nodules.
  - *CT:* Gland is asymmetric, multiple low, density area reflecting necrosis, cyst formation and areas of hyperdensity reflecting calcification, hemorrhage and colloid.
  - *MR-T1W:* Multiple foci of high SI neph. Cyst containing colloid/hemorrhage.
  - T2W diffuse heterogenicity may be present. Enhancement is visually inhomogeneous.

CT and MR are useful in evaluating secondary manifestation of goitre including compression and displacement of trachea, oesophagus and adjacent vessels along with substernal and mediastinal extension.

NEOPLASM OF THYROID GLAND

Benign	Malignant
↓	– Papilloma carcinoma (most common) (Figure 27.2)
Adenoma	– Follicular carcinoma
	– Anaplastic carcinoma.
	– Medullary carcinoma.
	– Metastasis.

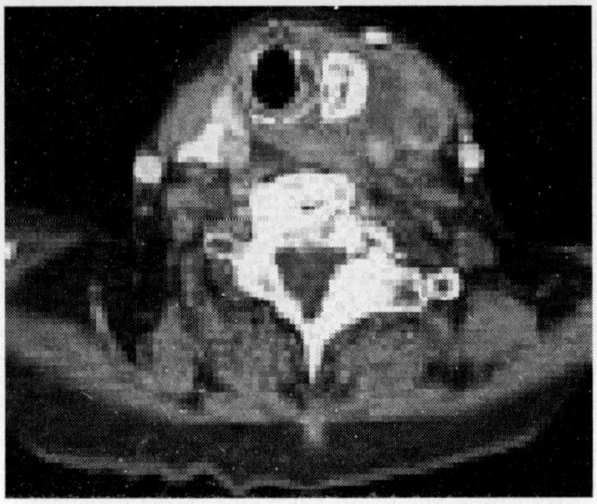

Fig. 27.2: CECT axial section of neck showing carcinoma left lobe of thyroid with heterogenous enhancement pattern

Adenoma

- These are true benign neoplasm with well-developed fibrous capsule, usually solitary and non-functioning.
- Toxicity is most commonly seen with large lesion.
- Sudden enlargement is due to spontaneous hemorrhage.

USG

- Mass with - or - echogenicity.
- *'Halo sign':* Complete hypoechoic ring surrounded isoechoic solid mass.

Color Doppler

- Study reveals nodule with peripheral vascularity.

Malignant Neoplasm

- History of neck irradiation.
- Rapid growth and stony hard module.

PAPILLARY CARCINOMA

- 60% of all thyroid carcinomas.
- Female > Males in 5th decade.
- Lymphatic spread to regional lymph node. May spread to lung and bone.
- The imaging app of papillary carcinoma is variable and may include dominant nodule, multifocal nodules, and diffuse infiltration of the gland that manifests as heterogenous hypodensity on CT.

NI

- Usually appears as cold nodule.

USG

- Tumor of ↓ echogenicity, purely solid/complex mass with areas of necrosis, hemorrhage, cystic degeneration and calcification (Figure 27.3).

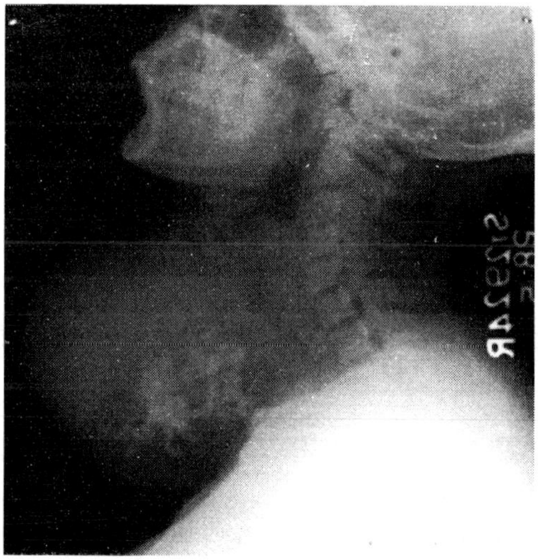

Fig. 27.3: Radiograph of the soft tissue neck shows a large thyroid mass with irregular calcification

X-ray

- Punctate, linear, psammamatous calcification at tumor periphery.

CT Scan

- Heterogeneous hypodense mass showing variable enhancement.
- Margins are ill defined and it may infiltrate adjacent soft tissue neck.
- Associated cervical lymphadenopathy may be present. Lymph nodes may be calcified, cystic, hemorrhagic, may contain colloid.

  Hemorrhagic and colloid containing nodes may be hyperintense on T1W MR images.

SUMMARY

- The major role of scintigraphy in assessing a dominant palpable thyroid mass is to determine whether the lesion is hot or cold as there is marked increase in risk in cold nodule.
- USG because of its availability, is the first modality used to assess a thyroid mass. It distinguish solid from cystic lesion and show cervical adenopathy, if any.
- Any nodule formation in enlarged thyroid, determine volume of nodule.
- Useful during follow up to distinguish nodular growth from intranodular hemorrhage.
- The main role of cross - sectional imaging is to assess findings related to a thyroid mass including invasion through the thyroid capsule and infiltration of adjacent tissue and str. In the neck and to detect cervical lymphadenopathy.

Color Doppler

- Most of the benign adenomatous module shows peripheral distribution of blood vessels while majority of thyroid malignancies show internal vessels with or without peripheral component.

  Doppler examination can also be used to monitor the response of therapy in Graves disease, as there is significant decrease in vascularity following treatment.

PARATHYROID GLANDS

- Imaging of parathyroid glands primarily focuses on the detection of adenomas in patients with primary hyperparathyroidism.
- Second focus is the detection of an unrecognised adenoma in patients with persistent/recurrent hypercalcemia after prior surgery of hyperparathyroidism.
- The number of parathyroid glands is usually four.

ANATOMY

- Upper parathyroid glands are post to the middle 1/3 of thyroid gland.
- Lower parathyroid glands are lateral to lower pole of thyroid gland.
- The normal parathyroid glands are each less than 9 mm in maximum dimension.

IMAGING OF PATHOLOGY OF PARATHYROID GLAND

1. Parathyroid Adenoma

USG

- High-resolution linear array transducer is used.
- Typical appearance of adenoma is that of a homogenous well-defined mass with echogenicity less than that of thyroid gland.
- Adenomas are typically encapsulated and solid may have cystic/hemorrhagic components.

Color Doppler

- May help to distinguish thyroid from parathyroid lesions. Specifically thyroid lesions tend to have some glands more often lack Doppler signal.

  USG has its limitation in identifying ectopic parathyroid adenomas.

CT/MR Imaging

- Allow detection of ectopic parathyroid adenomas.
- IV contrast must be used in CT to distinguish blood vessels from adenomas as 25% of these adenomas enhance.
- Sensitivity and specificity of HRCT improve over USG and being 70% and 90% respectively.
- MR allows excellent evaluation of mediastinum and is more sensitive than CT in identifying parathyroid adenomas.

  On T1W: These are iso to hypointense comp. to thyroid gland.

  On T2W: These are hyperintense and show enhancement after IV gadolinium.

  The MRR imaging has specificity over 95%.

NI

Is used to identify parathyroid adenomas performed with several nucleotide including Thallium-201, Tc-99m sestamibi subtraction imaging with I-123. Because no radionucleotide is taken up by the parathyroid glands alone, subtraction technique allow radionucleotide that are conc. in thyroid gland (Tc and I) to be subtracted from those that accumulate within both thyroid and parathyroid tissue (Thallium and Sestamibi).

After thyroid subtraction, parathyroid adenoma appears as a focus of thallium uptake.

Parathyroid Hyperplasia

Causes hyperparathyroidism in 50% difficult to evaluate with any imaging modality due to small size of hyperplastic glands. The sensitivity for detection is 30-50% with cross-sectional imaging while Tc-99 sestamibi has upto 80% sensitivity.

Solitary Pulmonary Nodule

- SPN is defined as a single, discrete pulmonary opacity that in less than 3 cm in diameter surrounded by normal lung tissue and not associated with adenopathy or atelectasis.

  Radiographically, a nodule is a lesion less than 3 cm and anything larger than 3 cm is termed as a mass.

Frequency

- In US SPN's is one of the most common thoracic radiographic abnormalities.

  Approximately 40-50% of these nodules are malignant. Most are bronchogenic CA but 10-30% are solitary metastases.

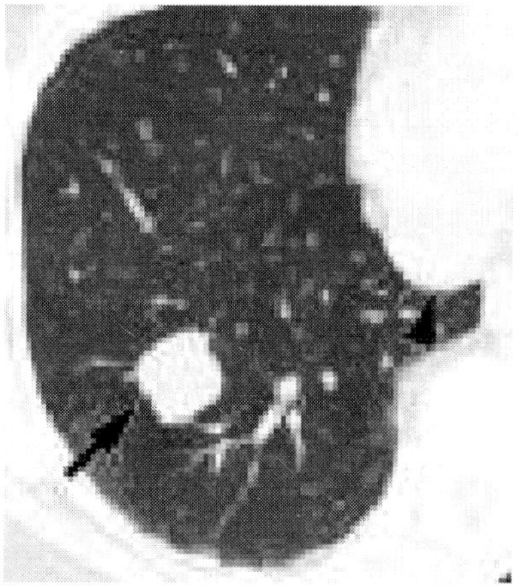

Fig. 28.1: Axial CT section of chest showing solitary pulmonary nodule. No internal fat density with normal surrounding lung parenchyma

Clinical Details

- Most SPN's are asymptomatic (Figure 28.1).
- Important features in the patient history include the following:
  1. Age–Risk of malignancy increases with age. It is 3% at 35-40 years, 15% at 40-50 years, 48% at 50-60 years and 50% in > 60 years.
  2. Smoking history.
  3. Prior history of malignancy.
  4. History of travel to areas of endemic mycosis or high prevalence of TB.
  5. Exposure to asbestos, radon, nickel, vinyl chloride etc.
  6. Previous history of TB or mycosis.

Causes

1. *Neoplastic*

Malignant

- Primary (bronchogenic Ca).

- Metastasis.
- Lymphoma.
- Plasmacytoma.
- Alveolar cell carcinoma.

Benign

- Hamartoma.
- Adenoma.
- Connective tissue tumor.

2. ***Inflammatory (infectious)***

   Granuloma TB, histoplasmosis, blastomycosis etc.

   Lung abscess.

   Round pneumonia.

   Hydatid cyst.

3. ***Inflammatory (non-infectious)***

   Rheumatoid arthritis.

   Wegener's granulomatosis.

   Sarcoidosis.

   Lipoid pneumonia.

4. ***Congenital***

   AVM.

   Sequestration.

   Bronchogenic cyst.

5. ***Pulmonary infarct***
6. ***Pulmonary hematoma***
7. ***Impacted mucus***
8. ***Pleural***

   Fibroma.

   Loculated fluid.

9. ***Skin and chest wall lesions***
10. ***Artefacts***

Investigations

- Chest X-ray is the initial examination and most SPN's are discovered as an incidental finding.
- CT scan detect much more smaller nodules as detected by X-ray.
- PET and SPECT are becoming important imaging tools in evaluating SPN.

Work Up

Medical History

- If there is a tumor elsewhere in the body there is 50% chance that the nodule is malignant.

  If there is no other tumor or any part history of benign or malignant tumors there is a 60-95% chance of the nodule being benign.
- Patient's history of smoking is important for SPN being bronchogenic CA.

  In countries prevalent with mycobacterial infection TB is an important cause.

LAB STUDIES

- Have a limited role in work up of SPN.
- Anemia or elevated ESR may indicate neoplastic or infectious process.
- Elevated liver enzymes, ALP or serum calcium indicate metastases from bronchogenic CA or extra pulmonary malignancy
- Patients with fungal injections have IgG and IgM Ab specific to these fungi.

Imaging

Chest X-ray

- The recent chest X-ray should always be compared with older X-rays if available because it indicates the rate of growth of the lesion and appearance of new lesions may be seen.

- The first step is to determine whether the nodule is pulmonary or extra pulmonary.

  Lateral films, fluoroscopy or CT help determine the location of the nodule.
- Usually nodules are identifiable by the time they are 8-10 mm in size. Occasionally may be seen at 5 mm.
- Chest X-ray provides information about nodule size, growth rate, margins, calcification pattern and these signs aid in differentiating malignant and benign lesions.

1. Nodule Size

Nodules >3 cm are more likely to be malignant while those <3 cm are likely benign. However, criteria of size have limited value and smaller nodules can be malignant and longer benign.

2. Growth Rate

Refers to doubling time of the nodule i.e. doubling in volume.

- 26% increase in diameter on chest X-ray represents one doubling. For e.g. increase from 1 to 1.3 cm is one doubling.
- Doubling time of most malignant nodules is 30 to 400 days.
- Benign nodules have doubling time of less than 30 or >400 days.
- Doubling time >400 days are typically benign.
- Absence of change in size of a nodule over 2 years is highly s/o benign lesion.

3. Margin Characteristics

Benign lesions have well-circumscribed smooth borders.

Malignant nodules have irregular, lobulated, speculated borders.

4. Calcification

Calcification in a nodule is more likely seen in benign lesions. 10% of malignant nodules demonstrate calcification.

In benign lesions the calcifications may be diffuse, concentric, laminar central or popcorn calcifications. Popcorn pattern is typical of hematoma.

Stippled or eccentric pattern is seen most commonly in malignant nodules.

5. Other Associated Features

Presence of air bronchogram makes bronchogenic carcinoma or metastasis unlikely, however, it may be seen in bronchoalveolar carcinoma or lymphoma.

Invasion of adjacent bone by the nodule is pathognomic of bronchogenic carcinoma.

Cavitation with thin smooth wall may indicate lung abscess or benign lesion, whereas thick walled eccentric cavitations implies an underlying malignancy.

COMPUTED TOMOGRAPHY

CT scan has many advantages over plain film and allows better assessment of nodules.

1. Better resolution – Nodules as small as 3-4 mm are detectable. Morphologic features of specific diagnosis are better visualized.
2. Areas that are difficult to assess on plain radiograph are better visualized such as lung apices, perihilar regions and CP angles.
3. Multiple nodules can be detected.
4. Malignancy can be staged.
5. CT can help guide needle biopsy.

CT Densitometry

- Measure the attenuation coefficients of a lesion and aids detection of occult calcification.
- A value >185HU has been suggested as a cut off for benign lesions.

CT Halo Sign

- I.e. ground glass attenuation surrounding a nodule most commonly indicates invasive aspergillosis. Other less common possibilities are T.B. CMV or herpes simplex infections.

CT Contrast Enhancement

- Malignant nodules are more vascular assessment of enhancement involves repeated measurement over 5 min periods. Enhancement <15 HU is s/o benign lesion and >20 HU is more likely ass with malignant lesions.

Feeding Vessel Sign

- This sign may be seen in hematogenous or vascular causes of nodules such as metastatic deposits of septic emboli.

Cavity Wall Thickness

- Thin walled cavity less than 1 mm is s/o benign lesion; a thick walled cavity is usually indeterminate.

MRI

- Provides better imaging for pleural, diaphragm and chest wall disease for staging. It is however, poorer than CT for assessing lung parenchyma because of poor spatial resolution.

U/S

- Has a very limited role, can be used only for percutaneous biopsy of large peripherally based lesions.

NUCLEAR MEDICINE

PET Imaging

- Malignant cells have a higher metabolic rate than normal cells, therefore glucose uptake is higher.
- Therefore fluorine 18-fluorodeoxyglucose shows increased uptake in most malignant tumors.
- PET scans are analysed using standardized uptake values (SUV) to normalize measurements for patients weight and injected dose of the isotope. SUV of less than 2.5 cm is indicative of benign lesion.
- It has better advantage of detecting mediastinal metastases.

SPECT Imaging

- Spect scanners have the advantage of being more readily available than PET scanners.
- Depreotide is a somatostatin analogue labelled with Tc99 m, which has been shown to bind to somatostatins receptors expression on now small cell carcinomas.

Intervention

- After clinical and radiological assessment of SPN, all patients can be divided into the following groups:

1. ***Patients with Benign Lesions***
   - Like patients <35 years without other risk factors, stability of SPN over 2 years or a benign pattern on chest X-ray patients should be followed with serial X-ray or CT every 3-4 months for the first year and every 4-6 months in the second year.
2. ***Patients with Malignant Lesions***
   - Progress to thoracotomy for removal.
3. ***Patients with Indeterminate Lesions***
   - Most patients fall into this category. Further evaluation with biopsy/FNAC.
   - Biopsy can be transbronchial or transthoracic percutaneous.

SALIENT FEATURES OF COMMON LESIONS

1. **Bronchogenic Carcinoma**
   - Peripheral or central mass speculated margins, eccentric cavitations may be present.

Section 3

Adjacent bone erosion or metastasis elsewhere may be present.

- Mediastinal invasion, lymph nodes and pleural involvement are better seen on CT scan.

2. Metastasis

- Most common primary tumors producing solitary mets are carcinoma colon, testes, kidney, breast, bone sarcomas and malignant melanomas. Metastases are often peripheral and subpleural.

  Metastases are usually spherical with well-defined margin.

3. Lymphoma

- May involve lung in 30% cases.

  Present as lymphangitis, solitary areas of consolidation, large confluent areas or miliary nodules. Pulmonary opacity may show air bronchogram and may cavitate.

4. Bronchial Adenoma

- Central well defined nodules bronchial obstruction may cause recurrent segmental pneumonia, bronchiectesis or air trapping.

5. Hamartoma

- Normally peripheral well circumscribed nodules. 80% show calcification and popcorn pattern is typical. CT may demonstrate fat within the lesion, which is diagnostic.

6. Tuberculoma

- Localized granuloma usually upto 5 cm in diameter. Calcification is common but cavitation unusual.

7. Lung Abscess

- When completely filled with fluid may appear as nodule. Air fluid level indicates communication with airway. Wall may be thick initially and become thinner later on due to further necrosis.

8. Hydatid Cyst

- Unilocular cyst, well circumscribed, round or oval, homogenous mass, may be upto 10 cm in diameter. Calcification rare.

9. Pulmonary AVM

- Large fistulas may be seen as homogenous masses with arteries and veins seen draining the lesion.

10. Pulmonary Sequestration

- Intralobar or extralobar.
- Usually seen as soft tissue mass lying in lower lung posteriorly, usually on left side.

11. Bronchogenic Cyst

- Usually mediastinal, less commonly intra-pulmonary. Seen as well circumscribed attenuation mass (0-10 HU) on CT.

12. Rheumatoid Nodules

- Uncommon lesions.
- Usually associated with subcutaneous nodules.
- Were circumscribed, rounded opacities, solitary or multiple.

13. Pulmonary Infarcts

- Usually peripheral wedge shaped opacities.

Section 3—Respiratory System

Chapter 29

Pulmonary Cavity

A cavity (Figure 29.1) is a gas filled space surrounded by a complete wall which is 3mm or greater in thickness. Thinner walled such lesions are called cysts or ring shadows. Cavitation occurs when an area of necrosis communicates with a patient airway.

Features of Importance

- Location.
- Outline.
- Wall thickness.
- Presence of fluid level.
- Contents of the cavity.
- Satellite lesion.
- Appearance of surrounding lung.
- Multiplicity.

Meniscus sign: It is seen when an intracavitatory body is surrounded by a crescent of air as seen in fungus balls such as an aspergilloma. There is movement of ball with change in patient position. Other such lesions can be inspissated pus, blood clot and cavernolith.

Differential Diagnosis

A. *Neoplasm*

Lung primary

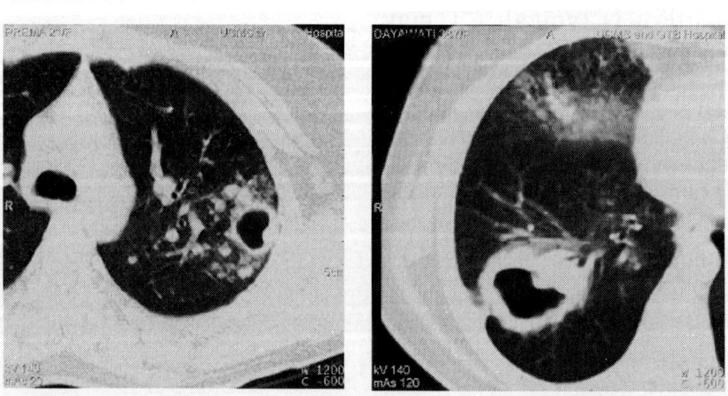

Fig. 29.1: Axial CT images show pulmonary cavities with secondary changes in the lung

- Squamous cell carcinoma.
- Adenocarcinoma.
- Bronchoalveolar carcinoma.
- Hodgkin's disease.

Metastases (4% cavitate)

- Squamous cell carcinoma (nasopharynx, cervix, esophagus).
- Adenocarcinoma (colorectal).
- Sarcomas: Ewing's, osteo, angio.
- Melanoma.
- Seminoma, teratocarcinoma.
- Wilm's tumor.

B. *Collagen Vascular Disease*

- Wegner's granulomatosis.
- Rheumatoid nodules.
- SLE.
- Polyarteritis nodosa.

C. *Granulomatous Disease*

- Histiocytosis X.
- Sarcoidosis.

D. *Vascular Diseases*

- Pulmonary embolus with infarction.
- Septic emboli (staph aureus).

E. *Infections*

- *Bacterial:* Pneumatoceles from Staph/ gram negative pneumonia.
- *Mycobacterial:* TB.
- *Fungal:* Nocardiosis, cryptococcosis, coccidio, aspergillosis.
- *Parasitic:* Echinococcosis (multiple in 20-30%).

F. *Trauma*

- Traumatic lung cyst after hemorrhage.
- Hydrocarbon ingestion.

G. *Bronchopulmonary Disease*

- Infected bulla.
- Cystic bronchiectasis.
- Communicating bronchogenic cyst.

Malignant Cavities (Figure 29.2)

- Squamous cell carcinoma is the most common primary lung carcinoma to cavitate as such the cavities are thus most commonly located centrally.
- Cavities are thick and shaggy walled with irregular ill defined margins.
- Patient is usually of old age and has history of cigarette smoking.

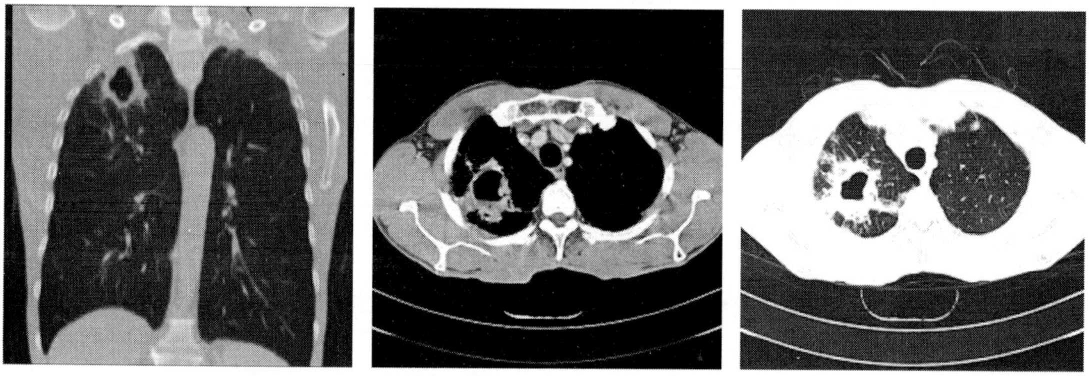

Fig. 29.2: Coronal MPR and axial CT images show a carcinomatous pulmonary cavity in the RUL

- In metastatic cavities a history of a primary can usually be elicited.

Wegner's Granulomatosis

- Multiple large to small pulmonary nodules are evident usually in lower lung fields and there may be areas of alveolar infiltrates.
- These are fairly well defined and often cavitate.
- May resolve spontaneously with new crop appearing at a different place.
- The cavities may have thick or thin walls.
- A generalized reticulo-nodular pattern may be seen.
- There may be associated paranasal sinuses opacification, small pleural effusions, reactive hilar or mediastinal adenopathy.

Rheumatoid Nodules

- Uncommon but characteristic and are usually associated with subcutaneous nodules.
- Well defined rounded opacities upto 7 mm in diameter, may be single or multiple and often cavitate.
- Pleural effusions are most common manifestation of rheumatoid disease.
- Fibrosing alveolitis presents as reticulo-nodular pattern progressing to honeycombing.

Histiocytosis X

- Ill defined transient patchy consolidation is the earliest manifestation.
- A fine reticulonodular pattern can be seen especially in the mid and upper zones.
- On HRCT there is a mixture of discrete nodules and cystic spaces sometimes with sparing of lung bases.
- Spontaneous pneumothoraces may develop.

Infected Cavity

- Tuberculosis is the most common infective etiology to cavitate.
- The cavities are thick or thin walled with shaggy inner lining.
- The surrounding lung may show areas of alveolar infiltrates and nodular shadows.
- There may be associated pleural effusions and hilar adenopathy.
- There may be fluid level in the cavity due to abscess formation.

Bronchiectasis

Bronchiectasis is an irreversible dilatation of one or more bronchi, and is usually a result of severe, recurrent or chronic infection. It may be localized or generalized. It is frequently basal but in tuberculosis and cystic fibrosis it usually involves the upper zones also.

Etiology

A. Congenital

- *Structural defects of bronchi:* Bronchial atresia, Williams Campbell syndrome.
- *Abnormal mucociliary transport:* Kartagener syndrome.
- *Abnormal secretions:* Mucoviscidosis (cystic fibrosis).

B. Congenital/Acquired Immune Deficiency (usually IgG)

- Chronic granulomatous disease of childhood, Alpha 1- antitrypsin deficiency.

C. Post Infectious

Measles, whooping cough, Sawyer James syndrome, allergic bronchopulmonary aspergillosis, tuberculosis.

D. Bronchial Obstruction

Neoplasm, inflammatory nodes and foreign body.

E. Aspiration/Inhalation Gastric Contents/ Inhaled Fumes.

F. Pulmonary Fibrosis

Traction bronchiectasis due to increased elastic recoil with bronchial dilatation and mechanical distortion of bronchi by fibrosis.

Symptomatology

- Chronic cough with copious sputum production.
- Recurrent infections.
- Shortness of breath.
- Hemoptysis.

Location

Posterior basal segments of lower lobes (50%), middle lobe/lingual (10%), central bronchiectasis in bronchopulmonary aspergillosis.

Classification

- **Cylindrical/fusiform/tubular bronchiectasis:** Square abrupt ending with lumen of uniform diameter and same width as parent bronchus.
- **Varicose bronchiectasis:** Beaded contour with normal pattern distally.

- **Saccular/cystic bronchiectasis:** Progressive ballooning dilatation towards periphery with diameter > 1cm.

Imaging

Plain Ski Gram Chest

- Normal radiograph in 7%.
- Increase in size of lung markings (retained secretions).
- Loss of definitions of lung marks (peribronchial fibrosis).
- Crowding of lung markings (if associated with atelectasis).
- Cystic spaces with or without air fluid levels <2 cm in diameter.
- Honeycomb pattern in severe cases.
- Compensatory hyperinflation of uninvolved ipsilateral lung.

Bronchography

- Until recently bronchography was the definitive investigation for the diagnosis of bronchiectasis and for assessing the extent of the disease. HRCT has now largely replaced bronchography.
- Occasionally it is still used to evaluate recurrent hemoptysis when all other investigations are negative and to demonstrate bronchopleural fistulae and congenital lesions such as sequestrations and agenesis.
- Approaches include cricothyroid puncture, nasal or trans oral drip, and tracheal intubations under LA or GA.
- Physiotherapy before and after procedure and atropine to reduce the secretions are essential.
- Films taken include AP, lateral, oblique and if necessary tomograms. Delayed films demonstrate distal filling.
- All the bronchi should be surveyed for narrowing; occlusion; intraluminal filling defects and dilated mucosal glands.

HRCT

- HRCT combines the use of thinly collimated CT slices that are 1 to 2 mm in thickness with a high spatial frequency algorithm that enhances edge detection and a fast acquisition time.
- On many CT scanners the high resolution algorithm is a bone reconstruction algorithm.
- Thin collimation decreases partial volume averaging and improves the ability to demonstrate small pulmonary lesions.
- High spatial frequency algorithm by decreasing the amount of smoothening of the image data, enhances edge detection and makes lung structure look sharper.
- Field of view should be reduced to cover the lung parenchyma only.
- Confusions caused by crowded pulmonary vessels and dependent lung edema/atelectasis is minimized if the scans are obtained at suspended end respiratory volume.
- If necessary prone views differentiate focal dependent edema/atelectasis commonly seen in lung bases of normal patients from early pulmonary fibrosis.
- The reconstruction algorithm used in HRCT makes detection of mediastinal adenopathy and focal liver lesions difficult.
- High resolution algorithm also tends to accentuate pleural thickness an important factor to keep in mind when evaluating patients with asbestos exposure for pleural disease.

Appearances on HRCT

- Lack of tapering bronchi (in 80% of cases and is the most sensitive finding).
- Internal diameter of bronchus larger than adjacent pulmonary artery.
- Bronchi visible within 1cm of pleura.
- *Signet ring sign:* This is because each bronchus is accompanied by a pulmonary artery, the dilated bronchus seen in cross-

section forms the ring, the accompanying artery forms the signet of the ring.

- Railroad track/tram track is seen in cylindrical bronchiectasis and is when the dilated bronchus is sectioned longitudinally and the parallel thick wall gives the above appearance.
- String of pearls is seen in varicose bronchiectasis when areas of dilatation are seen alternating with areas of constrictions.
- Cluster of grapes appearance is seen in cystic bronchiectasis when dilated bronchi are grouped together.
- Air fluid levels owing to retained secretions or superimposed infections are commonly identified in the dependent areas of cystic ally dilated bronchi.
- Mucous plugs are identified by the branching tubular nature of the opacity and is due to inspissations of mucous.
- Bronchiectatic cyst (Figure 30.1) is recognized by its connection to dilated proximal bronchus. And in contrast to blebs or bullae these cysts demonstrate discrete and thickened walls and may be multiloculated.

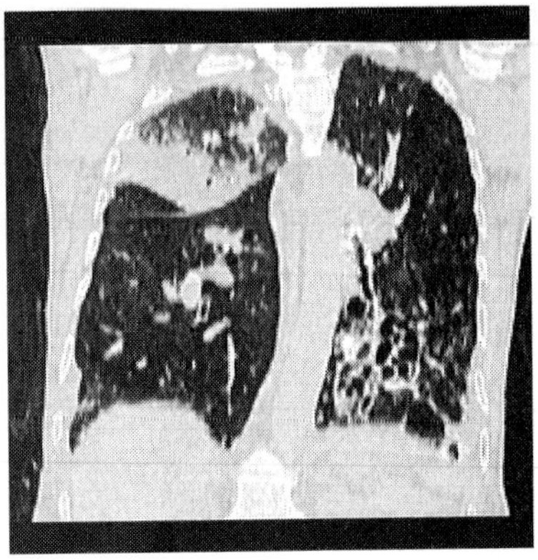

Fig. 30.1: Coronal MPR CT image shows cystic bronchiectasis in the lower lobe of the left lung with consolidation collapse in the right upper lobe

- In central bronchiectasis there is marked dilatation of proximal bronchi with relative sparing of more distal segments.

Bronchiectasis is more difficult to identify. The thickened peripheral bronchioles because of small size and short length may be mistaken for small nodules and if dilated may mimic small cavitating nodules.

Pneumoconiosis

- The term pneumoconiosis means dusty lungs. It is used to describe the non-neoplastic diseases of lungs due to inhaled dust particles. By definition, the term pneumoconiosis exclude asthma, bronchitis and emphysema.
- The characteristic and severity of the reactions of lung tissue are determined by following features:
  1. The nature of the dust.
  2. The duration and intensity of exposure.
  3. Time elapsed from initial exposure.
  4. Dust particle size and density (0.5-5μm most significant).
  5. Individual susceptibility.

CLASSIFICATION OF PNEUMOCONIOSIS

1. Due to dusts thought to be inert:

   Iron – siderosis

   Tin – Stannosis

   Barium – Baritosis

2. Due to dusts which cause interstitial fibrosis

   Beryllium – Berylliosis

   Aluminium – Aluminosis (Shaver's diseases)

   Asbestos – Asbestosis.

3. Due to dust causing reticulonodular dust deposits/and or fibrosis. May progress to massive fibrosis (PMF).

   Coal – Anthracosis, coal workers, pneumoconiosis (CWP)

   Silver – Silicosis

   Tale – Talecosis

   Kaolin – Kaolinosis

   Graphite – Graphitosis

RADIOGRAPHIC CLASSIFICATION OF PNEUMOCONIOSIS

Opacities due to dust inhalation.

Multiple small opacities upto 1 cm in diameter		Opacities larger than 1 cm in diameter
Small opacities definitely seen but few in number	Numerous small opacities with normal lung vasculature still visible	Very numerous opacities where the lung vasculature is partly or total obscured

Silicosis

- Amorphous
- Crystalline – quartz

Small size dust particles
↓
Deposition on alveolar wall
↓
Ingestion by macrophage
↓
Macrophage die
↓
Fibrosis

Chest Radiographs: Between 10 and 20 years exposure is usually necessary.

- Diffuse upper zone predominant nodular or reticulonodular infiltrates.
- Conglomeration of nodules in the upper lobes leading to PMF (it is defined as nodules greater than 1 cm in diameter).
- Development of emphysema with increasing fibrosis.
- Calcification in pulmonary nodules and hilar and mediastinal nodules.

Acute Silicoproteinosis

- Internal exposure to silver dust may result in lung damage after only weeks or months, so called acute scoliosis. In these cases, there is a marked cellular and exudative alveolar reaction and death may ensure within 2 to 3 years. The dominant feature is the presence of an alveolar proteinaceus exudate, hence the term "acute silico proteinous".

CXR

There is widespread alveolar shadowing that progress rapidly over a period of months.

- There is reasonable side to side symmetry but a tendency to central and upper zone is frequent.
- Air bronchogram and consolidation of the lungs (+).
- Peripheral air trapping, bulla formation, lung volume loss and distortion of mediastinal stroma all indicating fibrosis.
- Pneumothorax may occur.

COAL WORKERS PNEUMOCONIOSIS

Pathology

Excessive dust load
↓
Overwhelming of the clearance by the mucociliary excalator
↓
Fibroblasts lay down reticulin
↓
Coal macule
↓
Weakening the bronchiolar wall
↓
Proximal acini or focal emphysema

CXR

- Simple.
- Complicated form.
- Nodules appear in the upper 2/3rd of the lungs.
- A reticular pattern may be seen either in combination with the nodules or in isolation and septal (Kelley) lines may be seen.
- Typically PMF starts as a mass near the periphery of the lungs. The shape varies.
- It may be round or oval with lobular or irregular edges.
- There is often a well-defined lateral border that parallels the lateral chest wall. The medial border is frequently ill-defined. The depth of the mass is less than the side-to-side diameters

(lens shaped). It is usually bilateral and accompanied by widespread modulation in the remainder of the lung.

- If PMF is unilateral then the differential diagnosis is bronchial carcinoma.

1. PMF

   Lens shaped density in an upper lobe close to and parallel to the major fissure and has a well defined outer margin paralleling the chest wall.

2. PMF–Small irregular calcification.
3. PMF–It may cavitate.
4. MRI–Lung cancer, high signal intensity area on both T1W and T2W sequence.

   PMF–Low intensity.

5. PMF–Rate of growth takes year carcinoma–in diameter taking months.
6. PMF–Migrate towards the hilum, slowly taking 10 or more years to reach the hilum severe emphysema accompanies such migration.

CT IN THE EVALUATION OF SILICOSIS AND COPD

Micro nodules–Nodules upto 7 mm in diameters.

Nodules–Lesion 7 and 20 mm in size.

PMF–Lesions greater than 20 mm in size.

The findings on standard CT and HRCT are as follows:

1. *Centrilobular micro nodules – Micro nodules in a centrilobular location are the earliest features of silicon and CWP*
   - In silicosis the modules correspond to the periadventitial silicotic nodules and in CWP pneumoconiosis they correspond to the coal macule.
   - The lesions show a distinct tendency to involve the upper lung zones and posterior aspect of the lungs.
   - As the disease evolves, there is spread anteriorly and inferiorly.
2. *Subpleural micronodules and subpleural plaque formation*
   - Small nodules may be visualized on the pleural margin of the lung, particularly posteriorly and laterally.
   - Confluence of these nodules may lead to linear narrow subpleural densities or plaques.
3. *Nodular*

   Growth of the micronodules to exceed 7 mm in diameter occurs in the evolution of silicosis and CWP.
   - The nodules are set on a background of centrilobular and sub pleural micro nodulation and they are likely to be subpleural plaques.
4. *Emphysema*
   - It appears to be common with silicosis and CWP.
   - The deterioration of pulmonary formation correlate with the severity of the associated emphysema.
   - The emphysema may be centrilobular, panacinar or bulbous.
5. *Progressive massive fibrosis*
   - Growth and coalescence of nodule results in PMF, which usually develops in the periphery of the upper and posterior lung zones, and show a distinct tendency to central contractions towards the hilar regions with further growth of the nodules.
   - PMF may be rounded in contour but ovoid masses are more usual.
   - The outer margin of PMF often parallels the contour of he adjacent chest wall.
   - Large lesions (5 cm or greater in a diameter) often show irregular low attenuating regions indicative of vascular necrosis and cavitation may occur.

- Lesions may show irregular punctate calcification.

6. *Diffuse interstitial pulmonary fibrosis:* This leads to honey combing, may develop in silicosis and CWP.
7. *Lymphadenopathy and lymph node calcification*
   - Enlargement of the hilar and mediastinal nodes is a regular feature of silicosis and CWP.
   - Necrosis frequently occurs in the nodules and eggshell calcification is a characteristic finding.

ASBESTOS RELATED DISEASES

- Asbestos is composed of a group of fibrous silicates with differing chemical and physical properties but with the notable common property of heat resistance.

Fibrous Type	
• Serpentine • Long curly fibers composed of fibrillary nutrients e.g. chrysolite	• Amphibole • Straights shorter needle like fibers e.g. crocidite, amosite, anthrophyllite • Much greater fibrogenic and carcinogenic potential.

DELETERIOUS EFFECTS OF ASBESTOS EXPOSURE

1. Benign asbestos related pleural effusion.
2. Diffuse pleural thickening.
3. Pleural plaque formation.
4. Rounded atelectasis.
5. Asbestosis.
6. Malignancies
   - Lung cancer and other epi malignancies; Larynx and GIT.
   - Mesothelioma.
   - Pleural.
   - Peritoneal.
   - Pericardial.

Benign Asbestos Pleural Effusion

- Usually occurs within 10 years of initial exposure.
- Unilateral or bilateral.
- Often-asymptomatic otherwise fever, pleuritic chest pain or dyspnea.
- Usually small but may be >500 ml.
- Fluid exudative, often blood tinged.
- Usually resolve completely but may leave diffuse pleural thickening.

Pleural Thickening and Calcification Related to Asbestos Exposure

- Pleural plaques are identified more than 20 or 30 years after the initial asbestos exposure.
- Asbestos induced pleural plaques occur on the parietal pleura, esp. over the diaphragm and along the posterolateral chest wall. The apices, the costophrenic sulci and the mediastinal surfaces tend to be spared.
- The plaques are composed of hyalinzed fibrous tissue and frequently lie beneath the ribs.
- There is evidence that the widely used, more benign form of asbestos, chryoslite, is particularly associated with this transpleural migration while the more fibrogenic and carcinogenic amphiboles, crocidolite and amosite, tend to get held up in the lung parenchyma.
- On radiographic examinations, pleural plaques are irregular smooth elevations of the pleural most easily identified in profile along the margins of the lungs or over the diaphragm.
- Plaques seen on face are relatively flat in relation to their width and the density of the shadow projected over the lungs is therefore

less then could be expected for a parenchymal lesion of equivalent size.

- Furthermore, one margin of the lesion is likely to the indistinct as it smooth off into normal pleura.
- Plaques are multiple and there is reasonable side-to-side symmetry.

Asbestosis

- Pulmonary fibrosis related to asbestos exposure.
- A late result 30-40 years after initial exposure.

CXR

- Pulmonary fibrosis with basal and subpleural predominance.
- Coarse fibrous bands extending into the lung from the pleural surface.
- Benign asbestos related pleural changes and rounded atelectasis might be present.

CT (Figure 31.1)

- Ground glass density.
- Interlobular septal thickening and sub pleural modulation.
- Interlobular peribronchiolar thickening.

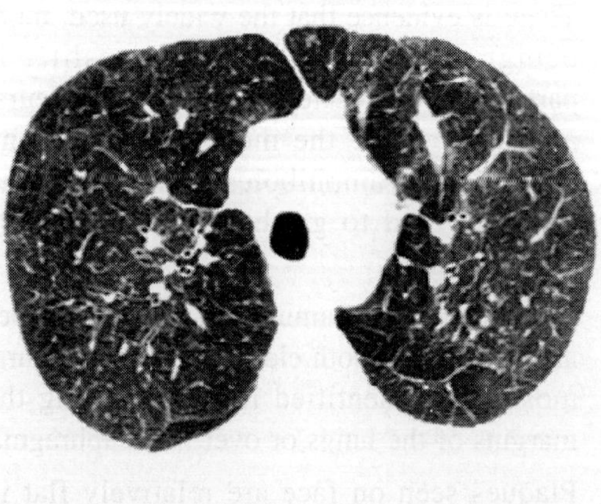

Fig. 31.1: Axial CT section of chest showing features of pneumoconiosis with paraseptal thickening

- Curvilinear line density paralleling the chest wall in sub pleural location.
- Coarse parenchymal bands of fibrous tissue extending into lung from the pleural surface.
- Honeycombing.
- Mediastinal adenopathy.
- Benign asbestos related pleural changes and rounded atelectasis might be present.

Berylliosis

- Causative agent – elemental beryllium.
- Use of beryllium – high-grade alloys (formerly used in the fluorescent light industry).
- Exposure – in the processing of pure beryllium.
- Effects of high intensity acute expose – acute trachobronchitis and pulmonary edema, possibly leading to death but may remove with variable long-term lung fibrosis.
- Effect of chronic exposure berylliosis
  - Hilar adenopathy.
  - Granulomatous pulmonary infiltration leading to fibrosis bulla formation and cor-pulmonale.
- Calcification is linear when seen on foci, the appearance in variable, and the most common type being "holly leaf calcification".
- Extensive pleural calcification in association with parenchymal fibrosis may be lace like.
- Enlargement and spreading of plaques results in thick irregular sheets of pleural thickening, which are often calcified.
- Pleural plaques do occur on the visceral pleural esp. in association with parenchymal fibrosis.
- Asbestos exposure has been associated with pericardial fibrosis and calcification.

D/D of Pleural Plaques

- Extra pleural fat deposition in obesity.
- Extra pleural thickening in relation to multiple rib fracture.

- Post inflammatory pleural thickening.
- Pleural metastases.
- Overprotected densities representing unusually prominent costal insertions of the serratus anterior muscle.

Rounded Atelectasis

Synonyms – Folded lung, atelectatic pseudo tumor.

Causes – Asbestos-related pleural fibrosis (70%).

T.A. pleuritis or any non-specific pleuritis Drasslers syndrome or chronic heart failure.

Radiographic Features

- Intra parenchymal mass.
- Juxtrapleural location.
- Subjacent pleural thickening.
- Convergence of broncho vascular bundles into the mass – "parachute cords", "comet tail" or "helical effect".
- Common location – posterior and basal.
- Single or multiple.
- Homogenous enhancement with CT.
- Indistinct margin towards hilum with CT.
- Ultrasound may identify a linear echogenic structure in the mass.
- Granulomatous skin rashes.
- Granulomatous infiltration of the liver and spleen
  - Hypercalcemia.
  - Nephrolithiasis.

Section 3—Respiratory System

Chapter 32

Interstitial Lung Disease

INTERSTITIUM

Concepts of Radiologic Anatomy

- It consists of continuum of connective tissue that provides support to the lung divided into three compartments:
  - Bronchoarterial interstitium.

    Is the sheath around the bronchovascular bundles extended from the hila to the lung periphery, as far out as the alveolar ducts and sacs.
  - Peripheral or subpleural interstitium.

    Surrounds the surface of the lung beneath the visceral pleural and penetrates the lung to surround the secondary pulmonary lobules.
  - Septal or parenchymal interstitium.

    Is the finer network of connective tissue fibres within the lobules and support the alveoli.

A. RETICULAR PATTERN

- Caused by thickening of interlobular septa due to infiltration by:
  1. Fibrosis–fibrosing alveolitis (FA).
  2. Abnormal cells–lymph carcinoma.
  3. Fluid– alveolar proteinosis (AP).
- Types
  1. Smooth – Pulmonary edema and A.P.
  2. Irregular – Pulmonary fibrosis.
  3. Beaded – Lymph carcinoma.
- Variety

  Fine
  - Early pulmonary fibrosis.
  - Cryptogenic fibrosing alveolitis (IPF).

  Course – End stage lung.

B. NODULAR PATTERN

- Are discrete opacities 2-10 mm in diameters.
- Nodular thickening of bronchovascular interstitium.

↓

Irregular: Interface between margins of bronchovascular (BV) bundles and the surrounding lung parenchyma

↓

Interface sign

- BV distribution of nodules

↓

Classic of sarcoidosis

- Miliary nodulation 3-7 mm
  1. TB.
  2. Pneumoconiosis.
  3. Pulmonary metastasis.
  4. Fungal.
  5. Talcosis.
  6. Mets of bronchoalveolar carcinoma.

C. GROUND GLASS OPACITY AND INCREASED LUNG DENSITY

Hazy increase in lung density without obscuration of vascular markings–GGO.

Black bronchus sign GGO makes airways more obvious.

Seen in:

• CCF	• Pulm. edema
• Pneumatosis carini pneumoconiosis	• Extrinsic allergic alveolitis
• Pulmonary hemorrhage	• Wilson Mikity syndrome
• ARDS	• Desqamative interstitial pneumonia
• Sarcoidosis	• Eosinophilic pneumonia
• Lymphoid Interstitial pneumonia	• Broncholitis obliterans organizing pneumonia (BOOP)

D. CYSTIC AIR SPACE

- Clearly defined air containing space with a definable wall.
- Seen in
  - Lymphangioleiomyomatosis (LLMM).
  - Histiocytosis –z.
  - End stage fibrosing alveolitis.
  - Pneumatosis, carini pneumoconiosis.
  - Lymphoid interstitial pneumonia associated with Sjögren's syndrome.
  - Advanced tracheo bronchial papillomatosis.
  - Tuberous sclerosis.
  - TB.
  - Systemic sclerosis.
  - Cystic bronchiectasis.
  - Mounier Kuhn syndrome.

Common Indications for HRCT – Suggested Protocols

A. *Obvious ILD /Abnormal CX-R*

Inspiratory supine narrow sections at 10-20 mm interval.

B. *Suspected ILD/Normal or Near Normal CXR*

Inspiratory supine marrow sections at 10-20 mm in with inter spaced (3 or 4 cm) prone sections.

Additional Imaging

Expiratory Sections (3-4 cm interval) for suspected sub acute extrinsic allergic alveolitis.

C. *Suspected or Obvious Airways Diseases*

Inspiratory supine narrow sections at 10 mm intervals only.

Additional Imaging

Expiratory Sections (at 23 cm interval 1 for suspected small airways do).

Marrow window settings for emphysema.

Clinical Approach to a Patient with ILD

1. Age and sex of the patient

LLMM	Asbestosis and CWP
↓	↓
Male	Female

Chapter 32

2. History of known underlying disease like – malignancy with chemotherapy/radiology.
   - Lymphoid carcinoma
   - Pulmonary injury
   - Opportunistic infections.
   - AIDS.
3. Drug history.

   Methotrexate.

   Bleomycin – Basilar ILD.
4. IV Drug abuser.

   Septic emboli talcosis AIDS related injury.

DISTRIBUTION OF DISEASE

Subacute extrinsic alveolar alveolitis	Mild and lower zones on X-ray diffuse involvement on CT
Fibrosing alveolitis	Lower zone and sub pleural distribution ↓ Pathognomonic of disease
UIP and DIP predominant	Lower zone and peripheral
Histiocytosis × Aspiration pneumonitis	Upper and mid zone Basal location
Sarcoiosis and lymphoid carcinoma	Bronchocentric distribution

INDICATIONS FOR HRCT

- To diagnose diffuse lung disease with normal or near normal chest.
- To narrow DD's or make a histospecific diagnosis in patients with obvious but nonspecific radio abnormalities.
- To investigate patients with unexplained severe Chronic Obstructive Airways Disease.
- To investigate patients presenting with hemoptysis.
- To evaluate disease reversibility, especially fibrosing alveolitis.
- To guide the type and site of lung biopsy.

CLASSIFICATION OF ILD'S (Figure 32.1)

- Chronic interstitial pneumonias
  – UIP (Usual interstitial pneumonia).
  – DIP (Desquamative interstitial pneumonia).
  – BOOP (Broncolitis obliterans organizing pneumonia).
- Granulomatous lung diseases.
  – Sarcoidosis.
  – Extrinsic allergic alveolitis.
- Neoplastic or proliferative diseases.
  – Lymphangitis carcinomatosis.
  – Lymphoma.
  – LIP.
  – Histiocytosis.

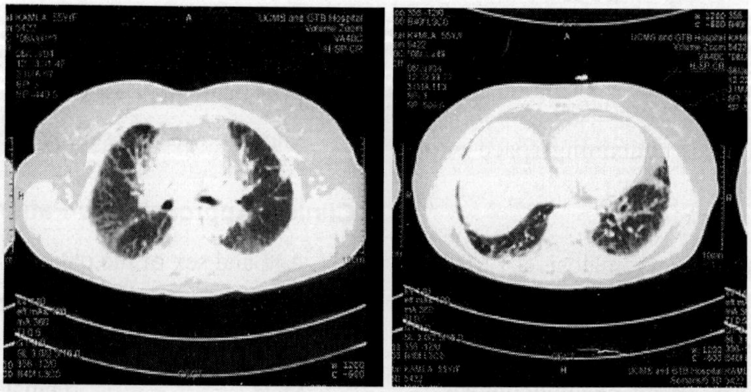

Fig. 32.1: Axial CT images show features of the interstitial lung disease

- Occupational lung diseases
  - Asbestosis.
  - Silicosis.
  - Coal workers pneumoconiosis.

SALIENT FEATURES OF COMMON ILD'S

UIP

- Patients usually have Interstitial Pulmonary Fibrosis (ILF) (Figure 32.2) and also associated with:
- Asbestosis.
- Collagen vascular disease
  - Rheumatoid arthritis.
  - Systemic sclerosis.
- Reticular opacities – subpleural regions of lung bases.
  - Fine.
  - Coarse.
- Basal and peripheral predominance.
- GGO.
- Honeycombing – late stages.

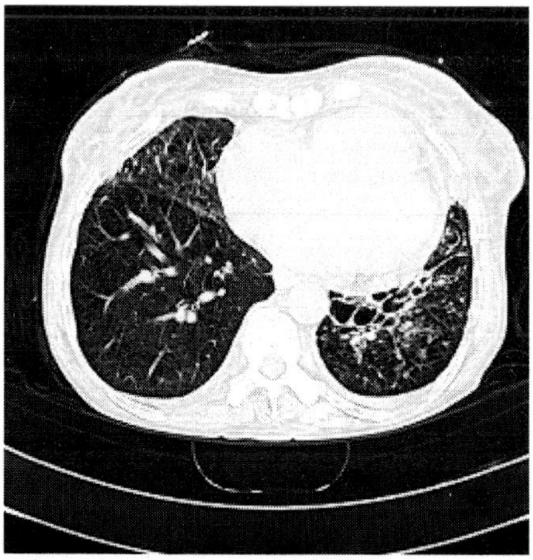

Fig. 32.2: Axial CT image shows honey comb cysts in the left lung base in case of idiopathic pulmonary fibrosis

DIP

- Represents the early stage of same disease process as of UIP-Imaging features:
  - Ground glass opacity with basal and peripheral predominance, cysts±. Combination of cysts and ground glass opacities suggests the diagnosis.
- Late stages–features suggestive of fibrosis and honeycombing:
  - Extensive parenchymal abnormalities.

Boop

- May be seen in:
  - Viral and bact. pneumonias.
  - EAA.
  - Chronic eosinophilic pneumonia.
  - Collagen vascular disease.
  - Idiopathic.
- Usually bilateral air space consolidation – patchy and asymmetric.
- Small nodular opacities.
- Sub pleural peripheral (may be migratory) distribution is evident.

Sarcoidosis

- Sarcoid granulomas – Hallmark.
- Mid and upper lobe predominance is an important distinguishing feature.
- 3 stages:

Stage I AP-Symmetrical, bilateral hilar and right paratracheal nodal calcification is seen in late stages.

II LAP + parenchymal opacity/ masses, pleural thicking.

III Parenchymal opacity
GGO nodules
Alveolar sarcoid.

Nodules are irregularly marginated (1-10 mm in size) and are typically

Chapter 32

found along bronchovascular bundles, interlobar septa and pleural surfices. Features suggestive of irreversible fibrosis e.g. cysts, nonseptal lines, traction bronchiectasis and architectural distortion is evident in advance stage of the disease.

- Cx fibrotic stage
  - Corpulmonale.
  - Mycetoma.
  - Pneumothorax.

Extrinsic Allergic Alveolitis (EAA)

- Hypersensitivity of the disease of lungs are due to inhalation of antigen.

Acute	Sub acute	Chronic
↓ Consolidation –diffuse and bilateral	↓ GGO-diffuse, bilateral with poorly diffused centrilobular nodules in mid and lower zones, focal areas of decreased attenuation is common associated findings.	↓ Fibrosis-predominantly in mid and lower zones.

LYMPHANGITIS CARCINOMATOSA

- Breast, lung, stomach and colon.
- Beaded uneven thickening of IL septa.

HISTIOCYTOSIS –X

Small nodules (<5 mm)	and	Cystic air spaces
Usually solid or sometimes small cavities within the infiltrates		↓ <10 mm in diameter
↓ Early stage		↓ Late stage of disease

Upper 2/3rd of lungs in predominantly.

LYMPHANGIO LEIOMYOMATOSIS (LLMM)

- Exclusively in females.
- Irregular opacities.
- Honeycombing over inflation.
- Recurrent pneumothoraces.
- Chylous pleural effusions.
- Cysts 2-5 cms.
- Diffuse lung involvement.

Miliary Shadowing of the Lungs

A miliary nodule is a pattern of small discrete nodules seen on chest radiograph. Miliary nodules are usually widespread in distribution and approximately equal in size. A miliary pattern has been described by the Fleischner Society Nomenclature Committee as consisting of nodules measuring 2 mm or less in diameter, but this criterion is arbitrary. The term micronodules or small nodules are usually used in describing similar HRCT findings.

Alveolar Microlithiasis

- Very rare disease of unknown etiology characterized by myriad of calcospherites or tiny calculi within alveoli.
- Striking discrepancy between striking radiographic findings and mild clinical symptoms.
- Very fine, sharply defined, sand like micronodulations (<1 mm).
- Diffuse involvement of both lungs.
- Intense uptake on bone scan.

Berylliosis

- Chronic granulomatous disorder as a result of beryllium specific cell-mediated immune response (delayed hypersensitivity reaction after exposure to acid salts of beryllium oxide) in fluorescent lamp factory workers.
- Latent period 5-15 years.
- Fine nodularity, alongwith irregular opacities, particularly sparing the apices and bases.
- Hilar and mediastinal adenopathy that may calcify.
- Emphysema in upper lobes with interstitial fibrosis.
- Pneumothorax in 10%.
- Bronchial wall thickening and pleural irregularities.

Broncholitis Obliterans (Constrictive Bronchiolitis)

- It is characterized by inflammation of bronchioles leading to obstruction of bronchiolar lumen.
- *Causes:* Toxic fumes, infections, drugs, connective tissue disorders, etc.
- Peak age is 40 to 50 years.
- Mosaic perfusion of lobular air trapping.
- Areas of decreased attenuation with vascular attenuation.
- Bronchial wall thickening and bronchiectatic changes.
- Tree in bud appearance of bronchioles.

Coal Worker's Pneumoconiosis

- Latent period of 10 years.
- Poor correlation between symptoms, physiologic findings and radiographic findings.
- Small round 1-5 mm opacities, frequently in the upper lobes.
- Nodularity correlates with the amount of collagen and not the amount of coal dust.
- No progression is seen in absence of further exposure.

Extrinsic Allergic Alveolitis (Hypersensitivity Pneumonitis)

- Characterised by inappropriate host response to inhaled organic allergens that are often related to patient's occupation.
- Markedly increased cell count with often >50% T-lymphocytes on bronchoalveolar lavage.
- Predominantly mid zonal involvement.
- Poorly defined centrilobular micronodules <5 mm.
- Widespread patchy ground-glass attenuation in >50%.
- Areas of decreased attenuation and mosaic perfusion.
- In chronic stages, irregular linear opacities, loss of lung volume and adenopathy may occur.

Histoplasmosis

- It is caused by inhalation of wind-borne spores which germinate within alveoli releasing yeast forms that are phagocytosed but not killed by macrophages; invasion of pulmonary lymphatics with spread to hilar and mediastinal nodes; hematogenous dissemination of parasitized macrophages throughout the RES.
- Miliary pattern is seen in disseminated histoplasmosis which rapidly progresses to diffuse airspace consolidation.
- There is associated hilar and mediastinal adenopathy and hepatosplenomegaly.

Langerhan's Cell Histiocytosis

- It is multisystem disorder characterized by granuloma formation containing Langerhan's cell.
- Ill-defined nodules, complex or branching thin-walled multiple cysts <5 mm equally distributed in central and peripheral lung zones and sub pleural blebs with intervening normal lung.
- Manifestations can also be noted in skin, bone, lymph nodes, brain, etc.

Lymphoma

- Parenchymal shadowing is seen in 20-30% during disease duration, most commonly nodular sclerosing type in HD; invariably subsequent to hilar adenopathy.
- Besides miliary nodulation, coarse reticulo-nodular pattern, subpleural nodules and massive pneumonic forms may also be seen.

Miliary Tuberculosis (Figure 33.1)

- It results from massive hematogenous dissemination of organisms anytime after the primary infection.
- Seen in 2-3% of the TB infections.
- Chronic focus is often not identifiable.
- Radiographically recognizable after 6 weeks post hematogenous dissemination.
- HRCT allows earlier detection.
- Associated necrotic mediastinal lymphadenopathy may be seen.

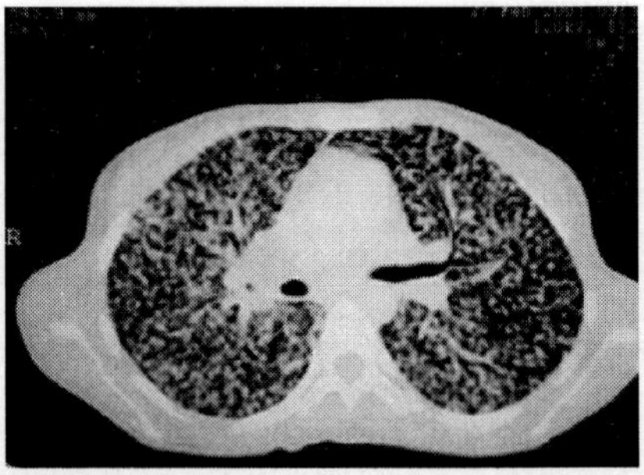

Fig. 33.1: Axial CT section showing milliary infiltrates in patient with pulmonary Kochs

Mycoplasma Pneumonia (Primary Atypical Pneumonia)

- Most common cause of nonbacterial pneumonia with a mild course usually lasts for 2-3 weeks and only 10% of the infected subjects develop pneumonia.
- Radiological findings often diverge from the clinical findings.
- Pulmonary infiltrates show a significant lag time.
- Fine miliary nodulation from hilum into the lower lobe is the earliest change.
- Left side is more commonly involved and the pattern is bilateral in 10-40%.
- Small pleural effusions is seen in 20%.

Nocardiosis

- It is commonly seen in the immunocompromised.
- Miliary nodules are seen with or without cavitation.
- Associated lobar consolidation.
- Empyema formation without sinus formation.
- Rarely SVC obstruction.

Respiratory Distress Syndrome of the Newborn (Hyaline Membrane Disease)

- It is an acute pulmonary disorder characterized by generalized atelectasis, intrapulmonary shunting, ventilation perfusion abnormalities and reduced pulmonary compliance due to immature surfactant production.
- Hypoaeration with loss of lung volumes.
- Pulmonary shadowing coincides with the onset of clinical disease. Prominent air bronchograms.
- The condition is bilateral and symmetrical in distribution.
- Spontaneous clearing is seen within 7-10 days (mild course in untreated survivors).

Sarcoidosis

- Immunologically mediated multisystem granulomatous disease of unknown etiology with variable presentation, progression and prognosis.
- Peak incidence 20-40 years and female outnumbers the males (M:F=1:3).
- Parenchymal disease is seen in 60% without adenopathy in 16-20%.
- There is predominantly midzone involvement.
- On HRCT, there is irregular septal thickening, perilymphatic, nodules, traction bronchiectasis, ground glass opacity, honeycombing and irregular/nodular bronchial wall thickening.

Siderosis

- It results from inhalation of inert iron oxide or metallic iron deposits.
- Occupational exposure is seen in workers involved in arc welding, cutting / burning of steel, foundry, grinders, felters, polishers.
- Miliary or reticulonodular pattern is seen which may disappear when the exposure is discontinued.
- No secondary fibrosis or hilar adenopathy is seen unless mixed dust inhalation as in siderosilicosis.

Silicosis

- It results from inhalation of silicon dioxide; most prevalent silicosis of progressive nature after termination of the exposure.
- At least 10-20 years of dust exposure is required before appearance of radiographic abnormality.
- Miliary nodulation begin in the upper and mid zones, which may calcify in 5-10%.
- Associated hilar adenopathy is seen, that may calcify in 5% (eggshell pattern).

- On HRCT, besides, micronodules, there is thickening of intra and interlobular lines, subpleural lines, ground glass pattern, parenchymal fibrous bands, pleural based nodular irregularities, traction bronchiectasis and honeycombing.

Viral Pneumonia

- Rhinovirus, RSV, parainfluenza and adenovirus are commonly implicated.
- There is hyperaeration with air trapping.
- There is peribronchial cuffing and perihilar linear densities.
- Interstitial or airspace pattern or both may be seen.
- Pleural effusion seen in 20%, hilar adenopathy in 3%.
- Radiographic resolution lags 2-3 weeks behind clinical resolution

Carcinoma Lung

Most frequent cause of deaths in males (35% of all cancer deaths) and females (21 % of all cancer deaths).

TWO TYPES

1. Bronchogenic carcinoma.
2. Alveolar cell carcinoma.

Bronchogenic Carcinoma (Figures 34.1 and 34.2)

- Age at diagnosis 55-60 years.
- Asymptomatic especially with peripheral tumors however they may present with pleuritic or local chest pain, pan coast syndrome, SVC syndrome and hoarseness.
- Central tumors present with symptoms of cough, hemoptysis, pneumonia.
- May also present with symptoms of metastatic disease.
- Paraneoplastic syndromes:
  a. Cachexia of malignancy.
  b. Clubbing and hypertrophic osteoarthropathy.
  c. Non-bacterial thrombotic endocarditis.

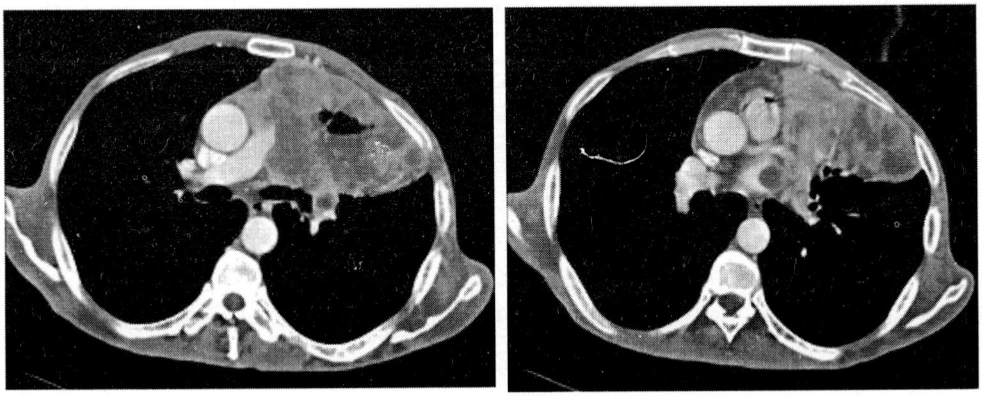

Fig. 34.1: Axial CT images show carcinoma bronchus with necrosis with pulmonary artery and pericardial invasion

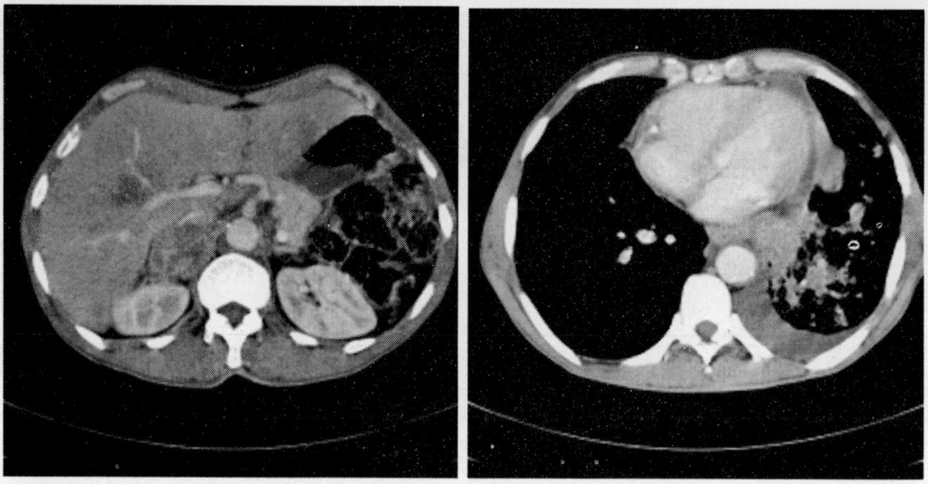

Fig. 34.2: Axial CT images show adrenal metastases on right side in a case of carcinoma bronchus

d. Migratory thrombophlebitis.

e. Ectopic hormone production as hypercalcemia, SIADH.

Cushing's syndrome, gynecomastia, acromegaly.

Pathological Types

Adenocarcinoma (50%): It is the most common type seen in women and non-smokers. Has intermediate malignant potential i.e. slow growth but with usually high incidence of metastases.

- Solitary peripheral subpleural mass or less commonly multiple nodules.
- May invade pleura or grow circumferentially mimicking malignant mesothelioma.
- Upper lobe distribution is most common.
- Rarely calcifications may be seen in the periphery of the mass.

Squamous cell carcinoma or epidermoid carcinoma (30-35%): Strongly associated with cigarette smoking and central necrosis is common. Slowest growth rate with lowest incidence of distant, metastases. It is the most common type that is diagnosed as radiologically occult.

- Hypercalcemia is common from tumor elaborated parathyroid like substance.
- Central location within main/lobar/segmental bronchus.
- Large central mass with or without calcification.
- Characteristic cavitation. Squamous cell carcinoma is the most common cell type to cavitate.
- Invasion of the chest wall and it is the most common cell type to cause pan coast tumor.

Small cell undifferentiated carcinoma (15%): Strongly associated with cigarette smoking. It has rapid growth and high malignant potential and presents with early metastases. Should be regarded as systemic disease irrespective of stage at diagnosis and is virtually never resectable.

- Typically large central hilar or perihilar mass often associated with mediastinal widening from adenopathy.
- Extensive necrosis and hemorrhage.
- Most common lung cancer causing SVC obstruction.
- Paraneoplastic syndromes include Cushing's syndrome and SIADH.

Undifferentiated large cell carcinoma (<5%): Strongly associated with cigarette smoking and has an intermediate malignant potential and rapid growth with early distant metastases.

- Large bulky usually peripheral mass.
- Large areas of necrosis.
- Pleural involvement.

Scar carcinoma: 7% of lung tumors is related to scars produced secondarily to lung infarcts or more commonly tuberculosis.

- Mostly adenocarcinoma (72%) or less commonly squamous cell carcinoma (18%).
- Tumor grows in the scar and subsequently engulfs it.
- Calcification is common.
- Location is most commonly upper lobes and 45% of all peripheral tumors originate in scars.

Radiological Presentation of Bronchogenic Carcinoma

- Solitary peripheral mass with corona radiata/ pleural tail sign/satellite lesion.
- Cavitation (16%) usually thick walled with irregular inner surface usually in squamous cell carcinoma.
- Central mass (38%) common in small cell carcinoma.
- Unilateral hilar enlargement (secondary to primary tumor/enlarged nodes).
- Anterior and middle mediastinal widening common in small cell carcinoma.
- Segmental, lobar, lung atelectasis (37%) secondary to airway obstruction (particularly in squamous cell).
- "S sign of Golden" seen on plain X-ray chest is incomplete lobar collapse with bulging contour and is produced by primary central tumor.
- Rat-tail termination of bronchus.
- Bronchial cuff sign is focal or circumferential thickening of bronchial wall imaged end-on.
- Local hyper aeration due to local check-valve type endobronchial obstruction, best seen on expiratory views.
- Persistent peripheral infiltrates secondary to post obstructive pneumonitis.
- No air bronchogram in consolidations produced distal to an obstructing endo bronchial growth.
- Pleural effusions seen should be treated as malignant unless proved otherwise.
- Bone erosions of ribs and spine.
- Involvement of MPA, lobar and segmental arteries may result in additional peripheral radio opacity secondary to lung infarcts.
- Calcification is seen in 7% on CT and 14% Histologically and is usually eccentric and finely stippled.

  a. Pre-existing focus of calcium engulfed by tumor.

  b. Dystrophic calcium within tumor necrosis.

  c. Calcium deposit from secretory function of carcinoma.

  (e.g. Mucinous adenocarcinoma).

- *Angio:* The bronchogenic carcinoma is supplied by bronchial circulation. Distortion, stenosis and occlusion of pulmonary arterial circulation may be seen.

Location: 60-80% arise in segmental bronchi.

- Central small cell and squamous cell carcinoma (sputum cytology positive in 70%), arises in central airways often at points of bronchial bifurcation, infiltrates circumferentially and extends along bronchial tree.
- *Peripheral:* Adeno and large cell carcinoma.
- Upper lobe lower lobe and right lung left lung ratio is 3:2.
- Most common site is anterior segment of RUL.

TNM Staging

TX Tumor proved by the presence of malignant cells, in bronchopulmonary secretions but

34 Chapter

not visualized radiologically or bronchoscopically.

TO	No evidence of primary tumor.
TIs	Carcinoma in situ.
T1	A tumor that is 3 cm or less in greatest dimension surrounded by lung or visceral pleura.
T2	A tumor more than 3 cm in greatest dimension or a tumor of any size that either invades the visceral pleura or has associated atelectasis or pneumonitis and is at least 2 cm distal to the carina.
T3	A tumor of any size with direct extension to the chest wall (including superior sulcus tumor), diaphragm, mediastinal pleura or pericardium without involving the heart and great vessels, trachea, esophagus or vertebral body or a tumor in main bronchus within 2 cm of carina.
T4	A tumor of any size with invasion of mediastinum involving the heart great vessels, trachea, esophagus, vertebral body or carina or presence of malignant pleural effusion.
NO	No nodal metastases.
NI	metastases to nodes in the peribronchial or the ipsilateral hilar region or both including direct extension.
N2	Metastases to ipsilateral mediastinal nodes and subcarinal nodes.
N3	Metastases to contralateral mediastinal nodes, contralateral hilar nodes, ipsilateral or contralateral scalene or supraclavicular nodes.
MO	No known distant metastases.
MI	Distant metastasis present.

Pan coast tumor; superior pulmonary sulcus tumor most commonly squamous cell.

- Atrophy of muscles of ipsilateral upper extremity due to brachial plexus involvement.
- Horner syndrome (enopthalmos, miosis, ptosis, anhidrosis) due to sympathetic chain involvement.
- Apical pleural mass or thickening ± soft tissue invasion or bone destruction.

3 Section

Pediatric Pulmonary Tumors

Most lung tumors that occur in childhood are metastatic. Primary malignant tumors of the lung, which include blastoma, mucoepidermoid carcinoma, bronchogenic carcinoma, hemangiopericytoma, and rhabdomyosarcoma, are extremely rare. The most common of these is pulmonary blastoma.

METASTASES

- It is the most common lung neoplasm.
- The incidence of pulmonary metastases varies with the primary tumor and the stage of the disease.
- The most common source of pediatric pulmonary metastases include rhabdomyosarcoma, osteosarcoma, Wilm's tumor, Ewing's sarcoma and testicular tumors are choriocarcinoma.
- Pulmonary metastases may result from spread by direct extension or seeding of body cavities such as the pleura. However, true metastasis to the lung occurs by one or more of three pathways hematogenous, lymphatic, and endobronchial. Hematogenous spread is the most common pathway.
- The hallmark of hematogenous pulmonary metastases is one or more pulmonary nodule predominantly distributed in the periphery of the lungs, most lying in close proximity to the pleura. The lung bases are more frequently involved than the apices. The pulmonary nodules vary in size from 12mm to many cm in diameter. They are usually multiple, distributed in both lungs and have well defined outlines. Occasionally, they show very irregular margins usually attributable to hemorrhage around the periphery of the metastatic nodules. Sometimes cavitation may occur. The thickness of the wall is variable and some cavitated nodules may have strikingly thin walls mimicking lung cysts. Occasionally, pneumothorax may be associated with cavitation of a subpleural metastatic nodule, particularly in osteosarcoma.
- Calcification in pulmonary metastases is very unusual except in metastases from sarcoma, particularly osteosarcoma, in which it is relatively common. Dystrophic calcification may be seen in areas of necrosis after therapy. Miliary nodulation resembling miliary tuberculosis is occasionally encountered. A minority of pulmonary metastases present as a solitary pulmonary nodule.
- CT is the most sensitive imaging technique available for the detection of pulmonary metastases. However, CT findings are

nonspecific. Granuloma and subpleural pulmonary lymph nodes can be indistinguishable from metastases. Volumetric acquisition using spiral CT scanning with overlapping reconstruction improves the detection of small lung nodules.

- After chemotherapy, many metastases decrease in size or completely resolve. However, some metastases after initial response to therapy become stable in size. Such nodules may only contain necrotic or fibrous tissue without viable tumor.

BLASTOMA

- It is an extremely rare lung tumor in children.
- It represents 0.5% of all primary malignant tumors of the lung and 25% present in childhood.
- Clinical presentation is variable, often presenting as respiratory tract infection or a pleural effusion.
- These are solitary masses located peripherally in the lung. As a result, they do not cause early symptoms and are frequently very large at presentation, occupying an entire lobe or hemithorax.
- The rare association of this tumor with Wilm's tumor and nephroblastomatosis has been described.
- It is a highly malignant neoplasm and often arises in pre-existing cystic lung disease.
- On chest radiograph, a mass lesion and pleural effusion are the most frequent findings, confirmed on CT, which may in addition show infiltration into the lung and chest wall. Calcification is uncommon. Definitive diagnosis is by biopsy.
- US of the thorax are helpful in distinguishing a massive pleural effusion from a complex echogenic mass occupying an entire hemithorax.

MUCOEPIDERMOID CARCINOMA

- It is an uncommon tracheobronchial neoplasm.
- The lesion occurs in two forms:
  - A tumor of relatively low grade malignancy with distinctive histological features, and a benign clinical course.
  - A neoplasm showing histological features of high-grade malignancy and an aggressive course.
- The majority of tumors are situated in the main or lobar bronchi; only rarely do they involve the trachea, and then usually in a supracranial location. Most grow within the airway lumen and produce a polypoid mass. Peripheral extension within the bronchial lumen may occur. The high-grade form may extend into the peribronchial tissue.
- Radiologically, they are seen as a perihilar nodule or mass, with obstructive pneumonitis. CT scan shows the polypoid endobronchial mass; it permits the assessment of endo- and exobronchial extension.

BRONCHOGENIC CARCINOMA

- Most patients with lung cancer present with clinical symptoms, and only a minority are asymptomatic.
- Patients with central tumors obstructing a major bronchus may present with cough, wheezing, hemoptysis and lung infection.
- Local intrathoracic spread may result in left laryngeal nerve paralysis, pleural or chest wall pain, symptoms related to superior vena cava obstruction.
- Sometimes symptoms resulting from distant metastases may reveal the lung cancer.
- A large variety of paraneoplastic syndromes may also be associated with lung cancer. They include skeletal abnormalities such as clubbing, hypertrophic pulmonary osteoarthropathy, endocrine and metabolic disorders such as

Cushing's syndrome from ACTH production, hyponatraemia associated with inappropriate ADH syndrome production, and insulin-like activity. A variety of neurological paraneoplastic syndromes may occur including neuromuscular dysfunction, carcinomatous myopathy, peripheral neuropathies, subacute cerebellar degeneration and encephalomyelopathy. Other—Paraneoplastic syndromes include various hematological, dermatological and vascular disorders, such as a migratory thrombophlebitis and arterial thrombosis.

- The radiological appearances of lung cancer depend on the location of tumor. Signs of intrathoracic spread include bone destruction, pleural effusion, hilar and mediastinal lymphadenopathy, lung nodule in the contralateral lung, mediastinal mass, or pleural nodularity or nodular thickening of the interlobular septa.

HEMANGIOPERICYTOMA

- It is a soft tissue tumor consisting of vascular channels of varying sizes from capillary to large sinusoidal spaces.
- It is very rare in children but has been reported in infants.
- It may be difficult to distinguish from other vascular neoplasms. 30 to 50% occur in the extremities. Clinically, there is a slow-growing painless mass.
- Associations include hypoglycaemia, osteomalacia and rickets.
- In children under 1 year the lesion is usually benign. In older children the lesion behaves as in adults and metastases can occur.
- The appearance on radiography and CT are of a non-specific soft tissue mass, occasionally with bone erosion.
- Ultrasound appearances are variable from cystic to mixed or solid.
- Angiography is more characteristic and demonstrates feeder arteries, radially arranged branching arteries in and around the lesion and a persistent tumor blush.
- MRI demonstrates a fairly well circumscribed mass of intermediate signal on T1- and high signal on T2-weighted images. Serpiginous low Signal may be seen on T2-weighted images.

BRONCHIAL ADENOMAS / CARCINOID

- Bronchial adenomas (tumors in the trachea or large bronchi, the large airways of the lung) are slow growing cancers.
- Central lesions are observed as well-defined masses that narrow, deform, or obstruct adjacent airways. Diffuse punctate calcifications are observed in 30% of cases and are characteristic but not diagnostic of carcinoid. Peripheral parenchymal atelectasis or bronchiectasis is common. Peripherally located lesions usually lie adjacent to the airway.
- Typical carcinoid is marked by homogeneous contrast enhancement.
- Atypical carcinoid is associated with less contrast enhancement and frequent irregular contours; regional adenopathy is common.
- Stromal osseous metaplasia due to tumor-induced necrosis of bronchial cartilage is observed on CT scan intra tumoral calcification.

Pathology of the Pediatric Chest

- Respiratory disorders most common cause of significant childhood illness.
- Different spectrum in neonates/infants and older children.
- Medical/surgical → Unilateral → from management point of view.

IMAGING MODALITIES

Plain Film

- CXR is the most frequent examination performed in most pediatric radiology departments.
- In neonates infants, young children:
  - Supine CXR – AP view.
  - Cross table lateral – may occasionally be required.
- In order children – erect view should be obtained whenever possible.
- As short exposure time as possible to be used with high KV and low mAs with fast film screen combination.

CT

- As in adults, CT is the most important adjunctive imaging modality.
- Contrast enhanced spiral CT/HRCT.
- For classification of equivocal or confusion CXR findings.
- For normal CXR with positive clinical findings.
- For non-resolving pulmonary lesion.
- Mediastinal/hibernation L.N.
- Detection – complicated bacterial pneumonia/ sequalae/immunocompromised.
- Chest masses–congenital/neoplastic/inflammation.
- Examination of abnormal airway/chest wall/ pleura.

HRCT

- Suspected ILD.
- Bronchiectasis.
- Cystic fibrosis.
- B.P.D.

MRI

- Currently MRI is recommended as first line investigation in suspected vascular lesions/ mediastinal masses/hilar/pleural/chest wall lesions.

USG

- Evaluation of pleural/mediastinal lesion.
- Opaque hemithorax.

Scintigraphy

- Masses of small parathyroid origin/enteric cysts with ectopic gastric mucosa/neuroblastoma/lymphoma.

  Angiography and Bronchography has no role in the present imaging era.

MEDICAL CONDITIONS

Neonatal Chest

- Most congenital and acquired lesions of respiratory tract in newborn present with respiratory distress.

Respiratory Distress in Newborn

- Pulmonary conditions:
  - Medical.
  - Surgical.
- Extrapulmonary causes:
  - Cardiac.
  - Upper airway obstruction.
  - Musculoskeletal obstruction of chest.
  - Lesions of diaphragm/abdomen.
  - CNS causes leading to hypoventilation.
  - Metabolic causes.

MEDICAL CONDITIONS

Transient Tachypnea of Newborn

Hallmark – Transient benign course, both clinically and radiographically.

(Wet Lung syndrome)–Tachypnea, rib recession, grunting.

  - Recovery in 48 hours.
- Due to retained fluid – lung filled with amniotic fluid.
- Pre-disposing condition – Cesarean Section prematurity, maternal diabetes (precipitous delivery), maternal fluid overload.

  Radiological Features – prominent pul. interstitial markings, fluid in inter lobal fissure, intrapleural space and slight overaceration.
- In severe cases pulmonary edema or reticular granular appearance may develop.

Immature Lung Disease

- Seen in premature infant – <1500 g.
- Feature of respiratory distress are absent for 1st 4-7 days.
- Surfactant present, but insufficient (accelerated maturation due to intrauterine stress).
- CXR diffuse granularity of lung with relative absence of air bronchogram and little or no under aeration of the lungs.
- Complication – Apnoea, bradycardia with persistent PDA may require ventilation.
- Prognosis much better than R.D.S.

RDS/HMD (Figure 36.1)

- A manifestation of pulmonary immaturity.
- Seen in newborn <36 weeks/<2.5 kg wt.
- Deficiency of pulmonary surfactant.

Hallmark

- Reticular granularity of lungs due to superimposition of multiple acinar nodules related to atelectatic alveoli and diffuse pulmonary under aeration (lung volume).
- Air bronchogram – Due to coalescence of areas of atelectasis around dilated terminal bronchioles.

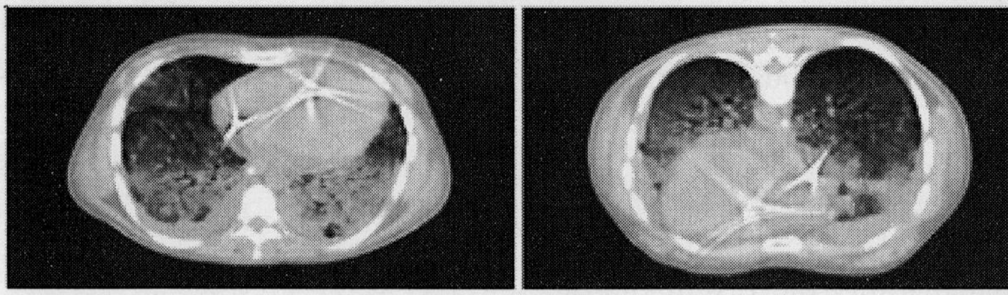

Fig. 36.1: Computed tomography scan of the lungs showing acute respiratory distress syndrome in supine (left) and prone (right) position

- In more severe cases – associated interstitial and alveolar edema with or without pulmonary parenchymal hemorrhage.

  ↓

  Loss of clarity of diaphragmatic and cardiac outline — White out lungs.
- Normal CXR at 6 hours of age excludes RDS.
- Treatment positive pressure ventilation (CPAP/IPPV), surfactant therapy.

Complication of Therapy

Early – due to air leak:

- Pneumothorax – usually under tension.
- Pneumomediastinum – can dissect subcutaneously into the neck, retroperitoneum, peritoneal cavity.
- Pulmonary interstitial emphysema:
  - Small bubbles of air radiating out (2-3 mm) from hilum, do not move with respiration, may become large.
  - If severe-over inflated lungs with cardiorespiratory embarrassment may occur.

Late-BPD – Effect of trauma due to PPV and O_2 toxicity.

- Defined as O_2 dependency with abnormal CXR at 28 days of age.

Pathologically

Areas of hyper expansion and atelectasis, intersperse with patchy areas of fibrosis.

Radiographic Appearance

- Patchy or linear strands of increased density with localized areas of unequal areas and generalized hyper aeration.
- Northney and Resin described classically 4 class stages in 1967:

I	Identical to RDS Reticular granular opacity are now rare.
II (4-10 days)	Bilateral white out lungs (interstitial edema).
III (1-20 days)	Bubbly appearance of lungs due to alveolar over distension and scarred acini.
IV (>1 month)	Classic appearance of BPD with bubbly appearance to lung with alternating cystic lucencies surrounded by curvilinear soft tissue stranding.

Pulmonary HTN with RVH may be seen.

HRCT

- Subpleural areas of extensive lung destruction.
- Parenchymal bands, areas of increased attenuation and perfusion.
- Bronchial caliber.

Wilson-Mikity Syndrome

- It is a type of pure O_2 toxicity.

Mechanical obstruction		Chemical pneumonitis	Surfactant inactivation
↓			Atelectasis
Air trapping			Intrapulmonary stenting
↓ Air leak	↓ Uneven ventilation	–Hypoxia –Acidosis	Persistent fetal circulation

- Radiological features similar to BPD with coarse interstitial pattern and the development of cystic changes.

Meconium Aspiration Syndrome

Pathophysiology

Meconium aspiration (Table 37.1).

Radiological Features

Bilateral patchy asymmetrical areas of opacification associated with marked overinflation complicated by pneumothorax and penumo mediastinum in 25% cases. Severe cases show more confluent widespread opacification than overinflation. Complicated by pneumothorax and pneumomediastinum in 25% cases. Severe cases show more confluent widespread opacification than overinflation.

- Due to chemical pneumonitis – slow clearing of radiological opacification and radiological clearance lagging behind clinical status.

  Treatment with antibiotics, ventilation, ECMO.

Neonatal Pneumonia

- Non-hemolytic streptococcus, gram-negative rods or stap aureus, viral – less common.
- Predisposing factors – prematurity, PROM, ascending infection, transplacental.

Radiological Features are – Varied

- Radiating parahilar streakiness, patchy parenchymal infiltrates, reticulonodular opacities.
- Hazy lungs, basilar infiltrates or diffuse granularity mimic RDS.

Differentiating Features from RDS

- Normal or increased lung volume.
- Asymmetry of reticulonodular pattern.
- Presence of pleural effusion.
- Lobar or segmental consolidation.

Pulmonary Hemorrhage

- RDS, BPD, aspiration pneumonia, heart disease, vit K deficiency, only congenital coagulation factor deficiency, thrombocytopenia, DIC.

Radiological Features

If mild, difficult to differentiate from underlying pulmonary disease.

If severe deterioration of clinical status-diffuse homogenous opacification.

SURGICAL CONDITIONS

Congenital Lobar Emphysema (CLE)

- Over distension of one or more lobes of a histologically normal lung.
- M>F, LUL (48%), RML (34%), RUL (21%).
- Associated cardiac anomalies.

Etiopathogenesis

- Cartilage under development with collapsed wall of bronchus with obstruction and air trapping.

- Focal bronchial obstruction (intrinsic/extrinsic).
- Poly alveolar lobe.
- Congenital hypoplastic emphysema (too few alveoli).
- Abnormal in alveolar structure (alveolar fibrosis).

CXR

- Over distended hyperlucent lobe with contralateral mediastinal shift and compression of ipsilateral uninvolved lobe.
- In infants presenting immediately after birth, the involved lobe may be opaque and not lucent.

CT

- Overdistended, hyperlucent with stretched and attenuated vascular structures with normal bronchial anatomy.
  - May demonstrate or exclude mass effect as a cause of obstruction.

  Pulmonary agenesis, aplasia, hypoplasia.

  Bilateral – Potter sequence (renal agenesis) PROM.
- Compression of lung:
  - Intrathoracic–CHD, C-CAM, pleural effusion.
  - Extrathoracic
    - ✦ Abdominal distension by mass.
    - ✦ Neuromuscular disease of chest.
    - ✦ Severe dysplasia A.T.D.
- Associated anomalies include – PDA, tracheo-esophageal fistula, and hemivertebra, associated skeletal anomalies.

Agenesis/Aplasia

- Opaque hemithorax with ipsilateral mediastinal shift.
- Compensatory emphysema of contralateral lung with herniation across midline.
- Absence of ipsilateral bronchus and pulmoanry artery – agenesis.
- Rudimentary ipsilateral bronchus – aplasia with small pulm. artery.

Hypoplasia

- Small hemithorax with hyperlucent lung and ipsilateral mediastinal shift and a small ipsilateral hilum.
- Arterial supply – usually from pulmonary artery (though systemic supply may also be present).
- Other associated anomalies errors in pulmonary location, bronchial branching, herniovertebras scoliosis.

Bronchopulmonary Sequestration

- Congenital mass of non-functioning lung tissue which contains both bronchial and alveolar elements but with lack of any communication with tracheo bronchial tree and receives most or all of its arterial supply from an anomalous systemic artery.

Intralobar	Extralobar
• Due to early development of supernumerary lung bud closes to normal lung bud	• Development later in embryonic life
• Recurrent pneumonia	• Co-incidental mass
• Venous drainage to left atrium	• To systemic veins
• Within normal pleural	• Separate pleural envelop
• Associated anomalies rare	• Common (associated diaphragmatic hernia in 30% patients).

Section 3

- Due to supernumerary lung bud development caudal to the normal lung bud.

CXR

- Intralobar sequestration occurs predominantly in lower lobes, most commonly on the left and in posterior basal segment.
- Oval, spherical, basal opacity with or without emphysema in normal surrounding lung due to collateral ventilation. OR
- Cystic parenchymal mass with multiple cysts of varying sizes simulating CCAM.

Congenital Cystic Adenomatoid Malformation

- Multicystic mass of pulmonary tissue in which there is proliferating immature bronchial structures at the expense of alveolar development.
- Usually unilateral and unilobar, occurs with equal frequency in both lung with slight predilection for the upper lobes.
- Normal trochobronchial communication, normal blood supply from normal pulmonary artery and vein.
- May be associated with hydramnios and fetal ascites.
- In neonate—It usually present with respiratory distress.
- Older children—Recurrent pulmonary infarction.

Three types:

I. Most common: 1-4 large cysts (3-10 cm); best prognosis > 2 cm.

II. Numerous small to medium sized cysts (0.5-3 cm).
   - May be associated with congenital anomalies.

III. Least common large solid lesion with numerous tiny (<2 mm) fluid filled cysts, worst prognosis.

Radiological Features

- Initial radiography within few hours of birth may show mediastinal shift by a soft tissue mass, which represents retained fluid within CCAM.
- Progressively the fluid is reabsorbed and the area is replaced by air filled cystic lesion.

Bronchogenic Cyst

- Usually presents after newborn period.
- Arises as a result of supernumerary swelling of the tracheal diverticulum of the foregut.
- Fibrous wall containing cartilage and is lined by respiratory epithelium and is filled with mucoid or serum fluid with or without air.
- M>F.
- Central mediastinal
  - Subcranial (Most common).
  - Paratracheal.
  - Hilar.
- Peripheral.

CXR

- Round or oral smooth sharply marginated, thin walled water density mass or air filled cyst with or without fluid level.

  Mass effect over the adjacent trachea, bronchus or oesophagus.

CT

- Iso/hypo/hyperdense.

Vascular Masses

- Congenital vascular malformation
  - Single
  - Multiple
    - More often as a part of syndrome.
    - Hereditary hemorrhagic telangiectasia.
    - Osler veber renaldo.

– Acquired
  - ♦ Liver disease
  - ♦ Cyanotic heart disease
  - ♦ Chronic pulmonary infection.
  - ♦ Emphysema.

– Multiple – 33-50%, B/L -8-20%.

– 60% in lower lobes.

– C/F
  - ♦ High out cardiac failure may occur.
  - ♦ Cyanosis, polycythemia, dyspnea, digital clubbing.

CXR

Pulmonary nodule with an associated linear opacity representing a feeding vessel.

- MSCT angio-diagnostic.
- Angio-embolisation – only safe agents – detachable balloon catheters of steel coils, carefully size matched, occlude as close to neck as possible.
- Radionuclide imaging – can be used to screened for the presence of R-L shunt.
  - – Tc^{99} labelled microspheres – normally does not cross pulmonary capillary bed.
- In shunt–activity detected in kidney.

Diaphragmatic Hernia

Congenital diaphragmatic hernia–Major surgical emergency in newborn, large hernias may come immediate and severe respiratory distress and cyanosis.

It is most common through foramen of Bochdalek *(Bochdalek hernia)*, located postero-laterally on (L) side, less common on right side. It is associated with ipsilateral pulmonary hypoplasia clinically shifted cardiac apex, scaphoid abdomen, RD, cyanosis.

- Antenatal USG – can diagnose as early as 18 months.
  - – Cystic or complete solid mass in hemithorax with mediastinal shift, failure to visualize stomach in the abdomen, abnormal position of abdominal viscera, hydramnios.

CXR

- Partial or complex opacification of hemithorax with clinically mediastinal shift in CXR obtained before air enters into bowel loops.
- Later air filled cystic lesions (loops of bowel) in hemithorax with clinically mediastinal shift and or abdomen devoid of gas.
- Barium/X-ray with nasogastric tube.

Morgagni Hernia

- Occurs through foramen of Morgagni.
- Anterio, unilateral medial or basal mass above diaphragm.
- Usually contain omentum – transverse colon may show upward hitch.
- Rarely may contain loops of bowel or liver.
- CT or coronal MRI – Useful to confirm herniation of liver, fat or omentum – with soft tissue opacities due to vessel. D/D–epicardial fat pad.

POST TRAUMATIC

Hiatus Hernia

Eventration

- Diaphragmatic muscle thin, absence or replaced by thin membranous sheet.

• Partial >	Complete	–	May be associated
↓	↓	–	Ipsilateral pulmonary hypoplasia
R>L	L>R	–	C/L mediastinal shift

CXR

- Elevated diaphragm/or smooth hump with upward displacement of underlying liver, spleen kidney or omentum.

  USG/Fluoroscopy – absent or paradoxical movement.
- May be difficult to differentiate from diaphragmatic paralysis.

Diaphragmatic Paralysis

- Congenital – Difficult delivery.
- Acquired – Unilateral surgery.
  - Neck
  - Chest

  Central line insertion in the neck.

  Mediastinal mass.

  Trauma.
- Bilateral Rare – birth trauma.
  - Neuromuscular disorders.
- Diagnosis USG/fluoroscopy.
- Movement best assessed using a transverse scan plane.

Inhaled Foreign Body

- Especially common in children <3 years.
- A clear history of possible inhalation of foreign body with sudden onset, wheeze is an indication for further investigation.
- Less obvious symptoms include – persistent cough, recurrent pneumonia, wheeze, stridor, and hemoptysis.
- Serial consolidation in different lobes – due to movement of foreign body.
- Peanut M.C. inhaled foreign body.
- Most bronchial foreign bodies do not cause symptoms unless they have been in place for long time and cause severe symptoms, organic foreign bodies cause more severe mucosal problems, present early as compared to non-organic foreign bodies.
- Opaque foreign bodies in only 10-15%.
- If foreign body inhalation is likely then bronchoscopy should be performed with or without delay. If there is possibility of F.B. ingestion, CXR should be perfomed only if immediate bronchoscopy is not available.
- More commonly lodge in right main bronchus.

Radiological Features

- Size, location, nature and duration of impaction of the foreign body.

Most Common Findings

- Unilateral hyperlucency due to air trapping and obstructive emphysema involving a lobe (Fig. 36.2) or entire lung.
- If complete blockage – atelectasis, ipsilateral mediastinal shift.
- In 16% normal CXR
  - Inspiration – expiration series.
  - Fluoroscopy – Clinically mediastinal shift during expiration.

CT Most Sensitive

Only indicated in problematic cases.

- Decubitus film with ipsilateral side down – hyper inflation of ipsilateral lung (of lack of partial deflation, normal seen in dependent lung).

Tracheoesophageal Fistula

- Dribbling of saliva, choking, coughing, and episodes of cyanosis on feeding.
- Association with VATER (VACTERAL) association.
- Trisomy 21 – ipsilateral esophageal atresia.
- Five types MC – esophageal atresia with distal fistula.
- Antenatal USG – absent gastric bubble.
- Distended esophageal pouch may be visualized.

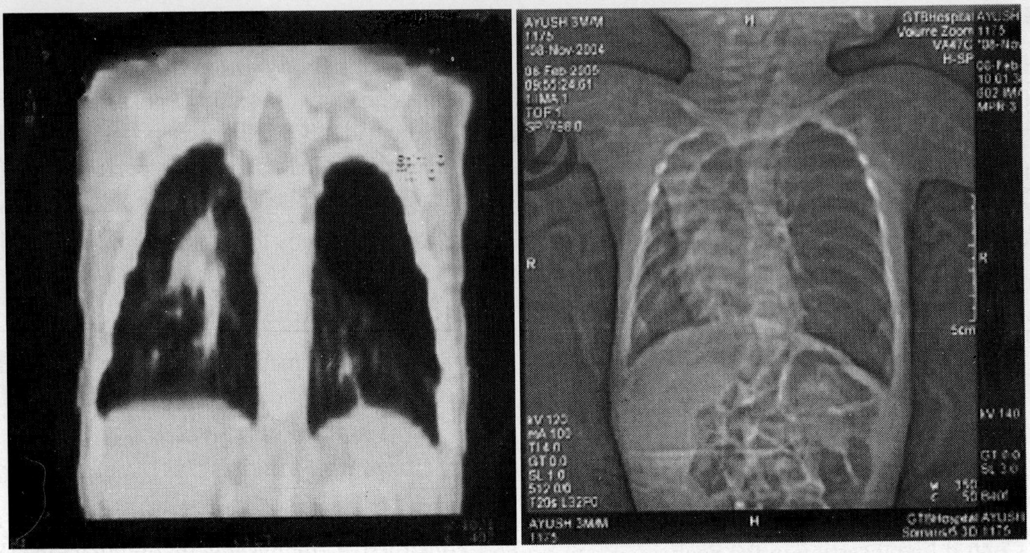

Fig. 36.2: Chest radiograph and coronal MPR CT image show congenital lobar emphysema of the upper lobe of left lung

- Polyhydramnios.
- CXR with nasogastric tube – tube coiled in proximal pouch – gas/air/contrast may be instilled.
- H type fistulas present later in infancy or childhood with episodes of choking or space during feeding or recurrent URTI – tube esophagogram – patient prone with horizontal beam fluoroscopy.

Tracheobronchial Stenosis

- Rare.
- Associated with aberrant left pulmonary artery.
- Anomalous completeness of tracheal ring.

  C/F Wheezing, R.D.

  CXR Obstructive emphysema or atelectasis.

  Bronchocele due to mucus impaction may be seen distal to narrowing as a round, oval or fan shaped opacity.
- Segmental stenosis may be seen on X-ray/CT/MRI.
- Normal neonatal tracheal diameter on CT should be >3 mm.

Tracheomalacia

- Atrophy or under development of tracheal cartilage resulting in soft tracheal wall, which undergoes focal calliper during expiration, leading to obstructive symptoms.
  - Primary.
  - Secondary.
    - In utero compression from extrinsic mass – vascular ring.
    - Chronic endotracheal intubation – Dilated – esophageal pouch in esophageal obstruction.

Pulmonary Abscess

- Staphylococcus.
- a and b hemolytic streptococci.
- Pseudomomas.
- Klebsiella.
- Aspirated anaerobic oral flora.
- Radiological features depend upon relative amount of consolidation, necrosis and presence of air.

Hydatid Cyst

- E. granulosus and E. mutlilocularis.

CXR – Well defined spherical or oval well defined homogenous opacity, single/ multiple/unilateral or bilateral.

- Rarely ever calcify.
- Meniscus/crescent sign.
- Air fluid level.
- Water lilly/camelote sign.

CT/MRI can detect signs of secondary infection (Figure 36.3).

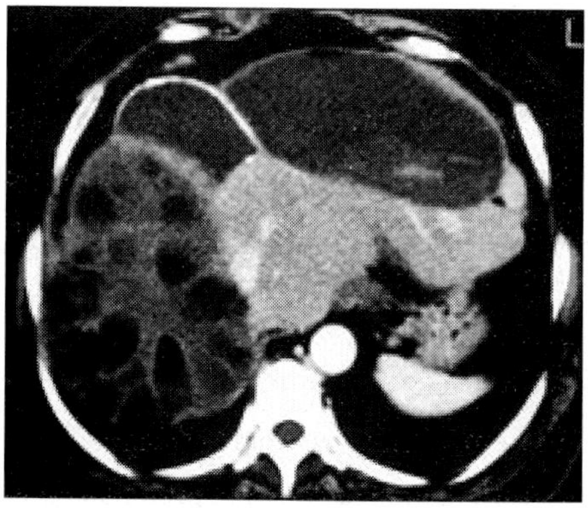

Fig. 36.3: Axial CECT scan showing multiloculated hydatid cyst in right lobe of liver

USG

- Floating membranes.

Pulmonary Neoplasms

- Pulmonary metastases: Most common cause of malignancy in children.
- Primary neoplasms are rare and has to be differentiated with benign lesions like hamartoma due to the presence of calcification (Fig. 36.4).
- Pleuropulmonary blastoma – arise from primitive pulmonary esenchymal blastoma, usually in adults 25% children.
- Solid or multicystic.
- Mesenchymal sarcoma may be associated with cystic lesion – bronchogenic cyst, CCAM, congenital pulmonary cyst.

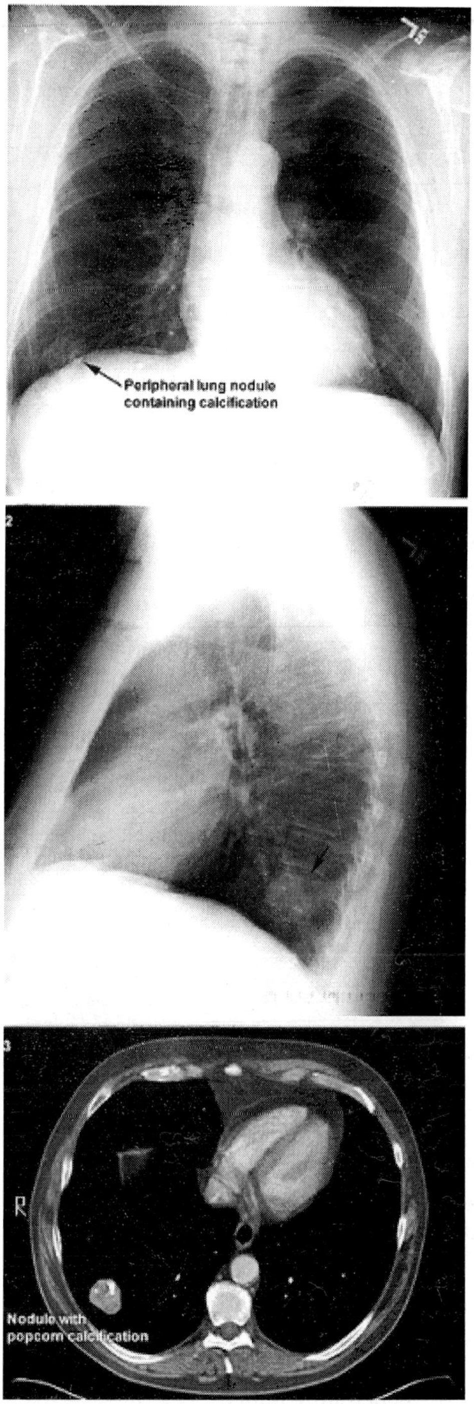

Fig. 36.4: Chest X-ray PA and lateral view and axial CT section of same patient showing pulmonary hamartoma in right lower lobe

Section 3—Respiratory System

Chapter 37

Empyema

Empyema (Figure 37.1) is an infected exudative pleural effusion containing pus (WBC count >5000/mm^3).

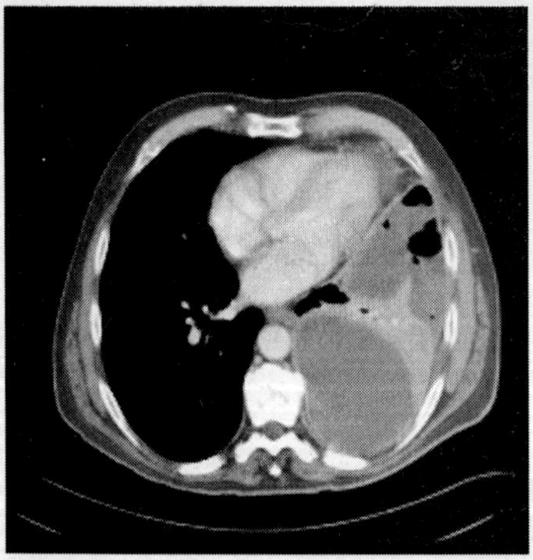

Fig. 37.1: Axial CECT showing left sided empyema with consolidation of underlying lung

CAUSES

1. Infected parapneumonic effusion – Most common cause.
2. Trauma
   - Penetrating injury.
   - Surgery.
   - Oesophageal perforation.
3. Extrapleural spread of subphrenic abscess.
4. Bone infection – osteomyelitis of ribs/vertebrae.
5. Infection following aspiration of pleural fluid of any etiology.

STAGES

1. Early empyema – exudative stage.
   - Inflamed pleura weeps proteinaceous fluid into pleural space.
   - Patient is profoundly toxic.
   - Hallmarks
     - Thin pus.
     - Mobile lung.
     - Thin pleura.
2. Established empyema
   - Fibrinopurulent stage.
   - Accumulation of neutrophils + fibrin deposition on pleural surface.
   - Adherent lung.
   - Inflamed and thickened pleura.
   - Thick pus in empyema space.
   - ± Multiple loculations.
3. Chronic empyema – organization stage
   - Fibroblasts infiltration leading formation of pleural ring.

- Limited chest expansion.
- Conditions predisposing to chronic empyema
  - Bronchopleural fistula
  - TB
  - Bronchiectasis
  - Lung abscess
  - Foreign body
  - Rib sequestration.

RADIOLOGICAL FEATURES

Plain radiograph of chest:

- Usually sufficient for diagnosing an empyema and for differentiating it from a peripheral pulmonary parenchymal lesion if empyema is in encapsulated form.
- Features of volume loss and pleural thickening are associated in cases with chronic empyema.
- Air may be present if:
  - Infected with gas forming organism.
  - Complicated by bronchopleural fistulae (BPT).
  - Introduced through ICD tube.

USG

- Helpful for diagnosis as well as for assisting in aspiration.
- Features of exudative pleural effusion:
  - Presence of internal echogenicities.
  - Presence of irregular, thick septations.

  Associated with nodular pleural thickening.

  Associated with pleural thickening of >3mm.
- Presence of pleural calcification favours diagnosis of empyema or TB as the cause.

CT

Pleural fluid is associated with:

- Thickening of parietal pleura.

  Seen in 60% patients on NCCT.

  Seen in 86% patients on CECT.
- Increased thickness and density of paraspinal and subcostal tissue due to inflammation of extrapleural fat.
- Curvilinear enhancement of chest wall boundary (in 96% patients) due to inflammatory hyperemia of pleura.
- 'SPLIT PLEURA SIGN' i.e. pleural fluid between enhancing visceral and parietal pleura.
- Gas bubbles in pleural space if there is gas forming organisms/bronchopleural fistula.

Complications of Empyema

1. BPF.
2. Empyema necessitans.
3. Predisposition to certain malignancies
   - NHL.
   - Squamous cell carcinoma
   - Mesothelioma.
   - Sarcoma.

BRONCHOPLEURAL FISTULA

BPF is a communication between the pleura and bronchial tree that results in persistent air leak.

Causes

A. Trauma
   1. Complication of resectional surgery e.g. pneumonectomy.
      - Lobectomy.
      - Bullectomy.
   2. Blunt or penetrating trauma.
   3. Barotrauma.

B. Lung necrosis
   1. Putrid lung abscess.
   2. Necrotizing pneumonia.
   3. Infarction.

C. Airway disease
   1. Bronchiectasis.

2. Empyema complicated by pneumonia or pneumothorax.

D. Malignancy.

Infective BPF

- Occurs in association with necrotizing pulmonary infection or empyema.
- Characterized by appearance of air fluid level in pleural space.
- It should be differentiated from:
  - Air introduced at thoracocentesis.
  - Infection with gas forming organism.
  - Pleuro esophageal fistula.
- Diagnosis is confirmed by:
  - Demonstration of fistula at thin section CT.
  - By introducing iodinated contrast in pleural space and demonstrating entry of contrast in bronchial tree.

THERAPEUTIC OPTIONS

- Surgical resection.
- Surgical or image guided occlusion of BPF with endobronchial vascular coils or glue.
- Antibiotics.

POST-SURGICAL BPF

- Usually develops 7-10 days following pneumonectomy.
- Should be suspected clinically when there is determination of patient e.g.
  - Pneumonia.
  - Hemoptysis.
  - Sudden expectoration of fluid.
  - Persistent large air leaks from pleural drain.
- In uncomplicated post pneumorectomy patient:
  - Residual space contains air and fluid with ipsilateral mediastinal shift with elevation of hemidiaphragm.
  - Air is resorbed over 2-4 months.
  - Later fluid is also resorbed – obliteration of space.
- Radiological signs in BPF:
  - Mediastinum returns to midline.
  - Increasing air and decreasing fluid in pneumonectomy space.
  - Contralateral aspiration pneumonia.
  - BPF may be directly visualized in 50% cases.
- Delayed onset (>6 months post pneumonectomy) BPF often indicate tumor recurrence:
  - Appearance of air in previously air free post pneumorectomy space.
  - Usually not associated with mediastinal shift as fibrosis has occurred by this time.

DIFFERENCE BETWEEN EMPYEMA AND LUNG ABSCESS

• Empyema usually has a venticular shape with oblong margins that taper and conform to the pleural space	Peripheral lung abscess usually has a spherical shape with non tapering ends.
• Forms obtuse angle with chest wall	Forms an acute angle with chest wall although concomitant pleural disease may cause angle to become obtuse.
• Unequal length of air fluid levels in different projections	Approx. equal.
• Contiguous with chest wall in at least one projection	Often separated on all aspects.
• Split pleura sign often present	Absent.
• Vessels and airways displaced	Contact margin.
• Wall thin, uniform, smooth on all aspects	Thick, non-uniform, irregular on both aspects.
	Multiple small side pockets may be present.
• Surrounding consolidation usually absent	Usually present.
• Extension into costophrenic angles may be present	Absent.
• May cross fissures	Does not cross fissures.
• Shape of space changes with change in posture	Does not change.

Section 3—Respiratory System

Chapter 38

Pleural Masses

- Primary neoplasms of the pleura are rare.
- The most common benign tumors involving the pleura are lipomas and fibrous tumors, the latter previously referred to as benign fibrous mesothelioma.
- Metastatic disease is the most common malignant neoplasm involving the pleura. Primary pleural tumors, such as mesothelioma, account for less than 5% of malignant pleural neoplasms and are usually associated with asbestos exposure.
- Computed tomography is useful in defining the location and extent of benign and malignant pleural tumors, and in assessing the underlying lung parenchyma and pleura in patients with a pleural effusion.
- Features suggesting a malignancy rather than a benign process include pleural thickening over 1cm, disseminated pleural nodules, and mediastinal pleural involvement.

BENIGN TUMORS

Pleural Lipoma (Figure 38.1)

- Benign lipomas of the pleura and chest wall are usually a symptomatic and incidental findings on a chest X -ray. Some lipomas may extend from the chest wall into the pleural space, protruding into the pleural surface; and simulating a pulmonary lesion on radiography.
- The radiographic appearance is of a well-defined rounded mass adjacent to the chest

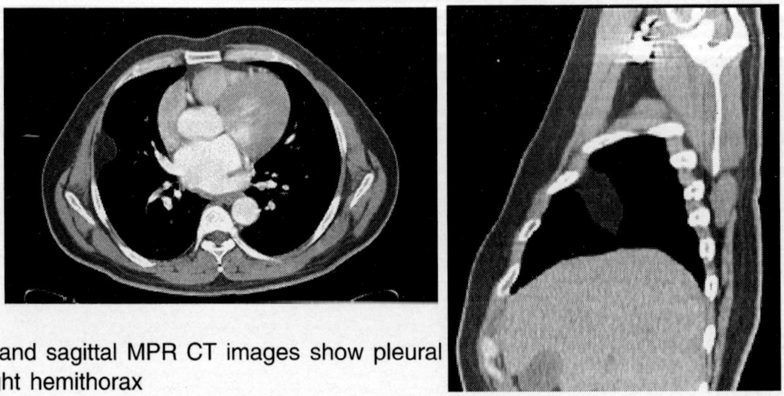

Fig. 38.1: Axial and sagittal MPR CT images show pleural lipoma in the right hemithorax

wall. They may change shape with respiration being soft tumors, and if large may erode adjacent ribs.

- CT allows a definitive diagnosis based on the characteristic fat attenuation, which is usually homogeneous. Although a capsule is sometimes identified, benign lipomas may have small bands of fibrous soft tissue which if more, prevents exclusion of liposarcoma.
- Liposarcomas are exceedingly rare and are typically more heterogeneous in their appearance. Inflammatory changes following infarction of a lipoma can produce a similar appearance.

Fibrous Tumors of the Pleura

- Fibrous tumors of the pleura are relatively rare, accounting for <5% of all pleural neoplasm's, but are most common benign pleural tumor.
- Previously called "benign mesothelioma" the name was changed because they do not arise from the mesothelial cells rather from the underlying mesenchymal connective tissue.
- They occur with equal frequency in men and, and are found in patients of all ages. They have no relationship to asbestos exposure.
- Fibrous tumors of the pleura usually are indolent and slow growing. Have been reported over periods as long as 13 years.
- Most are a symptomatic, discovered incidentally on routine chest radiographs. Patients with larger tumors may present with a cough, chest pain, or dyspnoea. Clinical findings may include hypoglycaemia, hypertrophic pulmonary osteoarthropathy, and clubbing.
- Most fibrous tumors arise beneath the visceral pleural layer and they may occur within a fissure, thus simulating a pulmonary nodule on radiographs.
- Pleural effusions are rare. Calcification occurs in approximately 10%.
- The radiographic appearance is of a well-defined lobulated mass adjacent to chest wall, mediastinum, diaphragm or a pleural fissure. The mass may be small or occupy most of the hemithorax.
- Computed tomography features suggesting the diagnosis of fibrous tumor of the pleura include a solitary, sharply defined, sometimes lobulated, soft-tissue pleural-based mass without evidence of chest wall invasion: tapering margins may be noted when the lesion is in the fissure.
- These tumors are usually sessile or lobulated but some are attached to the pleural surface by a pedicle or stalk. This allows mobility and they may change shape on inspiration and expiration, during fluoroscopy, or between examinations. Demonstration of a pedicle is pathognomonic and highly suggestive of the benign variety of the tumor.
- The vascularity of fibrous tumors typically results in homogeneous contrast. Enhancement, equal to or greater than other soft tissues. Although the smaller lesions typically appear homogeneous, the larger lesions may have low attenuation areas within them due to cystic necrosis or hemorrhage.
- Localized fibrous tumors have low signal intensity on Tl weighted images and high signal intensity on Tl weighted MR images.

Malignant Tumors

Pleural Metastases

- Metastases constitute the majority of malignant neoplasm's involving the pleura. Pleural metastases usually involve both the visceral and parietal pleural surfaces, and almost always cause an associated effusion.
- Adenocarcinoma is the most likely cell type to metastasise to the pleura. Over three quarters of pleural metastases are the result of lung and breast carcinoma and lymphoma.
- Both metastatic carcinoma and lymphoma can involve the abundant lymphatic channels and

lymphoid aggregates present just below the visceral pleura. Lung and breast cancer may invade the pleura by direct spread.

- Pleural metastasis also may occur as a result of hematogenous spread from tumor emboli lodged in distal branches of the pulmonary arteries.
- Invasive thymomas also may involve the pleura, by direct extension from the anterior mediastinum, resulting in discrete masses or diffuse pleural thickening. The mediastinal component of the tumor is not always large.
- Infiltration of the pleural surfaces usually results in a pleural effusion, which is the first manifestation in most cases.
- Computed tomography may reveal pleural-based nodules obscured by the pleural fluid. Pleural metastases usually appear as relatively small, lenticular masses having obtuse margins with the chest wall.
- As the disease progresses, they may encase the entire hemithorax and extend into the fissures. The soft-tissue component often enhances following contrast administration, allowing or improving differentiation from any adjacent no enhancing pleural effusion.
- Additional findings on CT, such as mediastinal lymph node enlargement, lung nodules, rib lesions, or a subcutaneous mass, support a presumptive diagnosis of pleural metastases.
- Metastatic adenocarcinoma of the pleura may be difficult to differentiate from malignant mesothelima; both may result in diffuse or nodular thickening, and, in some cases, encasement and modularity of the lung.

Pleural Lymphoma

- Both Hodgkin and non-Hodgkin lymphoma can involve the pleura. It is seldom the solitary initial manifestation of the disease but rather due to recurrence, or addition to thymic or mediastinal nodal and sometimes pulmonary parenchymal disease.
- A para spinal location is common. Lymphomatous involvement of the lymphatic channels and lymphoid aggregates found beneath the visceral pleura of the lung may present as sub pleural nodules.
- Lymphoma also may involve the pleura by direct extension from the mediastinum or chest wall. Enlarged mediastinal lymph nodes may cause lymphatic obstruction and lead to a pleural effusion, which occurs in upto 30% of patients with Hodgkin's disease at presentation. In addition to nodules and effusions, diffuse pleural involvement may occur.

Malignant Mesothelioma

- Mesothelioma (Figures 38.2, 38.3 and 38.4) is a highly malignant, locally aggressive tumor

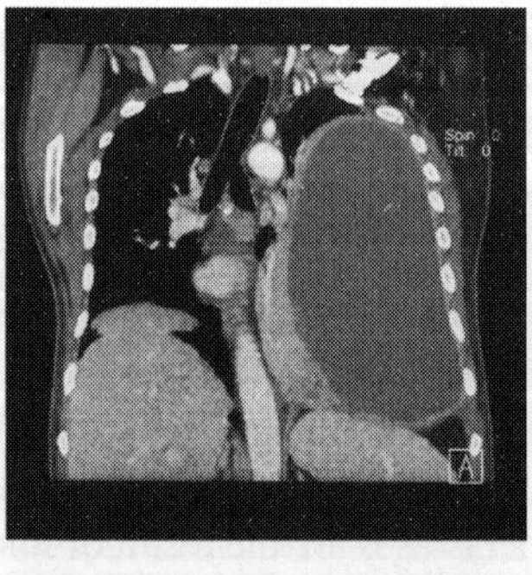

Fig. 38.2: Coronal MPR CT image shows loculated pleural effusion on left side

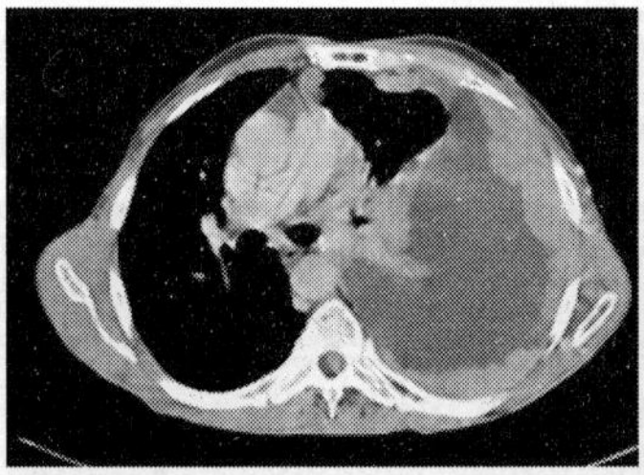

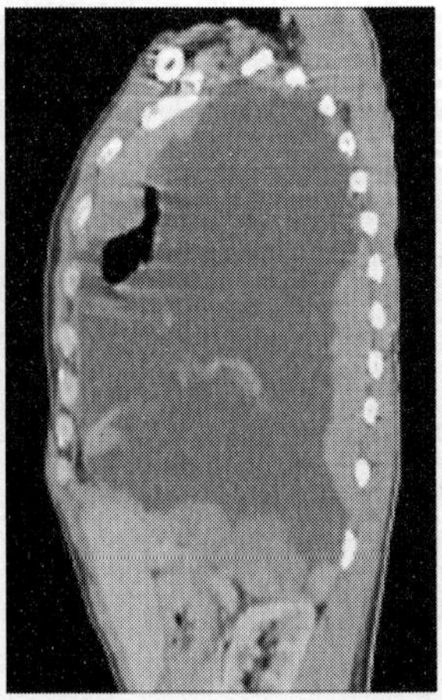

Fig. 38.3: Axial and sagittal MPR CT images show pleural effusion in case of pleural mesothelioma

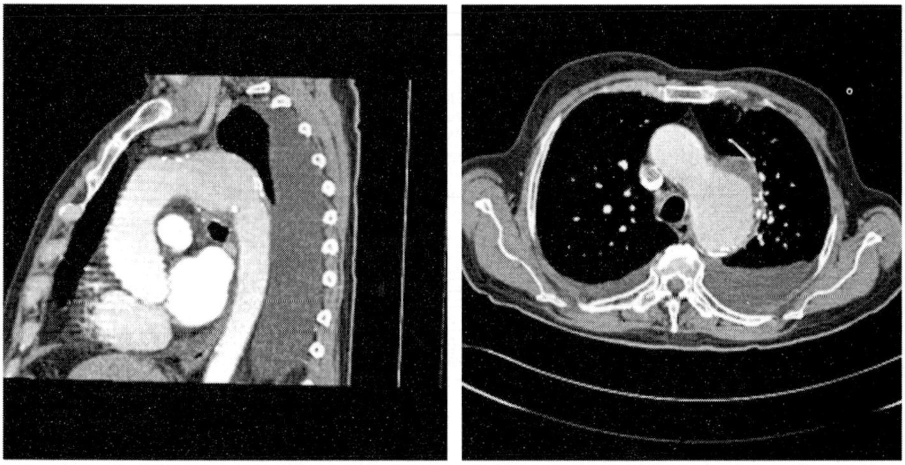

Fig. 38.4: Axial and sagittal MPR CT images show pleural effusion in case of pleural mesothelioma

of the pleura that is linked to asbestos exposure. This rare, rapidly growing tumor as an extremely poor prognosis and short mean survival time. It is three times more common in men than women, with a peak presentation in the fifth and sixth decades of life.

- Clinical symptoms are typically a late finding and include chest pain, dyspnoea, cough, weakness, and weight loss. Unlike the localized fibrous pleural tumor, hypertrophic pulmonary osteoarthropathy is unusual with malignant mesothelioma.
- Eighty percent of patients presenting with malignant mesothelioma have had occupational exposure to asbestos. Crocidolite is the most carcinogenic and fibrogenic form of asbestos. Chrysotile, anthophyllite, and tremolite are relatively more benign.
- The risk of developing a mesothelioma is unrelated to the duration or degree of exposure, which is often only mild to moderate.
- The usual appearance is nodular pleural thickening around all or part of the lung.
- Almost all patients will develop an, ipsilateral pleural effusion, and it is therefore the most common initial radiological manifestation of malignant mesothelioma. The effusion is usually exudative and often serosanguineous.
- It is variable in size, but may be large thus obscuring the pleural neoplasm. Often the mediastinum is central, despite the presence of a large effusion and this thought to be as a result from volume loss of underlying lung secondary to either ventilatory restriction by surrounding tumor or bronchial stenos is by tutor compression at the hilum.
- Rib involvement may occur, but is more likely to be due to metastatic bone tutor.
- There is often evidence of asbestos exposure in the contralateral hemithorax, including pleural thickening and pleural plaques in about half of the patients.
- Both CT and MRI are able to demonstrate the presence and extent of the pleural mass and pleural effusion. The fluid typically has a lower attenuation value than adjacent tumor. The tumor may present as diffuse nodular pleural thickening or focal masses between the lung and chest wall. Both the visceral and parietal pleura are involved and extension into the fissures and along the mediastinal pleural surface is common.
- As the tumor progress it may invade the lung, pericardium, mediastinum, ipsilateral chest wall, and occasionally the contralateral chest.

It may penetrate diaphragm and involve the peritoneal cavity or retroperitoneum.

- Malignant pleural mesothelioma slightly more common on the right side than the left, presumably due to the larger size of the right pleural space.
- Multiplanar MRI may be of use in assessing chest wall, diaphragm, and mediastinal involvement in patients with mesothelioma.
- Malignant mesothelioma has intermediate signal intensity on T1 weighted MR images and slightly high signal intensity. On T2 weighted images, loculated pleural fluid presents as areas of high signal intensity with T2 weighting.
- Malignant mesotheliomas have a very poor prognosis. The mean survival following diagnosis is < 1 year and < 10% survive over 3 years following the onset of symptoms.
- Surgical resection, either by a pleurectomy or extra pleural pneumonectomy, radiation therapy, and chemotherapy has all been advocated for treatment of malignant mesothelioma, but with little impact on survival, and operative morbidity is high. The rare patient with a potentially resectable tumor typically has normal extra pleural fat and muscle with preservation of intercostals spaces and normal signal characteristics in the chest wall on MR images.
- Rib displacement or extra pleural soft tissue infiltration suggesting chest wall invasion, infiltration of the mediastinal soft tissues with loss of normal fat planes, or even an extensive interface with the mediastinum is generally associated with unresectability.

Pulmonary Embolism

DEFINITION

Pulmonary embolism is defined as blockage of an artery in the lungs by fat, air, tumor, tissue or blood clot.

PREVALENCE

- Diagnosed in 1% of all hospitalised patients, in 12-64% at autopsy and in 9-56% of patients with deep vein thrombosis.

ETIOLOGY AND RISK FACTORS

Pulmonary embolism (PE) is caused by clots from the venous circulation, from the right side of the heart, from tumors that have invaded the circulatory system, or from other sources such as parasites, amniotic fluid, air, fat, bone marrow and foreign substances. Most (>90%) are caused from clots originating in the lower extremities called deep vein thrombosis (DVT) and many resolve on their own.

Risk factors include the following:

- Prolonged bed rest or inactivity (including long trips in planes, cars or trains).
- Oral contraceptive use
- Child birth
- Burns
- Stroke
- Heart surgery
- Surgery (especially pelvic surgery).
- Massive trauma
- Cancer
- Heart attack
- Fracture of the hips or femur

PATHOPHYSIOLOGY

The majority of clinically significant pulmonary emboli begin in a lower extremity vein as a collection of platelets that have attached to a venous valve. In the proper circumstances this platelet nidus will grow into a thrombus through the addition of other platelets and fibrin.

There are three factors that predispose a person to deep venous thrombosis:

- Venous stasis typically from bed rest or during a major operation.
- Injury to the intima of the vein; or
- A hypercoagulable state.

If the clot detaches from the lower extremity vein it will travel though the IVC, the right atrium, right ventricle and into the main pulmonary artery at which point it may end up in either the right or left lung. The result is usually an area of pulmonary hemorrhage and edema. In some cases that area of lung may infarct or dies.

The pathophysiologic changes that follow PE

involve derangement in pulmonary hemodynamics, gas exchange and mechanics. The change in cardiopulmonary function in proportion to the extent of obstruction, which varies with the size and number of emboli obstructing the pulmonary arteries, and to the patient's preembolic cardiopulmonary status, the resulting physiologic changes may include pulmonary hypertension with right ventricular failure and shock, dyspnea with tachypnea and hyperventilation, arterial hypoxemia and pulmonary infarction.

Pulmonary hypertension results from increased pulmonary vascular resistance. Consequently, the right ventricle must generate higher pulmonary arterial pressure to maintain normal cardiac output. Although some degree of pulmonary hypertension can occur after any PE, significant pulmonary hypertension (> 25 mmHg mean pressure) usually occurs in a previously healthy lung only when >30 to 50% of the pulmonary arterial tree is occluded.

If pulmonary vascular resistance increases acutely to the extent that the right ventricle cannot generate sufficient pressure to maintain cardiac output, hypotension develops and central venous and right atrial mean pressures increases. Cardiogenic shock occurs in persons without preexisting cardiopulmonary disease only after massive PE involving at least 50% and usually 75% or more of the pulmonary vascular bed. With severe hypotension and shock, mean central venous pressure tends to fall.

Tachypnea, often with dyspnea, almost always occurs after a PE. After occlusion of the pulmonary artery, areas of the lung are ventilated but not perfused, resulting in wasted ventilation – the physiologic hallmark of PE contributing to the hyperventilatory state. Depletion of alveolar surfactant within hours after the embolic event results in diminished lung volume and compliance. Diminished lung volume and possibly lowered airway PCO_2 may induce bronchoconstriction, leading to expiratory wheezing.

Arterial hypoxemia typically occurs with diminished arterial O_2 saturation (SaO_2= 94 to 85%), but SaO_2 may be normal. Hypoxemia is due to right to left shunting in areas of partial or complete atelectasis not affected by embolisation. Characteristically atelectasis can be partially corrected by deep breathing, either, voluntary or induced by a positive pressure ventilator.

Ventilation/perfusion / imbalance also contributes to hypoxemia. In massive PE, severe hypoxemia may result from right atrial hypertension that causes right-to-left shunting of blood through a patent foramen ovale. Low venous O_2 tension may also contribute to development of arterial hypoxemia.

Pulmonary infarction (PI) is hemorrhagic consolidation of lung parenchyma. When bronchial circulation is intact and normal, PI rarely develops (10% of cases). Collateral circulation from the bronchial artery probably keeps the lung tissue viable despite pulmonary artery blockage. However, patients with previously abnormal pulmonary circulation are prone to develop PI. Infarcts may heal by absorption and fibrosis, leaving a linear scar, or may resorb completely, leaving normal lung tissue (incomplete infarction).

Resolution of the pulmonary embolus through fibrinolysis and fragmentation is seen in 8% within 24 hours, in 56% by 14 days and in 77% by 7 months. The resolution is complete in 65%, partial in 23% and no resolution in 12%.

SYMPTOMS

It is important to note that the symptoms of pulmonary embolism may be vague or may resemble symptoms associated with other diseases:

- Classic triad is hemoptysis (25-24%), pleural friction rub and thrombophlebitis.
- Cough.
- Begins suddenly.
- May produce bloody sputum (significant amounts of visible/blood streaked sputum).
- Sudden onset of shortness of breath at rest or with exertion.
- Chest pain.

Class	Class I	Class II	Class III	Class IV
% Occluded PA	<20%	20-30%	30-50%	>50%
Symptoms	-	Anxiety, hyperventilation	Dyspnea, mild shock	Dyspnea, severe shock
Arterial PO_2	N	65-80 torr	50-65 torr	<50 torr
Arterial PCO_2	N	30-35 torr	<30 torr	<30 torr
CVP	N	N	Increased	Increased
Mean PAP	N	N	N	>20 mmHg
Systolic BP	N	N	N	<100 mmHg

- Under the breast, bone or on one side.
- Especially sharp or stabbing; also may be burning, aching or dull, heavy sensation.
- May be worsened by breathing deeply, coughing, eating, bending or stooping.
- Breathing, rapid.
- Rapid heart rate (tachycardia).

Additional symptoms that may be associated with this disease:

- Wheezing – Skin, clammy
- Skin discoloration, bluish – Nasal flaring
- Pelvis pain – Leg pain in one or both legs
- Swelling in the legs (lower extremities)
- Lump associated with a vein near the surface of the body (superficial vein) may be painful.
- Blood pressure, low – Pulse, weak or absent
- Lightheadedness – Fainting
- Dizziness – Sweating
- Anxiety

Signs and Tests

Tests to evaluate the function of the lungs:

- Arterial blood gases.
- Pulmonary function tests.

Tests to detect the location and extent of embolism:

- Chest X-rays.
- Lung scan.
- Pulmonary angiogram.

Tests to detect DVT (a common cause):

- Venography of the legs.
- Extremity arteriography.
- Blood flow studies.
- Doppler ultrasound examination of an extremity.
- Plethysmography of the legs.

An ECG may show abnormalities caused by strain on the heart.

This disease may also alter the results of the following tests:

- Pulmonary ventilation/perfusion scan.
- Febrile/cold agglutinins.
- Anti thrombin III.
- ACE levels.

CHEST RADIOGRAPHY

The chest X-ray is often the first imaging procedure that is obtained when a patient presents with dyspnea.

- In patients with pulmonary embolus the radiograph is often abnormal.

- A normal chest radiograph occurs in a minority of cases of pulmonary embolus. Only 14% of the chest X-rays are normal.
- Atelectasis and parenchymal densities are quite common, especially in the lower lobes.
- Parenchymal densities are caused by pulmonary hemorrhage and edema and can be confused with infectious infiltrates or malignant masses.
- Pleural effusions are common and most often unilateral. They are almost always small, occupying less than 15% of a hemithorax and rarely increase in size after 3 days. Any increase in size after 3 or 4 days should raise the suspicion of a pulmonary infection or re-embolization.
- Pleural based opacities with convex medial margins are also known as a Hampton's Hump. This may be an indication of lung infarction.
- Melting sign refers to regression of the opacity from periphery to center.
- Fleischner lines refer to fibrotic scars with invagination of pleura at the base of lung resulting in pseudofissure.
- A diaphragm may be elevated, reflecting volume loss in the affected lung.
- The central pulmonary arteries may be prominent either from pulmonary hypertension or the presence of clot in those arteries.
- A Westermark's sign implies an area of decreased vascularity and perfusion accompanied by an enlarged central pulmonary artery on the affected side.
- A Fleischner sign is local widening of the artery due to impacted embolus.
- A knuckle sign is abrupt tapering of an occluded vessel distally.
- Cardiomegaly is a non-specific finding but may imply an enlarged right ventricle as with large bilateral pulmonary emboli.
- Pulmonary edema is an uncommon finding in this group.

In conclusion, the chest X-ray can be normal in a minority of cases and abnormalities, when present, are often non-specific.

VENTILATION PERFUSION SCAN

Lung scintigraphy continues to be a useful procedure and is the logical imaging study to obtain after the chest radiograph.

Lung perfusion scans use IV injection of 20 to 50 μm particles of biodegradable albumin labeled with ^{99}Tc. These particles ultimately lodge in the small precapillary arterioles of both lungs. Nearly 100% of the particles remain in the lungs, except when right to left shunting is present, either at the cardiac or pulmonary level. Regional distribution of these particles is relatively homogenous in healthy persons and depends on the patient's position and pulmonary blood flow distribution at the time of injection. Visible activity is greatest at the base and gradually diminishes upto the apex, reflecting gravitational effects on perfusion when the patient is sitting.

The results of the test can be placed into one of 3 categories: normal, high probability and non-diagnostic.

- A normal perfusion scan is characterized by even distribution of radiotracer throughout both lungs.
- A high probability ventilation perfusion scan is represented by multiple segmental or larger defects with normal ventilation in at least one area of abnormal perfusion. This is also known as a ventilation/perfusion mismatch. Only a minority of patients with a pulmonary embolus has a high probability V/Q scan.

The differential diagnosis for a ventilation perfusion mismatch includes acute pulmonary embolus, previous pulmonary embolus, congenital vascular abnormalities, vasculitis, bronchogenic carcinoma, lymphangitic carcinomatosis and radiation therapy.

- When a ventilation/perfusion scan does not fit into either the normal or high probability category, then we consider the study to be non-diagnostic and further investigation is required. The majority of cases fall into this category which is characterized by scans with subsegmental defects of any size that match abnormalities on the chest X-ray or perfusion scan.

In conclusion lung scans are sensitive exams that essentially rule out the diagnosis of pulmonary embolus when they are normal. Patients with high probability lungs can often be treated without further workup. Those patients with non-diagnostic studies require further diagnostic investigation.

Perfusion deficit, with reduced or absent radioactivity, may result from vascular obstruction, displacement of a lung by fluid, chest masses, any condition causing pulmonary arterial or venous hypertension, or loss of lung parenchyma, as in pulmonary emphysema. Basal perfusion deficits, in which radioactivity is not concentrated at the lungs base, may develop without PE; they may be caused by any process leading to increased pulmonary venous pressure (e.g., heart failure, mitral valve disease, or veno occlusive disease), which can redistribute pulmonary blood flow.

A normal scan excludes life-threatening PE with a high degree of accuracy. Conversely, single or multiple wedge shaped marginal scan defects, especially in a segmental or lobar distribution, are highly suggestive of vascular obstruction. Acute airway diseases, including asthma or COPD may produce a pattern of focal perfusion deficits, but these deficits are typically accompanied by a corresponding lung ventilation defect not usually found with PE.

When differentiation between PE and COPD is difficult, the 133Xe lung ventilation scans may be useful. Inhaled radioactive gas distributes with the respiratory air. In acute PE with large perfusion defects, this scan usually shows relatively normal ventilation of affected areas, but with ventilation perfusion mismatches. Areas of parenchymal disease (e.g. lobar pneumonia) usually have abnormalities of both perfusion and ventilation (a matched defect) with delayed ventilation and trapping of radioactive gas. Matched ventilation perfusion defects may also occur with pulmonary edema. Sometimes matched / defects occur with PE as well, particularly if scanning is performed >24 hours after the event.

Results of scintigraphy are commonly reported as indicating various degrees of probability for PE and must be interpreted cautiously. If lung scans are entirely normal, the diagnosis of PE is virtually ruled out; if they are categorized as highly probable, the positive predictive value approaches 90%. However, although virtually all patients with PF have abnormal scans, <50% are placed in a high probability category.

COMPUTED TOMOGRAPHY

- Pulmonary infarcts are more readily identified on CT. The typical appearance of a pulmonary infarct on CT includes a pleural-based density with convex borders and linear strand at the apex of the triangle. The borders are bulging early in the process because the affected secondary lobule is filled with blood and edema fluid. The linear strand at the apex usually represents a distal pulmonary artery filled with clot. The apex of the triangle is often truncated and not wedged shaped which corresponds to the normal configuration of a secondary lobule in the lung periphery. Low attenuation areas within the infarct represents viable lung.

  The differential diagnosis for this abnormality includes infarct, hemorrhage, pneumonia, fibrosis, neoplasia and edema.

- In addition to visualizing the area of infarction we are often able to see the clot itself as an intraluminal-filing defect. Detection is poor in middle lobe and lingular branches.
- Spiral CT angiography is equal to angiography in detection of emboli within the proximal arteries (= 5th to 6th generation).

PULMONARY ANGIOGRAPHY

It should be performed within 24 hours, if the diagnosis is uncertain and the need to make the diagnosis with certainty appears urgent.

Pulmonary angiography requires the placement of a catheter from a peripheral vein through the right-sided cardiac structures, which include the right atrium, tricuspid valve and right ventricle into the main pulmonary artery. The catheter is then directed into either the right or left pulmonary artery using the ventilation perfusion scans as a road map. Iodinated contrast material is then injected which provides a detailed view of the pulmonary vasculature.

Despite the invasive nature of the procedure it is relatively safe with a reported morbidity rate of less than 1% and a mortality rate of less than 0.5%. Important complications include arrhythmia, endocardial injury, cardiac perforation, cardiac arrest and contrast reaction.

A negative pulmonary angiogram is associated with a good prognosis if a complete angiogram is performed. A complete study includes selective injections and magnified views.

The most reliable signs of pulmonary embolus are:

- An intraluminal filing defect (94%).
- An abrupt termination of a branch vessel.
- Other frequent but less conclusive findings include.
- Partial obstruction of pulmonary arterial branches with increased caliber proximal to and decreased caliber distal to the narrowing.
- Oligemic zones.
- Persistence of dye in the proximal portion of the artery during the late (venous) phase of the arteriogram.

  In lung segments with obstructed arteries, venous filling with contrast medium is delayed or absent.
- Wedge shaped parenchymal hypovascularity.
- Tortuous arterials collaterals.

Angiography is most accurate in segmental and larger sized arteries. The reproducibility of readings is subsegmental and a smaller vessel is poor.

In conclusion, angiography is a safe procedure that is most accurate when imaging emboli that lodge in segmental or larger arteries.

CONCLUSION

- The diagnosis of pulmonary embolus (Figure 39.1) is difficult despite advances in our understanding of the path physiology.

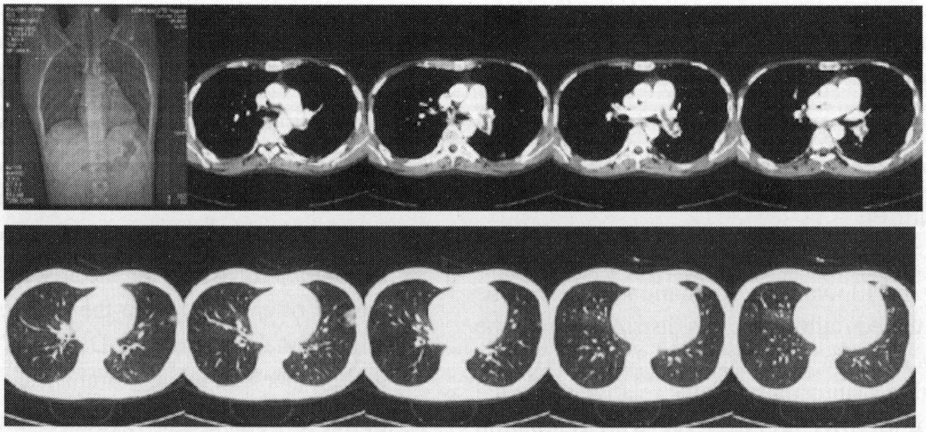

Fig. 39.1: Serial axial CT images in the mediastinal and lung window settings show left pulmonary artery thrombosis with changes in pulmonary ventilation and perfusion

Diagnostic Protocol

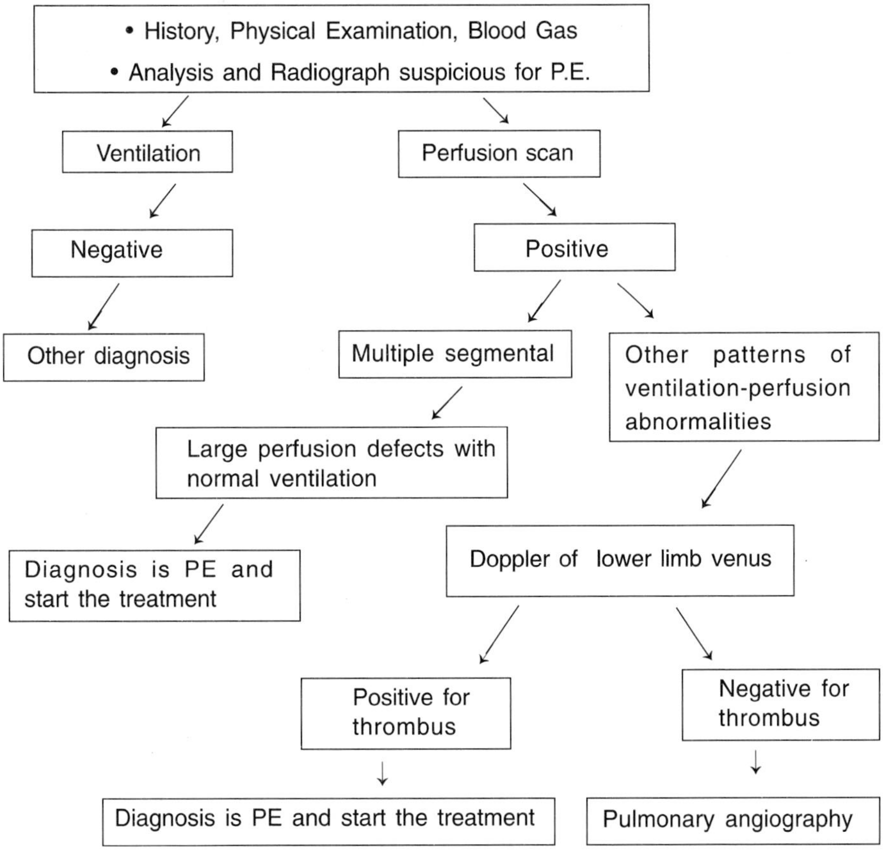

- The clinical diagnosis of pulmonary embolus is unreliable. Most patients present with dyspnea. However the signs and symptoms of pulmonary embolus are non-specific.
- The chest X-ray is abnormal in the majority of cases but the findings are often non-specific.
- Computed tomography provides information. The typical appearance of pulmonary infarction on CT can suggest the diagnosis when it was not previously considered.
- Ventilation/perfusion scanning is sensitive. A negative test essentially rules out the diagnosis. A high probability scan makes the diagnosis highly likely but is less specific when patients have suffered previous emboli. All other patterns of lung scanning are non-diagnostic.
- Angiography remains the "gold standard" for segmental or larger pulmonary arteries.

Section 3—Respiratory System

Chapter 40

Mediastinal Lymphadenopathy

MEDIASTINAL LYMPH NODES can be divided into:

1. Anterior mediastinal nodes or prevascular nodes in region of anterior mediastinum draining thymus and right heart.
2. Intrapulmonary nodes— along main bronchi.
3. Middle mediastinal nodes draining lung, bronchi, left heart, lower trachea and visceral pleura. Consists of 4 groups:
   a. Bronchopulmonary (Hilar) nodes.
   b. Carinal nodes.
   c. Tracheobronchial nodes.
   d. Paratracheal nodes.
4. Posterior mediastinal nodes including para-esophageal and retrotracheal nodes.
5. Parietal nodes consists anterior and posterior groups situated behind the sternum and posterior in intercostal region draining soft tissues and parietal pleura.

Clinical Presentation

Enlarged lymph nodes are often asymptomatic, but can produce cough, dyspnea and weight loss or may be associated with generalised lymphadenopathy.

Radiological Modalities used are:

1. Chest Radiograph.
2. Ultrasound (more useful in cases of abdominopelvic lymphadenopathy).
3. CT Scan (Plain + Contrast).
4. MRI.
5. Radionuclide scans.

CHEST RADIOGRAPH

The silhouette sign is often useful in localizing and recognizing lymphadenopathy. Obliteration of a segment of the descending aorta, right tracheal border, or pulmonary artery by large lymph nodes is common.

The **cervicothoracic sign** may be applicable to upper mediastinal node enlargement.Similarly anterior mediastinal node may obscure a segment of the border of the heart or ascending aorta.

CT SCAN

1. Is more accurate than chest radiograph in detection of mediastinal and hilar lymph nodes and showing their effect on adjacent structures.
2. Confirm findings on chest X-ray and to differentiate between normal or enlarged vascular structures from normal lymph nodes.

3. Detect occult lymphadenopathy in patients with suspected diseases (Bronchogenic Carcinoma, Lymphoma).
4. In detection of nodes in areas in which mild/ moderate nodal enlargement.
5. Information provided by CT scan can serve as a guide for subsequent nodal sampling as well as effect the choice of sampling method.
6. CT can be used to monitor response to treatment especially in case of lymphoma and metastasis.

Mediastinal Lymphadenopathy (Figure 40.1)

On CT individual lymph nodes are identified as discrete round or oval soft tissue attenuation structures within the mediastinal fat.

With increasing enlargement lymph nodes may become less sharply defined an adjacent fat may increase in attenuation secondary to extension of pathological process through nodal capsule or accompanying inflammatory or fibrotic reaction.

More progressive diseases is characterized by coalescence of multiple nodes to form a larger mass and more extensive cases causes diffuse, infiltration of mediastinum.

Measurement

Some advocate using the longest dimension with 1 cm as upper limit of normal while other consider 1 cm threshold measure along the short axis of nodes more accurate because lymph nodes are frequently oriented obliquely relative to scan plane (increase specificity but decreased sensitivity).

Size variation may occur in cases of subcarinal nodes with 12 mm threshold and cardiophrenic angle nodes, which are always less than 5 to 6mm.

Hilar Lymphadenopathy

NECT images frequently allow confident diagnosis however enlarge lymph nodes or other hilar masses are separated easily from normal hilar vascular structure using IV contrast media.

Size—Lymph nodes more than 5 mm is considered abnormal.

Findings are:

1. Focal or generalized hilar enlargement.
2. Alteration in normal hilar contour and anatomic interfaces (i.e. obliteration of space between left LL pulmonary arteries and descending aorta.

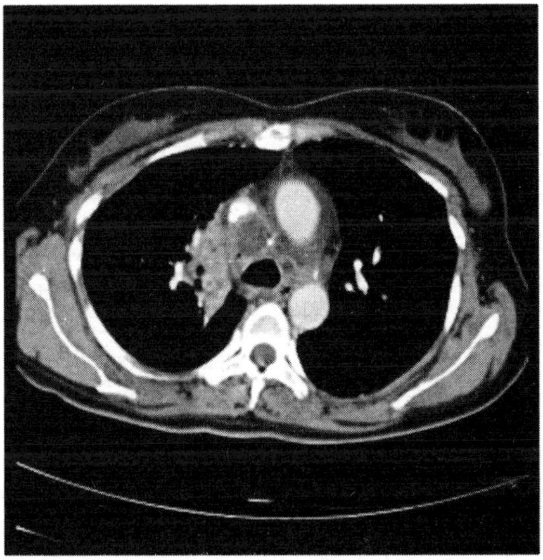

Fig. 40.1: Axial CT image show a mediastinal abscess secondary to mediastinal adenopathy in a case of tuberculosis

3. Thickening of posterior wall of RUL bronchus, bronchus intermedius or left main stem bronchi.
4. Bronchial compression or displacement.

CT Characterization of Lymph Nodes

Although most enlarged lymph nodes are of soft tissue attenuation, they can be:

1. Calcified.
2. Low attenuation.
3. Enhancing.

Low Attenuation Lymph Nodes

These are secondary to cystic degeneration or necrosis. May be seen in:

1. Tuberculosis or fungal infection (Areas of central necrosis surrounding by enhancing rim) may be seen secondary to cassation and liquefaction).
2. Metastasis due to bronchogenic carcinoma (sq. cell ca), testicular and ovarian cancer.
3. Lymphoma (esp. Hodgkin) either at the time of initial diagnosis or following radiotherapy or chemotherapy.

Enhancing Lymph Nodes

1. Vascular metastasis (RCC, papillary carcinoma thyroid).
2 Angioimmunoblastic lymphadenopathy.
3. Castleman disease (angiofollicular LN hyperplasia).

Calcified Lymph Nodes

1. Secondary to granulomatous diseases e.g. histoplasmosis, TB.
2. Disseminated pneumocystis carinii infection in AIDS patients specially who have received aerosolized pentamidine prophylaxis.
3. Inhalation disorders — Classical "egg shell" calcification however both central and peripheral calcification may be seen.
4. Treated lymphoma.
5. Sarcoidosis.
6. Amyloidosis.
7. Castleman disease (angiofollicular LN hyperplasia).
8. Metastasis (e.g. osteogenic sarcoma, mucinous ovarian or colonic carcinoma, papillary carcinoma thyroid or bronchogenic carcinoma).

MRI

It is useful as it has greater contrast resolution and multiplanar capability, which compensates for its slightly inferior spatial resolution.

It is most specific than CT in evaluating AP window and subcarinal spaces and to differentiate neoplastic and reactive hyperplastic nodes.

However it is less accurate than CT in evaluation of associated bronchial abnormalities and to identify calcification.

Sequences used are:

1. Cardiac gated TIW transaxial images (most commonly used).
2. Coronal and sagittal images helpful in detecting AP window or subcarinal lymph nodes.
3. GRE images used in cases in which there is uncertainty in delineation of vascular structures due to flow related artifacts.
4. A new lymphographic contrast agent using ultra small (<10 nm) super paramagnetic iron oxide preparation has been developed. Following IV administration, this compound bypass MNPS of liver and spleen and achieve widespread tissue distribution including LNs.The particles accumulate in normal nodes reducing their SI by super paramagnetic effect. Malignant tissue is spared, and metastatic nodes therefore appear more intense than normal nodes.

Lymph nodes are typically intermediate SI on T1WI in easily distinguishes from the higher intensity mediastinal fat and signal void mediastinal/ hilar vessels, however separation between nodes and fats are not as optimal on T2WI because there SI may be similar which are generally used in which further tissue characterization is needed (e.g. identification of suspected cystic mass or assessing disease activity in patients with lymphoma following treatment).

Untreated lymphoma appear homogeneous and show low SI (to muscle) on T1 WI, homogenous high SI (to fat) or heterogeneous high to low SI (due to fibrosis) on T2W images. Very high SI is suggestive of areas of necrosis and cystic degeneration.

MRI also useful in post treatment follow up for accurate assessment of clinical response and identification of sites of relapses of lymphoma as its SI decreases following treatment on T2WI images, so a residual mass that is of low SI on both T2 and T1WI is characteristic of inactive fibrotic tissue however residual mass containing viable tumor, inflammation and necrosis show high SI due to high water content.

Radionuclide Studies

Gallium-67 is also used in evalution of lymphoma particularly useful in differentiating residual disease from post treatment fibrosis as good correlation has been shown between uptake of Gallium-67 with residual mass and viable tumor and not by fibrotic or necrotic tissue.

SPECT Gallium-67 is 92% sensitivity and 97 % specificity.

PET scan with FDG in patients with lymphoma shows depletion on all sites of disease seen on CT.

COMMON DIFFERNTIALS

1. Infectious Granulomatous Diseases

A. Tuberculosis

Unilateral hilar and/or mediastinal lymph nodes enlargement. In tuberculosis characteristically in childhood primary tuberculosis. Although less common in adults similar findings may be seen as a manifestation of either primary or reactivation diseases.

60% of the patients with lymphadenopathy have pulmonary findings of active or healed TB. Rt paratracheal and tracheobronchial lymph nodes are involved most frequently.

CT pattern range from various degree of mild homogeneous enhancement (e.g. hyperplastic nodes) to lymph nodes with thin or thick irregular enhancing rims and focal/multifocal areas of low attenuation (e.g. nodes with central caseation and necrosis). Obliteration of adjacent mediastinal fat and low attenuation areas are more common with larger nodes.

B. Histoplasmosis

In most patients pneumonitis and associated hilar/ mediastinal LAP seen at the time of initial infection with histoplasmosis resolves with residual parenchymal and nodal calcification. Diseases spectrum includes clinically insignificant LAP to fibrosing mediastinitis.

Mediastinal granuloma (middle spectrum) though less common manifestation, represents a lobulated mass of caseous mediastinal lymph nodes, which on CT appear as low attenuation mass usually in right paratracheal and subcarinal region with or without compression-or-adjacent structures.

In fibrosing mediastinitis CT scan show hilar/ paratracheal/subcarinal masses which frequently contain multiple areas of calcification with associated findings of SVC obstruction, tracheobronchial narrowing, occlusion of oesophagus and pulmonary vessels.

CT and MRI are comparable in showing extent of mediastinal/hilar LAP however limitation of MRI is its inability to specifically detects calcification. Lymph nodes may appear relative low S1 on T2WI suggesting fibrosis or calcification.

CT is superior in showing the compressive effect of lymph nodes on adjacent bronchi.

2. Sarcoidosis

Characterised by non-necrotizing granulomatous inflammation.

75 to 85% have mediastinal/hilar lymphadenopathy on chest X-ray and half have associated parenchymal disease, however CT is useful in cases of atypical X-ray findings.

Symmetrical Bitateral hilar AP with or without paratracheal/AP window LAP is classical X-ray distribution of enlarged intrathoracic lymph nodes, however, they may be seen in other locations (subcarinal, anterior and posterior mediastinal nodes).

Unilateral hilar lymphadenopathy is seen only in 1 to 3% cases.

Lymph nodes calcification (occasionally "egg shell") is seen in 25% and is late manifestation.

In most cases diagnosis of sarcoidosis is made by bronchoscopy and transabdominal biopsy however in some cases mediastinal lymph nodes biopsy will be necessary.

3. Metastases

Most mediastinal and hilar lymph nodes metastases primary thoracic neoplasm, most commonly bronchogenic carcinoma. Generally unilateral (on the side of primary tumor).

Although identification of primary lung tumor on plain X-ray suggest diagnosis however in some patients the lung nodule/mass is only seen in CT examination.

In-patient with central sq. cell carcinoma or SCC the hilar/mediastinal mass may be the only abnormality seen in CT/chest X-ray in which mass represents central extension of primary tumor.

In patients with extra thoracic neoplasm intra pulmonary mets is 10 times more common than nodal mets and occur approximately 2% to mediastinal and hilar lymph nodes. The common tumor associated with intrathoracic nodal mets is

a. Renal and adrenal carcinoma–right hilar nodes.
b. Testicular carcinoma–paratracheal lymph nodes.
c. Head and neck carcinoma.
d. Breast carcinoma–internal mammary chain.
e. Esophagus carcinoma–posterior mediastinal nodes.

Isolated LAP is seen in 60% patients with asymmetrical hilar and right paratracheal nodal involvement most common.

CT is performed to assess the response to treatment in patients with mediastinal/hilar mets as enlargement of mass despite treatment is worrisome for treatment failure or reoccurrence.

4. Lymphoma

Primary neoplasm of lymphoreticular system has been classified into Hodgkin disease and non-Hodgkin lymphoma. CT is used to:

a. Determine extent of disease.
b. Assist in treatment planning.
c. Assess to response to treatment and evidence of possible relapse.

A. Hodgkin's Disease (HD)

Contiguous nodal spread common.

On initial presentation 65 to 80% patients with HD have abnormal X-ray with asymmetric bilateral widening of superior part of middle mediastinum or lobulated soft tissue mass in anterior mediastinum due to indentation by anterior ribs.

CT show additional site that may not be apparent on X-ray chest in additional to hilar abnormalities.

Involvement of superior mediastinum (Prevascular/paratracheal) lymph nodes is most common.

1/3 of patients presents with bilateral hilar LAP.

On CT involvement in HD disease ranges from enlarged. Discrete lymph nodes to large conglomerate masses. As apposed to carcinoma, masses from lymphoma are more likely to displace adjacent structure rather that constrict or invade them. Thymus involvement is seen in 70% cases of mediastinal HD.

On CT lymphomatous masses usually are soft tissue attenuation with slight to moderate enhancement after IV contrast however 20% show low attenuation areas.

Calcification is rarely seen prior to treatment.

Tumor may extent directly from mediastinum to invade the chest wall.

B. Non - Hodgkin Lymphoma (NHL)

In comparison with HD, patients with NHL often present with more advance disease, non-contiguous spread with extranodal sides. Intra thoracic disease is seen in 40 to 50% patients at the time of diagnosis. Superior mediastinum nodes are involved in less than 75% of those patients with intrathoracic lymphoma with involvement of other nodal group (posterior mediastinal, cardiophrenic angle, hilar nodes) and pleural involvement more common. CT may be performed at the time of initial diagnosis not only to define extent of disease but also to provide base line for monitoring treatment.

C. AIDS Related Lymphoma

Secondary to infection (most common myco bacterium) or neoplasm (lymphoma and less common due to bronchogenic Ca and Kaposi Sarcoma). Aggressive NHL of B cell origin and frequently involves extra nodal sites.

Pleural effusion and parenchymal nodules / infiltrates are most common manifestations with mediastinal/hilar lymphadenopathy occurring less commonly.

HILAR AND MEDIASTINAL LYMPH NODE ENLARGEMENT

	Etiology	Symmetry	GPS involved	Add. findings	Comments
Infectious	Bacteria TB	Unilateral 80%	Hilar 60% Hilar and Mediastinum – 40%	Parenchymal disease Always (+)	Low attenuation nodes with rim
	Fungi H. Capsulatum	Unilateral or Bilateral	Hilar or Mediastinum or both	May obstruct airway ↓ Obstructive Pneumonitis and/or atelectasis Parenchymal disease (+)	
	Coccidio-domycosis	Unilateral or Bilateral	Hilar or mediastinum or both	Parenchymal disease (+/-)	
	Virus EBV	Bilateral Sym	Hilar mostly	Lungs clear	Splenomegaly
Immunological	Sarcoidosis	Almost always Bilateral Sym	Paratracheal, tracheobronchial bronchopulmonary Groups	75-90% Mediastinal and Hilar LN 40% with diffuse lung disease	Sym. Appearance + ↓ Nodal size

Contd.

Contd.

					↓ With onset of diffuse lung disease ↓ characteristic D/D- Lymphoma TB
Neoplastic	Pulmonary Carcinoma	Usually Unilateral	Hilar or mediastinal or both	Pulmonary nodule/ mass, obstructive pneumonitis/ atelectasis, pleural effusion →Only enlarged med. lymph nodes	
	Hodgkin's disease	Typically Bilateral but often asymmetric, Unilateral adenopathy common, very unusual	Ant. Med. ↓ Most common	<30% → pulmonary invasion, Medias nodes++ 30% pleural effusion	
	Non-Hodgkin's lymphoma	Bilateral but asymmetric	Med. nodes are involved in most cases	Sometimes a/w pleuro pulmonary invasion	
	Leukemia	Usually sym	Med. and hilar	Both pleural and pulmonary involvement may be present	
	Metastatic carcinomas	Unilateral or Bilateral	Hilar or mediastinal or both	Pulmonary nodules often seen. Cyst, hemorrhage, calcification may be seen	RCC, breast, testis, lung, thyroid

Lymphoma

These are primary neoplasms of the immune system and arise within lymphoid tissue. Hodgkin's disease accounts for approx. 25% of the newly diagnosed lymphomas i.e. 1% of all malignancies. The histological type of lymphoma and the extent of involvement at the time of diagnosis have prognostic significance. The first and the most important distinction are between Hodgkin's disease and NHL.

HODGKIN'S DISEASE

- Bimodal presentation one peak in young adulthood and the second in old age.
- Slightly more common in males.
- Disease begins in the lymph nodes and slowly spreads by contiguity through the lymphatic system. Hematogenous dissemination is a late phenomenon and almost always follows splenic involvement.
- Involved lymph nodes usually emerge and eventually disease spreads extranodally into the adjacent tissues.
- Lymph nodes are enlarged often to a great extent, homogenous ill attenuation on CT with sharply defined often lobulated borders and may have central areas of necrosis, and may enhance on CECT.
- Lukas *et al.* divided Hodgkin's lymphoma into four histological subgroups:

1. *Lymphocyte predominant* (LP) is invariably present with a localized disease, often with palpable supraclavicular nodes. The patient is usually an asymptomatic young adult. The characteristic Reed Sternberg cells are Scanty.
2. *Lymphocyte depleted* (LD): The patient is usually older and polysymptomatic and have advanced disseminated disease at presentation. Reed Sternberg cells are numerous.
3. *Mixed cellularity* (MC) is most frequently seen. Common in young adults and patients are often symptomatic having the so called B symptoms i.e. unexplained weight loss of more than 10% of body weight in 6 months, unexplained fever, night sweats. These symptoms indicate that the disease may have involved abdominal lymph nodes or spleen. LP or MC variants may progress to LD or even to NHL.
4. *Nodular sclerosing* (NS) seen more commonly in female patients. Patient usually present in adolescence or early adulthood and almost always the mediastinal and supraclavicular nodes are involved. The nodes have a thick fibrous rim.

Staging of Hodgkin's disease (Ann Arrbor Staging system):

Stage I	Disease confined to single lymph node group on one side of the diaphragm.
Stage II	Disease involving two or more lymph node groups on the same side of diaphragm.
Stage III	Disease involving lymph nodes group on both sides of diaphragm.
Stage IV	Hematogenous (extra nodal) dissemination of disease.

NON-HODGKIN'S LYMPHOMA (NHL)

- Most frequently seen in elderly population.
- The working formulation divides NHL into low, intermediate and high-grade groups.
- They may also be divided into low grade nodular or follicular lymphomas and the high grade diffuse lymphomas.
- NHLs present as painless enlargement of lymph nodes, but the disease may also develop at a number of extranodal sites.
- The most common site is the neck and the Waldeyer's ring of lymphoid tissue is most commonly involved.
- A patient with NHL is much more likely to present with enlarged lymph nodes at unusual sites like the elbow or the knee.
- The secondary effects of adenopathy like limb swelling and SVC obstruction is not uncommon.
- Constitutional symptoms like weight loss, anorexia and fever are common.
- The Ann Arbor staging may also be used for NHL.
- Only about one third of the patients have clinically localized disease at presentation.
- The spread of NHL does not follow a contiguous pattern.
- Nodal disease previously treated may present extra nodally.
- The NHL may present primarily at an extra nodal site without obvious nodal disease.

Thoracic Lymphoma (Figures 41.1 and 41.2)

- CT is the current gold standard for evaluating the extent of thoracic involvement. CT sections should clearly demonstrate the extent of adenopathy. CT identifies abnormal lymph nodes by an abnormal increase in cross-sectional diameter, which is more than 1cm.
- Both pre and post contrast scans are warranted.
- Involvement of lungs is an uncommon feature of both HL and NHL.

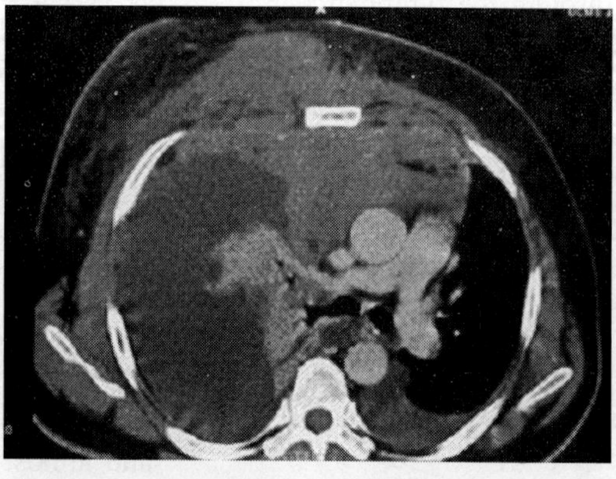

Fig. 41.1: Axial CT image shows thoracic lymphoma with sternal invasion

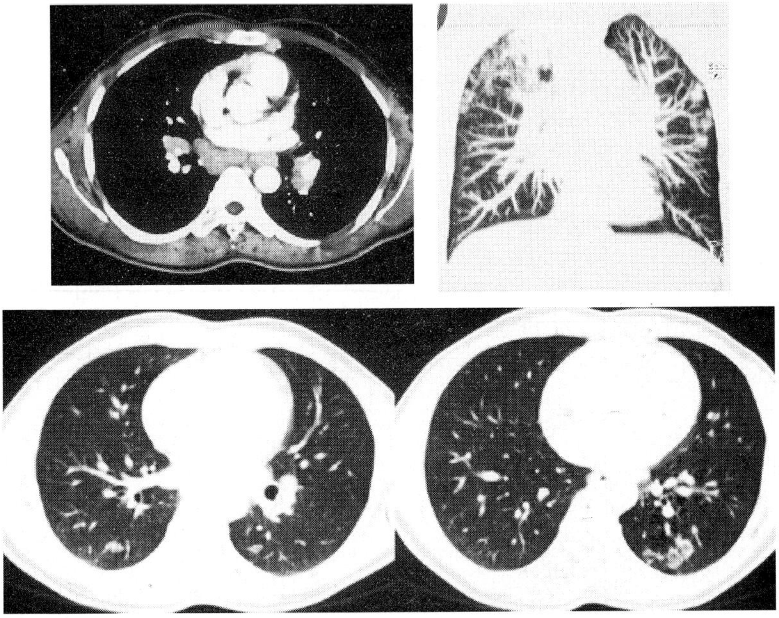

Fig. 41.2: Axial and coronal MPR CT images in the soft tissue and lung window settings shows mediastinal and pulmonary features of thoracic lymphoma

- In high grade NHL pulmonary involvement may be extensive, the radiological features often mimicking those of infection including patchy pulmonary shadowing, pulmonary consolidations and lobar collapse. However the most characteristic lung findings are the presence of one or more nodules within the parenchyma usually near the lung bases or near hila.
- Some of these arise in the bronchus associated lymphoid tissue.
- NHL involves the mediastinum less frequently than HL and mediastinal involvement in NHL typically reflects widespread disease dissemination.
- The anterior mediastinum is the focus from which HL of the chest appears to spread. It is extremely uncommon to have disease at other sites within the thorax in the absence of anterior mediastinal involvement.
- CT is ideally suited to demonstrate pleural and pleurally based lesions. These include solid plaques of tumor tissue and pleural effusions. It is however important to note that most pleural effusions in NHL are benign and are usually due to lymphatic obstruction. However the presence of pleural effusion in NHI, usually implies the presence of pleural tumor.
- The bones of the thorax including the ribs and vertebrae are involved due to their marrow content and usually in NHL. There is lytic lesion demonstrating permeative bone destruction, however sclerotic lesions may also be present. A large number of cases with bone involvement will show widely disseminated disease.

Abdominal Lymphoma

- CT is now the standard method of imaging the abdomen in patients with lymphoma.
- CT sections are taken following opacification of bowel either by oral contrast media or plain water may also be used. Both pre and post I/V contrast scans are taken.

- Abnormal lymph nodes are identified by sudden increase in size, the short axis diameter should be more than 1.5cm. Particular attention should be paid to retrocrural region where nodes greater than 0.6 cm are considered abnormal.
- Attention should also be paid to the retro peritoneum; the pelvic nodes and (esp. in NHL) the mesenteric nodes.
- Lymphomatous involvement of the liver and spleen most typically leads to enlargement, but there may also be focal lesions in the form of hypo dense areas, which are often large and well circumscribed.
- Miliary hypodense nodules may be seen in secondary hepatosplenic lymphoma.
- Hepatosplenic involvement is usually secondary and HI is the most common. Primary lymphomatous lesions are more commonly NHL.

Gastric Lymphoma

- Both Hodgkin's and NHL may involve the stomach either partially or diffusely.
- Stomach is the most common site of GI tract lymphoma especially NHL or extranodal Hodgkin's.
- The flexibility of gastric wall is preserved and mucosal folds and wall may be grossly thickened (4-5 cm) leading to linitis plastica like appearance.
- On CT there is homogenous overall attenuation and minimal enhancement after contrast administration. There may be diffuse retroperitoneal and mesenteric adenopathy.

Small Bowel Lymphomas

- Usually present with multiple sites of involvement and may present in children >6 years of age as intussuception.
- These arise from lymphoid tissues of peyer's patches with ileum being the most common site followed by jejunum and duodenum.
- May present as plaque like involvement of wall >5cm or more than 10cm ill length. There may be ulceration or desmoplastic response.
- Valvulae may be thickened with corrugated appearance.
- There may be aneurismal dilatation secondary to destruction of autonomic nerve plexus with muscle and tumor necrosis.
- There may be single or multiple polypoidal mucosal or submucosal, masses that may ulcerate or cause intussusception.
- There may be an endo or exophytic mass with small intramural component.
- Mesenteric or retroperitoneal adenopathy may be present displacing the bowel and forming ill-defined confluent masses.

Colonic Lymphomas

- Colon is less commonly involved than stomach or small bowel.
- Caecum is most commonly involved.
- It may present as a single mass, diffuse infiltration or polypoid lesion.
- There may be paradoxical dilatation, gross circumferential thickening (average size 5 cm).

CT of Blunt Chest Trauma

INTRODUCTION

Account for 100,000 hospital admissions a year in the United States and chest injuries are the third most frequent type of injury following high-speed motor vehicle accidents. With the advent of fast scanning with helical CT many institutions are screening trauma patients for aortic injuries using chest CT.

Frequency of injuries encountered in trauma patients referred for chest CT is as follows: Pneumothorax 69% (Figure 42.1), Lung contusion 67%, Rib fractures 66%, Hemithorax 28% (Figure 42.2), Flail chest 14%, etc.

AORTIC TRANSECTION

It is the cause of 16% of all deaths from automobile accidents. Of patients sustaining an aortic transection, 85% will die before reaching the hospital. Of the remaining short-term survivors, 50% will die within 24 hours.

Because of the high mortality rate associated with missed aortic injuries {4 months survival < 2%}. Traditionally, chest radiographic findings have been used to select patients to undergo aortography in the setting of high-speed blunt chest trauma.

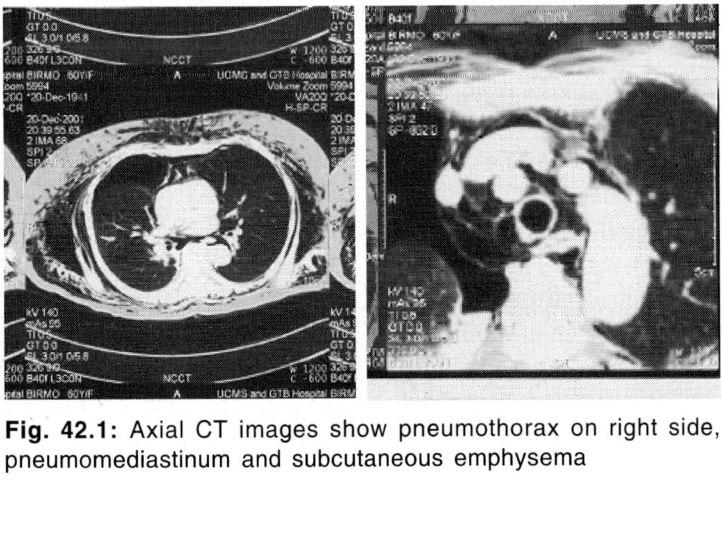

Fig. 42.1: Axial CT images show pneumothorax on right side, pneumomediastinum and subcutaneous emphysema

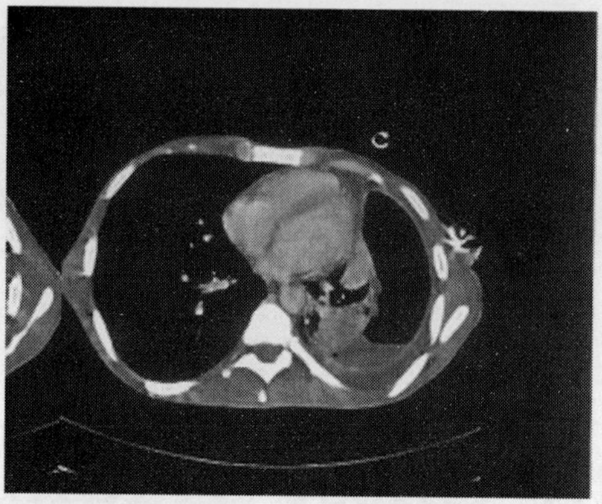

Fig. 42.2: Axial CT image shows hydropneumothorax with collapse of lung in left hemithorax

Chest Radiographic Findings Suggesting Aortic Injury include:

- Mediastinal widening — 8 cm.
- Loss of the aortic knob.
- Displacement of the nasogastric tube to the right of the T4 spinous process.
- Left apical pleural cap.
- Widened paraspinal lines.
- Widened right paratracheal stripe —5 mm.
- Loss of descending aorta line.

The Role of CT in Screening Patients for Aortic Injury is Controversial

The advantages of CT are:

1. A negative CT scan excludes a significant number of patients who might otherwise undergo an unnecessary and invasive procedure (mortality and morbidity risks for aortography are estimated at 1.7%).
2. In the course of evaluating the patient for possible aortic dissection with CT, many other unsuspected findings not identified by plain films are discovered including pneumothorax, pneumomediastinum, pneumopericardium, thoracic spine fractures, sternal and manubrial fractures and other skeletal lung trauma.
3. Using CT as a screening tool rather than the plain film to determine who needs aortography has potential health care cost savings.

The Disadvantages of Using CT to Screen Patients for Aortic Injury are:

1. Delay in obtaining the definitive aortogram or delays in taking the patient to surgery while pursing the CT may adversely affect prognosis in patients with aortic tears (With the increased speed of helical CT and the widespread use of abdominal CT to survey a majority of blunt trauma victims, this disadvantage is debatable).
2. Mediastinal hemorrhage is fairly common after blunt chest trauma. Most of these patients will not have an aortic injury, but a few will. These patients then undergo two contrast studies, a CT and an aortogram, both of which are likely to be negative.
3. Few, if any surgeons, will operate based on the CT findings of aortic injury without angiographic confirmation.
4. The utility of detecting branch vessel injury with CT is not known. Injuries to the great vessels occur in 1-2% of patients.

CT Findings of Aortic Injury Include:

- Mediastinal hemorrhage.
- Aortic contour deformity.
- Intimal flap.
- Thrombus protruding into the aortic lumen.
- Pseudo aneurysm.
- Abrupt change in caliber of the descending aorta compared with the ascending aorta (pseudocoarctation).
- And rarely contrast extravasation.

TRACHEOBRONCHIAL TEARS

Tears or fracture of the airways occur in approximately 1.5% of cases of blunt chest trauma.

They frequently go unrecognized on initial examination and delayed diagnosis is common. Bronchial fractures occur within 2.5 cm of the carina in 80% of patients.

Plain Film Findings of Bronchial Tear Include:

- Persistent pneumothorax despite adequate placement of one or more chest tubes.
- The fallen lung sign (it refers to the unusual appearance of a collapsed lung or lobe in the setting of bronchial injury and is thought to be due to disruption of the normal hilar attachments of the lung causing the collapsed lung to droop peripherally rather than centrally).
- Increasing subcutaneous emphysema.
- Pneumomediastinum and/or pneumothorax.
- Transection of the trachea particularly in the setting of neck trauma may also show– elevation of the hyoid bone on lateral c-spine films (hyoid bone above the level of the C3 vertebral body or greater cornu less than 2 cm from the angle of the mandible). This is, due to rupture of the infrahyoid muscles with unopposed action of the suprahyoid muscles.

CT Findings of Bronchial Fractures Include:

- A large pneumothorax despite adequate placement of one or more chest tubes.
- Massive pneumomediastinum and subcutaneous emphysema.
- Focal peribronchial collections of air.
- Discontinuity or irregularity of the bronchial wall.
- And a drooping, or collapsed lung or lobe of the lung.

  Another clue to tracheal tears on both plain films and CT is abnormality in the appearance or position of the endotracheal (ET) tube. These include:
- Overdistension of the ET cuff.
- Protrusion of the ET tube wall beyond the expected margins of the tracheal lumen.
- Extra luminal position of the tip of the tube.

DIAPHRAGMATIC RUPTURE

Disruption of the diaphragm occurs in 0.8-8% of cases of blunt trauma. Although the chest film is abnormal in 77% of these patients, the findings are nonspecific and the diagnosis is initially missed in the majority of cases. Early recognition and repair of diaphragmatic tears improves prognosis.

Diaphragmatic rupture is more common on the left side (77%-90%) that the right. Most tears are large (>10 cm) and occur in radical orientation in the posterolateral location. The diaphragm is the weakest at this location because this is where the pleuroperitoneal membrane finally closes during embryogenesis. Visceral herniation occurs in 32-58% of patients with diaphragmatic tears and the stomach is the most frequent abdominal viscus to herniate.

Chest Film Findings of Diaphragmatic Rupture Include:

- All elevated asymmetric or irregular diaphragm.
- Abnormal U shaped course of the nasogastric tube.
- Shift of the mediastinum to the opposite side.
- Herniation of bowel or abdominal organs into the chest.

CT Findings of Diaphragmatic Rupture Include:

- A discontinuity of the diaphragm (73%-82%).
- Herniation of peritoneal fat, bowel, or abdominal organ into the chest (55%).
- The collar sign or a waist-like constriction of bowel (27%).
- Identifying peritoneal fat, bowel or viscera

lateral to the lung or diaphragm, or posterior to the crus of the diaphragm.

- The absent diaphragm sign.
- Concurrent pneumothorax and pneumoperitoneum.
- Concurrent hemothorax and hemoperitoneum.

In stable patients or chronic cases, where CT is equivocal or nondiagnostic, MRI may also be valuable in documenting disruption of the diaphragm. With MR, one can directly acquire coronal and sagittal TI WI to trace the course of the diaphragm from its insertion sites to the dome of the hemi diaphragm on the suspected side. MR can be particularly helpful in the difficult case when the differential diagnosis is between diaphragmatic injury versus eventration or pre-existing elevation of the hemi diaphragm. The hemidiaphragm can be visualized with MRI as a hypointense band throughout its course, outlined by high signal abdominal and mediastinal fat on the left, and the liver on the right. Also, low tears involving the crust of the diaphragm are more convincingly displayed with coronal T1 images than with axial CT.

ESOPHAGEAL RUPTURE

Tears of the esophagus occur in an estimated 1% of patients experiencing blunt trauma and are far more common with penetrating or iatrogenic trauma. 82% of esophageal tears due to blunt trauma occur in the cervical and upper thoracic esophagus. Compression of the esophagus between the sternum and spinal column is one proposed mechanism of injury. Tears may also occur in the distal esophagus just above the GE junction along the posterolateral wall on the left side. The mechanism of injury in this setting is probably similar to spontaneous rupture in Boerhaave syndrome when esophageal pressure rises against a closed glottis. Esophageal rupture carries a high mortality rate secondary to rapidly developing mediastinitis. Survival improves dramatically if the esophageal injury is recognized and treated within 24 hours of occurrence.

Chest Film Findings of Esophageal Rupture Include:

- A large left pneumothorax.
- Extensive pneumomediastinum.
- Subcutaneous emphysema left pleural effusion.
- Left lower lobe atelectasis; and
- The "V" sign of Naclerio.

CT findings of esophageal rupture include all of the above and/or focal extra luminal and collections at the site of tear; mediastinal or esophageal wall hematoma. Occasionally a tract at the site of the tear can be identified on CT. In the setting of severe blunt chest trauma, the esophagus can also be obstructed and entrapped by fracture dislocations of the thoracic spine demonstrated on chest or thoracic spine CT examinations.

Diagnosis of esophageal rupture is usually confirmed with a swallow study using non-ionic oral contrast.

THORACIC SPINE INJURY

Fractures of the thoracic spine occur in 30% of blunt trauma cases. Spinal cord injury occurs in a high percentage of these patients. The most vulnerable portion of the thoracic spine is at the thoracoabdominal junction involving the T9-T11 vertebral bodies. Sternal fractures are often associated with T-spine fractures.

Plain film findings of thoracic spine fractures are often subtle and difficult to identify due to the limited quality of many trauma films. Only 51% of spine fractures could be identified on the initial chest radiography. Plain film findings include:

- Widening of the paraspinal lines.
- Mediastinal widening.
- Loss of height of the vertebral body or obscuration of a pedicle or pedicles.
- Left apical cap; and
- Deviation of the nasogastric tube.

On CT findings of vertebral body fractures include paraspinal hematoma; and disruption/ fracture of the vertebral body, pedicle, and/or spinous processes. Mediastinal hematoma confined to the posterior mediastinum is often a clue to a vertebral body fracture.

Compression fractures may be easily overlooked on axial CT scans of the chest unless bone windows are scrutinized. Supplementing axial images with reconstructed sagittal and coronal multiplanar images is often useful to confirm a simple compression fracture. One may also verify compression fractures by reviewing the lateral CT scout view. Further evaluation of thoracic spine injuries usually requires a dedicated T-spine CT examination of MRI.

CHEST WALL TRAUMA

Rib fractures occur in 60% of blunt trauma cases. Only 20% are detected by portable supine trauma chest films. Fractures of the first rib are an indication of severe blunt chest, trauma and may be associated with aortic tears, bronchial tears, and injuries to the subclavian vessels. The flail chest is present when there are 5 or more rib fractures in a row or 3 or more segmental (2 fractures in one rib) rib fractures. The significance of recognizing a flail chest is that respiratory failure may develop due to paradoxical movement of the flail segment.

Other chest wall trauma includes soft tissue hematomas and contusions. These are often evident on CT scanning of the chest and often indicate the region of primary impact. Overlying soft tissue edema or hematoma on CT, often indicates an underlying rib or other bony injury, which should be sought by reviewing the images using bone window settings. Lacerations of chest wall arterial vessels can result in massive chest wall hematomas.

SEAT BELT INJURIES

Seat belt injuries of the three point restraint type (combined lap and shoulder belt devices), if severe, produce bruises in the subcutaneous tissue and fat of the anterior chest wall identifiable on physical exam and on CT 30% of seat belt injuries severe enough to cause skin abrasions are associated with significant internal injuries. Evidence of seat belt contusions on CT should prompt a careful search for the following injuries in the chest.

- Fractures of the sternum.
- Ribs (bilateral along the diagonal course of the seat belt), and clavicles.
- Fractures of the transverse processes of C-7 or T-1.
- Aortic transection; cardiac contusions or ventricular rupture.
- Vascular injuries to the subclavian artery or superior vena cava.
- Tracheal or laryngeal tears; and
- Diaphragmatic rupture.

LUNG INJURY

Pulmonary contusions are common following blunt trauma and are due to hemorrhage into the alveoli. They appear quickly after trauma as areas of focal airspace consolidation on both chest films and CT. Typically, the air space consolidation due to contusion clears during the first week after trauma.

Pulmonary laceration is tears in the lung parenchyma. If the laceration fills with blood a spherical hematoma forms. If it fills with air, a traumatic pneumatocele or air cyst forms. If both blood and air are present, an air-fluid level may also be seen. In cases of severe blunt chest trauma, one may see 'pulverized' lung on CT, an area of airspace opacification with multiple small 5-10 mm air cysts disrupting the lung parenchyma. CT is more sensitive than plain films for detection of contusions and lacerations by a factor of 3 to 1.

Other causes of airspace opacification on chest films and CT scans of trauma patients are: aspiration pneumonia; atelectasis due to splinting or mucous plugs; cardiogenic and noncardiogenic pulmonary edema. After 24 hours, particularly in cases of severe trauma with long bone fractures, one must also consider fat embolism and developing Acute Respiratory Distress Syndrome.

PNEUMOTHORAX AND HEMOTHORAX

Small to moderate sized pneumothoraces that are not appreciated on plain films are frequently identified on Chest CT following blunt trauma. These are often in the anterobasilar location. CT is also more specific than plain films in characterizing pleural effusions.

Hemothoraces often show areas of high CT attenuation due to blood. A rapidly accumulating pleural effusion in the setting of trauma may be due to a hemothorax or a chylothorax due to a ruptured thoracic duct.

Persistent or increasing pneumothorax or hemothorax may be due to a variety of causes including bronchial tears, vascular injuries or malfunctioning or malpositioned chest tubes.

CHEST TUBE POSITIONING

Placement of thoracostomy tubes for chest trauma is often done in an emergency setting.

Malpositioning of chest tubes in extra thoracic, intraparenchymal, mediastinal, and intra-fissural locations is common (26%-58%). Complications of misplaced chest tubes include intercostal artery lacerations, liver lacerations, splenic injuries, and diaphragmatic tears. Extra thoracic, mediastinal and intraparenchymal chest tubes require immediate repositioning or cement. The significance of chest tubes within the fissure is controversial, though development of empyema within the fissural chest tubes has been reported. CT is much more accurate than portable AP chest films in identifying malpositioned chest tubes in the trauma patient.

CARDIAC INJURY

Cardiac injuries due to blunt chest trauma include cardiac contusions, cardiac rupture, pneumopericardium and hemopericardium, cardiac tamponade, and cardiac valve dysfunction.

Cardiac contusion is suspected when Electrocardiographic changes occur in the setting of blunt trauma. Pneumopericardium and hemopericardium are recognized on CT by the presence of air or high attenuation blood in the pericardial sac. Both may cause cardiac tamponade and may require emergent pericardial drainage. Constrictive pericarditis may develop as a long-term complication of hemo-pericardium. Echocardiography is often used at the bedside to evaluate for cardiac injuries, but hemopericardium in particular can be missed on echocardiograms due to the change in the echo properties of hemorrhagic fluid.

Embryological Development of Diaphragm

The diaphragm develops from following structures:

1. The septum transversum, which form the central tendon of diaphragm.
2. The pleuroperitoneal membranes.
3. Muscular components from lateral/dorsal body wall.
4. The mesentry of esophagus in which crura of diaphragm develops.

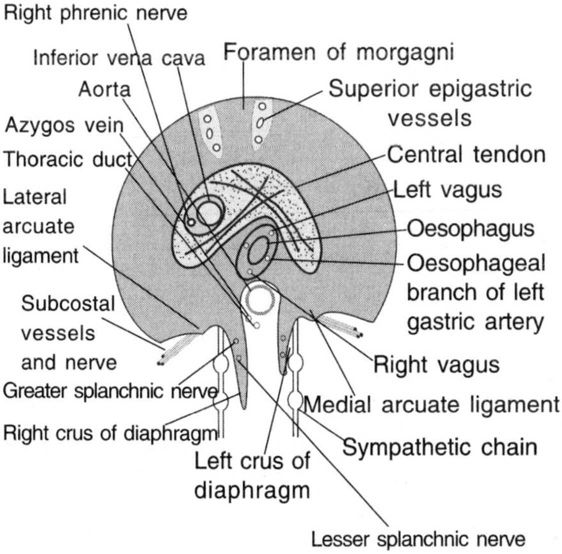

Fig. 43.1: The diaphragm as seen from below

APPLIED

1. Congenital Diaphragmatic Hernia:

- Tends to appear shortly after birth.
- Over 80% presenting on left side.
- There is respiratory distress, apparent dextrocardia, a scaphoid abdomen, and radiological appearance of bowel in the hemithorax.

Sites:

i. Foramen of Margagni: Anteriorly placed hernias with defect between the sternal and costal attachment of diaphragm. The most commonly involved viscus is transverse colon.

ii. Through Foramen of Bochdalek: This represents the persistence of the pleuroperitoneal canal with a posterolateral defect.

Most common diaphragmatic hernia in children and presents with classic triad of:

- Respiratory distress.
- Apparent dextrocardia.
- Scaphoid abdomen.

iii. Through oesophageal foramen.

The sternal part ↓	Costal part ↓	Vertebral part ↓	
Consist of two slips right/ left that arises from back of xaphoid process	Consists of broad slips one from inner surface of lower of each of six ribs	Right curves Larger Arises from bodies of L-1, L-2, L-3 vertebrae	Left curves Smaller Arises from bodies of L-1, L-3 vertebrae

2. **Eventration of the Diaphragm**

   This represents an abnormally elevated position of one or both diaphragm from paralysis or atrophy of muscle fibres.

   There may be some spontaneous improvement if the condition occurs in perinatal period but long standing cases with paradoxical respiration may benefit from surgery.

ANATOMY

The origin of diaphragm can be divided into: (see Fig. 43.1)

- The medial margin of the two arura is joined to each other to form median arcuate ligament.
- The medial arcuate ligament represents condensation of fascies over quadrant lumborum.
- The lateral arcuate ligament represents the condensation of fibres over psoas muscle. From its extensive origin the muscular fibre of diaphragm run upwards and converge to be inserted on the margins of large flat central tendon.

RELATIONS

- Superior surface lies in relation to 3 venous membranes.
- On each side pleura separates it from base of corresponding lung. Over the middle falcum of central tendon the pericardium is interposed between it and the heart.

Inferior surface: Mostly covered by peritoneum

Right side	-	Right lobe of liver Right kidney Right supra renal
Left side	-	Left lobe of liver Fundus of stomach, spleen Left kidney Left supra renal

APERTURES IN THE DIAPHRAGM

1. *Aortic aperture T12-L1 IV disc.*
   - Aorta
   - Thoracic duct
   - Azygos
   - Hemizygos veins.
2. *Aperture for oesophagus:* T10 formed by splitting of fibres of right crus.
   - Oesophagus.
   - Right/left gastric nerves.
   - Oesophageal branches of left gastric artery.
3. Opening for the inferior vena cava (IVC): Central tendon at the level of T8. The wall of IVC is adherent to the opening and this helps in its expansion during inspiration, also transmits whole part of right phrenic nerve.
4. The left phrenic nerves passes through the muscular part of the diaphragm.

RADIOLOGICAL ANATOMY

1. **X-ray:** Superior profile of diaphragm rises on each side of cardiac pattern to a smooth convex dome.

   Right dome is normally higher than the left by 2-2.5 cm on full inspiration, right dome crosses anterior part of 6th rib.

2. **USG: Specular Reflector:** A diaphragm is a large and relatively smooth surface that reflects sound like an interior reflects right. Thus the sound striking the diaphragm at nearly a 90° angle is reflected directly back to the transducer resulting in a strong echo sound while those striking the diaphragm obliquely reflects away from the transducer and an echo is not displayed.

Muscles of diaphragm are seen as thin hypoechoic line.

- The interface between diaphragm and liver appear as thin echogenic line.
- The interface between diaphragm and lung appear as a stronger and thicker echogenic band.
- Occasionally another thin echogenic line is present cephalad to diaphragm using interface. This is a mirror image artifact of diaphragm liver interface.
- The diaphragmatic slips refer to normal prominent muscular insertions. The cross-section they may appear as focal echogenic masses of various sizes/shapes that may be mistaken for focal liver/peritoneal lesion.

  The diaphragmatic crura may be seen as thin hypoechoic band anterior to upper abdominal aorta and posterior to IVC. They become thicker on deep inspiration.

CAUSES OF ELEVATED HEMIDIAPHRAGM

Thoracic Conditions

- Collapse
- Pneumonia
- Pulmonary infarction
- Adhesions
- Phrenic nerve palsy
- Pleural effusion.

Upper Abdominal Conditions

- Hepatomegaly
- Pancreatitis
- Subphrenic abscess
- Liver abscess.

CAUSES OF INCREASED SPACE BETWEEN GASTRIC FUNDUS AND DIAPHRAGM

- Normal space—3-11mm.
- Left lobe of liver/normal/enlarged
- Spleen
- Ascites
- Subphrenic abscess
- Tumors
- Tumors of kidney/adrenal/pancreatic/diaphragm.

CAUSES OF BILATERAL ELEVATION OF DIAPHRAGM

- Ascites
- Pregnancy
- Hepatosplenomegaly
- Large abdominal neoplasm/cyst.

Diaphragmatic Hernias

Normal Anatomy

Herniation of abdominal viscera into the thoracic cavity occurs through:

- The diaphragmatic hiatus–Sliding and paraesophageal hiatus hernia.
- Congenital defect.
- Bochdalek.
- Morgagni hernia.
- Diaphragmatic hernia.

SLIDING HIATUS HERNIA (Figure 44.1)

- Most frequent type of diaphragmatic hernia.

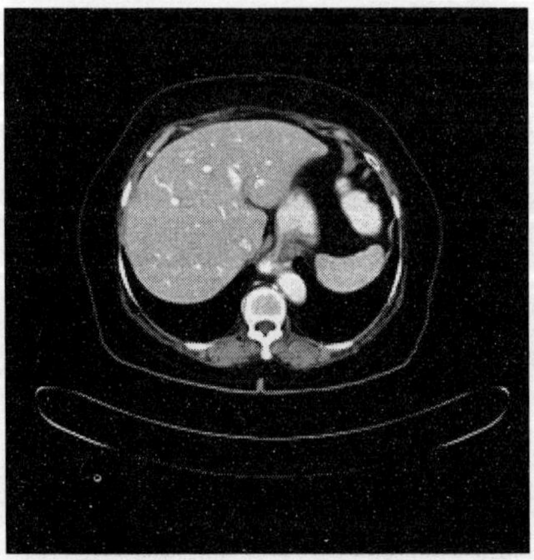

Fig. 44.1: Axial CT image shows hiatus hernia

- Phrenico oesophageal ligaments extend from the margins of the diaphragmatic hiatus to the lower oesophagus and it is the stretching with age or the rupture of these ligaments that allow a hernia to develop.

  Oesophagus normally shortens in length during swallowing and the elasticity of the phrenico-oesophageal ligaments allow the gastroesophageal junction to move up to 2 cm above the diaphragmatic hiatus.
- Small hernias appear only in lying down posture and they reduce spontaneously on standing or sitting. Larger hernia become fixed and predispose to gastroesophageal reflux and peptic esophagitis.
- A sliding hiatus hernia is a pouch of stomach that protrudes more than 2cm above the hiatus.
  - Three or more gastric folds may be identified passing from the stomach across the hiatus on barium study and the Z-line and area gastricae are located above the hiatus.
  - The hiatus is wide measuring more than 3 cm in diameter.
  - On CT the diaphragmatic crura are separated by more than 15 mm and the hernia produces a mass of soft tissue density that protrudes above the hiatus

and which may be surrounded by mesenteric fat.

Rolling Hiatus Hernia

- It is a rare type of diaphragmatic hernia in which the cardia remains below the diaphragm while the fundus herniate through a weakness or tear in the phrenico-oesophageal membrane to lie alongside the lower oesophagus.
- The most frequent complication is anemia from chronic bleeding with slight risk of peptic esophagitis.
- Most paraesophageal hernias are not reducible.
- Larger hernias increase the risk of volvulus, strangulation and infarction of the stomach.

Congenital Hernias

- These usually result from failure of closure of the pleuroperitoneal canal.

Two types:

- Bochdalek – congenital weakness or defect hernia in posterior aspect of one or both hemidiaphragm.
- Morgagni hernia.

  ↓

  Defect or weakness between the sternal and costal attachment of the diaphragm.
  Incidence — 1 in 2400 births.

  More common on the left side.

C/F: Usually seen as an emergency in the neonatal period.

Child is brought with a severe respiratory distress and scaphoid abdomen.

Usually associated with pulmonary hyperplasia.

CXR: A mass of water or mixed water or gas density in one hemithorax.

The diaphragmatic contour is lost.

The lesion is usually centred in the lower chest.

The mass effect may be considerable with obvious shift of the mediastinum to opposite side.

If a nasogastric tube is inserted, this may either be embedded in the region of the esophagogastric junction or turn up in the chest cavity.

In morgagni hernia, the hernia contents are usually extraperitoneal fat, omentum, liver and transverse colon, which make the diagnosis obvious on chest radiograph.

USG: It is useful in the diagnosis of congenital diaphragmatic hernia both prenatally and postnatally.

Peristalsis of bowel within the thorax may be observed and the normal uninterrupted contour of the diaphragm is not seen.

On the left side, there may be herniation of the spleen or kidney without herniation of the bowel.

Poor Prognostic Indicators

- Absence of aeration of the contralateral lung or the presence of a contralateral pneumothorax.
- Right-sided defect.
- Intrathoracic position of the stomach.

DIAPHRAGMATIC RUPTURE

Mechanism of Injury

- Penetrating injury.
- Blunt trauma usually high speed motor vehicle accidents or fall from a height.

Incidence

- Seen in 3% to 5% of patients admitted to major trauma centres.
- Mortality is approx. 20% to 25% mainly due to associated injuries.

- Over 90% have solid abdominal organ damage.
- 10% have associated aortic laceration.
- Pelvic fractures, spinal fractures and closed head injuries are common.

Plain Films

- Pleural fluid ± pulmonary contusion.
- Elevated hemidiaphragm.
- Stomach and bowel loops high in the chest.
- Abnormal course of a nasogastric tube.

USG

- Disrupted diaphragm.
- Floating portion of diaphragm – flapping of diaphragm on real time USG.
- Demonstration of liver or bowel herniation.

CT

- High position of the liver or the stomach in the chest with contralateral shift of the cardiac shadow (Figure 44.2).

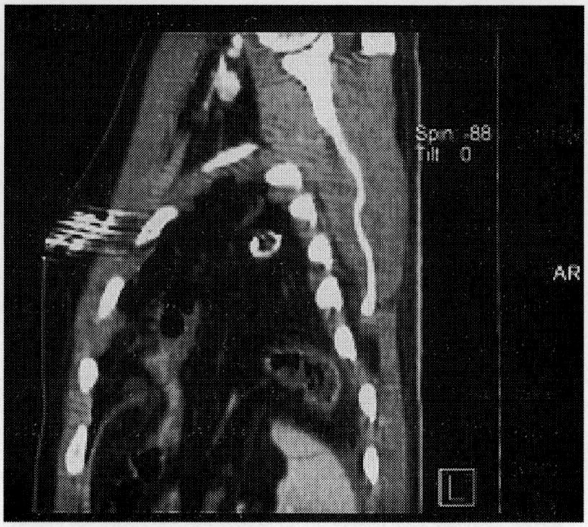

Fig. 44.2: Sagittal CT image shows traumatic diaphragmatic hernia

- Diaphragmatic defect may be directly seen.
- Absent diaphragm sign.

MRI

- Disrupted diaphragm may be seen.
- Herniation of liver, stomach or bowel clearly shown.

	Eventration	**Diaphragmatic hernia**
Cause	Weakness in the muscular portion of the diaphragm	Protrusion of contents through diaphragmatic hiatus
	Congenital	Congenital and acquired
Fluoroscopy	Sniff test paradoxical movement present	Not present
CXR lat.	The raised diaphragm appears as an even line with a superior convex curve running from the back of the sternum to the post chest wall round the defect.	The low line of the stomach will only occupy a part of thorax and will merge in front or behind with a more horizontal line caused by the remains of the diaphragm

Embryological Development of Great Vessels of Neck, Thorax and Abdomen

As the branchial arches develop during the 4th week of intrauterine life, they receive arteries from the heart. These bronchial arch arteries, called aortic arches, arise from the dilated region of truncus arteriosus known as the aortic sac and terminate in dorsal aorta of corresponding side. Although six pairs of aortic arches develop, they are not all present at the same time.

DERIVATIVES OF AORTIC ARCHES

- During the six to eighth weeks, the primitive aortic arch pattern is transformed into the basic adult arterial arrangement.

The First Pair of Aortic Arches

- These vessels largely disappear, but they form part of maxillary arteries. These may also contribute to development of external carotid arteries.

The Second Pair of Aortic Arches

- Dorsal portions of these vessels persist and form parts of stapedial arteries, they disappear during the fetal period leaving foramina in the stapes.

The Third Pair of Aortic Arches

- Proximal part—Common carotid arteries.
- Distal portion—Join with dorsal aortic to form internal carotid arteries.

The Fourth Pair of Aortic Arches

- Left fourth aortic arch forms part of arch of aorta. The proximal part of arch of aorta develops from aortic sac and distal part from the left dorsal aorta.
- The right fourth aortic arch becomes the proximal portion of right subclavian artery. The distal part of right subclavian artery derived from right dorsal aorta and right seventh intersegmental artery.

  Left subclavian artery forms from the left seventh intersegmental artery. As the development proceeds differential growth shifts the origin of left subclavian artery cranially.

The Fifth Pair of Aortic Arches

- In about 50% of embryos, the fifth pair of arches appear as rudimentary vessels that soon degenerates, leaving no derivatives. In rest, these arteries never develop.

The Sixth Pair of Aortic Arches

- The proximal part of left sixth aortic arch persists as proximal part of left pulmonary artery. The distal part which passes from left pulmonary artery to the dorsal aorta persist as a shunt called the ductus arteriosus.

  Right sixth aortic arch – proximal part persist as proximal part of right pulmonary artery's distal part degenerates.

  The distal parts of pulmonary arteries are derived from the buds of sixth aortic arches.

AORTIC ARCH ANOMALIES

Coarctation of Aorta

Post ductal	Pre ductal
Common	Less common
Constriction is below the level of ductus arteriosus which usually closes and forms ligamentum arteriosum	Constriction is above the level of ductus arteriosus. The ductus usually remains open
Better development of collateral circulation during fetal period	

Patent Ductus Arteriosus

- This common manifest is two to three times more common in females than in males. Failure of distal partition of left sixth arch to involute after birth and form ligamentun arteriosum.

Double Aortic Arch

- Characterized by a vascular ring which many compress tracheal oesophagus. The ring results from failure of involution of the distal partition of the right dorsal aorta. Thus both right and left aortic arch arise from the ascending aorta. The vascular ring is initially large but gradually decrease in size. Usually right aortic arch is larger and passes behind trachea and oesophagus.

Right Aortic Arch

- When entire right dorsal aorta persist and the distal segment of left dorsal aorta involutes a right aortic arch results.

Right aortic arch without a retroesophageal component No vascular ring formed asymptomatic Associated cardiac anomalies. E .g. Tetralogy of Fallot, Pulmonary atresia with VSD, double outlet right ventricle, transient arteriosus	Right aortic arch with retroesophageal component Vascular ring formed, compressing trachea and oesophagus

EMBRYOLOGICAL DEVELOPMENT OF GREAT VEINS OF NECK, THORAX AND ABDOMEN

In the fifth week of intrauterine life, three pairs of great veins can be distinguished:

1. Vitelline veins – carrying blood from yolk sac to sinus venosus.
2. Umbilical veins – Carrying oxygenated blood from placentae to the embryo.
3. Cardinal veins – Draining the body of embryo proper.

Vitelline Veins

- Before entering sinus venosus, the vitelline veins form a closure around the duodenum and pass through septum transversum. The liver cards growing into septum interrupt the course of veins and an extensive vascular network is formed known as hepatic sinusoids. With the reduction of left sinus harm, blood from left side of liver is rechanelled towards

Section 4

the right resulting in enlargement of right vitelline vein (right hepato cardial channel). Ultimately right hepato cardiac channel form the post hepatic partition of inferior vena cava. The proximal and distal parts of left vitelline vein disappears. The anastomotio network around duodenum develops into a single vessel, the portal vein. The superior mesenteric vein develops from right vitelline vein.

Vitelline Vein

- Post-hepatic partition of inferior vena cava portal vein superior mesenteric vein.

Umbilical Veins

The umbilical vein pass initially in each side of the liver but soon become connected to hepatic sinusoids. The proximal part of both umbilical veins, as well as remainder of right umbilical vein then disappear so that the left vein is the only one to carry blood from placenta to liver. With the increase of placental circulation, a direct communication is formed between left umbilical vein and right hepato cardiac channel, the ductus venosus. This vessel bypass the sinusoidal plexus of liver after birth left umbilical vein and ductus venosus are obliterated and form ligamentum teres hepatis and ligamentum venosum respectively.

Cardinal Veins

- Initially cardinal vein from the main venous drainage system of embryo.

  Ant. cardinal vein – cephalic part.

  Post-cardinal vein – remaining part of body.

During fifth to seventh week a number of additional veins are formed.

1. Subcardinal veins – which mainly drains kidneys.
2. The sacrocardinal veins – which drain lower extremity.
3. The supracardinal veins – which drain body wall by way of intercostal veins.
   - Anastomosis between anterior cardinal vein—left brachiocephalic veins.
   - Superior vena cava—Right common cardinal vein and proximal portion of right ant. card. vein.
   - Left renal vein—anastomosis between subcardinal veins.
   - Renal segment of IVC—right subcardinal vein.
   - Left common iliac vein—anastomosis between sacrocardinal veins.
   - Sacrocardinal segment of IVC—right sacrocardinal vein.
   - Azygous vein—right supracardinal and a portion of right posterior cardinal vein.
   - Hemizygous vein—left supracardinal vein.

DOUBLE INFERIOR VENA CAVA (Figure 45.1)

- Left vacrocardinal vein has fented to lose its connection with left subcardinal and left common iliac may/may not be present.

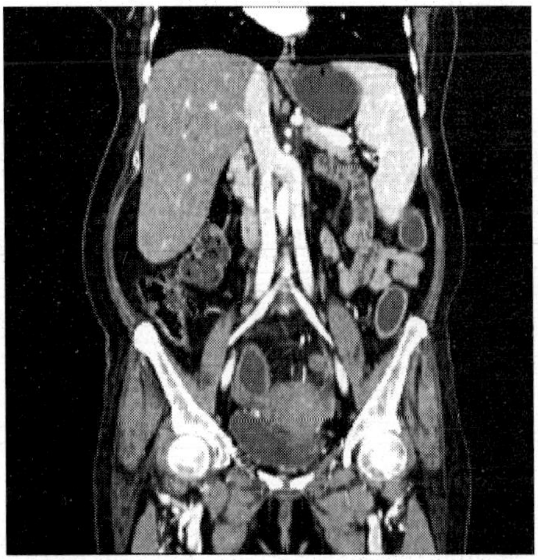

Fig. 45.1: Coronal MPR CT image shows infrarenal duplication of the inferior vena cava

Section 4—Cardiovascular System

Chapter 46

Carotid Artery Disease

EVALUATION OF CAROTID ARTERIES

- US.
- Colour doppler.
- MR angiograpy.
- Spiral CT an angiograpy (Figure 46.1).
- Intra-arterial DSA gold standard.

MANAGEMENT OF CAROTID ARTERY DISEASE

For Medical Management

- Asymptomatic stenosis <30%.
- Symptomatic stenosis <70%.

For Surgical Management

- Asymptomatic >80%.
- Symptomatic stenosis >70%.
- High risk with symptomatic stenosis >70% - unprove.

Indications of Intervention

- Stenosis of 80% and in combination with stenosis or occlusion of the contralateral carotid artery.

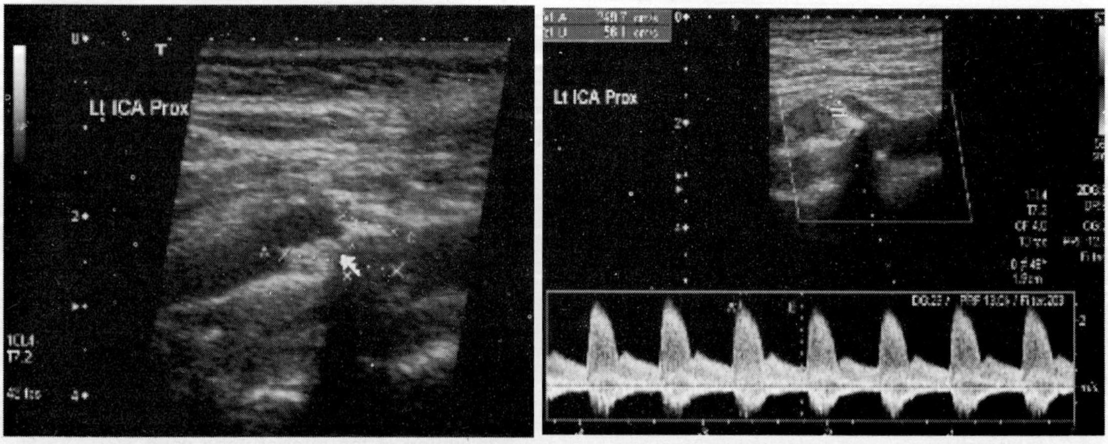

Fig. 46.1: Moderate amount of plaque at the origin of the left common carotid artery (arrow) extending into the internal carotid artery. Velocity measurements indicate stenosis in the order of 70%

- Incomplete circle of Willis decreasing the chances of adequate cross flow.
- Significant supra aortic multivessel disease.

ENDARTERECTOMY VS STENTING

Contraindications of Endarterectomy

- Short thick necks.
- High carotid bifurcations.
- Long lesions.
- Previously operated or irradiated neck.
- Lesions in non-cervical Intracranial Aneurysms (ICA).

Complications of Endarterectomy

- Neurological complications.
- Cranial nerve palsies.
- Hematomas, infections.
- Restenosis.

Advantage of Angioplasty

- Controlled injury to the vessel and plaque fracture, displacement, stretching and dissection.

Indications

- Symptomatic stenosis >70%.
  Asymptomatic stenosis >80%.
- Asymptomatic stenoses with unilateral Intracranial Aneurysm occlusion, necessitating of major surgery or degree of stenosis increasing >15% within 6 months.
- In patients with a hostile neck situation due to previous carotid surgery, radical neck dissection prior radiotherapy or inflammatory disease like lymph node TB.
- Patients with bilateral carotid disease, tandem lesions, and multiple vessel disease or in patients with poor cross flow or incomplete circle of Willis.
- Advanced age and increased operative risk factors.
- Postoperative recurrent stenosis or non-atherosclerotic carotid artery disease (FHO, Takayasu's radiation induced).

Procedure

- Aspirin 325 mg OD and Ticlopidine 300 mg IB are started 3 days prior.
- Intra operative monitoring of the patients BP, heart rate and activated clotting time performed.
- Patients are atropinised through an IV access prior to the procedure.
- PC access via the femoral artery is used.
  ASF sheath is placed in femoral artery.
- 5000 units of heparin are administered to raise the ACT around 200 sec.
- A diagnostic angiogram is performed.

A Guidewire is Used for Selective Angiography

- A long resistant sheath with its dilator is advanced over the wire.
- After crossing the stenosis a pre dilatation is performed with a low profile, small size shaft balloon catheter.
- Stents is placed across the stenosis.
- Post dilatation is performed.
- Angiography is done.

Implications

- Access site hematoma.
- Dissection.
- Acute thrombosis.
- Embolic occlusion of vessel.
- Hyperperfusion syndrome.
- Restenosis.
- Carotid artery rupture in the neck.
- Formation of carotico cavernous fistula.
- Rupture of carotid artery aneurysm.

INTRA - ARTERIAL THROMBOLYSIS IN STROKE

Local Intra-Arterial Thrombolysis

- A cranial CT is done to exclude an intracranial hemorrhage — a contraindication to thrombolysis.

- Diagnostic angiography is done to establish the diagnosis and the location of the occluding thrombus.
- A catheter is navigated through a guiding catheter placed in the affected ICA. The guiding catheter is irrigated with a continuous infusion of normal saline containing nimodipine and heparin.
- The tip of the catheter is wedged in the thrombus.
- Thrombolytic agent is infused.

Advantage of Intra-Arterial Thrombolysis

- High local concentration of thrombolytic agent.

Indications of Intra-Arterial Thrombolysis

1. Occlusion of the distal ICA.
2. Occlusion of the M1 or M2 segment.
3. Occlusion of the large branch of the MCA at the trifurcation with associated significant neurological deficit.
4. Occlusion of the basilar artery tip.

Complication

- Intracranial hemorrhage.

RUPTURED INTRACRANIAL ANEURYSMS

Techniques for Management

- Endovascular coiling.
- Surgical clipping.
- Electrically detachable plastinum coils.

Indications for Platinum Coils Use

1. Multiple aneurysms.
2. Resurgery for a 2nd aneurysm.
3. Pre an anticoagulation treatment.
4. Associated vasospasm.
5. Unsuccessful clipping.

Contraindications

- MCA bifurcation aneurysm.
- Giant/very large aneurysm.
- Very small aneurysms (<2-3 mm).
- Large associated parenchymal hematoma.
- Aneurysm with a wide neck.
- Branch wiring from the neck of aneurysm.
- Grossly tortuous vascular anatomy.

Procedure

- A preliminary angiography is done.
- A baseline ACT is performed.
- The procedure is carried out under GA.
- A bolus of 5000 units of heparin is administered with 1000 units every hour.
- The heparinization is monitored by frequent ACT check.
- A suitable 5F or 6F guiding catheter is placed in a parent artery.
- A micro catheter is then advanced with a micro guide wire.
- A coil is placed in the largest aneurysm and is allowed to form a basket.
- The aneurysm is then packed with coils of progressively smaller size till no further spaces in the coil mark are appreciated.
- A chest angiogram is then performed.

Technical Problems and Solutions

1. Spasm of parent artery—infusion of 50-100 ugms of NG with addition of nimodepine.
2. Aneurysm perforation—reversal of heparin and continued coiling.
3. Coil stacking—the coil is withdrawn and a larger diameter coil is used.

Communicating HC—lumbar CSF drainage and subsequent lumboperitoneal or ventriculo peritoneal shunt is done.

Aortic Pathologies

1. Root of aorta – from aortic valve to sinotubular junction.
2. Ascending aorta – from sinotubular junction to origin of innominate artery, passes superiorly and to the right.
3. Arch of aorta – from origin of innominate artery to origin of left subclavian artery (SCA).
   - Passes posteriorly to left anterior to trachea.
   - Gives 3 branches – BCA, Lt. CCA and Lt. SCA.
4. Descending aorta – beyond the origin of Lt. SCA.
   Passes inferiorly in posterior mediastinum anterolateral to spine and posterolateral to esophagus continuing into abdominal aorta at level of diaphragm.
5. Abdominal aorta (Figure 47.1).

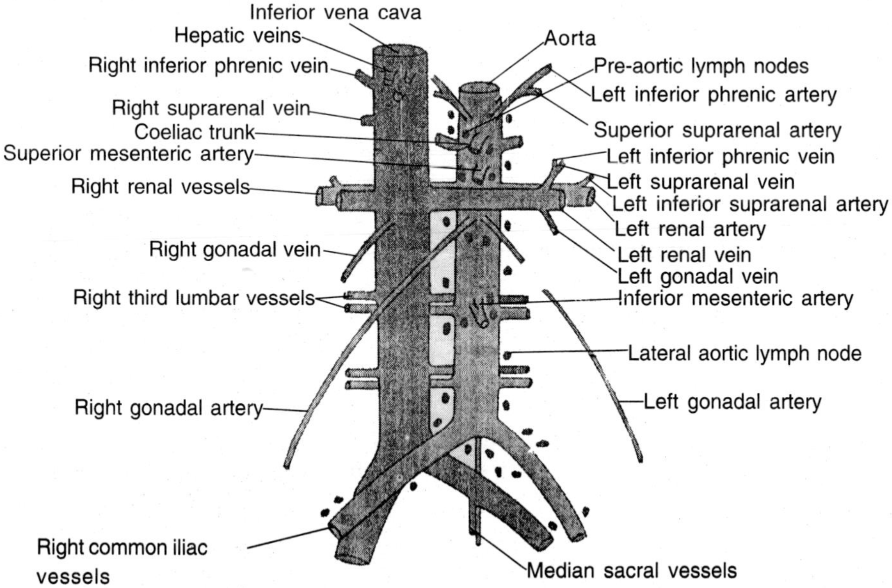

Fig. 47.1: The abdominal aorta, and inferior vena cava and associated lymph nodes

NORMAL DIAMETERS

Mid ascending aorta – 3.3±0.3 cm.

Arch of aorta – 1.5±1.2 cm.

Descending aorta – 2.2±0.3 cm.

- Ratio of ascending to descending aorta – 1.5:1. This ratio decreases with age because the descending aorta increases in diameter more quickly with age.
- In measuring aortic aneurysm the largest short axis diameter should be measured.

Causes of Enlarged Aorta

1. **Volume overload**
   a. AR.
   b. PDA.
2. **Post stenotic dilatation**
   a. In valvular AS.
3. **Intraluminal pressures**
   a. Systemic HT.
   b. Coarctation.
4. **Mural weakness**
   a. Cystic medial necrosis.
   b. Congenital.
   c. Infective/mycotic.
   d. Atherosclerotic.
   e. Traumatic.

Thoracic Aortic Aneurysms

- Aneurysm represents a permanent dilatation of the aortic wall.

Types

1. *True aneurysm*
   - Dilatation of all layers of weakened but intact wall.
2. *False aneurysm*
   - Focal perforation of vessel wall with escaped blood contained by adventitia, perivascular connective tissue and organized blood.

Fusiform

- Involve entire circumference of wall.

Saccular

- Involve only a portion of the wall.

Etiology

1. *Atherosclerotic aneurysm*
   - Most true aneurysms of thoracic aorta (70-90%) are caused by atherosclerosis.
   - Usually fusiform (80%).
   - Most frequent in proximal descending aorta.
2. *Degenerative*
   - Cystic medial degeneration – most common cause of ascending aortic aneurysms.
   - Seen with Margan's or Ehler's Denlos syndrome or with age and hypertension.
   - There is typically fusiform enlargement of ascending aorta which decreases in size as it approaches the arch. The arch is usually normal. (In atherosclerosis commonly ascending aorta and arch both are involved).
3. *Mycotic*
   - Due to intravenous drug abuse.
   - Bacterial endocarditis.
   - Aortic injury.
   - Typically saccular.
   - Commonly involve ascending aorta.
4. *Aortitis*

Infective or Non-infective aortitis

Infective	Non-infective aortitis
↓	↓
Syphilis	Takayasu arteritis
	Giant cell arteritis

5. *Post traumatic*
   - Most common type of aneurysm in young patients.
   - They are pseudo aneurysms.
   - Most occur near aortic isthmus, are usually saccular.
   - May calcify, contain thrombus and progressively enlarge.

Clinical Presentation

- Mean age =60 years
  M: F = 3:1
- Most patients are asymptomatic and aneurysm is detected as incidentally on plain chest radiograph.
- Substernal/back/shoulder pain 26%.
- Dysphagia from esophageal compression.
- Dyspnea from airway compression.
- Hoarseness of voice from recurrent laryngeal nerve compression.
- SVC syndrome due to venous compression.
- Fever in mycotic aneurysm.

Diagnosis

1. *Chest Radiograph*
   - Widening of the mediastinum.
   - Round or oval soft tissue mass with a well-defined outline, in close proximity to aorta.
   - Wide tortuous aorta.
   - Curvilinear peripheral calcification in mass (75%).
   - Pressure erosion of sternum or anterior scalloping of one or two vertebral bodies.
2. *CT Scan*
   - It can accurately show the size and extent.
   - There is usually sacular or fusiform dilatation of aortic segment.
   - Transverse diameter >4 cm indicates aneurysm.

Calcification in the aortic wall

- It is typically peripheral (in dissection it may be displaced centrally).
- Dystrophic calcification can be seen in mural thrombus.

Intraluminal thrombus

- May be crescentic or circumferential.
- Thrombus is more common in aortic arch and descending aorta than in ascending aorta.
- Intraluminal thrombus may cause irregular lumen.

Displacement of adjacent mediastinal structures

E.g. displacement of trachea, esophagus, bronchial tree, SVC, pulmonary artery.

- Bony erosion is easily identified.
- CT easily shows decreased lung perfusion due to compression of pulmonary artery.

Evaluation of impending or suspected rupture

- Rapid increase in aortic diameter.
- High attenuation crescent (i.e. acute bleeding) within the aortic thrombus – are suspicious for imminent rupture.

Aortic Rupture or Leak is Suggested by:

a. High attenuation periaortic hematoma.
b. Aortic drape sign
   - Is highly suggestive of a contained leak.
   - The posterior aspect of aortic wall cannot be identified as a distinct line from adjacent structures and if the posterior aorta is closely applied to the spine and follows the contour of the vertebra on one or both sides.
   - Thoracic aneurysms most commonly rupture into the left hemithorax or mediastinum.

- Aorto bronchial and aorto esophageal fistula may occur.

3. *MRI*

It is an excellent alternative to CT especially in patients in whom IV contrast cannot be administered.

- Advantage of multiplanar imaging.

Disadvantage

- Limited ability to detect calcifications.
- Patients with pacemakers, aneurismal clips cannot be examined.

Cardiac gated, spin echo sequences, gradient echo sequences – transaxial coronal oblique parasagittal views.

- MRI also depicts important features of aortic aneurysm like diameter, extent, configuration, size of residual lumen, mural thrombus, relationship to branch vessels and adjacent structures and peri aortic hematoma.

4. *Aortography*

Allows direct identification of aorta and lumen of the aneurysm.

Disadvantages:

- Invasive.
- Non-diagnostic if a mass on chest X-ray is not an aneurysm.
- Only defines the aortic lumen and thrombus is not directly imaged.

Angiography is normally performed if CT/ MRI is inconclusive or for pre operative assessment.

5. *Transthoracic Echocardiography*

- Can evaluate most ascending aortic aneurysms.
- Limited value for aortic arch and descending aorta because of increased distance between transducer and aorta and obscuration of U/S window bylung, fat etc.

Post Treatment Evaluation

1. *Graft interposition technique*

Aorta is completely transected proximal and distal to the aneurysm and direct end-to-end anastomosis is performed between Dacron graft and native aorta.

2. *Graft inclusion technique*

Dacron graft is placed within the opened aneurysm and then anastomosed to the native aorta.

Dacron graft, Teflon buttressing material may be seen on CT as a high attenuation ring.

Postoperative complications like anastomotic leak, perigraft hematoma, and pseudo-aneurysm formation and graft infection are easily seen on CECT or MRI.

Imaging in Congenital Heart Diseases with Normal Pulmonary Vasculature

A. Right Ventricle Predominant

- Pure pulmonary stenosis.

B. Left Ventricle Predominant

- Coarctation of aorta.
- Aortic or subaortic stenosis.
- Intraventricular septal defect (small).
- Primary myocardial disease, glycogen, storage disease.
- Primary endocardial fibroelastosis with or without associated valvular abnormalities.
- Patent ductus arteriosus with left to right shunt.

Pulmonary Valve Stenosis (PVS)

Pulmonary valve cusps are fused and thickened forming a diaphragm perforated by an orifice, which varies in size from pinhole to substantial one and in location of central to eccentric.

Conventional Frontal Radiograph

- In post stenotic dilatation of main pulmonary artery extending into left pulmonary artery, it produces a large dilated hilum but rarely involves right pulmonary artery and causes a smaller than normal right hilum.
- Heart more slightly enlarged but may have a right ventricular shape with flattened apex raised above the diaphragm.
- Right atrium may cause a prominent convex right heart border especially if cardiac septa are intact.
- Aortic arch not as prominent as usual as it tends to be rotated by hypertrophied right ventricle.

2D Echocardiography

- In moderate/severe pulmonary valve stenosis, there is thickening of the leaflets and cloning during systole in RV outflow tract long axis or parasternal short axis planes with post stenotic dilatation.

Pulses and Continuous Wave Doppler

- Estimation of peak systolic gradient along with increasing RV anterior wall thickness.

Angiocardiography

- Demonstrates diagnostic doming of pulmonary valve cusp in ventricular systole.
- The right ventricle is heavily trabeculated proportionate to degree of PVS and the crista

may be especially prominent and hypertrophied imposing obstruction to RV outflow.

MRI Imaging

- Gradient echo acquisition through right ventricular outflow and proximal main pulmonary artery shows a systolic jet of signal void due to turbulence extending into main or left pulmonary artery.

Coarctation of Aorta (CoA)

The typical coarctation occurs in the aortic isthmus. The coarctation consist of an obstructing membrane on the greater curvature of the aorta opposite the ductus or ligamentum arteriosum.

If coarctation is distal to ductus arteriosus, blood flow is initially from aorta to pulmonary artery in treatment → right treatment direction. If later, the pulmonary vasculature resistance increases because of an Eisenmenger reaction, the shunt may become bidirectional or reversed.

If coarctation is proximal to ductus arteriosus, the flow through the ductus will depend on the size of ductus and difference between pulmonary and systemic vascular resistance, if the blood flow is from pulmonary artery to descending aorta, produces cyanosis in lower ½ of body. Oxygenated blood from left ventricle goes to aortic arch arteries, which deoxygenated blood from right ventricle goes through ductus to lower blood.

Chest Film Abnormalities

- The figure 3 sign is the undulation in the distal aortic arch at site of coarctation. The distal convexity in this region represents post-stenotic dilatation.
- Rib notching is result of enlarged and tortous intercostal arteries that serve as collateral channels.

  The notches are an exaggeration of the neurovascular groove in the inferior aspect of the rib.
- A barium esophagogram is useful to outline the medial side of aorta. The barium in esophagus when fully distended has a reversal of the figure 3 sign. The sharp lateral out-pouchings represents the site of coarctation and inferior area of constriction represents post-stenotic dilatation of aota.

Ultrasound in Infant

- In suprasternal plane, echo dense tissue narrows the aortic isthmus from its posterior aspect.

Angiography

- To image coarctation, for investigation of associated cardiac abnormalities and measurement of pressure gradient across lesion.

MRI Imaging in CoA

- For demonstration of the location and length of coarctation segment, the status of aortic isthmus and degree of arterial collateralization present.
- MRI examination as follow up after balloon dilatation and repair of CoA as to assess residual stenosis and early demonstration of post-operative pseudoaneurysm formation.

Aortic or Subaortic Stenosis

- The aortic sinuses are usually normally formed but there is fusion and asymmetry of two of the aortic valve leaflets producing a slit like orifice. The fused leaflets are joined by a thickened raphe that represents the missing commissure.

Chest X-ray

- Prominence of left ventricular outline.
- Lateral film shows—LV enlargement, aortic

valve calcification and enlargement of ascending aorta.

Echocardiography

- Identifies restriction of cusp movement and thickening of aortic valve leaflets.

MRI Imaging

- The shape and size of signal void jet as well as its variable expression into ascending aorta depend on shape of orifice and degree of narrowing.
- Valvular calcification appears as a filling defect on gradient echo examination.

INTERVENTRICULAR SEPTAL DEFECT (SMALL)

Chest X-ray

- Small shunts that represent <2:1 shunt to pulmonary artery. Chest film is usually normal.

Angiography

- Small muscular defect as thin streams into right ventricle visible throughout most of systole.
- If defects are tiny, contracting trabeculations may close these holes so that they are visible on ventriculography only during early part of systole.

Glycogen Storage Disease of Heart

- In cardiac type, glycogen is deposited in ventricular wall and interventricular septum. The atrial walls are ordinarily not thickened.

Radiographically

- Heart markedly increased in size and volume with a globular shape due to thickening of both the ventricles.

Diagnosis

- Confirmed by somatic muscle biopsy and detection of specific enzyme deficiency.

Primary Endocardial Fibroelastosis

- It is one of the common causes of cardiomegaly during infancy and may occur either isolated or in combination with various valvular and vascular lesions.

  It is characterized by a glistening opaque endocardium throughout the heart.

Radiologically

- Generalized enlargement usually affecting all chambers.
- ECG—Left ventricular preponderance.
- An enlarged left atrium with Ba filled esophagogram can be seen.

Patent Ductus Arteriosus

Imaging

- If the shunt is small, appearance on conventional radiograph of the heart and lungs may be normal.
- The most specific radiological feature in the filling in of the normal angle between the aortic arch and the main pulmonary arteries on PA chest radiograph.
- Occasionally a closed ductus may exhibit a little calcification on frontal film, which tends to disappear in later life.

Echocardiography

- Demonstrates left atrial and left ventricular enlargement, which reflects the size of shunt.

Doppler

- Pulsed Doppler of main pulmonary artery shows normal systolic flow from the pulmonary valve towards its bifurcation and reversed diastolic flow from the bifurcation of pulmonary artery towards pulmonary valve.

Angiocardiography

- Demonstrates anatomy of the ductus.

MRI Imaging

- An hourglass like narrowing may be found in its midportion of the duct.
- The duct usually has a tunnel shape, where there is a broad base on aortic side and a narrow attachment to pulmonary artery.
- In coronal section, communication between underside of distal aortic arch or proximal aorta with superior aspect of left pulmonary artery seen.

Cardiac Masses

BACKGROUND

- Cardiac neoplasms may be primary or secondary, they may be related to the heart muscle or the pericardium, or they may occur by means of direct extension of primary tumors or by means of metastases from adjacent structures.
- The most common intracardiac mass is thrombus.
- Benign primary tumors are more frequent than primary malignant tumors.
- Secondary tumors are accepted to be more common than primary tumors by a factor of 20-30.
- Metastatic tumors to the heart and pericardium are more common than primary neoplasms and occur in as many as 1.5% of patients with malignancies.

Primary Cardiac Tumors

- Myxoma, fibroma, lipoma, rhabdomyoma, plasma cell granuloma, sarcoma, lymphoma, thymoma, hemangiopericytoma, fibro-elastoma, mycosis fungoides, hamartoma/angiomyolipoma, hemangioma, angioma, lymphangioma, and pheochromocytoma.
- In general, primary cardiac tumors are of mesothelial or epithelial origin.

Myxomas

- Overall, myxomas account for approximately 30% of all primary cardiac neoplasms. Of atrial myxomas, 90% occur on the left 90% are solitary and occur more often in women than in men.
- They are characteristically attached to the interatrial septum adjacent to the edge of the fossa ovalis in approximately 85% of patients.
- Myxomas can invade the interatrial septum and the opposite atrium. Tumors may be pedunculated or polypoid.
- Firm, oval masses are associated with dyspnea and show small vessels, tortuous vascularity, hemorrhage and fibrosis. Soft papillary tumors tend be associated with neurologic symptoms and brain infarcts. Almost one half may have surface thrombus, and almost one half may have fibrosis.
- Lipomas are the second most common benign cardiac tumor and account, for approximately 10% of all cardiac neoplasms. They have no sex predilection.
- Endodermal tumors also can be found. For example, atrioventricular (AV) nodal tumors

may contain neuroendocrine cells, and thus they may be of endodermal origin.

- Primary tumors of the cardiac valves and chordae are uncommon. However, when they do occur, most often, they are fibroelastomas.
- Fibroelastomas are small tumors that may be an incidental finding at autopsy. They can be mistaken for valve vegetation.
- Lipomatous tumors of the heart valves also have been described.

Primary Cardiac Sarcomas

- Angiosarcoma, osteosarcoma, fibrosarcoma, malignant fibrous histiocytoma, leiomyosarcoma, myxosarcoma, synovial-sarcoma, neurofibrosarcoma, liposarcoma, lymphosarcoma, reticulum cell sarcoma, and undifferentiated sarcoma.
- **Angiosarcomas** are the most common primary cardiac malignant tumor—Account for 33% of all malignant primary cardiac neoplasms, and leiomyosarcomas are the second.
- Angiosarcomas tend to be located in the right heart. Angiosarcomas are more common in males. They have a high mortality rate and patients do not survive beyond 6 months of the diagnosis.
- Leiomyosarcoma frequently invades the mitral valve and pulmonary veins, and it frequently involves the left atrium.
- Osteosarcomas tend to calcify and are usually found in the left atrium.
- Other common sarcomas include rabdomyosarcomas and fibrosarcomas. Fibrosarcoma is frequently necrotic and favors the left atrium.
- Primary cardiac liposarcoma has been reported it is extremely rare and part of the differential diagnosis of a mass with fat signal intensity on MRIs. Most liposarcomas involving the heart either arise from the pericardial or are metastatic. All are rare.
- Patients have been aged 1-75 years at presentation and may present with symptoms secondary to distal metastases.

Metastatic Tumors

- Bronchogenic carcinoma, breast carcinoma, lymphoma, leukemia, carcinoid tumor, melanoma, cervical carcinoma, and germ cell tumors.
- Metastatic disease may result from contiguous extension, lymphangitic spread, or hematogenous spread.
- Metastatic cardiac tumors are frequently bronchogenic carcinomas, breast carcinomas, lymphomas, leukemias, carcinoid tumors, or melanomas.
- Metastases to the heart tend to involve the myocardium rather than the valves and endocardium.
- Alternatively, contiguous extension of tumor may come from primary or metastatic disease. For example, metastases to the lung can invade the mediastinum by means of local extension, such as by a malignant thymoma.
- Liver cancer, such as hepatocellular carcinoma, can extend cephalad via the inferior vena cava into the heart.
- Other abdominal tumors can affect the heart: extension of tumor thrombus via the inferior vena cava into the right atrium is a well-recognized complication of advanced renal cell carcinoma, also can occur with cervical carcinoma and renal angiomyolipoma.
- Benign uterine leiomyomatosis also affect the heart intravenously.
- Germ cell tumors (e.g., testicular teratomas) and embryonal cell carcinomas can metastasize to the heart, as choriocarcinomas.
- Thyroid metastases have been seen. Musculoskeletal tumors, such as hemangiopericytomas, also can metastasize and grow in the heart. Mortality rates are high, especially

in those with metastases, which tend to involve the heart late in the course of malignant disease.

Primary Pediatric Cardiac Tumors

- Rhabdomyoma, intrapericardial teratomas, myxomas, fibromas, hemangiomas, mesotheliomas, multicystic hamartomas, epicardial lipomas, and rhabdomyosarcomas.
- Rhabdomyomas are the most common pediatric cardiac tumor, and most children with rhabdomyomas have tuberous sclerosis.
- Rhabdomyomas can affect all 4 cardiac chambers. Rhabdomyomas frequently resolve spontaneously. Most primary pediatric tumors are diagnosed in the first year of life.
- Rhabdomyosarcoma is the most common pediatric malignant cardiac primary neoplasm. Compared with other primary cardiac sarcomas, rhabdomyosarcomas are more likely to involve the valves.
- Primary pediatric cardiac tumors present with murmurs and arrhythmias. Intrapericardial tumors can cause airway compression and dyspnea. In utero, fetuses can present with abnormal sonogram findings.
- The tumors can cause conduction abnormalities. Conduction abnormalities can be evaluated by electrophysiology testing and may be amenable to radiofrequency ablation.
- Primary pericardial tumor includes malignant spindle tumor, localized fibrous tumor (also called localized fibrous mesothelioma), pericardial cysts, liposarcoma, lipoma, and teratoma, direct extension of primary cardiac tumors, or lung cancer.
- Cardiac angiosarcomas tend also to involve the pericardium secondarily and to produce hemorrhagic pericardial effusions.
- Pericardial mesotheliomas frequently are associated with asbestos exposure. Most specimens have identifiable asbestos fibers, particularly crocidolite and amosite fibers, as well as chrysotile to a lesser extent.
- Lymphomas frequently are found in patients who are immunocompromised and frequently involve the pericardium.
- Liposarcomas are rare tumors, they tend to be extracardiac, and they tend to form large infiltrating masses.
- **Non-neoplasms or Pseudotumors** include thrombus or variants of cardiac anatomy, e.g., prominent pulmonary vein orifice, right atrial Chiari network or crista terminalis, valvular vegetation, thrombus within a left ventricular aneurysm, lipomatous hypertrophy of the interatrial septum, rheumatoid nodule, pulmonary collapse, ruptured chordae tendineae, intracardiac varices, tumors outside the heart and pericardium (can resemble a cardiac mass, e.g., phrenic nerve tumor), and anatomic structures, such as hiatal hernia.

EVALUATION OF THE CARDIAC MASSES

Age

- Patients with primary cardiac sarcomas have presented at age 1-75 years. Cardiac lipomas occur in patients of any age.
- Most primary pediatric tumors are diagnosed within the first year of life.
- *Pediatric tumors:* In children aged 15 years or younger, the most common benign primary cardiac tumors are as follows: rhabdomyoma (the most common benign primary tumor in those <1 year of age and associated with tuberous sclerosis in 30-50%), fibroma, hemangioma and teratoma.
- In children aged 15 years or younger, the most common malignant primary cardiac tumors are as follows: rhabdomyosarcoma fibrous histiocytoma, angiosarcoma, fibrosarcoma and myxoid sarcoma.

- *Adult tumors:* Angiosarcomas tend to be found in patients aged 20-50 years. About 70% of myxomas occur in middle-aged patients, usually those aged 50-70 years.
- In adults, the most common benign primary cardiac tumors are as follows (in approximate order of frequency): Myxoma (>50%), fibroma, hemangioma, granular cell tumor, lipoma, paraganglioma, hamartoma, histiocytoma, and hemangioendothelioma.
- In adults, the most common malignant primary cardiac tumors are as follows: Angiosarcoma, fibrous histiocytoma, leiomyosarcoma, osteosarcoma, fibrosarcoma, myxoid sarcoma, rhabdomyosarcoma, and liposarcoma.

Clinical Details

- Patients with left heart disease may present with mitral valve obstruction or apparent subacute bacterial endocarditis.
- Patients with right heart disease may present with tricuspid valve disease, pulmonary embolism, or hypertension.
- Atrial myxomas can cause breathlessness, fever, weight loss, syncope, hemoptysis, peripheral emboli and sudden death.
- Angiosarcomas frequently involve the right heart and result in right-sided heart failure. Patients may also present with cardiac tamponade secondary to bloody pericardial effusions or with pleuritic chest pain.
- Intrapericardial masses can cause dyspnea as a result of compression of airways.
- Patient with cardiac fibromas may present with congestive heart failure, arrhythmias, sudden death, cyanosis, or chest pain, although one third of patients may be asymptomatic.
- Patients with intracardiac pheochromocytomas may present with chest pain, palpitations, and flushing. Catecholamine release can cause irregular heartbeats, which can be detected by the patient as palpitations Blood pressure can rise with an increased pulse rate, resulting in more work for the heart.
- Lipomatous hypertrophy of the interatrial septum—frequently is found in people with obesity.
- Most children with rhabdomyomas also have tuberous sclerosis, which is associated with adenoma sebaceum seizures, and mental retardation.

Preferred Examination

- Initially, intracardiac tumors are often best evaluated by using echocardiography.
- Differentiation of left atrial masses from thrombus may best be achieved by using transesophageal echocardiography.
- Owing to a larger field of view with a better opportunity to assess contiguous extracardiac involvement or the presence of metastatic disease, MRI, magnetic resonance angiography (MRA), and CT are preferred over echocardiography for less-straight forward cases or for cases in which acoustic access is restricted.

Limitations of Techniques

- Chest radiography may show the effects of intracardiac obstruction with features of pulmonary edema, but otherwise, they may contribute little. Echocardiography is easily accessible, but it is limited by restricted acoustic access.
- CT scanning is accurate, but it requires radiation and contrast material. In suitable patients, MRI has the fewest limitations proved that the patient can remain motionless during the examination.

X-ray

- *Findings:* Plain radiography is not an effective method for screening for cardiac neoplasms or evaluating the extent of tumor. The degree of confidence is limited.

- Plain radiographic changes in cardiac tumors are nonspecific.
- Cardiac myxomas may be calcified, and hence, they may be visible on lateral chest radiographs.
- Left atrial enlargement may be noted this may result from mitral valve obstruction.
- Disease that expands the cardiac silhouette, by either bulk or secondary effusion, may be suggestive of pericardial involvement.

Ultrasound

- Ultrasonographic findings are accurate for identifying tumors inside cardiac chambers provided acoustic access is adequate.
- Ultrasonography is less helpful if acoustic access is poor or if tumors extend outside the heart or into the great vessels.
- Although it is more invasive, transesophageal echo imaging is best for imaging left atrial and left ventricular tumors.
- Unlike CT or MRI, echocardiography is somewhat operator dependent, and it has a more limited field of view. Area behind the sternum, ribs, or lung cannot be visualized adequately, and acoustic windows limit the structures imaged on any single plane or view.
- The benefit of echocardiography is its portability and ease of use for a first-peak approach to cardiac pathology.

Findings

- In many patients, especially those with myxomas, echocardiography may be all that is required to make the diagnosis and stage the tumor.
- In patients with poor-quality transthoracic echocardiograms, transesophageal echocardiography usually provides better images, especially of masses in or adjacent to the left atrium.
- Characteristic findings on M-mode and 2-dimensional echocardiography of the most common primary cardiac tumor demonstrate an echogenic mass in the left atrium during ventricular systole, which is seen prolapsing through the mitral valve during diastole.
- The mass may be mobile or relatively sessile.
- Myxomas may demonstrate variable echogenicity and can cause atrial enlargement.
- Other tumors may invade the myocardium or project into the affected cavities. Often, pericardial effusion is associated with malignant tumors. Prenatal ultrasonography can identify intracardiac mass and brain lesions of tuberous sclerosis and intrapericardial tumor such as teratoma.

CT Scan

- The degree of confidence is high for detecting tumors on contrast enhanced CT scanning.
- Tissue characterization is limited.
- ECG gating improves image quality and precision.

Findings

By virtue of its larger field of view, CT scanning is better than echocardiography in many situations in which mediastinal involvement or restricted acoustic access is suspected. Both the heart and contiguous structures can be assessed.

Cardiac function and the effects of a tumor on function can be evaluated using ECG-gated multiring detector spiral scanners or electron-beam scanners. Such functional imaging is at par with functional MRI.

These techniques also can be used to detect the motion of a pedunculated tumor, such as an atrial myxoma.

Using CT scans, with excellent depiction of calcific attenuating areas, can also image tumors that calcify, e.g., myxomas.

Tumor tissue tends to have an attenuation of approximately 40-100 HU. Cardiac or pericardial lipomas are identified easily by low attenuation (-100 HU) and look similar to the fat of the mediastinum.

Angiosarcomas appear as a right atrial mass with associated hemopericardium.

MRI

MRI probably offers the most accurate noninvasive test in patients who can hold their breath.

Findings

Both MRI and MRA are superior to echocardiography in detecting or excluding cardiac tumors, the precise location of cardiac tumors (i.e., paracardiac, mural, or intracavitary), the extent of disease, the presence of effusions, and the presence of metastases. Other effects and complications of tumors are demonstrated well.

MRI has advantages over CT, because:

- Intravenous contrast material is not required for imaging.
- Extracardiac disease is demonstrated well, as is the cardiac morphology. Cardiac contractility can be evaluated.
- MRI may be better than CT at providing superior depiction of tumor morphology via soft-tissue contrast resolution.

Using MRI/MRA via cine and tagging techniques can assess effects of the disease on cardiac function.

Contrast-enhanced MRI can be used to differentiate areas of slow flow from solid material.

Contrast-enhanced MRI may define the extent of the tumor, but it is limited in discerning benign from malignant disease.

Based on signal-intensity characteristics, an estimate of the tissue type may be possible. Fatty masses demonstrate high signal intensity on T1-weighted spin-echo images and medium signal intensity on T2-weighted spin-echo images.

Lipomatous hypertrophy of the interatrial septum, which is a transformation of tissue rather than a neoplasm, high, signal intensity on T1-weighted images and can extend to the free wall.

Myxomas tend to have low signal intensity on breath-hold, cine images, and they are visually conspicuous against surrounding bright (hyperintense) blood.

Similarly, turbo short-tau inversion recovery images demonstrate a hyperintense tumor enveloped by hypointense blood within the atrium. However, myxomas have variable amounts of calcification and fibrous and myxomatous tissue (which is bright on T2-weighted images).

Water-rich myxomatous tissue tends to have signal intensity higher than that of normal myocardium on T2-weighted images.

Angiosarcomas often have high signal intensity on T1-weighted images.

Angiography

Findings: The need for angiography is limited. Tumor vascularity may be seen with selective angiography. Generally, angiography is required only if information concerning coronary artery anatomy is required or if percutaneous intervention is planned.

Neovascularity of myxomas may be seen on selective angiography.

Section 4

Section 4—Cardiovascular System

Chapter 50

Diagnostic Imaging in Lower Limb Deep Venous Thrombosis(LLDVT)

LLDVT is a common clinical disorder that can lead to fatal pulmonary emboli and post phlebitis syndrome. The clinical evaluation for DVT has been found to be useful in non-hospitalized patients but a low cost, easily available technique to confirm the presence of LL thrombi is still needed.

Doppler ultrasound with compression has emerged as the diagnostic imaging study of choice. Contrast venography, MRI or radionucleide scintigraphy may be useful in selected patients.

Prevalence

DVT (Figure 50.1) affects 1-2% of hospitalized patients. If untreated, may progress to life threatening pulmonary emboli. Most of these emboli originate from thrombi in veins located in proximal lower limb or the pelvis.

Pathogenesis

Thrombosis formation originates as a 'clot nidus' in the setting of:

- Stasis.
- Endothelial injury/Virchows triad.
- Hypercoagulable state.

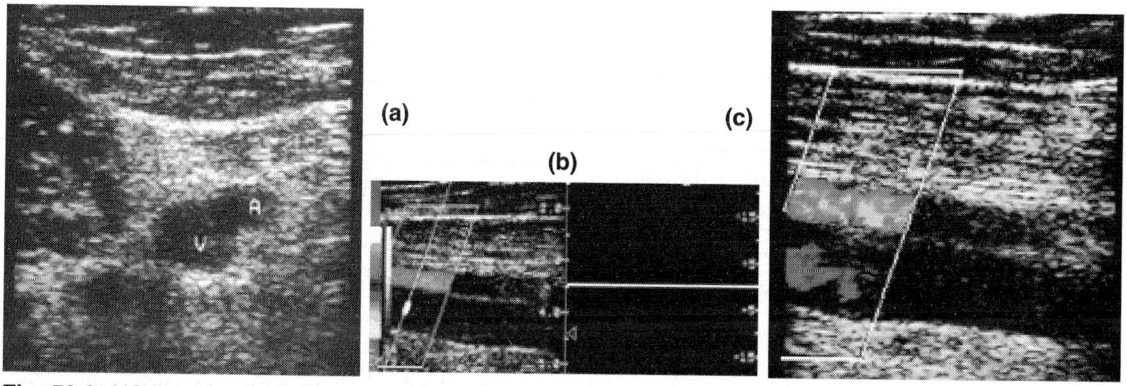

Fig. 50.1: US images of acute proximal DVT. (a) Transverse image of the superficial femoral artery (A) and vein (V) shows noncompressible vein due to acute thrombus. (b) Longitudinal image at the same level demonstrates lack of spontaneous venous flow. (c) Doppler image during augmentation demonstrates flow (blue) around the acute thrombus.

For e.g. patients who have undergone surgery may be immobilized

↓

Inactivity of calf muscles

↓

Blood pools in the LL and eddy current deposit thrombi on the cusps of vascular valves

↓

Clot nidus then propagates into thrombus that fills the venous lumen

Predisposing Conditions and Risk Factors for the Development of Venous Thrombosis

1. Immobilisation.
2. Oral contraceptives.
3. Pregnancy.
4. Previous DVT.
5. Obesity.
6. Heart disease (except hypertension).
7. Malignancy.
8. Trauma.
9. Coagulopathy.
10. Venous coagulation.
11. Surgery.

Since the thrombus is initially attached only at its origin and may float freely in the blood stream, embolization may occur.

Clinical Evaluation of DVT

History and clinical examination are useful for estimating the probability of DVT in ambulatory patients.

Prediction criteria can be used to place the patients in one of the three probability groups for DVT i.e.:

1. Low risk group (5% probability).
2. Medium risk group (33% probability).
3. High risk group (85% probability).

Major Factors

- Active cancer.
- Paralysis/recent casting of lower limb (LL).
- Recently bed ridden for more than three days and/or major surgery within four weeks.
- Localized tenderness along the deep venous system.
- Swollen thigh or calf.
- Strong family history of DVT.

Minor Factors

- Hospitalization in the previous six months.
- Leg trauma in the past 60 days.
- Findings in symptomatic legs.
  - Pitting edema.
  - Dilated superior veins.
  - Erythema.

High Probability

$\geq$ 3 major factors OR

$\geq$ 2 major factors + $\geq$ 2 minor factors.

Medium Probability

Includes all patients without a high or low probability of DVT.

Low Probability

1 major factor + 1 or no minor factors OR no major factor +2 or fewer minor factors.

While these probability assessments can be used to classify a patient's risk, they are not sufficiently exact to exclude or confirm DVT. Therefore, they should be used in conjunction with other diagnostic techniques in patients with suspected DVT.

ESTABLISHED DIAGNOSTIC IMAGING TECHNIQUES

1. Contrast Venography

- Considered the gold standard for the detection of deep venous thrombosis.
- Performed on a fluoroscopic table with the patient in a semi upright position and bearing weight on the leg that is not being examined.

- Radiographic contrast material is infused into the deep venous system via a catheter placed in the foot.
- Venographic criteria for diagnosis of thrombosis is — intraluminal filling defect in the deep venous cont. column.
- *Less specific finding:* Abrupt cut off of a deep vein with the development of collateral circulation.

2. Limitation of Contrast Venography

- Inadequate visualization of the deep venous system in 20-25% patients b/o previous thrombosis.
- Dilution of contrast medium in the proximal lower limb.
- Difficulty in venous access relates to obesity, severe edema or cellulitis.

Complications

- Reaction to radiographic contrast material like allergic reactions, ARF, venous thrombosis.

Advantages

- Available in most hospitals.
- High sensitivity and specificity.
- Direct imaging of clot.
- Can determine the extent of thrombi in the calf, proximal LL and pelvis.
- Relatively inexpensive.

Disadvantages

- Invasive.
- Difficult to perform in critically ill patients.
- Not portable.

DOPPLER US WITH COMPRESSION

- Ultrasound examination is performed with a 3 to 7 MHz real time transducer:
  - Appropriate gain settings are made so that normal vessels are free of internal echoes.
  - Venous anatomy is evaluated in both the transverse axis (for optimal compression) and the longitudinal axis (to localize the vein).
  - Moderate transducer pressure will collapse the normal venous lumen, whereas deep venous thrombosis prevents venous wall coaptation.
  - Examination is performed from the level of the inguinal ligament to the trifurcation of popliteal vein.

    Life threatening pulmonary emboli usually arises in the deep venous system of the proximal limb. Thus in most patients with higher risk proximal DVT this technique detects most clots, so that assessment of the tibial and peronial vein is not necessary.
- Duplex and color Doppler US examination are often used to verify the findings obtained by compression technique.
- Also in areas where compression is difficult to apply like the adductor canal or inguinal ligament. Color and duplex Doppler can confirm the patency.

DVT

- Acute thrombosis.
- Subacute thrombosis.
- Chronic thrombotic scarring.

ACUTE THROMBOSIS

Refers to thrombus that is days to perhaps 1-2 weeks old characterized by:

1. Low echogenicity to low level echoes, which is, difficult to visualize on gray scale images but is seen as flow void or color Doppler images.

2. Venous distention occurs except when the thrombus is small non-occlusive.
3. Loss of compressibility.
4. *Free floating thrombus:*

   The proximal end of an acute thrombus may not adhere well to the vein wall, in such cases the thrombus is said to float freely within the lumen.
5. *Doppler signal abnormalities:*

   When thrombus of any age substantially occludes the vein lumen – flow augmentation is diminished or absent in veins proximal to the thrombosed segment.
6. *Collateralization:*

   Collaterals may be located either adjacent to the thrombsed vein or more distant.

SUBACUTE THROMBOSIS

Refers to a thrombus that is weeks to 1 to 2 months old. It presents as area of increased echogenicity characterized by:

1. *Echogenic intraluminal material*
   - Overall echogenicity is greater than that of adjacent muscle.
   - Seen as focal plaque like thickening of the vein wall.
   - If the vein lumen does not recanalize, the vein may be reduced to an echogenic cord.
2. *Valve abnormality*

   Valve damage is seen as:
   - Thickening of the cusps.
   - Adherence of cusps to the vein wall.
   - Restricted cusp motion.
   - Failure of opposition of the cusp in the center of the valves.

   Consequences of valve damage are:
   - Reflux and persistent venous distension.
   - Varicosities.
   - Chronic edema, skin changes and ulceration (post thrombotic syndrome).
3. *Doppler flow abnormalities*
   - Lack of spontaneous flow.
   - Lack of phasicity.
   - Absence of valsalva response.
     – Subnormal or absent augmentation.
4. *Decreased thrombus size*

   Retraction and lysis may noticeably reduce the size of thrombus.
5. *Reduced vein size*
   - Vein becomes less distended and returns to normal caliber.
   - If vein does not recanalize, it may shrink to a subnormal size as the thrombus retracts and becomes a scar.
6. *Adherence of thrombus*

   Free-floating acute thrombus becomes attached to the wall.
7. *Resumption of flow*

   With retraction and lysis, blood flow obstruction diminished and recanalization occurs.
8. *Collateralization*

   Collaterals form in the acute phase and persist in the subacute phase.

CHRONIC THROMBOTIC SCARRING

The term chronic thrombosis is a misnomer and the proper term is chronic thrombotic scarring. Refers to a phase months to years after the acute episode.

During this phase a thrombus that is not lysed is invaded by fibroblasts and becomes organized as a fibrous tissue that persists indefinitely. Complete lysis occurs only in 20% cases.

Limitations

- Even with color Doppler US, the DVT in the calf usually remains undetected. Therefore, in high risk patients with a negative examination, a follow up US examination in 4-6 days is recommended to detect 20-40% clots that originate in the venous plexus of the calf and propagate to the level of popliteal vein or higher.

- For six months after the acute episode, upto 50% patients have compression ultrasound abnormalities that are indistinguishable from the original findings of DVT.

Advantages

- Available in most hospitals.
- Non-invasive.
- Lacks ionizing radiation.
- No radiographic contrast material is required.
- Equipment is portable.
- Test can be usually performed in 15-30 mts.
- Can be performed serially on the same patient.

CONTROVERSY IN VENOUS ULTRASOUND

Is calf vein examination necessary?

Previously argued – no need to examine calf vein because:

1. Isolated calf vein thrombosis does not pose a risk for pulmonary embolism.
2. Some physicians feel that isolated calf vein thrombosis does not warrant anticoagulant therapy.

But, the newer concept is:

1. Referring physician wants to know the cause of calf symptoms.
2. Isolated calf vein thrombosis may cause long-term disability – valvular incompetence, venous stasis.
3. Calf vein thrombosis may propagate in a cephaloid direction or embolize (20-30% cases).

Recent literature also shows that colour Doopler ultrasound is accurate (with specificity of 60-90%) for the diagnosis of acute calf venous thrombosis in symptomatic patients when the calf veins can be seen adequately.

MRI

- Because of the limitations of contrast venography and US with compression, several investigators have advocated the use of MRI for detection of DVT.
- MRI is able to detect filling defects in the entire deep venous system of the LL, including calf veins (peroneal and tibial veins), which are not evaluated by compression US.

  MRI also visualizes pelvic veins, which are difficult to examine using contrast venography or compression US.

Limitations

- MRI is highly operator dependent and an experienced examiner must be present to restudy areas comprised by MRI related artifacts.
- Expensive.
- Not available in emergency situations.

RADIONUCLIDE SCINTIGRAPHY

- Various radiopharmaceuticals have been used to detect LLDVT.
- Radionuclide venography with ^{99}TC labelled RBC or macro-aggregated humen serum albumim can be performed in DVT. Venography using labelled macro aggregated humen serum albumin can be performed in conjunction with lung perfusion scanning.

Limitations

- Does not provide direct information as to the cause of venous obstruction.
- Unreliable in calf because of the presence of multiple vessels.
- Cannot differentiate intrinsic from extrinsic obst.
- Accuracy of this imaging technique decreases markedly in patients with previous DVT.

  Radionuclide scintigraphy using labelled peptides that attach to activate platelets is currently being evaluated for detection of Ac DVT.

Section 4—Cardiovascular System

Chapter 51

Vascular Interventional Techniques

VASCULAR INTERVENTIONAL RADIOLOGY

- Is a medical speciality which uses image guided minimally invasive techniques for the diagnosis and/or treatment of variety of medical conditions and often represents a viable alternative to surgery.

Interventional Methods

- Disobliteration techniques.
- Embolization techniques.
- Foreign body retrieval.
- Inferior vena cava filter insertion.

Disobliteration Techniques

- Vascular dilatation (Transluminal angioplasty).
  - Percutaneous transluminal angioplasty (PTA) refers to dilatation of stenotic vessels as well as dilatation and recanalisation of occluded vessels. It encompasses procedures such as balloon dilatation, atherectomy, stent replacement, and laser therapy and percent aspiration.

Technique of Balloon PTA

- The fundamental technique is to position a balloon catheter in the region of vascular stenosis and carefully dilate the balloon under fluoroscopic control to distend the stenotic segment and improve flow.

Procedure

1. The basic method consists of passing a guiding catheter to a site from which a guide wire can be negotiated through the site of narrowing.
2. An injection of contrast medium is made through the guiding catheter to delineate the extent of the stenosis and radio-opaque markers mark it.
3. Guide wire and catheter are manipulated through the lesion and the guide wire is positioned distal to stenosis.
4. Guiding catheter is withdrawn and replaced by balloon catheter of appropriate dimension without altering position of wire and is then manipulated to stenotic site.
5. Balloon is then inflated by a pressure pump at pre-selected pressures or manually by syringe filled with dilute contrast medium.
   - Some use one or two successive dilatations lasting 30 sec or more, others use short bursts of multiple inflations.

Mechanism of Action

- There is some change in mechanical structure of vessel wall rather than simple flattening and redistribution of atheroma.
- There is splitting, desquamation and cracking of plaque.
- Actual increase in calibre of vessel is due to overstretching and or rupture of tunica intima media adventitia irreversibly.

Application of PTA

1. *Lower Extremity*
   - Vascular occlusive disease is a common clinical problem in which PTA along with balloon dilatation and/or stenting has proved to be valuable.
   - Short focal stenoses respond better to PTA
   - Isolated stenoses of iliac vessels respond well to angioplasty either performed by retrograde ipsilateral approach or contralateral approach across aortic bifurcation.
   - Occlusion of common iliac artery (Figure 51.1) was previously contraindication to PTA; however use of stents is now more applicable and less expensive than bypass of aortoiliac occlusion.
   - Localized stenosis of superficial femoral and popliteal criteria is also suitable for PTA and up to 10 cm length can be successfully dilated.
2. *Renal PTA*
   - It is a useful technique for management of renovascular HT.
   - It can be used in both atherosclerotic stenosis or fibromuscular dysplasia.
   - Stenting is used in situations of inadequate primary balloon dilatation or generation of intimal flap.
3. *Percutaneous Transluminal Coronary Angioplasty*
   - PTCA employs a guiding catheter introduced through groin or anus and an inner balloon catheter that passes co-axially through the guiding catheter into the coronary artery.
4. *PTA at Miscellaneous Sites*
   - Aortic stenosis – can be dilated using two balloon catheters inflated simultaneously or through modern large diameters balloons.
   - Internal iliac PTA may cure impotence.
   - Coeliac or mesenteric vessels dilatation can relieve visceral angina.

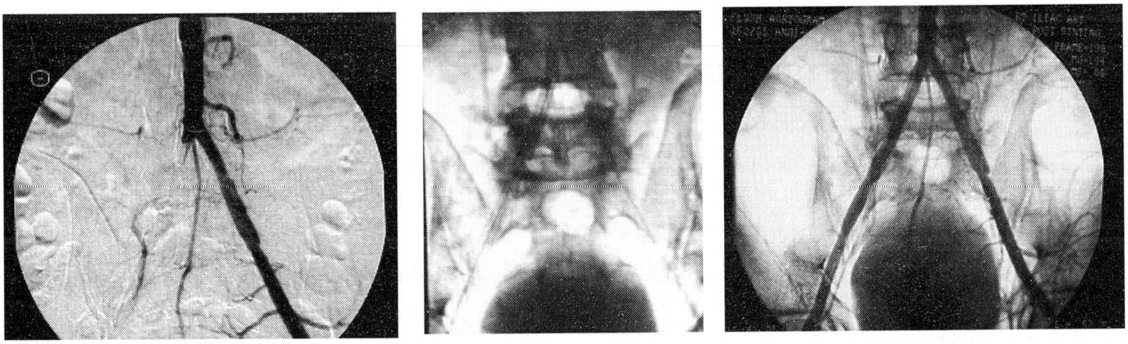

Fig. 51.1: DSA images showing occlusion of the right common iliac artery, stent during placement and post-procedural patent right common iliac artery

- Venous narrowing.
- For dilatation of graft and anastomotic stenosis.

Complications of PTA

- At puncture site – hemorrhage, thrombosis, pseudo aneurysm.
- In target vessel and its territory – embolization, thrombosis, dissection, perforation, occlusion.
- With catheter – Balloon rupture.
  - Irregular margins of ruptured balloon may damage vessel wall.
  - Fragment of balloon may detach and embolize.
  - Balloon may fold over itself and may stuck in vessel requiring arteriotomy for removal.
- Peripheral embolisation of atheromatous deposits.

VASCULAR STENTS

- It is a cylindrical meshwork splint most commonly of stainless steel that is placed across a stenosis to maintain patency of the vessel.
- For insertion it is placed on or within a catheter precisely positioned across the stenosis under fluoroscopic control and released.

  Within 2 weeks the device becomes covered with endothelial cells, becoming incorporated in vessel wall.

Thrombolysis

- Local low dose intra-arterial thrombolysis in which a catheter is embedded in thrombus is an established therapeutic option.
- Fibrinolytic agents are plasminogen activators, converting it to its active form plasmin, which breaks down fibrin.
- E.g. of fibrinolytic agents are streptokinase, urokinase, prourokinase and tissue plasminogen activator.
- Indications are MI, peripheral arterial thromboembolis, after vascular angioplasty, renal and gastrointestinal thrombosis, focal DVT and pulmonary embolism.

Intravascular Ultrasound

- Catheters with small ultrasound transducers may be used to visualize vessel wall and intra-luminal abnormalities especially branch vessel involvement in aortic dissection and results of angioplasty and stenting.

Embolization Techniques

- It includes deliberate occlusion of arteries, veins or abnormal vascular spaces by embolic materials injected through a selectively positioned catheter.

Embolic Materials and Techniques

- Metallic coils, detachable balloons, absorbable gelatin sponge, polyvinyl alcohol foam, sodium tetradechyl sulphate, absolute ethanol and N-butyl 2-cyanoacrylate.
- Embolization is preceded by high quality angiography to define the vascular territory under consideration and its anastomotic communications.
- Embolizing catheters are then sited selectively and embolic material is injected.

Indications

- *Acute bleeding*:
  - Can be used to prevent acute bleeding in surgically inaccessible lesions.
  - GI bleeding, bleeding from renal arteries can be controlled. It has been used in post biopsy, hemorrhage, postoperative bleeding, renal trauma and bleeding tumors.

- Sometimes it is the only alternative to nephrectomy when only single functioning kidney is present.
- Bronchial embolization can be done in control of hemoptysis.

Tumors

- Embolization (Figure 51.2) can be used in three principal ways to assist in management of neoplasms.

Definitive

- Benign tumors can sometimes be successfully treated by embolization alone. E.g. endocrine tumors such as parathyroid adenomas and benign bone tumors.

Operative Embolization

- Used extensively for renal adenocarcinoma. The vascular tumor is embolized hours or days before surgical resection to reduce operative blood loss, shortens the duration of operation, reduce the risk of dissemination of malignant cells and possible stimulate an immune response to tumor.

  Nasopharyngeal tumors, hepatic tumors, glomus juglase tumors, meningiomas, chemoductomas and vagal neuromas can also be embolised pre operatively.

Palliative embolization in inoperable malignancy e.g. embolization of metastatic deposits can increase survival time.

Vascular Abnormalities

- Vascular malformations, AV shunts, benign tumors of vascular origin and aneurysms can be treated by embolization.
- Treatment of femoral artery pseudoaneurysms using direct injection of thrombin is successful in almost all cases.

CNS

Embolization can be used to treat AVM and aneurysms e.g. endovascular costing for aneurysm and glue for AVM.

Spleen

Splenic artery embolization may be performed to control or prevents hemorrhage.

Proximal embolization is done by embolizing splenic artery or one of the branches by steel coils or balloons in order to stop bleeding, occlude aneurysms or reduce flow as preop measure.

Distal embolization is performed by particulate material with deliberate interruption of infarcting splenic tissue. This is done when surgical splenectomy is indicated but poor general condition of patient or impaired coagulation preclude surgery.

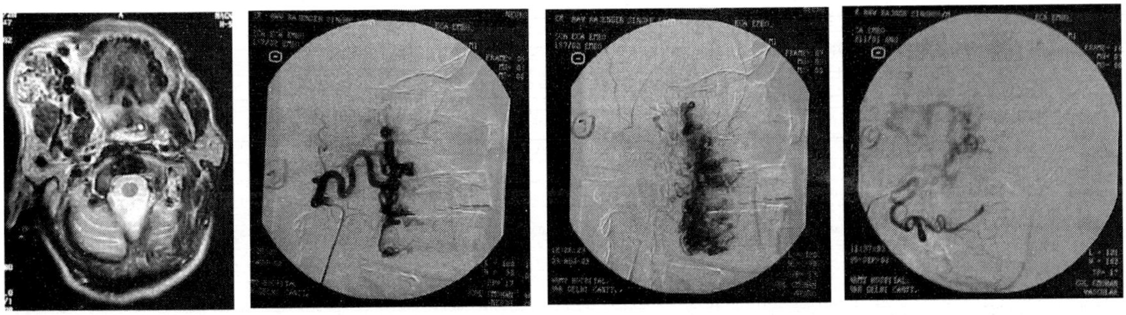

Fig. 51.2: Axial MR image shows AVM of the right cheek; DSA images show that the AVM being fed by the internal maxillary artery; pre and postembolisation images show the success of the procedure

Priapism

When secondary to trauma an AV fistula is often present and will respond to embolization.

Complications

1. General	Hazards of arteriography Contrast reactions.
2. Specific	Pain, nausea. Inadvertent embolism of normal structures. Loss of embolic devices in vascular system. Adhescence of catheter tip to vessel wall by liquid adhesives. Injection. Tissue necrosis. Renal failure. Death.

3. Foreign body retrieval

   Most common intravascular foreign body requiring percutaneous removal is portion of a central venous catheter.

   Many retrieval devices like looped wire snores tip deflecting wires, dormia wire baskets, biopsy forceps, fragment graspers are available.

Inferior Vena Cava Filter Insertion

In cases of recurrent or threatened pulmonary embolization from lower extremities and pelvis IVC filters can be inserted. Especially useful in patients who already have complications due to anticoagulation like GI hemorrhage or heparin induced thrombocytopenia.

Indications

Absolute

1. Recurrent pulmonary embolism despite anticoagulants.
2. Prophylaxis in high risk patients e.g. those with compromised pulmonary vascular bed and free-floating clot in veins.
3. Prophylaxis after successful pulmonary embolectomy.
4. Prevention of paradoxical embolism in patients with right to left shunts.

Relative

1. Free floating emboli in iliac or femoral veins on in IVC.
2. Prophylaxis in patients with risk of hemorrhage with anticoagulation.
3. Prophylaxis prior to pelvic surgery in high-risk patients.
4. Prophylaxis in polytrauma victims.

   Percutaneous interruption of IVC is done through right IJV or femoral vein, filter normally being placed below renal veins.

   Complications are IVC thrombosis, migration of occluding device to heart or lungs, and continued recurrent pulmonary artery embolisation.

Intravascular Radiological Iodinated Contrast Media

- Iodine (whose atomic No. (27)) is the only element, which has provided satisfactory for general use as an intravascular radiological contrast media (RCM).
- In RCM – Iodine – provides radio opacity.

  Rest of the molecule acts as a carrier of iodine, greatly increase solubility and markedly reduce the toxicity.
- For carrier, organic compounds are used. It is based on a fully substituted benzoic acid (6 'C' ring) with 3 atoms of iodine replacing 'H' at C. 2, 4 and 6 on the benzene ring.
- Intravascular organic iodinated RCM were introduced into clinical practice in 1928-29 by MOSES SWICK, a urologist from Berlin. He produced the 1st IVU using non-ionic selecton neutral and ionic uroselecion both were pyridine (5 atom 'c' and 1 atom 'N' to the 6th pointed ring) containing 1 atom of N2/molecule.
- Presently, there are 4 varieties of iodinated ROM in clinical use (Table).

Ionic Monomers

- Of all above, diatrizoate and iothalmate are most frequently used.
- All are salts of Na^+ or maglumine as non-radioopaque cation and tri iodo-benzoic acid as anion.
- Dissociates Iodine: Particle ratio is 3:2.

Non-Ionic Monomers

- 1st non-ionic triodinated monomer – metrizamide was introduced in 1990's however, metrizamide has a serious disadvantage of being unstable at high temperature, making it impossible by autoclave.
- This was replaced by more stable, less toxic, less expensive 2nd generation non-ionic monomers: iohexol, iopamidol etc.
- Each has 3 iodine atoms and one osmotically active particle produced an iodine: particle of 3:1.

Ionic Dimers

- Ioxaglate (Hexabrix) is the only compound in this group.
- It's a mixture of Na and meglumin salts of monoacids double benzene ring.
- It has 6 iodine atom and dissociates into two ions prevailing iodine: particle ratio of 6:2 (3:1).

Classification	Iodine atom molecule	Osmotic particles for molecule	Iodine particle ratio	LD50 Iodine/kg wt this use at 2ml/min I/V
Ionic monomers	3	2	3:2	7
• Diatrizoate (urograffin) • Iokalamate (conray) • Metrizoate (Isoopaque) • Ioxithalamate				
Non-ionic monomers	**3**	**1**	**3:1**	**22**
• Ishexol (omnipaque) • Iomeron • Iopamidol • Iopromide • Ioversol • Toxilan • Xenitix				
Ionic dimmers	**6**	**2**	**6:2 (3:1)**	**12**
• Ioxaglate				
Non-ionic dimers	**6**	**1**	**6:1**	**>26**
• Iodixanol (visipaque) • Iotrolan (Isovist)				

Non-Ionic Dimers

- Iodixanol (Visipaque) and Iotralon (Isovist) are non-ionizing chemicals containing 2 non-ionizing tri iodinated benze rings linked together.
- Each has 6 iodine atoms with a single particle i.e on iodine: particle ratio of 6:1.
- Iotrolan has been recently withdrawn because of unexpected delayed reactions usually allergic and skin manifestation, which seems to be more severe and frequent in Japanese ionic monomers: are the conventional HOCM and Rest: **are the LOCM.**

Adverse Reaction to RCM

- Like any other drug in the clinical medicine, RCM also has certain adverse effects.
- RCM should be administered only when there are clear and defensible clinical indications and when the benefit outweighs the risk and discomfort.

4 Section

- RCM should be used in smallest concentration of smallest total dose. Never compensate an inadequate radiological technique by increasing the dose of contrast medium.
- Although RCM's are exceptionally safe drugs, they are not entirely without risk and may cause severe and even fatal complication.

The American College of Radiology has divided these adverse areas into:

1. Idiosyncratic anaphylactoid reactions.
2. Non-syncratic reactions.
3. Combined 1+2.

IDIOSYNCRATIC ANAPHYLACTOID REACTIONS

- These are the most dreaded and the most frequent serious and fatal complication of RCM as they occur without warning, cannot be reliably predicted and am not preventable in the proper stage of knowledge.
- Occur during or immediately after the injection of contrast and about 85% occur within 5 minutes of the injection.
- In contrast to normal subjects, they are most frequent in patients.
  - Who had a previous adverse risk to RCM (4-6 times).
  - Asthmatics (8 times).
  - Allergic and atopic (5 times).
  - In patients with impaired CVS and renal system.
  - Patients on beta-blockers and possibly NSAID's.
- These reasons vary greatly in severity.
- Possible mechanism carry these reactions are:
  1. Inhibition of enzyme such as cholinesterase with hydrolysis ach. This produce symptoms of vagal over-estimation e.g. CV collapse, bradycardia and bronchospasm.
  2. Release of vasoactive substance such as histamine, 5-HT, or bradykinen which may result in vaso motor collapse.
  3. Activation of physiological cascade system: including complements cascade, kinin system with bradykinin release, the coagulation system (inducing i/vascular coagulation and (+) n of Rb view type system) and optimal platelet aggregation.
  4. Immune system disturbance.
  5. Anxiety apprehension and fear by activation of hypothalamic system resulting in CV collapse and respiratory collapse.

Side effect include:

Ionic HOCM ADR%		Non ionic LOCM ADR%
4.58	Nausea (HC)	1.04
2.29	Heat	0.92
2.97	Vomiting	0.45
3.16	Urticaria	0.47
1.12	Flushing	0.16
0.40	Venous pain	0.05
0.58	Coughing	0.15
0.17	Dysnoea	0.04

- Reactions are non-dose dependent and death has been known to occur following a 1ml of intravenous test dose or often full dose.

NON-IDIOSYNCRATIC REACTIONS

These are divided into: Chemotoxic, osmotoxic, and vasomotor regions:

1. Chemotoxic

- Toxicity to contrast medium molecule as a whole, not its iodine content as iodine is firmly bound to benzoin ring.

- Chemotoxic side effects include, cardiac, neurological and renal toxicity as well as vascular manifestation.

2. Osmotoxic (Hyper Osmolar) Reactions

- Osmolality of the ionic HOCM is 5-8 times of physiological osmolality (~300 mosm/kg water) degree of hyperosmolality reduced if non-ionic 3:1 LOCM is used and even none of 0:1 LOCM non-ionic LOCHM dimers are used.

  Hyperosmolality causes:

  Erythrocytic damage: Loss of intracytoplasmic water leading to rigidilization and reduction of the essential deformability of red cell which is necessary for RBCs to pass through capillaries.

- *Endothelial damage*

  Endothelial damage of capillary wall is damaged.

  ↓

  ↑ Permeability with passage of toxic substances into extravascular tissue.

  Endothelial cells are also increased to produce active substance like factor XII, arachidone acid, PL's and prostacyclin etc. which effect vasodilatation and coagulation.

- *Blood brain barriers*

  Endothelial lining of BBB is damaged.

  ↓

  Passage of RCm into the extravascular hematological tissue fluid and exerts a direct toxic effect in the delicate nerve tissue cells.

- *Vasodilatation*
  - Vasodilatation of arteriolar and capillary bed

    ↓

    Rapid increase in blood flow several times the physiological flow rate

    ↓

    Feeling of warmth, heat, discomfort or severe pain during peripheral angiography.
  - Systemic generalized vasodilation causes severe systemic hypotension, peripheral vein pooling, ↓ VR to heart and CY shock which may be extremely severe and fatal.

- *Hypervolemia*
  - Osmotic attraction extravascular fluid into the circulation.

    ↓

    ↑ Blood volume by ~ 10-20 % within few minutes and ↓ Hb count.

    ↓

    ↑ CO and stress on the left ventricle.

- *Cardiac depression*
  - Due to hypotension, ↓ VR, myocardial ischaemia and direct depression of myocardial contractility, particularly after coronary angiography.

- All of the above reasons are related to hyperosmolality and therefore depends upon close concentration and volume of RCM and are reduced by substituting LOCM for HOCM.

3. Vasomotor Reaction

- May follow after idiosyncratic or non-idiosyncratic reactions or may develop independently.
- May be severe hypotensive, tachycardia or bradycardia with apprehension, sweating and disturbed conciousness.
- Depressed myocardial contractility with markedly decreased CO.
- Vasovagal reaction caused bradycardia and vasomotor collapse is accompanied by tachycardia.

4 Section

COMPLICATIONS

Divided into four groups:

A. Minor Reactions

- Include nausea, flushing, burn pain, pruritis, vomiting, headache and mild urticaria.
- Those symptoms are mild, of short duration, self-limiting.
- Clinically no treatment is required. Reassurance and restoration of the patients confidence is enough. Occasionally, oral antihistamines for urticaria, a tranquillizer (diazepam, 5 mg) or a mild analgesic may be helpful.
- Incidence: ~ 5-15%.
- Pain is less frequently seen with LOCM as compared to HOCM.

B. Intermediate Reactions

- Include serious degrees of above minor symptoms plus moderate degree of hypotension and bronchospasm.
- Respond readily to appropriate therapy – reassurance, antihistaminic (orally I/M or I/V) for urticaria, diazepam for anxiety, salbutamol inhalation for bronchospasm, hydro cortisone 100-500 mg I/M or I/V, Adrenaline 0.3-1.0 ml of 1/100 sole I/M or S/C (children 0.01 ml/kg) for more severe bronchospasm.

  Incidence: ~0.5-2% of I/V injection of HOCA and probably ¼ times of this, following I/V LOCM.

C. Severe Life Threatening

- Severe manifestation of all the above symptoms + convulsion, consciousness, laryngeal edema, severe bronchospasm, pulmonary edema, severe cardiac dysrhythmias, cardiac arrest and CV and pulm. collapse.
  - Treatment is urgent and its response is unpredictable.
- Airway secure. $+O_2$.
- Artificial respiration.
- External cardiac massage + DC defibrillation.
- I/V access
  - Fluids to resolve blood volume.
  - Drugs.
- Frusemid I/V or I/M for pulmonary edema.
- Diazepam and barbiturates – convulsion.
- Aminophyllin – for bronchospasm.
- Antihistaminic – anaphylaxis.
- Vasopressors – hypotension.
- BP monitoring.
- $NaHCO_3$ – acidosis.
- Atropine – vasovagal shock and bradycardia.
- *Adrenaline:* 0.3-1.0ml 1/100 soln deep S/C or I/M repeated at 10-20min interval. It can precipitate ventricular fibrillation, so it should be given preferably under ECG cautre.

Incidence: 0.2% with I/V HOCM and reduced to 0.04% with LOCM.

Deaths:

- Adverse reactions may not respond to the treatment and patient may die.
- Usually due to intractable cardiopulmonary collapse, severe pulmonary edema or intense bronchospasm.
- Median mortality is around 1 in 40,000 I/V injection (range: 1/14,000 to 1/170,000).
- Recent analysis as per the studies done in many places around the world suggests that DEATHS due to LOCM are no fewer than those due to HOCM.

FACTORS PREDISPOSING TO ADR'S

- *Previous adverse region:* ↓es risk factor of a severe HOCM by about 6-10 times.

- *History of asthma or bronchospasm:* 5-10 times–than the usual rates: 2nd RCM injection in such patients may be extremely severe and even fatal.

Above two is the most dangerous predisposing factor:

- *History of allergy or atrophy:* 5 times ↓ed risk to normal individual of severe ADR's.
- *Cardiac allergy or atrophy ↓ed by 2 times:* Much greater of patient in severe/unstable heart failure or with dysrhythmias.
- Overload with large volume of high osmolar contrast media may precipitate cardiac decompensation.
- *Dehydration:* Patient should be well hydrated specially diabetic, renal and myeloma patients.

Hematology and Metabolic Condition

- *Sickle cell anemia:* Particularly HOCM causes ↓ed sickling and fatal complication. Biliary cerebralcoronary angiography.
- *Patients with thrombotic tendency:* ↓ed risk especially with non-ionic RCH.
- Myelomatosis develop renal failure.

Now less frequent – Use of trioiodinated contrast agents + adj hydration maintained.

Phaecochromatosis: May develop hypertensive crises so precautionary alpha and beta blockers should be done if phaecochromocytomas is suspected (before the procedure).

Renal disease: In pre-existing said disease or diabetes induced renal complication, there is ↓ed risk of renal failure. In LOCM it is said to be less.

If for diabetes metformin is given, it should be discontinued 48 hours before and 48 hours after the RCM injection (as it is exposed by kidneys and may cause lactic acidosis if renal parenchyma get impaired due to RCM).

Others: Neonates, elderly and infants patients are at increased risk probably because of associated morbid condition.

Anxiety and apprehension: Predisposes to increased adverse reaction.

Delayed adverse: Idio synergetic and non-dis dependent – delayed for few days – Reactions are uncomfortable but not dangerous.

More Common in Females

- Include arm pain, delayed rash, flu like symptoms, salivary gland swelling (iodide mumps).
- Few deaths reported due to delayed vasculitis, SLE, Stevens-Johnson syndrome.
- Delayed reactions are more frequent with LOCH than with HOCM.
- Iotrolan known to cause this has now been withdrawn.

Principle for Investigating Patients at ↓ed Risk

- Always weight the advantages of the diagnostic procedure against the small but even present severe ADR.
- It possibly replaces the procedure by different imaging modalities (USG, MRI).
- Referring clinician should be informed of the ADR's and the risk factors and avoid giving RCM. If still clinician insists, both radiologists and clinician should document it to the patient notes. Patient should be informed and reassured as necessary.
- Smallest dose, lowest concentration and smallest number of injection that gives reliable and comprehensive diagnostic results should be used.
- Do not leave patient unattended for the 1st 20 minutes after injection.
- Premedication should be strongly considered with previous history of adverse reactions, asthmatic and diagnostic patient with history of allergy/atrophy who should be given 24 hours of steroid and antihistamines. Location should be send and if possible other

investigation not requiring RCM administration should be done.

- In patients with increased note, LOCM should be used in preference to HOCM and non-ionic LOCM should be preferred to Ionic LOCM or HOCM.
- Basic RCM administration, emergency trolley should be checked, ECG, suction apparatus and defibrillator should be in hand.

Note: It has been said that selective use of LOCM is best justified in patients with adverse asthma or allergy at least 67% of adverse reactions can be prevented.

CONTRAST MEDIA RELATED TO SPECIFIC CLINICAL AREAS

1. Renal tract

- High dose of contrast media, cause decrease urine output, dicreased serum creatinine and urea, dicreased creatinine clearance and dicreased GFR peaking at 3-5 days. Some may proceed to renal failure and even death.
- Important administrative factors are: Severe and deteriorating pre-existing renal failure and oliguria, diabetic nephropathy. Poor hydration and high dose at RCM.
- Nephrotoxic drugs may enhance the adverse effect of RCM like antibiotics, NSAIDS, cytotoxic agents etc. These should be stopped or reduced before RCM are given.
- After early uncertainty, it now appears that HOCM are more nephrotoxic and LOCM are preferred for all patients to be at risk, especially those with diabetic nephropathy.

Renal Arteriography

Future albuminuria may occur after selective renal angio with HOCM and metrozamide (1st non-ionic LOCM). This occurs much less with 2nd junction LOCH< which is preferred for renal arteriography.

2. Nervous system

- LOCM were comfortable than HOCM, but if later are used meglumine salts are preferred.
- DSA preferred over conventional radiography as it provide good contrast with low RCM dose.
- However, this is now slowly being replaced by MR angiography.

  S/E – Dilatation of ECA and tertiary caring pain and heart.
  - Damage to blood brain barrier carry cerebral edema.
  - Bradycardia and hypotensive.

  Myelography
  - Now replaced by MRI/CT.
  - Non-ionic LOCH must be used as ionic CM (both HOCM and LOCM) is toxic in the subarachnoid space.
  - Myelography with oily products such as iophendylate (myodil/pentopaque) must be abandoned, as it is known to cause chronic adhesive arachnoiditis.

3. Cardiovascular System

Peripheral Angiography

- LOCM preferred over HOCM as it causes less warmth, discomfort, pain and undesirable movements.
- If HOCM are to be used meglumine salts should be used as it cause less vasodilatation.
- Peripheral venography.
- Mx. conc. of HOCM should be about 200 mg I/ml but this may be increased to 3000 ugI/ml if LOCM is used.
- Whatever the control is used endothelial contact times should be reduced by way out the contrast with saline, massaging or by exercising the leg.
- *Intracardiac injection*

  LOCM preferred as it causes less disturbances

of cardiac function, less depressive of myocardial contractility, less vasodilatation, less hypertensive, less systemic hypotensive and fewer conductive ECG changes them HOCM.

- *Pulmonary angiography*

  LOCM preferred as it causes less elevation of pulmonary artery pressure, coupling and this discomforts.

- *Aortography*

  LOCM instead of HOCM, as iodine concentration are preferred as they cause less discomfort and less vasodilatation.

- *Coronary angiography*

  LOCM preferred over HOCM as they cause less marked hemodynamic, myocardia and physiological changes.

- If ionic are used, Na^+ content should be near the physiological level of 140mg/L.

PTCA

- Ionic dimer ioxaglate is regarded as the optimal RCM because of its anticoagulant and low osmotic properties.
- Selective use of LOCM should be accorded to the following specific patients.
- Those undergoing painful procedure e.g. peripheral angiography cardiac angniography, without DSA.
- Any high risk procedure e.g. Spinal angio, coronary or renal angiography/angioplasty, pulm. angio in PTE and pulmonary hypertension.
- Greater than usual risk of an ADR's.
- Those examination requiring very high doses of RCM.

MEDICOLEGAL ASPECT OF RCM

Some of the following issues are of particular medicolegal importance:

1. *Clinical indication:* It is imperative to have a sound defensible clinical indication for any RCM.
2. *Patients of increased risk:* If RCM administration is essential the discussion of the risk factors with the patient and the clinical should be documented in the notes, prophylactic oral steroids (12-24 hours before Radiological Contrast Media administration) and LOCM should be used and patient should be carefully monitored at least 30 minutes after the procedure to the resuscitation instruments and personal should be checked and readily available.
3. *Informed consent:* Patient should be informed of all ADR's.

   Informed consent should be taken and even offering the patient to choose between cheaper but more uncomfortable, more toxic HOCM or more expensive less uncomfortable and less toxic LOCH.
4. *Dosage:* It is recommended to keep within the recommended dose of all drugs including RCM.

Section 5—Hepatopancreatobiliary System

Chapter 53

Cystic Hepatic Lesions

DIFFERENTIAL DIAGNOSIS OF CYSTIC LIVER LESIONS

1. Simple cyst.
2. Polycystic liver and kidney disease.
3. Hydatid (or echinococcal) cyst (Figure 53.1).
4. Liver abscess.
5. Hematoma or biloma.
6. Choledochal cyst.
7. Biliary cystadenoma and cystadenocarcinoma.
8. Primary and metastatic liver tumor.

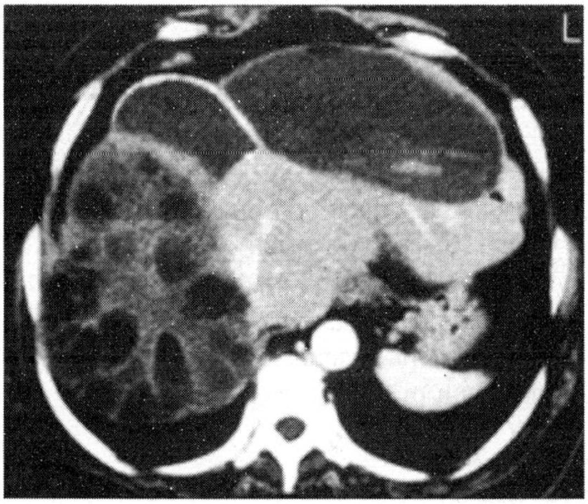

Fig. 53.1: Axial CECT scan showing multiloculated hydatid cyst in right lobe of liver

HEPATIC (BILE DUCT/SIMPLE CYST)

- Simple hepatic cysts are benign developmental lesions that do not communicate with the biliary tree.
- The current theory regarding the origin of true hepatic cysts is that they originate from hamartomatous tissue.
- Hepatic cysts are common and are presumed to be present in 2.5% of the population.
- They are more often discovered in women and are almost always asymptomatic.
- Simple hepatic cysts can be solitary or multiple, with the latter being the more typical scenario.
- At histopathological analysis, true hepatic cysts contain serous fluid and are lined by a nearly imperceptible wall consisting of cuboidal epithelium, identical to that of bile ducts, and a thin underlying rim of fibrous stroma.
- On all imaging modalities, uncomplicated simple liver cysts have thin, imperceptible wall.
- On US, they are seen as anechoic masses with smooth borders and posterior acoustic enhancement.
- A hepatic cyst appears as a homogeneous and hypo attenuating lesion on nonenhanced CT scans, with no enhancement of its wall or

content after intravenous administration of contrast material. It is typically round or ovoid and well defined.

- At MR imaging, hepatic cysts have homogeneous very low signal intensity on T1-weighted images and homogeneous very high signal intensity on T2-weighted images. Owing to their fluid content, an increase in signal intensity is seen on heavily T2-weighted images. This increase allows differentiation of these lesions from metastatic disease. No enhancement is seen after administration of gadolinium chelates. In cases of intracystic hemorrhage), a rare complication in simple hepatic cysts, the signal intensity is high, with a fluid-fluid level, on both T1- and T2-weighted images when mixed blood products are present.
- As majority is asymptomatic, so they do not require treatment.
- Complications of these cysts include hemorrhage and infection.
- Large cysts may cause symptoms resulting from mass effect.

POLYCYSTIC HEPATIC DISEASE

- Hepatic cysts (Figure 53.2) can also be part of polycystic liver disease, an autosomal dominant disorder often found in association with renal polycystic disease.
- Although hepatic cysts are found in 40% of cases of autosomal dominant polycystic disease involving the kidneys, they may be seen without identifiable renal involvement at radiography.
- Usually, patients with autosomal dominant polycystic liver disease are asymptomatic and liver dysfunction occurs only sporadically.
- However, advanced disease can result in hepatomegaly, liver failure, or Budd-Chiari syndrome. In these more severe cases, percutaneous interventional alcohol ablation has been useful as an alternative to partial liver resection or even transplantation.

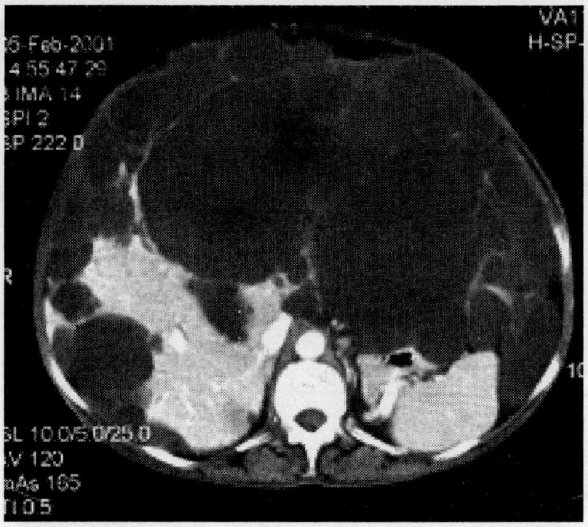

Fig. 53.2: Axial CT image shows multiple hepatic cysts in a case of polycystic liver disease

- Polycystic liver disease typically appears as multiple homogeneous and hypoattenuating cystic lesions with a regular outline on nonenhanced CT scans, with no wall or content enhancement on contrast enhanced images.
- At MR imaging, hepatic cysts in polycystic liver disease have very low signal intensity on T1-weighted images and do not enhance after administration of gadolinium contrast material. Owing to their pure fluid content, homogeneous high signal intensity is demonstrated on T2-weighted and heavily T2-weighted images. In patients with polycystic liver disease, signal intensity abnormalities indicating intracystic hemorrhage are more frequently encountered than in cases of simple hepatic cysts due to the great number of cysts. Although the diagnosis of polycystic liver disease is easily made with both CT and MR imaging, MR imaging is more sensitive for the detection of complicated cysts.

HYDATID CYST

- Hydatid (or echinococcal) cysts represent the

larval stage of the echinococcus tapeworm in which humans are the accidental intermediate host.

- The definitive host is a carnivore, usually a dog.
- The adult tapeworm lives in the jejunum of the dog. Its eggs pass through the dog faeces and when eggs are swallowed by the intermediate host, embryos are freed in the duodenum and pass through the mucosa to enter a branch of the portal vein, most of which arrest in the hepatic capillaries. Some embryos pass through the liver to the lung and less frequently to other organs.
- Gharbi *et al.* classified the ultrasonographic findings of liver hydatid cyst into 5 patterns, namely:
  - Type I: Pure fluid collection.
  - Type II: Fluid collection with a split wall.
  - Type III: Fluid collection with septa.
  - Type IV: Heterogeneous echo patterns; and
  - Type V: Reflecting thick wall.
- The type I was the most common variety of hydatid cyst.
- These variable ultrasonographic findings of liver hydatid cysts may make it difficult to distinguish these cysts from other disease processes.
- The differential diagnosis varies with the type of echographic patterns.
  - The types II and III patterns are characteristic of hydatic cysts.
  - Types V and I pattern are suggestive of hydatid cyst in endemic countries.
  - Type IV is the most difficult to diagnose and may easily be confused with a primary or secondary liver tumor.
- Crescentic or ring-shaped calcification of the walls or linear calcifications of the septa are more frequently visualized on CT (Figure 53.3) than on the plain film of the abdomen. On CT E. granulosus cysts appear as well-demarcated thin or thick walled hypoattenuating structures, which can be uni- or multilocular. Daughter cysts are usually visible as small structures with their own walls in the interior of the mother cyst. Sometimes the daughter cysts are confined only the peripheral area of the mother cyst. Typically, the fluid in the daughter cysts has a lower attenuation value than that in the mother cyst. Thin linear structures within the fluid represent free-floating membranes following wall rupture.

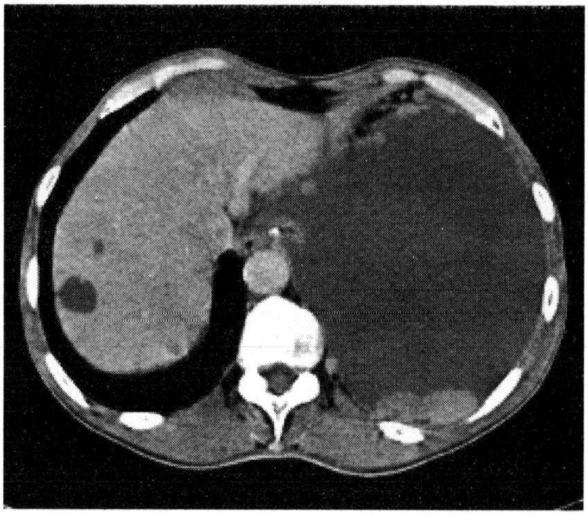

Fig. 53.3: Axial CT image shows an incidental hepatic cyst in a patient with hydrothorax of left side

Dilatation of the bile ducts either due to external compression or to intrabiliary rupture with obstruction may be present. In case of intrabiliary rupture, small daughter cysts or high attenuation material can be observed within the larger bile ducts. Septa and cyst walls enhance following intravenous contrast medium administration. The CT appearance of E. multicolaris is different from that produced by E. granulosus. Lesions appear hypoattenuating but inhomogeneous and with unsharp borders. There is no evidence of septation. Calcifications are punctiform or amorphous. The masses enhance poorly or not at all. Distinction between hydatid cysts and primary or secondary malignant neoplasm may be difficult on CT alone.

Most hydatid cysts are hyperintense on T1-weighted and hyperintense on T2 weighted images. The visualization of a peripheral rim of low signal intensity both on Tl-weighted and on T2-weighted images is considered to be typical. The internal structure of the cyst can be displayed well on MRI.

HEPATIC ABSCESS (Figure 53.4)

- Abscesses can be classified as pyogenic, amoebic, or fungal.
- Hepatic abscesses can result from infection by five different routes:
  a. Biliary, due to ascending cholangitis.
  b. Portal venous, due to bacteraemia from intra-abdominal sepsis.
  c. Arterial, due to septicaemia.
  d. Local extension, due to suppuration involving neighbouring tissues.
  e. Traumatic, due to blunt or penetrating injuries.
- Patients are usually symptomatic, commonly presenting with fever, malaise, and abdominal discomfort.

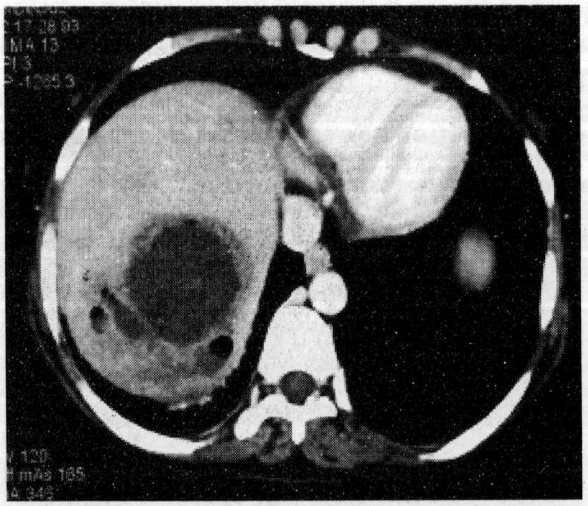

Fig. 53.4: Axial CT image show a typical hepatic abscess

- Most hepatic abscesses are pyogenic or fungal in origin; where as amoebic abscesses predominate in endemic areas.
- Escherichia coli is the organism most commonly isolated in culture in most reported series.
- The ultrasonographic appearances of liver abscess are varied, often nonspecific. Differentiation of a pyogenic abscess from an amoebic abscess or other complex cystic lesions is generally not reliable. Ultrasonogrphically guided needle aspiration in helpful for an accurate diagnosis.
- Five characteristic ultrasonographic features of amoebic abscesses have been described, namely:
  1. Absence of significant wall echoes.
  2. Oval or rounded shape.
  3. Hypoechoic lesion that is homogenous and has low-level internal echoes.
  4. Location near to or touching the liver capsule; and
  5. Enhanced acoustic through transmission deep to the lesion. However, only 30% of proven amoebic abscesses demonstrate all five features. A blinded comparative study of ultrasonographic findings in amoebic and pyogenic abscesses showed that the two most statistically reliable features of amoebic abscesses were a rounded or oval shape and a hypoechoic appearance with homogeneous low-level internal echoes.
- Pyogenic liver abscesses may be classified into either micro-abscesses or larger confluent lesions. Micro-abscesses may be seen as either discrete hypoechoic nodules or ill-defined areas.
- The sensitivity of CT for detecting hepatic abscess is as high as 97%.
- At CT, hepatic abscess appears as a single or multiloculated mass with low attenuation (0-45HU). Abscesses frequently have a peripheral

rim or capsule that demonstrates contrast enhancement.

- At MR imaging, hepatic abscesses, show prolonged Tl and T2 relaxation times, which correspond to decreased Tl signal and increased T2 signal. Contrast enhanced MR images reveal enhancement of the peripheral rim relative to the necrotic center.

HEPATIC BILOMA

- Rupture of part of the intrahepatic bile ducts enables bile to leave the biliary tract and accumulate, so forming a fluid collection of variable size (biloma). Whether this occurs and the size to which it develops depends on the extent of damage and bile flow rates.
- The most common underlying cause is hepatic trauma.
- Sonography reveals a well-defined fluid collection within the liver, which may contain internal echoes from debris or hemorrhage.
- Differentiation of a biloma from other forms of liver cysts requires either aspiration of bile from it, or scintigraphic demonstration of communication with the biliary tree using Tc99m labelled HIDA.
- Most bilomas will resolve spontaneously, though persistent enlargement or complications such as infection may necessitate intervention.
- CT findings of a post-traumatic biloma demonstrate a cystic structure of low attenuation in or around the liver. Bilomas may contain debris or septa.

CHOLEDOCHAL CYSTS (Figure 53.5)

Choledochal cysts can present from birth to old age but most commonly manifest early in life.

- Presenting symptoms include jaundice (80%), abdominal mass (50%), or abdominal pain (50%).

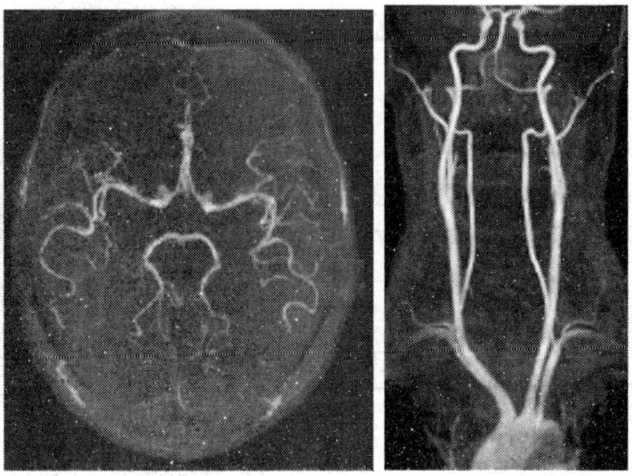

Fig. 53.5: Magnetic Resonance Angiography (MRA) show the vessels known as the Circle of Willis in the brain and neck vessels

- On CT and US, a choledochal cyst is seen a cystic mass in the region of the porta hepatis separate from the gallbladder but which communicates with the intrahepatic ducts.
- Hepatobiliary scintigraphy can be used to demonstrate radiotracer uptake within the cyst, confirming the diagnosis.

CAROLI'S DISEASE

- Named after Jacques Caroli, French Physician), it is a condition comprising multiple congenital liver cysts, which communicate with the bile ducts and overlaps with choledochal cyst type IV.
- Clinical findings include hepatomegaly, a right upper quadrant mass, jaundice and symptoms related to infection, bile stasis and calculi.
- Ultrasound demonstrates multiple spherical anechoic cystic structures throughout the liver.
- Complications such as cyst hemorrhage and infection may result in low level echoes within the cysts and debris fluid levels.
- Similar findings are evident on CT and MRI.
- Hepatobiliary scintigraphy shows that these cysts communicate with the bile ducts. In the parenchymal phase they appear as photophenic defects, which subsequently fill

in and persist after the parenchymal phase has passed.

- Complications such as calculi and malignant change may be detected by sonography but require more detailed imaging (PTC, ERCP) for complete evaluation.

HEPATOBILIARY CYSTADENOMA AND CYSTADENOCARCINOMA

- Rare cystic neoplasms of the liver occurring predominantly in women.
- They represent less than 5% of hepatic cysts of biliary origin.
- The large majority arises in the intrahepatic bile ducts whereas the remainder originates in the extrahepatic bile ducts.
- It is believed that all hepatobiliary cystadenomas are premalignant.
- Cholangiography reveals intraluminal-filling defects of varying size and is most useful for cystadenoma, which develops within the larger bile ducts.
- The cross-sectional radiological imaging methods accurately depict the morphological features of these neoplasms.
- Ultrasound demonstrates the multiseptated appearance and nodularity of the wall.
- CT demonstrates a well-defined multilocular large mass with attenuation values between 0 and +20 HU. The attenuation in the different locules may vary depending on the composition of its contents (mucinous, proteinaceous or hemorrhagic). Small stippled calcifications situated in the septa and the walls are best displayed on CT. The thickened septa, tile wall and the nodular components will enhance following intravenous contrast medium administration.
- MRI visualizes a complex multiseptated mass with predominantly high signal intensity on T2-weighted images and mixed high and low signal intensity on T1-weighted images. If hemorrhagic fluid is present, increased signal intensity may be noted on T1-weighted images. A low signal intensity rim on T2-weighted images has been observed and is probably due to hemorrhage in the wall of the lesion.
- On angiography the mass is predominantly hypovascular with the exception of the solid nodules that may show some degree of tissue blush.
- The different imaging findings do not allow in most instances the differentiation between hepatobiliary cystadenoma and cystadenocarcinoma although the presence of nodularity. Calcifications or hemorrhage is seen more frequently in the malignant form. However, because the treatment for both benign cystadenoma and malignant cystadenocarcinoma is similar and consists of total surgical excision, the preoperative distinction has little therapeutic implications.

OTHER CYSTIC HEPATIC TUMORS

- Cystic metastases includes: Sarcomas specially leiomyosarcoma of gastrointestinal origin, cystadenocarcinoma ovarian; cystadenocarcinoma pancreatic, mucinous carcinoma, colorectal, squamous cell carcinoma.
- A sonolucent pattern is seen in metastases that are partially or totally cystic. However, commonly mural thickening, mural nodules or internal low-level echoes due to septation, debris or a fluid-fluid level are present and will help to distinguish these lesions from simple hepatic cysts.
- On CT, their attenuation values may be below 20 HU and their appearance may resemble hepatic cysts.

5 Section

- Most hepatic metastases are hypo intense on T1-weighted and hyper intense on T2-weighted images relative to the liver parenchyma. This is based on the prolonged T1 and T2 relaxation times due to the increased intracellular water present. Metastases occasionally appear and bright lesions on T1-weighted images due to subacute hemorrhage, to melanin accumulation in metastases from melanoma, or to high protein (mucin) content.
- Cystic degeneration can also be seen in hepatic tumor due to necrosis.

Calcified Hepatic Masses

INFECTIONS

- Tuberculosis, histoplasmosis, gumma, brucellosis.
- Echinococcal cyst.
- Old pyogenic or amoebic abscess.

VASCULAR

- Hepatic artery or portal venous aneurysms.
- Portal vein thrombosis.
- Hematoma.

BENIGN TUMORS

- Congenital cysts (usually show curvilinear calcification).
- Cavernous hemangiomas.
- Capsule of regenerating nodules.
- Infantile hemangioendothelioma.

PRIMARY MALIGNANT TUMORS

- Hepatoblastoma.
- Cholangiocellular carcinoma.
- Fibrolamellar carcinoma.
- Epithelioid hemangioendothelioma.

METASTATIC TUMORS

- Mucinous carcinoma of colon, breast, stomach.
- Ovarian carcinoma.
- Melanoma, pleural mesothelioma, osteosarcoma, carcinoid, leiomyosarcoma.

HEPATIC HEMANGIOMAS

- Most common benign liver tumor and second most common liver tumor after metastasis.
- May have central areas of necrosis if large.
- Calcifications are extremely uncommon but when present may be nodular or amorphous. Phleboliths are also uncommon.
- Uniformly echogenic on USG when small, may be heterogenous when large.
- On CT they are spherical, ovoid or round masses of low attenuation on non-contrast images.
- They show early peripheral enhancement with delayed centripetal filling with central non-enhancing regions seen in large masses due to fibrosis or hemorrhage.
- Centripetal filling alone is not characteristic as it can be seen in other hepatic neoplasm. The

pattern of peripheral filling coupled with delayed filling and persistence of enhancement constitute the diagnostic triad of hemangiomas.

INFANTILE HEMANGIOENDOTHELIOMA

- Solitary mass is less commonly seen. It usually presents as multiple nodules of varying sizes.
- Areas of hemorrhage, thrombosis, fibrosis and calcifications are common.
- Most common liver tumor during the first six months of life, females being affected more commonly than males.
- Appearance on CT is similar to hemangiomas and on precontrast scans it appears as low density lesion with calcification and may show peripheral enhancement with delayed central enhancement.

Epithelioid Hemangioendothelioma

- Primary malignant vascular tumor of liver, soft tissues, bone or lung seen in adult age group.
- Probably associated with oral contraceptives or exposure to vinyl chloride.
- Multiple nodular form is more common and the nodules may coalesce to form large masses, calcification is seen in 15% of tumors.
- Low attenuating on NCCT and may become isoattenuating on CECT.

HEPATOBLASTOMA

- Most common primary malignant liver neoplasm of childhood usually seen in first three years of life.
- Large solitary well circumscribed mass with a nodular or lobulated surface and may contain areas of fibrosis, calcifications and osseous matrix.
- On CT they appear as low attenuation large solid masses that contain areas of calcifications and show exuberant contrast enhancement on CECT.

CHOLANGIOCELLULAR OR INTRAHEPATIC CHOLANGIO CARCINOMA

- Usually presents as a mass 5-20 cm in diameter.
- Satellite nodules are seen in 65% of cases.
- Contains punctate or chunky calcification in upto 18% of cases.
- Single predominantly homogenous round to oval mass with irregular borders.
- Peripheral wash out sign is seen on CECT — there is early minimal to moderate rim enhancement with progressive concentric filling and clearing of contrast material in rim on delayed images.
- Marked-homogenous delayed enhancement may be seen in 74% of cases.

Fibrolamellar Carcinoma

- Slow growing malignant tumors of hepatocellular origin that arises in non cirrhotic liver.
- Satellite lesions are often seen.
- The tumor is present as partially to completely encapsulated solitary mass 5 to 15cm in diameter.
- There is a prominent central stellate fibrous scar that may show calcification.
- On NECT it appears as a mass of low attenuation with variable contrast enhancement on CECT.

Metastasis

- There is usually a history of known primary.
- The hepatic metastasis enhance strongly during the arterial phase as they are supplied by the hepatic artery with negligible supply by the portal venous system.

Chapter 55

Vascular Scar Tumors of Liver

1. Focal nodular hyperplasia.
2. Hepatic adenoma.
3. Giant cavernous hemangiomas.
4. Fibrolamellar HCC.
5. Well differentiated HCC.
6. Hypervascular metastasis.
7. Intrahepatic cholangiocarcinoma.

FOCAL NODULAR HYPERPLASIA

- Rare benign congenital hamartomatous malformation or reparative process in the areas of focal injury.
- Oral contraceptives do not cause FNH but exert a trophic effect on its growth.
- Often asymptomatic may present with vague abdominal pain or as an abdominal mass when very large.
- Size usually <5 cm (85%) more common in right lobe.
- It is well circumscribed, non-encapsulated, mass in otherwise normal liver, shows no calcification, may be multiple in 20% of cases and may be pedunculated (5%) when situated at the surface of liver.

USG

- Iso/hypo/hyperechoic (33%) homogenous mass may have a central hyperechoic scar and causes displacement of hepatic vessels.

Doppler

- Enlarged afferent blood vessel with central arterial; hypervascularity with centrifugal filling to the periphery in "spoke wheel" pattern, similar pattern seen on angiography.

NECT and CECT

- Iso to slightly hypoattenuating homogenous mass which may show an even more hypoattenuating central scar.
- Transient intense hyperdensity (after 30 - 60 seconds) on bolus injection followed rapidly by isodensity so that the lesion may be missed without pre contrast study.
- The fibrous scar may show early enhancement of vessels traversing it with accumulation of contrast on delayed images. This sign is described as highly indicative of FNH.

HEPATIC ADENOMA

- Rare benign neoplasm more commonly seen in young women after oral contraceptive use.
- No true capsule seen. Pseudocapsule forms due to compression of adjoining liver tissue.

- More common in right lobe and is subcapsular with average size of 8-10 cm.

USG

- Small well demarcated solid echogenic or complex echotexture mass with anechoic areas if large.

CT

- Hypoattenuating rounded mass with areas of necrosis.
- Hyperdense areas of fresh intra tumoral hemorrhage.
- Transiently enhancing on arterial phase with centripetal filling similar to hemangioma, and iso to hypoattenuating on delayed phase images.

GIANT CAVERNOUS HEMANGIOMAS

- Most common benign liver tumor and second most common liver tumor after metastasis.
- More common in females.
- May be associated with FNH, Rendu-Osler-Weber disease.
- Asymptomatic if small, may present with spontaneous life threatening hemorrhage if large, hepatomegaly, Kasabach-Merritt syndrome.
- Size usually less than 4 cm (90%) when larger than 10cm they are known as giant hemangiomas.
- May have central areas of fibrosis forming a central scar, necrosis of cystic spaces especially when giant.

USG

- Uniformly hyperechoic (60-70%) when small giant hemangiomas may be hypoechoic to mixed echotexture.
- May show acoustic enhancement.
- May have no Doppler signals to signals with peak velocity of <50 cm per sec.

CT

- Well circumscribed spherical to oval low density mass.
- May have areas of higher or low density within them especially when giant.
- Typical triad of early peripheral filling coupled with centripetal delayed filling and persistence of enhancement 3 to 30 min after bolus characterize hemangiomas from other similar tumors.
- Central areas of fibrosis may not show any enhancement at all.
- Angiography (gold standard) historical in importance now.

FIBROLAMELLAR HCC

- Seen in otherwise normal livers and is alpha fetoprotein negative.
- Seen in relatively young age group 5-35 years and M: F is 1:1.
- Well circumscribed strikingly desmoplastic tumor with calcifications and a central fibrous scar and is partially to completely encapsulated.
- On CT it is of low attenuation with varying degree of enhancement on CECT.

WELL-DIFFERENTIATED HCC

- Most frequent primary visceral malignancy of the world.
- Diverse etiology ranging from cirrhosis to chronic hepatitis B/C to carcinogens and inborn errors of metabolism.
- Most commonly solitary but may be multi-centric to diffuse.
- Vascularity is hepatic arterial but in 6% of cases it may be portal venous.

- Portal venous invasion is common with tumor thrombus.

CT

- Sensitivity of 63% in cirrhotic livers and 80% in non-cirrhotic hypodense mass to hyper-dense in fatty livers.
- A dominant mass is seen with satellite nodules.
- Mosaic pattern multiple nodular areas with differing attenuation on CECT 63%.
- Diffusely infiltrating neoplasm.
- There is enhancement during hepatic arterial phase.
- Decreased attenuation during portal venous phase with inhomogenous areas of contrast accumulation.
- Isodensity on delayed scans (10%).
- Wedge shaped areas of decreased attenuation in liver due to portal venous thrombus.

INTRAHEPATIC CHOLANGIOCARCINOMA

- Second most common primary hepatic malignancy.
- Average age 50-60 years more common in males.
- Satellite nodules are seen in 65% of cases and the mass may show punctate or chunky calcification.
- Calculi may be seen in biliary tree.

USG

- Dilated IHBR.
- Predominantly homogenous mass may show areas of heterogeneity.

CT

- Single predominantly homogeneous round to oval hypodense mass with irregular borders.
- Peripheral wash out sign = early minimal to moderate rim enhancement with progressive concentric filling and clearing of contrast in rim of lesion on delayed images.
- Marked homogeneous delayed enhancement in 75% of cases.
- May encase portal and hepatic veins similar to HCC but without tumor thrombus.

Section 5—Hepatopancreatobiliary System

Chapter 56

Hepatobiliary Injury

Blunt Trauma

- Approximately 5-10% of blunt trauma has a liver injury.
- Steering wheel injury, direct blow, and rapid deceleration in motor vehicle accidents (shearing forces).
- Most frequent site – posterior segment of right lobe.
- Left lobe less common associated with retroperitoneal injury.
- Major hepatic venous injury -13%, can be suggested by multiple lacerations around the IVC and porta hepatis.
- Injuries of bare area of liver, no peritoneal signs or findings on diagnostic peritoneal lavage.

Penetrating Injuries

- Stabbing, gunshot or shot gun injury.

Iatrogenic Injuries

- Needles, wires, cannular and catheters. External cardiac compression, low insertion of chest tube.

Spontaneous Rupture

- Eclamptic or preeclamptic women in 3rd trimester, spontaneous hemorrhage, sickle cell anemia, hepatoma, adenoma.

EVALUATION OF THE HEPATIC INJURY

Diagnostic Peritoneal Lavage

Plain Film

- Neither specific nor sensitive fracture of lower ribs.
- Hemoperitoneum – loss of inferior liver fat interface.
- Hepatomegaly, irregularity of liver margin.
- Pul. contusion, pneumothorax, pleural effusion, hemothorax.

Ultrasound

- Ultrasound is much more accurate in the detection of hemoperitoneum than in diagnosis of specific parenchymal or hollow viscus injury.
- FAST (Focussed abdominal sonogram for trauma) – free fluid.
- Can demonstrate a number of traumatic lesions.
- Subcapsular hematoma – Lentiform or curvilinear fluid collection initially anechoic, progressively echogenic by 24 hours.
- By 4-5 days – hypoechoic. Internal echoes and septations develop in 1-4 weeks.

Contusions

- Hypoechoic, transiently become hyperechoic and then hypoechoic.
- Lesions posteriorly in right lobe or over the spine within left lobe are usually not sonographically demonstrable.

Parenchymal tears with or without hematoma, irregular defects with abnormal echo architecture relative to surrounding normal tissue.

Intraparenchymal hematomas as small as 3.5ml round, echogenic foci.

Biloma–Rounded or ellipsoid, anechoic, lobulated structures with sharply defined margins close to the liver and bile ducts. Scintigraphy is an important adjacent to show communication.

- Fluid aspiration.

COMPUTED TOMOGRAPHY (Figure 56.1)

- Imaging technique of choice for hepatic trauma.
- Can reliably diagnose and stage significant hepatic and extra hepatic injury.
- Major CT findings are branching linear lacerations, which most often parallel branches of hepatic and portal vein, parenchymal and subcapsular hematomas and periportal tracking.

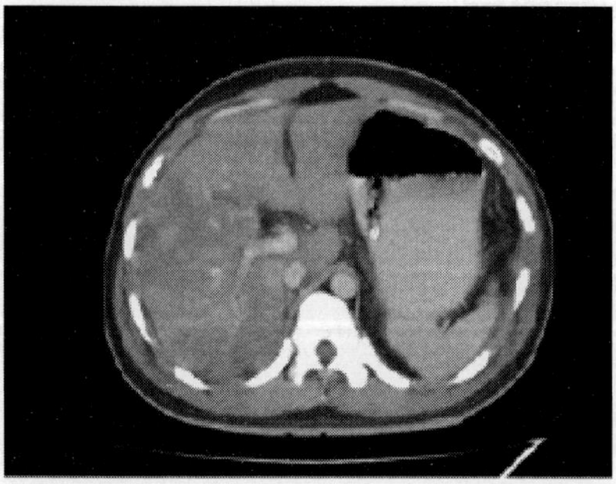

Fig. 56.1: Axial CECT scan in a patient with blunt abdominal trauma showing laceration of right lobe liver (grade III/IV injury)

Lacerations

- Superficial = 3cm.
  Deep > 3cm.
- Deep central parenchymal injuries – unrecognized at laparotomy, ESP if surface is normal.
- Associated with hematoma.

Periportal tracking – may be the only manifestation.

- May represent collections of blood or dilated periportal lymphatics.
- Usually seen due to rapid fluid resuscitation.

Intraparenchymal gas, in the absence of infection has been described in sterile resolving lacerations.

Hematoma

- NCCT – hyperdense.
- CECT – unclotted blood and bile are hypodense.
- Active hemorrhage – contrast extravasation (85-350 HU), hematoma (40-70-40).
- Fatty infiltration – Hematoma may appear isodense – marrow CT window settings.

CT BASED CLASSIFICATION OF BLUNT HEPATIC TRAUMA

Grade Criteria

1. Capsular avulsion superficial lacerations <1cm deep, subcapsular hematoma (<1cm) maximal thickness, periportal blood tracking only.
2. Lacerations 1-3 cm deep, central/subcapsular hematomas 1-3 cm.
3. Laceration >3 cm deep, central/subcapsular hematomas >3 cm diameter.
4. Massive central/subcapsular hematoma >10 cm/lobar-tissue restriction (maceration) or devascularization.
5. Bilobar tissue destruction (maceration) or devascularization.

MRI

- Gd. enhanced MR can depict complex hepatic

injuries in patients with contraindications of iodinated contrast media.

- Longer imaging time, metallic life support not accommodated.

Angiography

- Now performed only to investigate severe hemorrhage and post-traumatic fistulas.
- Demonstrates smaller arterial psuedoaneurysms than CT.
- Traumatic pseudoaneurysms, arteriobiliary fistulas, arteriovenous fistulas and portobiliary fistula – major sources.
- Amenable to transarterial embolization with gianturco coils or detachable balloons.

BILIARY TRACT INJURY

- Gallbladder and bile duct are rarely affected by blunt abdominal trauma because they partially embedded in the liver and shielded by rib cage.
- Nevertheless, contusion or rupture when forceful blow to the RUQ. Concomitant lacerations of bile ducts, liver or pancreas may also occur.
- Gallbladder perforation accounts for 80-85% injuries.
- Thin wall normal gallbladder more prone to rupture.
- Discharge of its contents into peritoneal cavity can occur.
- Avulsion of gallbladder – 10-15% of cases of biliary injury.
- Partially torn from the liver bed or deteched completely.

Diagnosed by finding a ruptured gallbladder with hematoma in its fossa and lumen on CT.

Contusion of the gallbladder lead to discrete blurring or intramural bleeding without significant signs and symptoms. If blood supply compromised – necrosis and delayed rupture.

- Acute hemorrhagic cholecystitis – cystic duct blockage caused by occult injury or secondary hemophilia and formation of intraductal clots.
- Extrahepatic bile duct – disruption occurs near the hepatic bifurcation in the liver hilum and leads to profuse bile leakage or peritonitis.
- Intrahepatic branches – can be injured. Difficult to recognize by inspection at surgery.
- Cholangiography and hepatobiliary scintigraphy – most sensitive.

PENETRATING INJURIES

- Patients with liver injuries may have associated lacerations of the bile ducts and gallbladder.
- Co-existing trauma to liver, pancreas or other viscera dominates.
- Biliary trial injury suspected – jaundice, acholic stools, abdominal pain, and distension associated with bile stained peritoneal fluid.
- Post-traumatic disruption of intrahepatic branch result in localized bile leak. Usually present weeks to months after injury as simple thin walled cysts with low attenuation contents.

Hemobilia

- Due to communication with vascular tree, also usually present as a delayed manifestation with pain, jaundice and GI bleeding.
- CT may demonstrate – high attenuation blood in dilated biliary tree.

Biliary peritoneal leak may result in biliary peritonitis following secondary infection. Suspicious of leak – low attenuation of peritoneal fluid 0-20 HU.

PANCREATIC INJURY

- Blunt pancreatic injuries are relatively uncommon, occurring in 3-12% of abdominal trauma.
- Compression of the neck and body of pancreas against the vertebral column.

- Associated with injuries in duodenum spleen, kidneys or lumbar spine – 90%.
- Most of deaths occur within 48 hours injury, due to hypovolumic shock and major hemorrhage that result from vascular injury.

Clinically

Classical triad of acute pancreatic trauma of upper abdominal pain, leucocytosis and hyper amylasias are of limited value in the diagnosis of pancreatic injury.

Amylase levels may be normal in if obtained within 3 hours.

Hyperamylasemia – non specific finding.

Ultrasonography

- Acute assessment by US hampered by the presence of air in the stomach and small bowel secondary to aerophagy due to pain, also the retro peritoneum is poorly assessed.
- Findings may be subtle, usually demonstrating nonspecific gland enlargement caused by pancreatitis or contusion.

Computed Tomography

- CT is the most accurate available modality for the detection and gradation of pancreatic injury. However, even using optimal CT techniques pancreatic injury is often missed on intial appraisal. Upto 40% of pancreatic injuries may not be visible on CT obtained within 12 hours of trauma.
- Pancreatic contusions – mostly isodense but occasionally hyperdense masses because of intra parenchymal hemorrhage.
- Pancreatic fracture – well demarcated lucent defects traversing the gland generally including the neck perpendicular to long axis with little or no separation of fragments with subtle density changes.
- Direct injury to pancreas itself is not easily visible so ancillary secondary signs include presence of localized oedema.
- Retroperitoneal hematoma or fat infiltration.
- Localized collections of fluid in the lesser sac.
- Ant pararenal fascia thickening.
- Tracking of fluid between splenic vein and pancreatic body.

CT GRADING (BLUNT PANCREATIC INJURY) (OIS CLASSIFICATION)

Grade	*Criteria*
I	Minor contusion or laceration without duct injury.
II	Major contusion or laceration without duct injury.
III	Distal transection or parenchymal injury without duct injury.
IV	Proximal resection or parenchymal injury involving ampulla.
V	Massive disruption of pancreatic head.

Grade I and II can be conservatively managed.

- Pancreatic duct trauma – can't be reliably excluded on CT, the deeper the laceration the more likely.
- 80% of major laceration (>50% thickness) is associated with ductal injury.

Grade III-V – Higher complications – pseudocysts, fistula, absesses.

- A surgical approach is mandated and with deeper lacerations duct injury should be excluded by ERCP or peroperative pancreatography.

Delayed imaging: After initial delay in diagnosis of pancreatic injuries may often become more prominent owing to development of localized odema and auto digestion due to pancreatic enzyme leakage.

- So vigilance required – when persistent pain, and discomfort or an elevated amylase level, a repeat scan may be rewarding within the first 24 hours.

Anomalies and Anatomic Variants of the Gallbladder, Biliary Tract and Pancreas

- Many congenital anomalies of gallbladder and bile duct are seen and excluding biliary atresia and choledochal cysts, anemia are of much clinical/functional significance.

Embryology

- Along the anterior margin of the primitive foregut, a bifid bud forms.

  Bifid Bud
  - Cephalad part – gives rise to liver and intrahepatic bile duct.
  - Caudal part – gives rise to gallbladder and extrahepatic bile duct.
- These originally hollow primordium of gall-bladder and CBD becomes occluded with endoluminal cells but soon get revoluted.
- If recanalization is incomplete - compart-mentalized multiseptated gallbladder results:
  - Single transverse septum– Phrygian cap.
  - Longitudinal septum – bifid or triple gall-bladder

Agenesis of Gallbladder

- Caused by failure or development of the caudal division of the primitive hepatic bud/ diverticulum or failure of revascularization after the solid phase of development.
- Atresia/hypoplasia of the gallbladder also represent aborted development.
- Other congenital anomalies are seen in 2/3rd of cases including:
  - Congenital heart disease.
  - Imperforate anus.
  - Absence of one or more bones.
  - Polyplenia.
  - RVF (Rectovaginal fistula).
- Surgical incidence of gallbladder agenesis is approx. 0.02%.
- Pre operative diagnosis of gallbladder agenesis is difficult. USG/CT may suggest diagnosis but this disorder is usually diagnosed at surgery.
- Intra operative USG may be helpful in establishing diagnosis and excluding completely intrahepatic gallbladder.

DUPLICATION OF GALLBLADDER

- Occurs in 1 in 4000 people.
- Due to persistent longitudinal septum that divided the gallbladder lengthwise.
- Diagnosis, USG can diagnose this condition easily. To establish the diagnosis, two separate gallbladder cavities each with its own cystic duct, must be present.

- The two cystic ducts can enter the gallbladder in many ways:
  A. Form Y-configuration.
  B. Enters separately.
  C. One in CBD and other in intrahepatic duct.
- Most reported cases of gallbladder duplication have a clinical picture of cholecystitis with cholelithiasis in at least one the gallbladders.

Differential Diagnosis

- No of entities mimic double gallbladder at USG.
- Folded gallbladder.
- Choledochal cyst (Figure 57.1).
- Gallbladder diverticulum.
- Focal adenomyomatosis.
- Bilobed gallbladder.
- Pricholeocystic fluid.
- Vascular band along gallbladder.

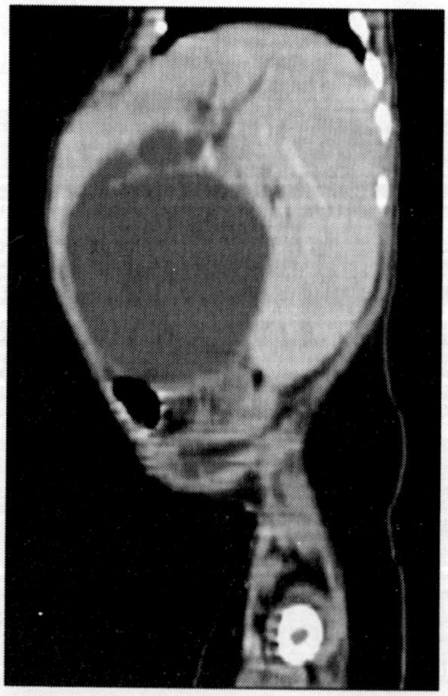

Fig. 57.1: Sagittal MPR CT image shows a large choledochal cyst with mild intrahepatic biliary dilatation

Complications

- Torsion.
- Development of papilloma, carcinoma, CBD obstruction and secondary biliary cirrhosis.

ANOMALITIES OF GALLBLADDER SHAPE

Phygian Cap

- Most common abnormality of gallbladder shape.
- Seen in 6% of population.
- Characteristized by a fold or septum of the gallbladder between the body and the fundus.

Two types:

- Retroserosal/concealed type.
- Serosal/Visible type.

This anomaly is of no clinical significance.

Diagnosis: Can be established by USG or oral cholecystography.

Multiseptate Gallbladder

- It's a solitary gallbladder characterized by multiple septa and various sizes internally and a faintly bisected surface externally.

These Septations Cause Stasis of Bile and Gall Stone Formation

USG: Multiple communicating septations and locules are seen bridging the gallbladder lumen.

Oral Cholecystography

- Reveals the honeycomb multiticystic character of gallbladder.

D/D in USG

- Desquamated gallbladder mucosa.
- Hyperplastic cholecystosis.

Diverticula

- Rare condition and is usually clinically silent.

- Congenital diverticulae are true diverticula, contain all the mucosal layers as compared to pseudo diverticulae of adenomyomatosis, which have little/no submucosal muscle layer in their walls.

ABNORMALITIES OF GALLBLADDER POSITION

Wandering Gallbladder

Occurs when gallbladder has an unusually long mesentry. The gallbladder can show any or more of the following features:

- Disappear in pelvis.
- Wander in front of the spine.
- To the left of the abdomen.
- Herniate through foramen of Winslow into the lesser sac.

In cases when gallbladder herniate through the Winslow's foramen:

- Oral obleosystography shows.
- Unusual angulation of gallbladder.
- Gallbladder lying parallel and adjacent to duodenal bulb with fundus pointing to the left upper quadrant.
- Best seen using barium meal and oral cholecystogram.

Ectopic Gallbladder

- Gallbladder can be located in a variety of anomalous position.
- Intrahepatic.
  - Gallbladder is completely surrounded by hepatic parenchyma.
  - May complicate diagnosis of acute cholecystitis because of paucity of clinical peritoneal signs.
  - Cause difficulty in coli cholecystectomy.

Diagnosis

- USG.
- Sulphur colloid scans, seen as a cold hepatic defect.
- Suprahepatic.
- Retrohepatic.
- Supra diaphragmatic.
- Retroperitoneal.
- Left sided gallbladder – seen in situs inversus.

BILIARY TRACT ANOMALIES

- Most common anomaly is an aberrant intrahepatic duct draining a circumscribed portion of liver. This duct can join the common hepatic duct, CBD, cystic duct or low right hepatic duct. Rarely it run through the gallbladder fossa or into the gallbladder which predisposes to its injury at cholecystectomy.

Cystic Duct Anomalies

- Absent cystic duct.
- Low insertion in CBD.
- Insertion into right hepatic duct.
- Conjoint segment with CBD.
- Proximal insertion at the confluence of right and left hepatic duct.

CHOLEDOCHAL CYSTS

- Congenital cystic dilatations of any portion of extrahepatic bile ducts, most commonly the main portion of CBD.

Pathogenesis

- Begin with an anomalous junction of the CBD and pancreatic duct proximal to the duodenal papilla. High pressure in the pancreatic duct combined with absent ductal sphincter allows free reflux of enzymes into CBD, weakening the wall of CBD.

- Male: Female = 3:1.
- 60% of patients present <10 years of age.

Association

- Biliary anomalies.
- Congenital hepatic fibrosis.

Complication

- Rupture → bile peritonitis.
- Secondary infection → cholangitis.
- Biliary cirrhosis.
- Portal H/T.
- Calculus formation.
- PV thrombosis.
- Liver abscess.
- Hemorrhage.
- Transformation into cholangio carcinoma.

C/F: Newborn and infants: Presents with obstructive jaundice.

Older childrens/Adults: Triad of (R) upper quadrant pain, intermittent jaundice and palpable (R) upper quadrant mass.

Imaging

USG

- Demonstrates, fluid filled structure beneath porta hepatis separate from the gallbladder that communicate with hepatic ducts. An abrupt change in the caliber is seen at the site of the cysts.
- It assesses the full extent of the ductal dilatation and identifies its connection with the biliary tree.

The presence of stones, strictures or tumors also can be detected with sonography.

Cholangiography

- Useful for fully defining ductal anatomy.
- It is necessary to confirm the diagnosis.
- Demonstrate cystic structure 2-15 cm in diameter that communicates with hepatic ducts.

Barium Study

- Shows a soft tissue mass in the right upper quadrant that causes anterior displacement of the 2nd part of the duodenum and antrum or inferior. Displacement of the duodenum or widening of the duodenal 'C' loop.

CT and MRI

- Appears as a right upper quadrant, fluid filled structure in contiguity with EH bile duct.
- Coronal imaging is helpful in delineating the communication of the cyst with the biliary tree. This can be done with CT using multiplanar reconstruction with or without the use cholangiographic contrast agents. Similarly, MRI with or without the use of MR cholangiography allows direct imaging of the cyst.
- The cyst can be differentiated from other cystic lesion such as pseudocysts of pancreas and enteric duplication cysts.
- Wall thickening, mural nodularity and wall enhancement in the choledochal cyst, in the absence of previous surgery, stress or cholangitis, raises the possibility of presence of tumor.

PTC/ERCP

- Best method of complete evaluation.
- Should be alone after detection of the cyst by USG/CT/MRI before operative treatment.
- It is the most reliable method to diagnose the presence of an anomalous pancreatobiliary junction.

Types: Choledochal Cyst

Original classification given by ALONZO-LEJ, and has been modified by TODANI *et al.* who described 5 types of choledochal cysts:

Type I (80-90% of cysts)	IA	Cystic dilatation of CBD
	IB	Focal, segmental dilatation of distal CBD
	IC	Fusiform dilatation of both CBD and CHD
Type II (2% of cysts)		True diverticula arising from the CBD
Type III (1.5% of cysts)		Cystic dilatation of intraduodenal portion of CBD (Choledochocoele)
Type IV (10% of cysts)	IVA	multiple intra and extra-hepatic cysts
	IVB	multiple extrahepatic cysts only
Type V		Generally involves only the intrahepatic ducts and may be single Or multiple (multiple are known as Caroli's disease).

CHOLEDOCHOCELE

- It's a type III choledochal cyst.
- It's the protrusion of dilated CBD into the duodenum.
- Manifestation in adulthood, no sex predilection.
- Presents as nausea, vomiting and episodic abdominal pain. It has sludge and stones and patients may also present with biliary colic, intermittent jaundice and pancreatitis.
- There is no increased risk of malignancy.

Cholangiography

- Smooth club like or sac like dilatation of intramural segment of CBD.

Barium Studies

- A mass does not fill with oral GI contrast but is seen as a smooth, well-defined intraluminal duodenal filling defect.

MRCP

- They have a high signal intensity, 'COBALT HEAD' appearance bulging into the duodenum.

CAROLI'S DISEASE

- It is a communicating, multifocal cancerous ectasia of the biliary tract, which is described as:
  a. Segmental, saccular dilatation of IH bile ducts.
  b. High incidence of bile duct stones, ascending cholangitis and liver abscess.
  c. Congenital hepatic fibrosis.
  d. Renal cystic disease (medullary sponge kidney, auto reverse polycystic kidney and cortical cysts). Most common association is medullary sponge kidney.
- Usually asymptomatic, however, if they develop symptoms, depends upon the predominant lesion.
  - IHBRD – episodic abdominal pain, fever, jaundice, secondary to biliary stone disease, ascending cholangitis and liver abscess.
  - Hepatic fibrosis – postal H/T with hematomas and lower GI bleeding.
- Male: Female = 1:1.

Imaging

- Before cross-sectional imaging studies, diagnosis was made at the time of surgical exploration and intraoperative cholangiography or at autopsy.

USG

- Multiple cystic areas in the liver which are communicating with the EH biliary ducts.

CT Scan/MRI

- Non-obstructive saccular or beaded dilatation of the intrahepatic bile ducts. This is displayed as multiple, intrahepatic, rounded cystic spaces of varying sizes communicating with the branching, dilating intrahepatic ducts. These IH cystic spaces contain calculi and/or amorphous debris. A pathognomonic features of Caroli's disease on CT scan is Central DOT SIGN.
- Central Dot Sign

  NCCT: Small dot of slightly high attenuation in the dependent portion of the dilated bile duct.

  CECT: Those dots enhance intensely. The central dot is representative of portal venous radicles that enveloped by (but not naturally inside of) the markedly dilated bile duct.
- Patient with hepatic fibrosis has HSM and dilated portal and splenic veins because of portal H/T.

DIFFERENTIAL DIAGNOSIS (ON CT AND MRI)

1. Polycystic Liver Disease

The cystic spaces in Caroli's are irregular in shape and communicate with the biliary tree, the cysts of polycystic liver disease are smoothen and rounded, do not communicate with the bile ducts (instead they deform the bile ducts).

2. Obstructive Bile Duct Dilatation

In this condition, the dilatation is more marked centrally, tapers towards the periphery in an organized pattern and lacks focal areas of cystic dilatation.

Patients of Caroli's disease are at high risk for developing cholangio carcinoma.

ANOMALIES AND ANATOMIC VARIANTS OF PANCREAS

Embryology

- Develops from two buds originated from endodermal lining of the duodenum.

Dorsal Bud

- Grows into the dorsal mesentery.
- Ventral bud – appears as an invagination at the biliary duodenal angle close to the bile duct.

Duodenum then falls on the right side.

↓

Ventral bud comes +ve on → and then dorsal on the (L)

- Ventral bud now, rotates posterior to the duodenum and comes in contact with the dorsal pancreas. And finally fuse.
- In mature organs.

Ventral primordium forms → inferior portion of head + uncinate process.

Dorsal primordium forms – rest of the head + body + tail.

New duct formation between distal part of dorsal bud and main duct of Wirsung — proximal dorsal duct. It usually atrophies and disappear or it may persist as accessory duct of Santorini.

Congenital Anomalies of Pancreas

Pancreas Divisum

- Pancreas is divided into the separate parts as a result of an absent or incomplete fusion of the vental and dorsal enlarge.
- Due to this.
  - Head and uncinate process.
    - Drain by duct of Wirsung through the major papilla.
  - Body and tail.
    - Drain by accessory. Duct of Santorini

5 Section

though minor papilla (2-3 cm above the major papilla).

- This anomaly is seen in 4-11% of autopsy series in 3-4% of ERCP series.

Clinical Features

- Most cases are asymptomatic.
- May cause idiopathic pancreatitis in young patients with no risk factors. About 12-28% of patients with idiopathic recurrent pancreatitis have this anomaly, as opposed to 3-6% in the general population.
- Mean age of presentation is 30-50 years.
- In pancreas division, duct of Santorini and its acceossory ampulla is too small to adequately drain the secretion produced by pancreas body and tail. Pancreatic studies showed increased pressure in dorsal duct (as compared to ventral duct) → postulated that chronic stasis of pancreatic fluid → increased risk of pancreatitis.

Imaging

ERCP

- It is essentially the only effective modality for confirming diagnosis of pancreas divisum.
- Contrast material when injected into the duct of Wirsung is met with resistance and pain. After opacification, the duct is short and gradually tapering and sends branches into the pancreatic head.
- Minor papilla, when the accessory duct opens, is difficult to cannulate. If possible, the full length and the accessory duct of Santorini is seen without communication to smaller ducts.

Sonographic Secretin Test

- In this, the main pancreatic duct is sonographically monitored before and after the IV administration of secretin (IU/kg/bw). ↓ ed HCO_3- secretin induced by secretin will not be able to cross the papilla, which is functionally inadequate.
- If pancreatic duct is normal and are before and 20 minutes after secretin – patient does not have ampullary stenosis.
- If duct dilates 1mm in diameter in only one segment – grade 1 response.
- Dilation >2 mm over 2 segments of pancreas (head and body) – grade 2 response.
- Dilates >2 mm over 3 segment of pancreas (head+body+tail) – grade 3 response.

CT Scans

- Contour abilities of the head and neck of pancreas have been identified on CT in some patients of pancreatic divisum.
- Can suggest diagnosis, when two distinct moieties or ductal system is identical on twin collimation.
- Fat cleft may separate the two moieties.

MRCP

- Heavily T2W images, two dimensional, fast spin echo sequences using a body coil accurately depict the pancreatic ductal anomaly that makes the diagnosis of pancreatic divisum.

Annular Pancreas

- In this, flat bond of pancreatic tissues completely encircles the 2nd portion of duodenum.
- Theories concerning the formation of the annular pancreas are:
  - Movability of both the ventral and dorsal ducts resulting in complete ring.
  - Adherence of ventral duct to duodenum before rotation.

Clinical Findings

- It's a uncommon anomaly.
- Clinically manifestation in neonates (52% or may be asymptomatic till adulthood (48%).

- Symptoms related to duodenal obstruction: vomiting on 1st day of life, associated history of polyhydramnios.
- Associated anomalies include duodenal atresia, interstinal malrotation and cardiac anomalies.

Imaging

- *Plain film*
  Shows double bubble sign: proximal bubble is due to gastric distension and the distal bubble by a dilated duodenal bulb.
- *Barium studies*
  It is characteristic and is best demonstrated when duodenum is maximally distended. Stenosis is demonstrated in the periampullary region associated with eccentric defect on the medial margin of the 2nd part duodenum. The mucosa is intact.
- *ERCP*
  Diagnosis of annular pancreas is most commonly suggested by ERCP, which shows typical features in about 85% of cases. This shows, abnormally located main pancreatic duct is seen in the body and tail that communicates with the small duct and pancreatic head, which encircles the duodenum.
- *CT scans*
  Findings are often non-specific showing enlargement of pancreatic head with a central region of high attenuation representing contrast material within the narrowed duodenal segment.
- *USG*
  Non-specific enlargement of the pancreatic head is the major abnormality in annular pancreas. Endoscopic USG is most accurate in accurate diagnosis.
- *MRI*
  Fat supposed T1 weighted images show a normal appearing pancreatic tissue encircling the duodenum.

Ectopic Pancreatic Tissue

- Seen mainly in the gastric antrum (25.5%) or proximal portion of the duodenum (27.7%). Infrequent sites include jejunum (15.9%), ileum Meckel's diverticulum , colon, appendix, mesentry, omentum, liver, gallbladder, spleen, bile ductus, esophagus mediastinal cyst, fallopian tube and broncho esophageal fistula.
- Ectopic tissues are located mainly sub-mucosally (73%).

Clinical Findings

- Majority of cases asymptomatic. When symptomatic, present as/or simulate duodenal ulcer, gallbladder disease or appendicitis.
- In stomach, it may simulate tumor-causing symptoms such as pyloric obstruction.

Radiological Findings

- Characteristically appears broad based, smooth extra mucosal or intramural lesion either along the greater curvature of gastric antrum of proximal duodenum.

Barium Study

- Small collection of barium appearing as a central umbilication, which is diagnostic. This represents the orifice of the rudimentary duct which ectopic pancreas empties.

Differential Diagnosis

- Peptic ulcer disease.
- Bruman gland adenoma.
- Leiomyosarcoma.
- Metstases to stomach.
- Gastric polyp.
- Leiomyoma.
- Lymphoma.

Section 5—Hepatopancreatobiliary System

Chapter 58

Acute Cholecystitis

- 1/3 patient of gallstones.
- Associated with cholelithiasis in 90-95%.

PREDISPOSING FACTORS

- ↑ Incidence with age, female.
- Chronic liver disease.
- Diabetes.
- Hemolytic disease – SCA, HS
- Congenital anomalies of biliary tree.
- IgA deficiency.
- Ileal resection.

* Infants
TPN
Phototherapy
Infection.

CLINICAL PRESENTATION

- Mild to dramatic according to presentation.

SEQUELAE

- Obstruction of cystic duct – bile stasis – distension of gallbladder.

Vascular compromise → mucosal infl. and necrosis →.

Bacterial contamination of bile.

INVESTIGATION

USG – Diagnostic

Primary signs	Secondary signs
Calculi as echogenic intraluminal foci (Figure 58.1)	Gallbladder Dilatation
Focal tender gallbladder 'Murphy sign'	Echogenic sludge
Impacted gall stone	Mural thickness >3 mm with halo of low reflectivity

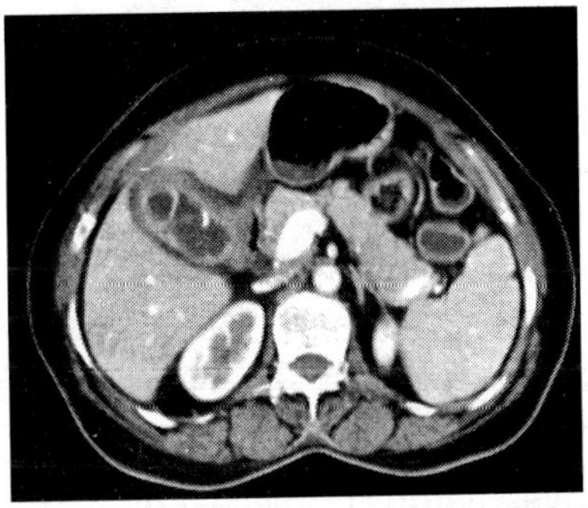

Fig. 58.1: Axial CT image shows calculus cholecystitis

CT

1. Distention of gallbladder (>5 cm in transverse or AP).
2. Gallbladder wall modularity.
3. Poor definition of gallbladder wall at interface with liver.
4. Inflammatory change in pericholecystic fat.
5. ↑ Density of bile (>20 HU).

CHOLESCINTIGRAPHY

90-95% sensitive and 38% specific.

- Persistent non-visualization of gallbladder.
- RIM SIGN and CYSTIC DUCT sign.

MRI

- Gd enhanced spin echo images – hyper intense gallbladder wall.
- ↑ SI on T2WI of gallbladder wall – intramural infiltration.

COMPLICATIONS OF ACUTE CHOLECYSTITIS (Figure 58.2)

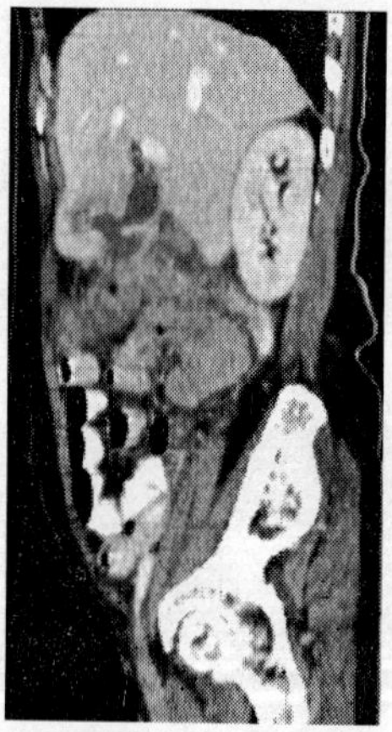

Fig. 58.2: Sagittal MPR CT image shows ruptured gallbladder secondary to cholecystitis (complicated cholecystitis)

1. Emphysematous Cholecystitis

Gas present gallbladder lumen or wall, may be seen in bile ducts.

- Elderly and diabetic men (38%) M/F – 7:3.
- Gas forming coliform bact. ischemia.
- Surgical emergency.

USG

- Intraluminal gas – non-dependent hyperechoic foci with ring down artifact.
- Intramural gas – semi circular/arc like configuration.
- Large gas – simulate gallbladder calcification/ gall stones.

CT

- AIR in the wall as well as lumen of gallbladder D/D/gallbladder carcinoma.

2. Gangrenous Cholecystitis

- 2 × 38% patients of acute cholecystitis.
- Associated with gallbladder perforation in 10% cases.
- 50% patients present as diffuse abdominal pain.

USG Findings

1. Marked irregular/assymetrical gallbladder wall thickening – 50%.
2. Multiple striations within thickened gallbladder wall.
3. Intraluminal membrane – fibrous strands, exudate, necrosis and sloughing of gallbladder mucosa.

CT

CECT

- Gallbladder wall thickening with high attenuation – intraluminal stones and debris.
- High attenuation fluid collection in pericholecystic fat.

PERFORATION

- Complicates 5-10% of acute cholecystitis (Figure 58.3).

NIEMEIER CLASSIFICATION

Acute – Generalized biliary peritonitis.

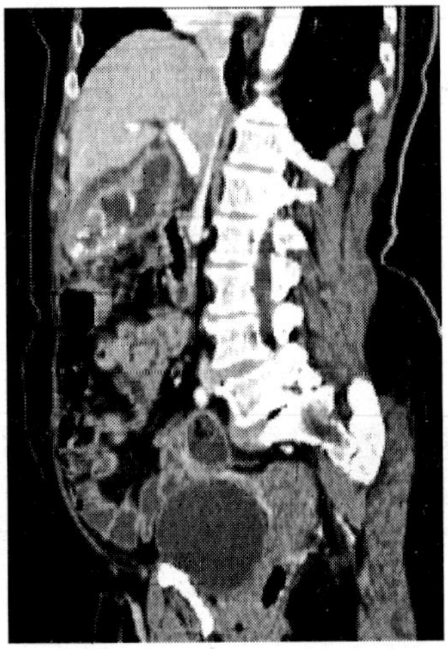

Fig. 58.3: Oblique MPR CT image shows GB mass with cholelithiasis and pericholecystic collection

Subacute – Pericholecystic abscess – Most common.

Chronic – Internal biliary fistula.

Fundus most common site.

USG

- Complex echogenic pericholecystic fluid collection with septations may encompass the gallbladder.
- Thick hypoechoic gallbladder wall and cholelithiasis.

Doppler

- Echogenic pericholecystic mass containing internal vascularity s/o inflammation.

CT

- Superior to USG.

Findings

1. Focal collection in gallbladder wall, liver, pericholecystic soft tissue.
2. Gas in gallbladder and or bile ducts.
3. Free fluid in abdomen with enhancing peritoneum.

Gallbladder Carcinoma

- 90% associated with gall stones.
- F/M 3.
- 40-50% history of chronic cholecystitis.

PREDISPOSING FACTORS

- Porcelain gallbladder.
- Sclerosing cholangitis.

Types

- Scirrhous.
- Local infiltrating.

MC

- Adenocarcinoma 80-90%.

CT AND USG FINDING ON VARIETY

1. Discrete intraluminal mass.
2. Mass replacing gallbladder – Most common.
3. Asymmetrical or diffuse gallbladder wall thickening.

ADDITIONAL FINDINGS

- Gallbladder wall calcification.
- Liver mets.
- Direct invasion of liver or adjacent structures.
- Adenopathy.
- Bile duct dilatation.
- On CT gallbladder carcinoma show ↓ attenuation on NE scans with heterogenous enhancement after IV contrast.

XANTHOGRANULOMATOUS CHOLECYSTITIS

- Rare complication.

- Associated with gall stone (Figures 58.4 and 58.5) and chronic infection → bile stasis.
- Degeneration and necrosis of gallbladder wall – replaced by inflammatory cell and xanthogranulomas → gallbladder wall thickening.

CT

- Marked irregular wall thickening simulating soft tissue mass.

May rupture through wall with pericholecystic spread.

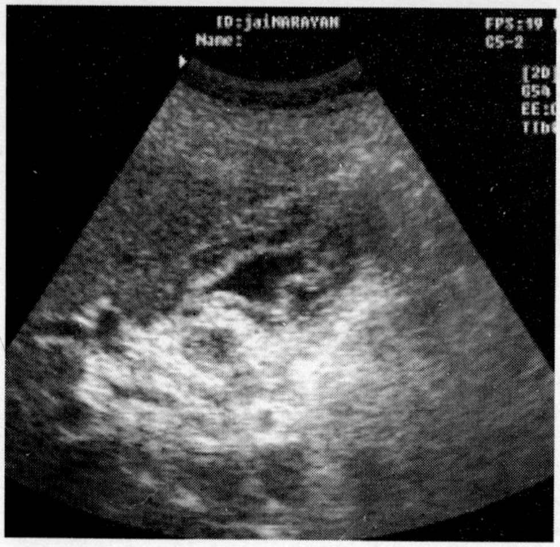

Fig. 58.4: US scan shows acalculous cholecystitis in a patient with enteric fever

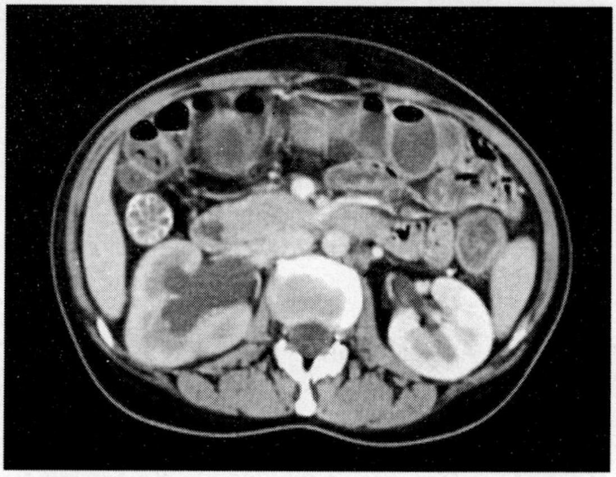

Fig. 58.5: Axial CT image shows calcified gallstones with incidental hydronephrosis on right

Cholangiocarcinoma

- 1/3 to 1/4th the incidence of gallbladder carcinoma Male >Female.

Average age of diagnosis – 65 years.

Risk factors – PSC.

- Choledochal cyst.
- Familial polyposis.
- Cong hepatic fibrosis.
- Exposure to thorium dioxide.

PATHOLOGY

- Scirrhous infiltrating neoplasm – causing stricture – most common.
- Exophytic bulky mass – most common in intrahepatic peripheral location.
- Polypoidal intraluminal ductal lesion – distal.

Classification

1. Intrahepatic (peripheral) lesions.
2. Hilar lesion (Klatskin tumor).
3. Distal duct tumor.

A. Intrahepatic cholangio Ca 20-30% (Figure 59.1).

USG mixed echogenicity or hypo or hyper.

Usually no bile duct obstruction.

Unenhanced CT – hypodense.

- Solitary.
- Satellite lesion.

Enchanced CT – variable.

Arterial phase – Not strongly enhancing but showing patchy and peripheral enhancement during the art. port. phase.

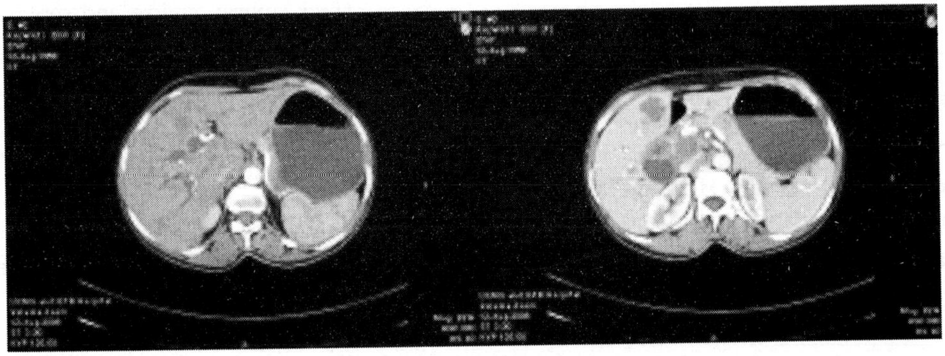

Fig. 59.1: CECT axial sections of abdomen showing cholangiocarcinoma involving common bile duct and causing dilatation of intrahepatic biliary radicals

Tumors with fibrous content → chronic late eq. phase E pattern with delayed marked retention of contrast at 6-20 minutes.

This delayed retention D/D mets.

Mucin producing tumors low attenuation on CT.

DIRECT CHOLANGIOGRAPHY to evaluate the extent Ch. stenosis of central, right and left hand with smooth shoulders or irregular tapering of the ducts. MRCP with 3D MIP recon with contrast MR are very helpful in complete tumor staging.

MRI

T1 – low SI than liver.

T2 – mod. higher than liver.

Area of fibrous tissue – low SI on both T1 and T2

G. D enh. Same enhancement pattern as seen on CT.

High mucin content – on T2WI.

Associated atrophy of liver parenchyma with retraction of the overlying capsule.

HILAR CHOLANGIO CARCINOMA.

Most common location.

USG Duct dilatation.

Isolation of RT and left bile duct segments.

Mass of BD wall thickening at the hilus.

Lobar atrophy with crowded, dilated bile ducts.

- Mass poorly defined and echogenic (submucosal scirrhous nature of this fibrotic neoplasma).

PV thrombosis – occasionally seen.

CT – mass seen is 40-90% of cases.

Less dense than liver on both NE and CE.

Most lesion shows + enhancement 8-15 min. after contrast administration.

MR – T1 = low, T2 ↑↑

High fibrous content = ↓ on T2

GDE – similar to CT.

- Liver parenchyma and HD lig. Commonly invaded by the Klatskin tumor.
- Lymph mets portocaval sup. PI and post PD L.N.S.

DISTAL DUCT TYPE

- Usually small and have better prognosis.
- Cholangiography – short structure of polypodial mass with almost always cause bile duct obst. Sonography can demonstrate the lesions at this level.
- Intra pancreatic portion of CBD – low signal intensity masses against the background of high SI head of pancreas on T1W fat suppressed I.

D/D of Cholangiocarcinoma

1. Intrahepatic mets – does not show chlangio late eq. phase E pattern with delayed marked retention of contrast.
2. Excessive mucin producing papillary intrahepatic cholangiocarcinoma lay resemble biliary cystadeno carcinoma appear hypoechoic on USG which might be associated with septations – middle aged female.
   - Mural nodules can be seen.
   - Thick, mural, coarse and septal ca^{++}.
   - Biliary dilation is usually not seen.

   CT – Uniloculated, multiloculated cystic mass.
3. Lymphoma, leomyosarcoma, carcinoid T, meta, sarcoidosis – rare.
4. PSC thickening of the duct wall with mural nodularity and contrast E – thickening in PSC – mild (<5 mm).

Section 5—Hepatopancreatobiliary System

Chapter 60

Acute Pancreatitis

Acute pancreatitis is an acute inflammatory process of pancreas with variable involvement of other regional tissues or remote organ systems.

Etiology

- Alcohol.
- Biliary tract disease.
- Hyperlipidemia.
- Hypercalcemia.
- Hereditary.
- Trauma.
  - External.
  - Operative.
  - Retrograde pancreatography.
- Ischemia.
  - Hypotension.
  - Cardiopulmonay bypass.
  - Atheroembolism.
  - Vasculitis.
- Pancreatic duct obstruction.
  - Neoplasms.
  - Cysts.
  - Pancreas divisum.
  - Duodenal diverticulum.
  - Ampullary stenosis.
- Duodenal obstruction.
- Infectious causes – viral, parasitic, fungal, bacterial.
- Drugs e.g. steroids, thiazide, diuretics.
- Idiopathic.

Pathogenesis

Endotoxins, Exotoxins, Viral infections, Trauma, Ischemia etc.

↓

Activation of proteolytic enzymes e.g. trypsinogen, chymotrypsinogen proelastase within the pancreas

↓

Digestion of pancreatic and peripancreatic tissues

↓

Proteolysis, edema, hemorrhage, necrosis (Autodigestion of pancreas)

Pathologic Spectrum

1. *Acute edematous pancreatitis*:

   Usually mild and self-limiting:

2. *Necrotising pancreatitis*:

   Pancreatic necrosis is defined at a diffuse or

focal area of non-viable pancreatic parenchyma, which is typically associated with peripancreatic fat necrosis. The degree of pancreatic necrosis correlates with the severity of attack.

3. *Hemorrhagic pancreatitis*:

Fat necrosis + interstitial hemorrhage.

Clinical Features

1. Abdominal pain:
   Steady and boring in character, located in epigastrium and para umbilical region, radiates to back. Most intense in supine and reduced by sitting.
2. Nausea, vomiting, abdominal distension.
3. On examination:
   Distressed and anxious patient with low-grade fever tachycardia, hypotension and shock.

DIAGNOSIS

1. Laboratory Determinations

A. Serum amylase

>60 units/L – suspicious.

>180 U/L – more likely.
Three fold or more - clinches the diagnosis.

B. Serum lipase

More accurate indicator of acute pancreatitis than S. amylase because lipase is purely of pancreatic origin.

C. Leucocytosis, hypocalcemia, hyperbilirubinaemia.

2. Radiographic Procedures

Plain X-ray

- X-ray abdomen

A. Colon cut off sign

– Dilated transverse colon with abrupt change to a gasless descending colon.

– Inflammation via sprenico colic ligament causes spasm and obstruction at the splenic flexure impinging on a paralytic colon.

B. Sentinel loop

– Localized segment of gas containing bowel in duodenum, terminal ileum or caecum.

C. Renal Halo sign

– Left kidney is displaced downwards and has a surrounding halo due to edema.

D. Gasless abdomen

– Due to fluid filled bowel associated with vomiting.

E. Mottled appearance of peripancreatic area due to fat necrosis.

F. Absent left psoas shadow.

G. Intrapancreatic gas from abscess formation or enteric fistula.

3. Chest X-ray

a. Pleural effusion usually left sided.
b. Left sided diaphragmatic elevation.
c. Left sided basal atelectasis, parenchymal shadowing.
d. Pulmonary oedema, pericardial effusion.

Barium Studies

1. Widening of retrogastric space, the inflammatory mass displaces the stomach anteriorly.
2. Enlarged, tortuous, edematous rugal folds along antrum and greater curvature.
3. Widening of C-loop of duodenum.
4. Jejunal and ileal fold thickening.

Ultrasound – Indications

1. Confirmation of diagnosis.

2. Detection of gall stones or CBD calculi.
3. Survey of possible complications and their follow up.
4. Guidance of interventional procedure.

U/S Signs of Acute Pancreatitis

1. Pancreatic Swelling

a. Massive swelling – thickness of the gland is three or four times than normal.

Normal shape of pancreas is lost and takes an ovoid cross-section.

b. Global harmonious swelling.

Shape is preserved but pancreas is swollen through out.

c. Segmental isolated swelling either at the level of head or isthmus.

There may be compression of IVC or SVC.

2. Contour

- The contour remains well defined, regular in cases of global swelling or there may be localised projections that may result in irregular contour.

3. Echotexture

a. Pancreas is usually hypoechoic because of interstitial edema in almost all cases.

b. The echotexture may be heterogenous with intense hyperechoic nodules alternating with semisolid areas and even liquid.

- Necrotic areas are the fluid collections, which may appear intensely echogenic due to numerous interfaces.
- Hemorrhagic areas also appear hyperechoic.
- Pancreatic fluid is either clear or septated as a result of associated hemorrhage or infection.
- Fluid collection may be inhomogenous and solid looking as a result of inflammatory nature of the edematous retroperitoneal tissues.
- Extrapancreatic fluid collection occurs within 4 weeks from the onset of acute attack.

4. Ascites, thickening of adjacent stomach, duodenum and colon

Thickened gall bladder wall with or without pericholecystic fluid.

CT Scan – Indications

1. In patients with an uncertain diagnosis.
2. For detection of complications.
3. For showing the morphologic changes in this disease.
4. To predict prognostic value.

CT Findings (Figure 60.1)

1. Normal appearing gland in one third or more of patients.
2. Diffuse or focal glandular enlargement.
3. Contour irregularity with blurring of outline caused by oedematous changes in contiguous peripancreatic fat.

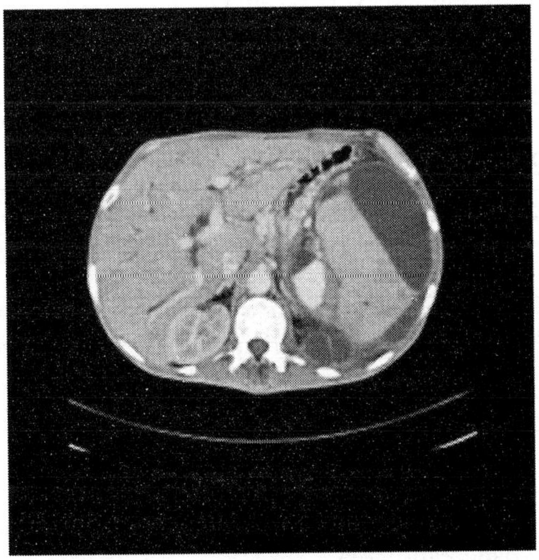

Fig. 60.1: Axial CT image shows pseudoaneurysm of the splenic artery, multiple fluid collections and minimally dilated IHBR in a case of acute pancreatitis

4. Focal irregular areas of non-contrast enhancement and decreased attenuation secondary to edema or necrosis.
5. Edema and thickening of peripancreatic fat and parietal peritoneal planes.
6. Dissection of fluid in anterior pararenal space resulting in thickening of Gerota's fascia.
7. Pancreatic "phlegmon" is boggy edematous soft tissue mass composed of admixture of inflammatory exudate and retroperitoneal fat and it may suppurate, liquefy and resolve spontaneously.
8. Hyperdense ares 50-70 HU in hemorrhagic pancreatitis.

MRI

1. Edema of pancreas causes diffuse signal intensity reduction on T1W images and reduced enhancement after I V gadolinium.
2. Peripancreatic edema appears as areas of low signal extending into peipancreatic fat on T1.
3. Exudates and fluid collections within and around the pancreas appear hypointense on T1 and hyperintese on T2.
4. Gas within pancreas produces areas of signal void.

Complications

1. Pancreatic Hemorrhage

- In 2.5%

  Clinically–falling hematocrit, hypocalcemia and failure to respond to resuscitative measures.

Mortality: 33 to 100%.

USG – Shows hyperechoic areas.

CT – Collection of high attenuation >60 HU in pancreatic area.

2. Vascular

Intrapancreatic and peripancreatic arteries and veins may be eroded or thrombosed by direct effect of pancreatic enzymes.

Pseudoaneurysm formation – due to erosion by histiolytic enzymes in vessels like splenic, gastroduodenal or hepatic arteries.

CT–shows highly enhancing perivascular structures usually within or adjacent to pseudo cysts. Definitive diagnosis requires angiography.

3. GI Involvement

- GIT is frequently involved by direct extension of the inflammation from pancreas resulting in edema, necrosis or perforation of the wall of stomach or duodenum.
- Secondary involvement of bowel by release and tracking of pancreatic enzymes through mesenteric attachment may result in bowel ischemia.

4. Infected Pancreatic Lesions

- Bacterial contamination of necrotic pancreatic tissue and fluid rises to a significant rate (71.4%) after 2 weeks of acute necrotic pancreatitis.

Pancreatic Abscess

- Occurs in 4% of all patients with AP.

  It is a localized collection of pus surrounded by more or less distinct capsule.

  Ultrasound shows a thick walled mostly anechoic containing debris with bright echoes from gas bubbles.

  CT shows pancreatic or peripancreatic gas and an inflammatory mass or fluid collection.

5. Pancreatic Pseudocysts (Figure 60.2)

- Collection of pancreatic juice enclosed by a wall of fibrous or granulation tissue.
- It is generally spherical in shape.

Section 5

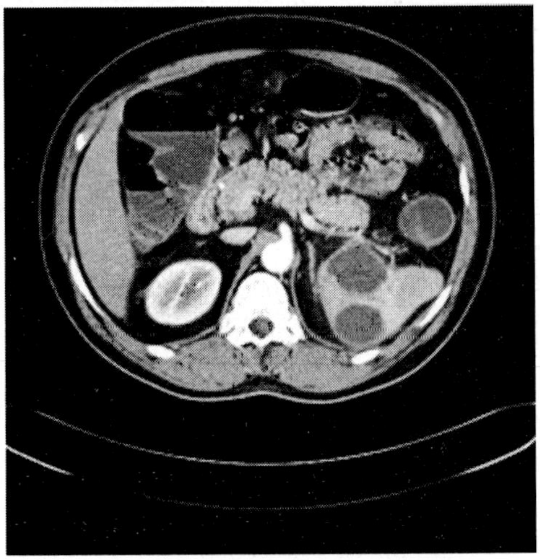

Fig. 60.2: Axial CT image showing multiple pseudocyst in a case of pancreatitis

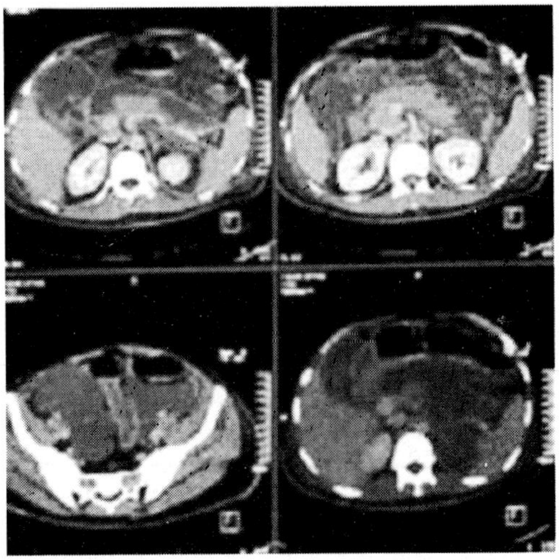

Fig. 60.3: Axial CT images show acute pancreatitis with its sequelae

- 4 to 6 weeks are necessary for a fluid collection to enclose itself by forming a wall composed of collagen and vascular granulation tissue.

USG

Well defined smooth walled, anechoic structure with acoustic enhancement.

There may be internal debris with hemorrhage or infection.

It may be multiloculated with calcification in walls.

CT

Shows a thick walled cyst with homogenous or heterogenous attenuation.

- Pseudocysts can dissect into adjacent liver, spleen, and kidney and even into the mediastinum.
- If large may cause obstruction of stomach, small bowel, colon or bile ducts, latter causing obstructive jaundice/ cholangitis (Figure 60.3).
- Pseudocysts may erode into stomach and cause GI hemorrhage. There may be variceal bleeding secondary to local portal hypertension caused by portosplenic venous thrombosis.
- Acute peritonitis can ensue with rupture of pseudocyst into peritoneal cavity.
- Pseudocysts that persist >6 weeks require decompression.

Criteria for Decompression

1. Persistence >6 weeks.
2. Size >5cm without evidence of ongoing regression on follow up Ultrasound or CT.
3. Smaller pseudocysts causing symptoms.
4. Presence of complications such as injections, hemorrhage or intra abdominal perforation.

6. Pancreatic Ascites

Results from slow leakage of pancreatic enzyme into the peritoneal cavity from disruption of main pancreatic duct or pseudocyst.

Anterior enzyme leakage enters the lesser sac to peritoneal cavity causing ascites.

Table 60.1: CT grading of pancreatic lesions

CT Features	*Score*
I. Grade	
• Normal gland	0
• Focal diffuse enlargement	1
• Peripancreatic inflamm. change	2
• Single pancreatic fluid coll.	3
• Two or more fluid collection or abscess	4
II. Necrosis	
• None	0
• <30%	2
• 30 to 50%	4
• >50%	6

Table 60.2: Morbidity and mortality of pancreatic lesions

Score	*Morbidity %*	*Mortality %*
0-3	3	3
4-6	35	6
7-10	92	17

Posterior enzyme leak moves cephalad into the mediastinum or pleural space resulting in pancreatic pleural effusion.

Assessment of Disease Severity on Imaging CT severity index (Balthazar).

MANAGEMENT

1. Non-operative

a. Supportive intravenous fluid or electrolyte therapy.

b. Pancreatic exocrine secretion suppression.

c. Elimination of toxic intraperitoneal compulsory peritoneal dialysis.

2. Operative

a. Drainage of injected pancreatic collections by percutaneous route.

b. Surgical debridement.

c. Correction of biliary tract disease.

Pancreatic Neoplasm

- The majority of pancreatic neoplasms are ductal adenocarcinoma.
- Extremely rare before 40 years. 3rd after 60 years.

Location

60-70%–Head, 15-20% – Body.
5%–Tail, 20% – Diffusely (Figure 61.1).

Clinical Symptoms

Early – Vague abdominal pain, weight loss.
Pain.
Ca –Head – Obstructive Jaundice.

Others – Unexplained venous thrombosis and pancreatitis.

Pathology

- Arise in ductal epithelium – 99%.
  Focal lesion.
  Invasion of adjacent structures.
  Distant metastasis.

Imaging

X-rays

- Do not calcify.

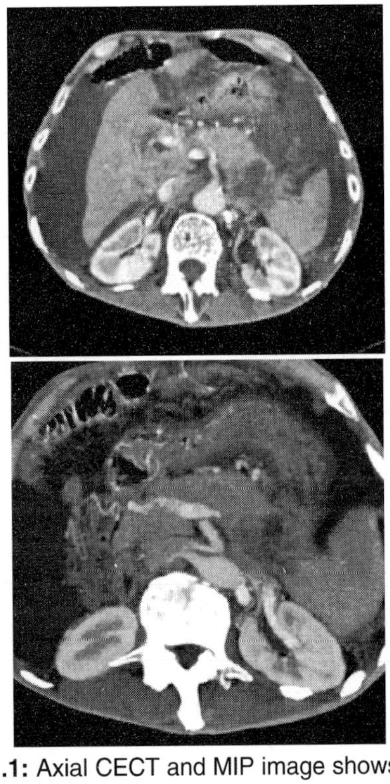

Fig. 61.1: Axial CECT and MIP image shows a mass in the tail region of the pancreas

- Sunburst calcification 10% of cystic tumors.
- Large pancreatic masses → soft tissue mass displacing gas shadows of stomach or bowel.
- Evidence of splenomegaly – malignant occlusion of splenic or PV.

BARIUM STUDY

Finding depends on the location of tumor. Large pancreatic tumors displace the stomach superiorly and anteriorly with widening of the reterogastric space.

Head –Pyloric antrum and duodenal loop.

Body –Distal duodenum, the Duodeno-Jejunal flexure and body of stomach.

Invasion results in mucosal irregularity, ulceration with fixation of the gastric wall.

Tail – Intraabdominal esophagus.

– Elongation and straightening → horizontal lie.

Invasion – obstruction.

Splenic vein occlusion – varices in gas fundus.

Duodenal Loop

- Widening loop with mucosal irregularity, speculation and nodularity of folds.
- Localized stricture.

  Double contour to medial border frostberg 'reversed 3' sign.

USG

Good for head, not so for body and tail.

Direct signs

Mass lesion – homogenous or heterogenous poorly defined mass – aMC.

Indirect signs

1. Dilatation of M.P.D. → Loss of its nature → tortuous or tapers abruptly → small ca can be detected.
2. Bile duct dilatation
   - Invasion.
   - Lymph node.

   DOUBLE DUCT SIGN
3. Displacement and involvement of adjacent structures.
4. Associated pancreatitis.
5. Liver metastasis.
6. Regional lymphadenopathy.

CT Scan

Important imaging modality for diagnosing and staging.

DIRECT SIGN

Mass → MC → focal hypovascular mass.

Other

1. Change in size of pancreas
   - Focal or diffuse.
   - More common.
   - Confined to anatomical area.
   - Non-specific—cannot be used as sole criterion
2. Change in shape and contour of pancreas
   - Frequently more important than actual size.
   - Head – most difficult area.
   - Tail ant surface or pancreatic body – readily detected.
3. Obliteration of peripancreatic fat
   - ↑ CT number.
   - When no fat plane is seen separating p. mass from adjacent structures → usually it is assumed that invasion has occurred → not above.
4. Dilatation of MPD and CBD.
5. Involvement of vessels and regional lymph nodes.
   - Using bolus injection.
   - Abrupt obstruction, narrowing or displacement of peripancreatic vessels.
   - Venous – dilatation proximal to obstruction → multiple venous collaterals.
   - Lymph nodes
   - Frequently detected by CT.
   - MC – Celiac and superior mesenteric, para aortic, pericaval, reterocraval, porta.

Metastasis

Liver 17 to 55%.

Hypovascular lesions best seen in portal venous phase, usually small.

Criteria for unresectability:

i. ≥ 5 cm diameters.

ii. Invasion of adjacent < tissues and organs except duodenum.

iii. Occlusion, encasement, stenosis of vessels.

iv. Distant nodal mets.

v. Hematogenous mets.

Magnetic Resonance

- Helps to distinguish tumors from inflammatory mass.
- Determine local extent.
- Carcinoma–low signal on fat suppressed T1 images: margins more distinct.
- In contrast enhancement, more marked.
- T2 – Iso or slightly hypointense.

  Lympha nodes and hepatic mets →↑ed signal on T2.
- After Gd administration.

MRCP

Non-invasive.

Advantages

- Patient with total obstruction.
- Gastric/pancreatic surgery.

Disadvantages

- Therapeutic maneuvers not possible.
- Stent and metal clips → image disturbance lower resolution.

ERCP

Further assessment in cases not clarified by USG/CT.

CHRONIC PANCREATITIS

- Diffuse/focal enlargement of pancreas.
- Focal – difficult to differentiate from carcinoma pancreas.
- CBD occlusion rare.
- Calcification – half with alcoholism.
- Chain of lakes of pancreatic duct.
- Diffuse signal reduction on fat suppressed T1 weighted images.

CYSTIC NEOPLASMS

- Muncionous macrocystic neoplasm.
- Usually malignant.
- ♀ < ♂ Younger patients; more common in tail.
- Usually large; unilocular or multilocular.

Large cystic spaces having thick mucoid substance.

CT

Cystic mass with enhancing walls and internal septation, mural papillary projection in otherwise unilocular cyst.

Serous Microcystic Neoplasm

- Benign, ♀ < ♂ 1.5:1, middle aged and elderly.
- Small uniform, well circumscribed, round ovoid, multilocular masses, fibrous band with central calcified scar.

CT

Encapsulated, hyperdense, lobulated mass.

Section 5—Hepatopancreatobiliary System

Chapter 62

Imaging of Obstructive Biliopathy

Various Uses

- Modalities, which are used for its detection USG, cholangiography.
- CT.
- MRI including MRCP.
- ERCP.
- PTC.

USG

- Usual screening modality in patients with jaundice.
- EHBRD precedes intrahepatic duct dilatation therefore; meticulous attention is paid on screening CBD.
- The CBD diameter upto 0 to 7mm is considered normal in adults (Figures 62.1 and 62.2).
- Finding of parallel intra hepatic channel of bile ducts anterior to the portal vein is considered diagnostic of IBRD and obstruction.
- Normal IHBD should not measure more than 2 mm and should not be greater than 40% of the accompanying portal veins.
- Dilated intrahepatic biliary ducts appear as too many tubes or give "Swiss cheese" appearance.

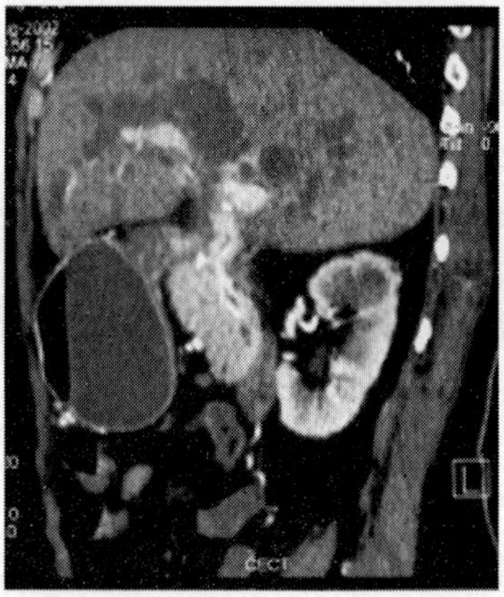

Fig. 62.1: Oblique MPR CT image shows diffuse cholangiocarcinoma of the common bile duct with proximal biliary obstruction

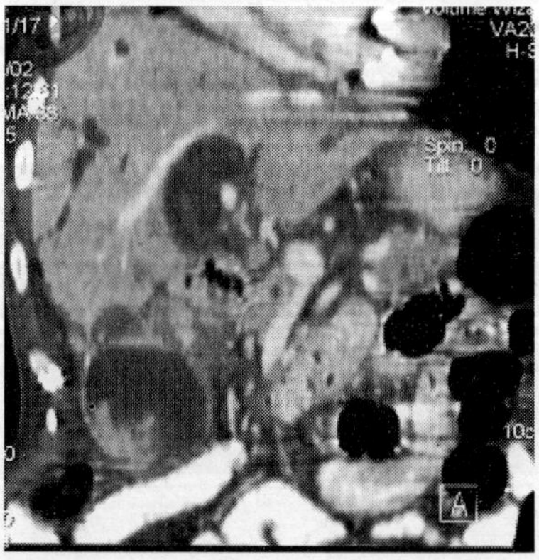

Fig. 62.2: Oblique MPR CT image shows a gallbladder mass with proximal biliary obstruction

CT

- On CT, dilated intrahepatic bile ducts are depicted as linear, lead branching or circular structures of near water density which enlarge and become confluent as they approach to porta hepatis. As one scans down from porta hepatis to the pancrease, dilated extrahepatic ducts appear as a series of low-density rings.
- On CT scan, upper limit of normal for the common hepatic duct diameter is considered to be 6 mm and the common bile duct 9 mm. Intrahepatic ducts more than 2 to 3 mm or duct visualization becoming confluent rather than scattered is considered abnormal.

Hepatobiliary Scintigraphy

- It is useful in the work up of a jaundiced patient, particularly a postoperative patient. The agents commonly used for hepatobiliary imaging are immuno-diacetic acid (IDA) derivative, which are accumulated by hepatocyte and secreted into the bile and subsequently into the small bowel.

MRI

- The acceptance of MR is related to technical refinement such as advances in hardware and software, which have greatly improved image quality and shortened examination times.
- The technical refinement include development of breathing independent sequences that suppress artifacts associated with surgical clips, stents and bowel gas and allow image acquisition at section thickness of 2 to 5 mm.
- MRCP is performed with heavily T2W sequence that depicts the biliary and pancreatic duct as high signal intensity structures.

Advantages of MRCP over ERCP and PTC

1. It avoids the complications of MRCP like pancreatic GIT perforation and hemorrhage.
2. MRCP does not expose patients to ionising radiation or iodinated contrast material.
3. MRCP is also useful in patients who had incomplete or failed ERCP attempt.
4. It is also useful in patients in whom the performance of ERCP is difficult due to surgical alterations of the G.I.T.

Disadvantages of MRCP over ERCP

- MRCP is entirely diagnostic whereas ERCP provides diagnostic information as well as access for therapeutic interventions.

ERCP

- ERCP is useful in clarifying complex ductal anatomy is the setting of an equivocal or non-diagnostic MRCP and identifying the bile duct and cystic duct leaks.

BENIGN LESIONS CAUSING OBSTRUCTIVE BILIOPATHY

- Choledocholithiasis.
- Benign stricture
  - Post operative/traumatic.
  - Post inflammatory.
- Choledochal cyst
- Primary sclerosing cholangitis.
- Parasitic diseases.
- Infections e.g. T.B.
- Ampullary stenosis
  - Choledochal varices.
  - Kemibilia.
  - Benign tumors of the biliary tract.

Choledocholithiasis

- It occurs in about 15% of patients with cholelithiasis.

Cholangiography

- Calculi within the bile ducts are readily detected as rounded or faceted filling defects within the contrast column. These defects are usually mobile.

- If the stone is impacted in any part of the CBD, a typical convex border of the contrast column in the distal CBD is seen outlining the proximal stone margin.
- Air bubbles are differentiated from CBD stones by their smooth, round appearance and their tendency to group together and rise to the non-dependent surface as compared to stones which are usually faceted or elliptical and tend to fall at the dependent portion of the biliary tree.

USG

Echogenic nodule with acoustic shadowing seen in dilated CBD.

CT

- Thin collimation scans of 3 to 5 mm obtained at close intervals in the region of transition zone of the distal bile duct may be required.
- High attenuation stones can be easily seen on CT contrasted with lower attenuation of bile.

MRCP

- It provides a non-invasive means of detecting bile duct stones.
- MRCP shows sensitivity of 90 to 100% and specificity of 92 to 100% for desection of CBD stones.

Benign Stricture

Causes

- Surgery.
- Trauma.
- Chronic pancreatitis.
- Gallstones.
- Duodenal ulcers.

Postoperative Biliary Strictures

USG

1. Smooth tapering stenosis with proximal dilatation of CBD (41%).
2. Abrupt cut off of CBD (18%).
3. Presence of echogenic nodule without acoustic shadowing.

RCP/ERCP/PTC

- In addition to confirming the presence of CBD stricture can also show the extent level of stricture. These are classified into 5 types:

Type I

- Low common hepatic duct strictures, the hepatic duct stump being longer than 2 cm.

Type II

- Middle, common hepatic duct stricture, the hepatic duct stump being less than 2 cm.

Type III

- High stricture or hilar stricture with preservation of the biliary confluence but no communication with CHD.

Type IV

- Hilar stricture interrupting the confluence, communication between right and left ducts no longer demonstrable.

Type V

- Strictures involving an anomalous distribution of the segment branch.

Post-Inflammatory Strictures

- Chronic pancreatitis, gallstones and penetrating or perforating duodenal ulcers can cause stricture other than cholangitis.

Cholangiography

- In chronic pancreatitis, these strictures appear as about 3 to 5 cm, smooth, concentric, often tapered narrowing of the intra pancreatic portion of the CBD.

- Strictures associated with gallstone are often short and some time weblike. These may be multiple and may involve any portion of the CBD.
- US, CT and MRI primarily demonstrate biliary dilatation but may also reflect the primary pathology leading to strictures.

Mirrizi's Syndrome

- Intrabiliary fistula between the gallbladder and CHD/BD secondary to an eroding stone located in the neck of the gallbladder or cystic duct is called Mirrzzes syndrome.

US

- Cholelithiasis in a small contracted gallbladder with an echogenic nodule or calculus either in the neck of the gallbladder or adjacent CBD with mild to moderate dilatation of proximal biliary radicles and a normal sized CBD distal to the calculus.

Cholangiography

- On cholangiography confluent filling defects (calculi) are seen involving the gallbladder neck/ cystic duct and CHD/CBD.
- A definite diagnosis of fistula is established by ERCP/PTC.

Choledochal Cysts

- These usually manifest in childhood and present as triad of jaundice, right upper quadrant pain and a palpable subcostal mass.

USG

- USG is the preferred imaging modality. It is classified into five types:

Type I

- Fusiform cystic dilatation of extrahepatic CBD within the porta.

Type II

- An eccentric fluid filled cyst, which may appear separate from CBD, as its neck may be narrow.

Type III

- Localized cystic dilatation of the distal intramural duodenal position of the CBD.

Type IVa

- Multiple cysts involving the intrahepatic and extrahepatic bile ducts.

Type IVb

- Multiple cysts involving the extrahepatic duct only.

Type V/Caroli's Disease

- Single or multiple intrahepatic bile duct cysts.

CT and MRI

- These are useful in evaluating choledochal cyst by accurately showing the extent of involvement.

MRCP and ERCP

- These are useful in detecting and defining the morphological characteristics of choledochal cysts and in detecting the presence of anomalous union of the pancreatic and bile ducts.

Primary Sclerosing Cholangitis

- It is a chronic progressive hepatobiliary disorder of unknown origin that occurs commonly in young man.
- Associated with IBD (UC), orbital pseudo-tumor and retroperitoneal fibrosis.

USG

- Diagnosis is difficult unless biliary ductal dilatation is present.

CT

- May show characteristic features in the form of saccular and interrupted dilatation of the intrahepatic biliary radicles especially close to the hepatic hilum.

MRCP/Cholangiography

- Both show the typical features of the alternate dilatation and narrowing of the intrahepatic biliary radicles with areas of sacular dilatation as well.

Biliary Ascariasis

Ascaris lumbricoides is very common worm infestation in the tropical countries like India. This parasite commonly harbors in the upper small intestine and can sometimes enter into the biliary tree through the ampulla of Vater, giving rise to signs and symptoms related to the biliary tree.

Cholangiography

- The worms are seen as smooth cylindrical translucencies.

USG

- The worms are recognized as tubular, nonshadowing, echogenic, structures in the dilated biliary ducts.
- When worms are alive, movements of worms can be seen and it is usually possible to see a sonolucent inner tube with the echogenic tubular structure representing alimentary canal of the worm.

CT

- On unenhanced scan they appear as hyper-attenuating tubular site surrounded by less attenuated bile.
- In TS on both US and CT, a "bulls eye" image may be seen caused by the worm inside a dilated bile duct.

Chonorchis Sinensis

Chlolangiography

- The small flukes may be seen as filling defects in contrast columns. The defects are usually multiple, short and curvilinear in appearance.

US

- A small echogenic forms without distal shadowing. Mild intrahepatic duct dilatation may be seen on CT or US.

Biliary Hydatid

- US, CT and cholangiography are helpful in arriving at a correct preoperative use – ERCP:
    1. Filiform linear material in the CBD due to laminated hydatid membranes.
    2. Rounded filling defect due to hydatid daughter cyst.
    3. Amorphous debris in the CBD due to mixture of hydatid membranes and daughter cysts.

Hemobilia

- Bleeding into the biliary tree most frequently due to trauma.

Cholangiography

- It may show clotted blood as a cast like filling defect in the bile ducts and may reveal a bile duct leak or a biliary vascular communication.
- Blood may be seen as echogenic material in gallbladder or CBD on US.

CT

- Blood is seen as high attenuating area (>30 HU) in the gallbladder or BD. Liver laceration, hematoma or other sources of blood may be detected.

Selective Hepatic Arteriography

- It may demonstrate extravasation of contrast material in the biliary tract or a pseudo anuerysm may be occluded by embolisation.

Malignant Lesions Causing Obstructive Biliopathy

- Carcinoma gallbladder.
- Cholangiocarcinoma.
- Carcinoma head of the pancreas.

CARCINOMA GALLBLADDER

- It is the most common biliary tract malignancy.
- Risk factors include:
  - Cholelithiasis.
  - Chronic cholecystitis.
  - Anomalous pancreatobiliary ductal union.
  - Chronic typhoid infection.
  - Porcelain gallbladder.

C/F

- Usually occurs in elderly females.
- Pain in right upper abdomen, nausea, vomiting, weight loss and jaundice.

USG

- Three major patterns are seen:

Type I

- Gallbladder is surrounded or replaced by a hypoechoic or heterogenous mass.
- Cystic areas may be seen within it representing necrosis or residual bile.

Type II

- There is focal or diffuse, irregular and asymmetric wall thickening.

Type III

- A polypodial, fungating intra luminal mass is seen.
- Gallstones are seen in 75% of the patients with carcinoma gallbladder.
- The lack of a distinct margin between the gallbladder mass and liver suggest liver invasion.
- Hematogenous distant metastases may be seen in the liver.
- Enlarged lymph nodes may be seen at the porta hepatitis, peripancreatic and para aortic region.
- Biliary obstruction in the form of dilated intrahepatic biliary radicles and CBD may be seen because of direct extension via hepato duodenal ligament or compression by lymphadenopathy.

CT

- Mildly enhancing mass that partly or fully replaces the gallbadder.
- Direct extension to the liver is seen as an ill-defined margin initially and then as a low-density lesion in the contiguous liver parenchyma.

- Less common CT manifestations are irregular wall thickening and intra luminal mass. The masses exhibit mild and variable contrast enhancement and improve visualization of the intra luminal component.
- Ancillary findings on CT include gallstones, wall calcification, dilated biliary radicals, hepatic metastasis, lymphadenopathy, ascites and extension into stomach, duodenum or colon. The lymph nodes may show necrotic center.

Cholangiography

- It shows infiltration, encashment and obstruction of the CBD in the region of cystic duct with no filling in the gallbladder.

MRI

- It shows a mass in gall bladder fossa, which is hypo intense on T1W images and hyper, intense on T2W images.

CHOLANGIOCARCINOMA (Figure 63.1)

Uncommon Tumor

- Commoner in males with peak incidence in 6th or 7th decade.
- Higher incidence is associated with sclerosing cholangitis, Caroli's disease, choledochal cysts, liver fluke infection and ulcerative colitis.
- Patients usually present with jaundice, weight loss and anorexia.
- Distally placed tumors are more likely to be resectable than those at the hilum.
- Patients usually die of hepatocellular jaundice and infection, which occur secondary to biliary obstruction.
- Metastasis involve regional lymph node, peritoneum, liver, gallbladder and diaphragm.
- Histologically majority of these tumors are adenocarcinomas with cuboidal or columnar epithelium and abundant fibrous stroma.

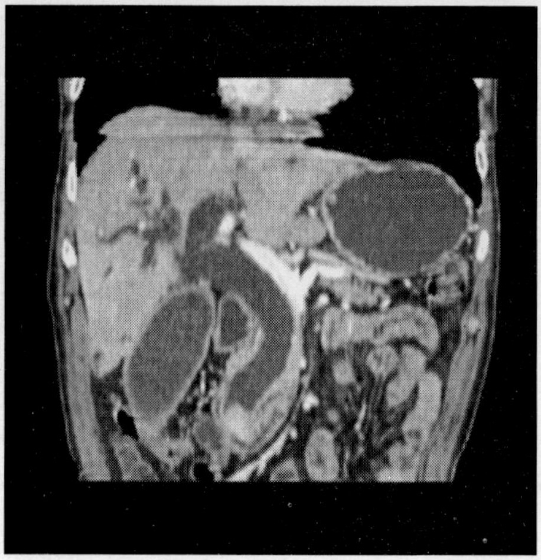

Fig. 63.1: Coronal MPR CT image shows extrahepatic biliary obstruction secondary to a small cholangiocarcinoma at the distal end of common bile duct

- Cholangiocarcinomas can be classified as:
  1. Intrahepatic tumors (peripheral lesions).
  2. Hilar lesions (the most common location) referred to as Klatskin tumor.
  3. Distal ductal tumor.

Intrahepatic (Peripheral) Cholangiocarcinoma

- These are usually large at presentation because they are rarely symptomatic early in their course.

USG

- There are non-specific and may be seen as hypo or isoechoic masses.

On Contrast Enhanced CT Scans

- The tumor shows mild and peripheral enhancement.
- On multiphase CT scan, the enhancement is peripheral and delayed. The central area of the tumor which contains fibrous tissue, does not enhance during early phase, but becomes hyperdense during the delayed phase 4 to 20

5 Section

minutes after injection, a feature which may help to differentiate it from HCC.

- The mass contains high-density mucin containing areas as well as areas of necrosis, which gives it a heterogenous appearance.
- Focal intrahepatic biliary ductal dilatation and atrophy of the segment of the liver drained by these ducts with retraction of overlying liver capsule may also be seen.
- On MRI, intrahepatic cholangiocarcinoma is seen as irregular, heterogenous mass with low signal intensity (SI) on T1 weights image and high SI on T2 weighted images.
- Mild to moderate rim enhancement is seen on contrast enhanced MRI.

Hilar Cholangiocarcinoma (Klatskin Tumor)

- The most common location is either at the confluence of right and left hepatic ducts or the proximal common hepatic duct and has been termed Klatskin tumor.
- On imaging biliary dilatation is seen with or without patency of the confluence.

USG

- Usually these are moderately echogenic reflecting cirrhous and fibrous nature of the tumor.
- There are dilated intrahepatic ducts without any evidence of extrahepatic dilatation and blocked confluence.

CECT

- There is an ill-defined mass with delayed enhancement at the confluence.
- Exophytic type of tumors are seen as hilar masses that spread into adjacent liver parenchyma.
- Polypoid tumors are rare and seen as intraluminal polypid masses on CT and US.
- Hilar cholangiocarcinoma may occasionally involve the portal vein, mostly the left branch, resulting in left lobe atrophy with findings of characteristic crowding of dilated bile ducts in small left lobe.
- Ancillary findings include infiltration of the liver, gallbladder, pancreas or duodenum and lymphadenopathy involving peri pancreatic or celiac group of nodes.

MRI

- Spoiled gradient echo sat T1W sequences obtained at 2 to 5 min after gadolinium injection demonstrates the tumor.
- Cholangiocarcinoma is seen as a moderately enhancing lesion with this technique.
- MR (T2W1) shows proximal hilar cholangiocarcinoma as moderately high signal intensity thickness duct wall or ill-defined tumor mass.
- The intensity of the thickened duct wall is higher than adjacent liver, but is of lesser intensity than intra luminal bile.

Cholangiography/MRCP/ERCP

- The Klatskin tumor is seen as an irregular stricture at the confluence, with prestenotic dilatation. Either one or both of the hepatic ducts may be obstructed in addition to the common duct.

Bismuth Classification

Type I	Involves common hepatic duct only.
Type II	Involves right and left hepatic ducts at the confluence.
Type III	First order branches of either of the hepatic ducts are involved.
Type IV	First order branches of both the hepatic ducts are involved.

DISTAL DUCT CHOLANGIOCARCINOMA

- The least common location for cholangiocarcinoma is the distal duct.

USG

- It demonstrate biliary dilatation proximal to an abrupt obstruction.
- Abrupt obstruction of distal duct is seen without visualization of a mass or calculus and the pancreas is normal.

CT

- It demonstrates biliary dilatation till the level of obstruction and less commonly mass.
- The diagnosis is suggested by abrupt cut off without a mass or calculus.
- Diffuse, enhancing wall thickening may be seen.
- If a mass is seen, it is hypodense in pre contrast scans and shows delayed enhancement on post contrast scans.

Cholangiography

- It reveals obstructive, stenotic or protuberant lesion.
- Most common is the obstructive lesion which appear as U or V shaped occlusion with nipple rat tail, smooth or irregular termination.
- The stenotic type is seen as a rigid, narrowed lumen with irregular margins and prestenotic dilatation.
- The protuberant type is seen as modular or polypodial intraluminal filling defects attached to the walls.
- The diffuse sclerosing type of cholangiocarcinoma causes widespread strictures of both intra and extrahepatic ducts resembling sclerosing cholangitis.

CARCINOMA HEAD OF PANCREAS

- Pancreatic adenocarcinoma.
- Serous cystadenoma.

Pancreatic Adenocarcinoma

- Seen in middle aged and elderly patients.
- M: F = 2:1.
- Risk factors – cigarette smoking, alcohol high intake of animal fat in diet and hereditary pancreatitis.

Imaging

Conventional Radiography

- Tumor calcification is not usually seen.
- Local invasion of D12 to L3 vertebrae may be seen.

Barium Studies

Barium Meal Upper GI Studies

1. Widening of the C loop with speculated duodenal wall with traction and fixation of the wall.
2. Antral pad sign.
3. Frostberg's or reverse 3' sign.
4. An increase in the retrograstic space >5 cm on lateral views.

Barium Enema

- It reveals localized haustral flattening or narrowing with serrated contour at the inferior aspect of the transverse colon.

USG

- Pancreatic carcinoma is usually hypoechoic as compared to normal parenchyma.
- Neurotic tumors may show heterogenous echopattern.
- Ductal obstruction and dilatation.
- Vascular involvement is seen on ultrasound as thickening of periarterial tissues in which normal echogenic fat immediately adjacent to the artery is replaced by tissue of lower echogenicity.

Endoscopic Ultrasound

- It uses a 7-12 MHz 360° radial scanner, the tip of which is placed in the 2nd part duodenum for the pancreatic head, portal vein and papilla, in the duodenal bulb for the head, neck and distal CBD and through the stomach for imaging of body, tail and pancreatic duct.

- EUS is especially sensitive for small (<2 cm) solid tumors.
- EUS criteria for nodal involvement are circulaty homogeneity, relative hypoechogenicity and proximally to the vascular lesion.
- For vascular involvement the criteria are loss of the hypo echoic vessel wall/tumor interface, direct presence of tumor in the vascular lumen and non-visualization of a major portal vessel in the presence of collateral vessels.

CT

- The most common abnormality is a small form hypovascular mass in the pancreas.
- Other findings include focal contour changes with or without definite disaster mass; a focal lesion of soft tissue density in an otherwise fatty replaced gland; spherical enlargement of the head and convex rounded borders of the uncinate process.
- The main pancreatic and CBD are often dilated proximal to the mass.

Criteria for tumor irresectability include the presence of one or more of the following CT findings:

1. Tumor diameter of 5 cm or greater.
2. Extrapancreatic invasion of adjacent tissue and organs with the exception of the duodenum.
3. Occlusion, stenosis and encasement of vessels including the portal venous system, superior mesenteric artery and major branches of the celiac trunk (cases of noncircumferential tumor vessel abutment or invasion of only one vessel of the portal system without other signs of unresectability are considered possibly resectable.
4. Distal nodal metastasis.
5. Hematogenous metastasis.

Vascular Involvement

- CT findings of perivascular infiltration and/or vascular encasement include change in caliber or contour deformity of the vessel and soft tissue infiltration of the perivascular fat.
- Venous involvement is more difficult to use than arterial involvement because vein lie immediately adjacent to the pancreatic parenchyma and are not surrounded by fat.
- Venous occlusion is suggested by distention of the affected veins proximal to the site of obstruction.
- Venous encasement or obstruction frequently produces multiple venous collaterals. They develop in the hepato duodenal ligament after occlusion of the portal vein and in the shorter gastric and gastric epipolic varices after splenic vein occlusion.

Lymph Node Involvement

- Lymph nodes are considered positive by CT criteria when the diameter of a distinct lymph node exceeds 1.0 to 1.5 cm.
- Gradient who and T1 weighted spin echo sequence are used to evaluate vascular invasion.
- T1 weighted spin echo sequences are employed to assess lymphadenopathy.
- T2W sequences are preferred for detecting hepatic metastasis.
- On T1W images most lesions are of low signal intensity relative to normal pancreatic parenchyma.
- On T2W images signal intensity is variable.
- On dynamic gadolinium enhanced images, these hypovascular lesions show poor or no enhancement, improving tumor to pancreas contrast.

ERCP

It is used:

1. In-patient in which the CT or USG findings are unclear.

2. In cases where ductal dilataton is seen without definite identification of a mass.
3. To differentiate duodenal or ampullary tumors from periampullary tumors in the pancreatic head.

MRCP

- MRCP identifies the presence and level of neoplastic obstruction of the pancreatic biliary tract.
- MRCP with abdominal MR and MRA yields a comprehensive examination that permits not only diagnosis, but also staging of maligant neoplasms of the pancreatic biliary tract.
- MRCP identifies not only the dilated ducts located proximal to the obstruction but also the ducts that are narrowed and enased by the tumor.
- The double duct sign represents dilatation of the biliary and pancreatic ducts.
- The duct penetrating sign refers to a non-obstructed main pancreatic duct penetrating an inflammatory pancreatic mass unlike its obstruction by pancreatic carcinoma.

Hepatobiliary Interventions

A. PERCUTANEOUS BIOPSY

Types

- Brush, scrape, needle or atherectomy.
- Cholangioscopic biopsy.
- FNAC.
- Plugged biopsy.

Pre-requisites

- Informed written consent.
- Patient preparation
  - Short fast.
  - Analgesia.
- Materials required
  - Chiba or Frausen needle.
  - 20cc syringe and tap.
  - 18G Invent needle spring loaded.

B. PERCUTANEOUS BILIARY DRAINAGE TECHNIQUES

Types

- External.
- Internal – external.
- Internal.

Pre-requisites

- Baseline CBC.
- Coagulation profile.
- Liver function tests
  - Consent and premedication.

Baschine PTC also performed to assess the level and nature of obstruction.

PTC————A – Endoscopically–ERCP.
B – T-Tube.
– Transhepatic.
– Biliary Cutaneous Fistulae

A. Carey Coon's Stent

- Length – 19 cms.
- 12F or 14F tube with multiple side holus and gradual 90° behind in its most distal aspect.
- 3.0 nylon sutures is attached to proximal shaft extending to silastic button.

B. Ring Kerlan Stent

- 12F made of percuflex.
- 8-10 cms long, perforated.
- Mallecot mushroom tip is positive at the trailing end.

OBSTRUCTIVE JAUNDICE

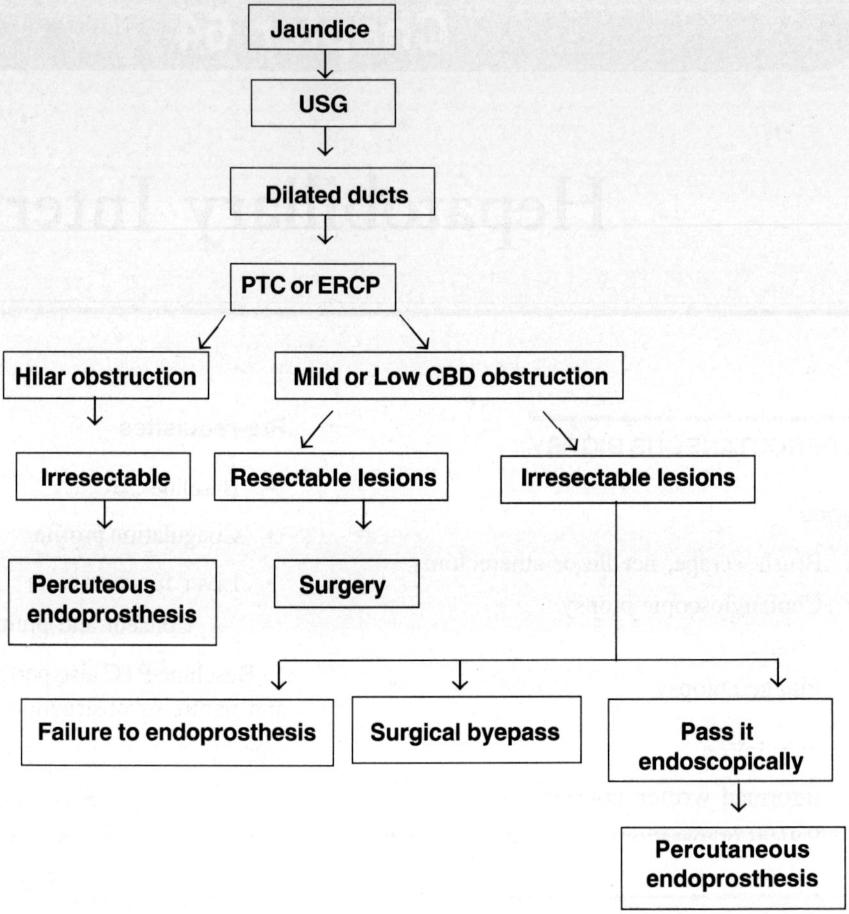

5 Section

A. Z- Stent

- Constructed of round 0.016 or 0.018-inch stainless steel wire with 6 zigzag bands. An interrupted suture connects the urine at the bend points, limited the luminal diameter.

  Diam – 6-12 mm.

  Length – 1.5 to 9 cms.

B. Wall Stent — Self-Expanding Stent

- Composed of 18 stainless steel monofilaments braided into a helical spring like mesh tube.

  Diam – 8, 10, 12 diameters.

  Length – 20-94 mm.

C. Palmaz Stent Balloon Expanded Stent

- Delivered third sheath, inflexible and short in length.

  Diameter – 4-12 mm.

  Length – 10-39 mm.

Endoscopic stent placement – 95% success rate in low bile duct strictures 10 and 2% - 67%.

For high strictures 17 and 8% morbidity and mortality.

MALIGNANT BILIARY STRICTURES

- External drainage.
  Baseline cholangiogram obtained – US guidance for duct selection:
  - Co-axial cope catheter used.
    Initial puncture with 21 or 22G needle following sequential changes of increasingly larger catheters.
  - Finally, placement of catheter with several side holes lying above the level of obstruction.
  - Connection to plastic bag.
  - Graduated biliary drainage.
  - Disadvantage.
  - Pain management.
  - Bile salt and electrolyte replacement.
  - Ab Rx.
  - Routine catheter replacement 2-4 months.

EXTERNAL INTERNAL DRAINAGE (Figure 64.1)

- Catheter crosses the obstruction with several side holes and below it.
- Can be external capped for complete internal flow.

Advantage

- Easy access for future interventions:
  - Brachy therapy.
  - Internal stent placement.

Disadvantage

- Need for regular flushing and dressing.
- Routine catheter checks.
- Treatment related to prolonged biliary intubation.
  - Cholangitis.
  - Bleeding.
  - Skin infection.
  - Bile leak.
  - Ascites.
  - Catheter fracture and dislodgement.
- Rib erosion/ostiomyelitis.
- Seeding of tumor cells along tract.

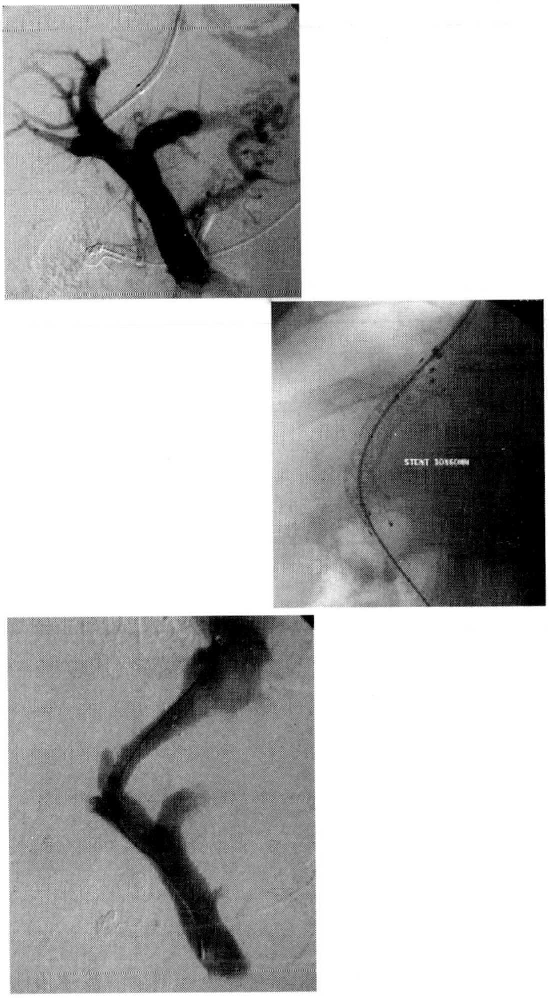

Fig. 64.1: DSA images show the portal vein branch with multiple collaterals; TIPS stent placed between the hepatic vein and the portal vein and post-TIPS angiogram through the stent shows no collaterals

INTERNAL DRAINAGE

- Endoprosthesis/biliary stent.

  Lies totally within the biliary tract.

Advantage

- Improved quality of life.
- No bile salts/electrolyte replacement.

Disadvantage

- No ready access to biliary system in the event of stent dysfunction.

ENDOPROSTHESIS

Plastic

- Carey Coons stent.
- Ring Kerlan stent.

Metallic

- Gianturco Rosch Z stent.
- Wall stents.
- Palmaz stent.

BENIGN BILIARY CIRRHOSIS

Etiology

- Iatrogenic
  - Surgery.
  - Radiation.
  - Chemotherapy.
- Primary sclerosing cholangitis.
- Recurrent pyogenic cholangitis.
- AIDS-related cholangitis.

Morphology

Smoothly tapering lesions.

Though surgery promises the best long term result but with higher morbidity and mortality.

Indication

- Patients who are not candidates for surgery.
- With more distal primary strictures.
- Recurrent strictures despite surgery.

Management

- Balloon dilatation.
- Stenting.

Complications

- Sepsis and pain.
- Bleeding and pseudo aneurysm.

C. NON-OPERATIVE REMOVAL OF BILIARY CALCULI

Gallbladder calculi and percutaneous cholecystostomy.

Indication

- Surgically high-risk patients.
- Postoperative residual calculi.

Efficacy

- PC can lead to dramatic resolutions of acute cholecystitis – is a safe procedure performed under US.
  - Transhepatic
  - Transperitoneal - 2 approaches

  Trocar

  Seldinger - 2 techniques

Complications

- Bleeding.
- Hepatic laceration.

BILIARY CALCULI

Indications

- Retained stones (5-15%).
- Primary intra hepatic stones.

Non-Surgical Techniques

- ERCP sphincterotomy and stone removal.
- Percutaneous mechanical techniques.
- Cholangioscopy.
- Laparoscopic common duct exploration ESWL.
- Catheter directed infusion pharmacotherapy with mono octanion.
- Laser photocoagulation.
- Dissolution – MTBE.

D. MANAGEMENT OF BILE DUCT INJURIES

0.6-0.8% prevalence.

Complications

- Obstructed biliary system.
- Abnormal fluid collection.

Aim

- Define the nature and extent of the biliary injury.
- Render definite treatment for biliary leaks and bilomas.
- Provide temporary drainage in patients.

E. PERCUTANEOUS HEPATIC DRAINAGE

Indications

- Deterioration during medical treatment of at least one week duration.
- Pain and impending rupture.

Drainage of:

- Abscess
  - Pyogenic.
  - Amoebic.
- Cysts
  - Congenital simple.
  - Acquired hepatic.
    a. Parasitic.
    b. Post traumatic.
    c. Inflammatory.
    d. Neoplastic.

Technique

↓ US guidance and ab cover with LFT and coag. profile.

8 F or more catheters placed using trocar or seldinger technique.

Left in place with curled up end and gravitated drainage.

F. LIVER TUMOR TREATMENT

- Chemical ablation with ethanol –95% (PET) or acetic acid (PAI).

Mode of Action (PEI)

- Coagulative necrosis and fibrosis by promoting denaturation of primary and small vessel thrombosis.
- Consistency and vascularity → rationalise the treatment.
- Alcohol injected decreased radio guidance in multiple session.

Using Long Needle

Started from deep to superficial portion.

Total amount of alcohol injected= $\frac{4}{3}\pi\,(r+0.5)^3$ ml

r= radius of lesion in cms.

PAI

Total amount of acetic acid injection – 3 × diam of lesions.

DO NOT INJECT IN VESSELS

Radiofrequency ablation – RFA.

- For small tumors and metastasis.

Mode of Action

- Necrosis of tumor by deposition of thermal energy around the tip of the electrode inserted in the tumor.

  Size upto 5 cms.

  No upto 5.

Complications of the Procedure

- Severe pain post procedural.
- Local hemorrhage.
- Peritonitis.
- Cholecystitis.
- Colitis.
- Vascular injury or thrombosis.

Response

RFA response × 1/tumor size.

<2 cms – 85% response rate.

3 cm – 35% response rate.

TRANSCATHETER ARTERIAL CHEMOEMBOLISATION (TACE)

- Mainstay of therapy for unresectable HCC.

Mode of Action

Intra-arterial delivery of high concentration of chemothorax agent emulsified in lipiodol combined with an embolic agent directly to the tumor.

Agents are:

1. Adriamycin.
2. Epirubicin.
3. Mitomycin-C.
4. Cisplatain.

Contraindications

1. Poor hepatic function.
2. S. bilirubin > 2.0 mg%.
3. Portal perfusion <50%.
4. Thrombosed main portal vein.

TRANSCATHETER ARTERIAL EMBOLISATION OF THE TUMOR

- As an emergency procedure to ↓ GI hemorrhage – as in varices.
- Direct tumor invasion of duodenum, transverse colon and stomach.
- Using radioisotopes.

Treatment of Benign Tumors

- Hemangioma.
- FNH.
- Adenoma.
- Other vascular tumors.

G. TRANSJUGULAR LIVER BIOPSY (TJLB)

Indications

1. Coagulopathy (PT>115 sac, Platelet < 60,000/ml).
2. Massive ascites.
3. Obesity, small liver, right pl. effusion, FUC liver transplant and cavernous hemangioma.

CI

1. Bleeding.
2. PSVT.
3. Cholangitis.
4. Intraperitoneal bleed.

   Plugged biopsy preferred.

5 Section

Section 6—Alimentary Tract

Chapter 65

Normal vs. Abnormal Appearance of Oesophagus

- Normal wall thickness – 3 mm when adequately distended; 5 mm when incompletely distended.
- Abnormal–greater/eccentric thickness, AP diameter of esophagus > 16 mm. Lateral diameter of esophagus > 24 mm.
- Normally no air is seen in cervical oesophagus, small amount of air may be seen in thoracic esophagus in 65% people.
- Abnormal air fluid level or fluid filled lumen is due to either obstruction or motility disorder.

ESOPHAGEAL TUMORS

Table 65.1: Types of tumors

Benign		**Malignant**
Mucosal	*Submucosal*	
• Papilloma • Glycogen acanthosis	• Leiomyoma • Fibrovascular polyp • Hemangioma	• Carcinoma • Leiomyo sarcoma • Malignant spindle cell tumors • Primary malignant melanoma • Metastases

LEIOMYOMA

- Most common among benign submucosal tumors (>50% of all).
- Location

  Distal third of oesophagus (60%)

  Middle (30%)

  Proximal (10%)
- Single or multiple (3-4%)
- Multiple associated with Alport's syndrome.
- CT appearance:
  - Smoothly marginated intraluminal mass or eccentric or concentric esophageal wall thickening of homogeneous soft tissue attenuation.
  - Calcification may be treated.
  - Mediastinal fat planes are intact.
  - May simulate localized malignant tumor.
- In leiomyomatosis–marked wall thickening of distal esophagus with soft tissue attenuation.

FIBROVASCULAR POLYP

- Composed of fibrous tissue, adipose tissue and vascular structures.
- Site of origin: Upper 1/3rd of esophagus near cricopharyngeus.

- Common in elderly man.
- CF Long standing dysphagia.
  Weight loss.
  Vomiting.
  Respiratory difficulty.
  May cause sudden death.
- CT Attenuation varies depending on content of fat. Oral contrast surrounds the mass.
- MR Shows lipid containing substances Mucoid secretions.
  Sometimes acute blood within tumor.

T1W Bright signal.

T2W Soft tissue and muscular component show low signal.

Hemangioma

- Rare (<5%)

  MC symptom Dysphagia; hemorrhage.

  CT Well defined homogeneous mass with soft tissue attenuation phleboliths may be +ve.
  Marked contrast enhancement.

  MRI Isointense on T1W.
  Hyperintense on T2W.

ESOPHAGEAL CARCINOMA (Figure 65.1)

Table 65.2: Types of esophageal carcinoma

Squamous cell carcinoma >90% of oesophageal malignancy	Adenocarcinoma Associated with Barrett's oesophagus
Risk factors – Tobacco, Alcohol, Achalasia, Lye stricture, Head and neck tumors, Celiac disease, Plummer Winson syndrome, Tylosis and Radiations	40% cases with Barrett's oesophagus. Progress to adenocarcinoma
	Site – Distal oesophagus (2/3rd) Tend to invade gastric cardia and fundus
	550% of gastrooesophageal junction tumors are Barrett's carcinomas
Clinical Features – Dysphasia when lumen↓ by 50% 2/3rd circumference invaded by tumor	Clinical Features — Dysphasia; weight loss
Odenophasia – when ulceration occurs in tumor	By the time dysphasia occurs, tumor is quite advanced
Chest pain related with swallowing when mediastinal invasion in + weight loss	Unresponsive to RT and CT

Contd.

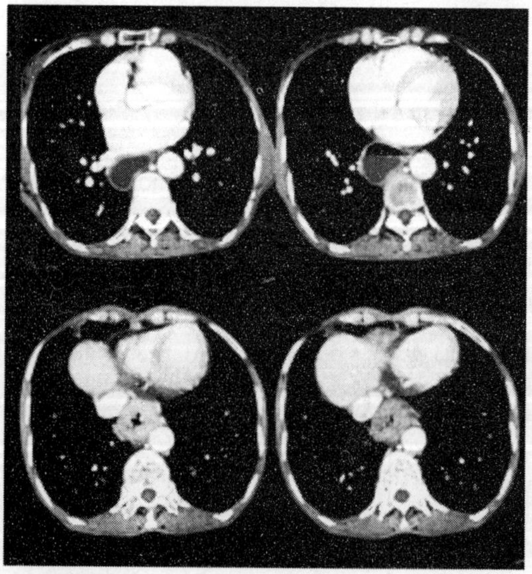

Fig. 65.1: Axial CT images show intraluminal narrowing and proximal dilatation secondary to midesophagus carcinoma

TNM STAGING FOR ESOPHAGEAL CANCER

Table 65.3: Staging of tumor

T – Primary tumor	N – Regional L.N.
TIS – Carcinoma in situ	N_1 – No regional nodes
T_1 – Tumor invades mucosa and submucosa	N_2 – Regional nodal mats
T_2 – Tumor invades muscularis propria	Include cervical mediastinal and perigastric L.N.
T_3 – Tumor invades adventitia	Celiac L.N. mets are
T_4 – Tumor invades adjacent structures	N_1 in adeno ca M_1 in sq. cell ca

M – Distant metastasis.

M_o – No distant mets.

M_1– Distant metastases +ve.

Stage I	$T_1N_oM_o$
Stage IIA	$T_{2\text{-}3}\ N_oM_o$
Stage IIB	$T_{1\text{-}2}\ N_1M_o$
Stage III	$T_3N_1M_o$, T_4 any NM_o
Stage IV	$T_{any}\ N_{any}\ M_1$

IMAGING FEATURES

Barium Swallow

- Stricture with nodular elements.
- Ulcerative lesion with firm irregular rim.
- Polypoid lesion.
- Early stages – Stiffening of mucosa
Failure to collapse completely after peristaltic wave.
- Varicoid – Tortuous thick folds.
- Infiltration of myenteric plexus – achalasia like picture.
- Fistulisation to trachea/aorta.
- Endoscopic USG – Depth of tumor invasion is elated and prognosis.

5 Layers of esophagus are seen with alternating echoes

Mucosa	I	T1
Muscularis mucosa	I	
Submucosa	I	
Muscularis propria	I	T2
Adventitia	I	T3

- Accuracy 75-100%.
- False positive in cases with peritumoral inflammation, associated lymphadenopathy can be assessed.

CT and MRI

- Tumor staging.
- CA appears as a mass or wall thickening (>5 mm) of soft tissue attenuation with irregular or eccentric oesophageal lumen.

  On MRI, esophageal CA is

  Isointense on T1W

  Hyperintense on T2W

Periesophageal fat invasion – seen as strand like areas of soft tissue attenuation in periesophageal fat on CT.

MRI shows it as an ill-defined irregular margin; regional absence of bright jet signal; tumor mass in adjacent mediastinal fat and sometimes resulting in abscess formation (Figure 65.2).

Peri oesophageal fat invasion affects prognosis but is not a contraindication to en block curative resection of tumor.

Usually surgical resection is contemplated even when nodal mets are present for palliation.

Involvement of tracheobronchial tress, great vessels and bone are contraindications to surgical resection.

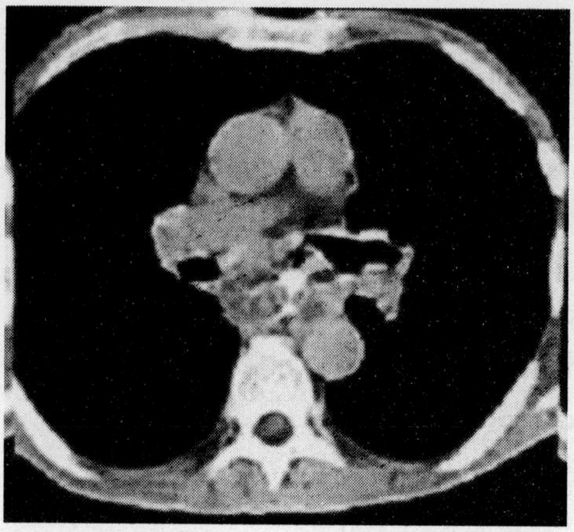

Fig. 65.2: Axial CT image shows a large esophageal mass with mediastinal abscess formation

Tracheobronchial Invasion

MC Sites Distal trachea
Left main bronchus

Criteria

- Displacement/indentation of posterior wall of trachea or bronchus by tumor mass.
- Direct tumor extension in lumen of airway.
- Extension of mass between trachea and aortic arch.
- Extension of mass between left main bronchus and descending aorta.

Absence of fat planes alone does not indicate invasion. Posterior concavity of trachea or main bronchi alone is a non-specific feature.

Aortic Invasion

- 90° criteria is 90% accurate when fat planes above and below tumor are maintained.
- If arc is $<45^o$ – aortic invasion is unlikely between 45 to 90° indeterminate.
- Fat planes may be lost in cachectic patients without invasion.
- Displacement of aorta.
- Deformation of aortic lumen.
- Obliteration of fat plane is diagnostic between oesophagus, descending aorta and spine.

Pulmonary vein invasion – Amputation or lack of opacification of pulmonary vein.

Bone invasion – Bone destruction and replacement of bone by soft tissue.

Pleural, pericardial, diaphragmatic and gastric invasion are not contraindication for surgery as they can be removed in blue.

Pericardial Invasion

- Pericardial thickening contiguous with tumor.
- Pericardial effusion.
- Inward deformity of heart with loss of intervening fat planes at the level of tumor with intact fat planes above and below it.

Gastric Invasion (Figure 65.3)

- Soft tissue mass extending from oesophagus into proximal stomach under adequate distention.
- More common with adenocarcinoma.

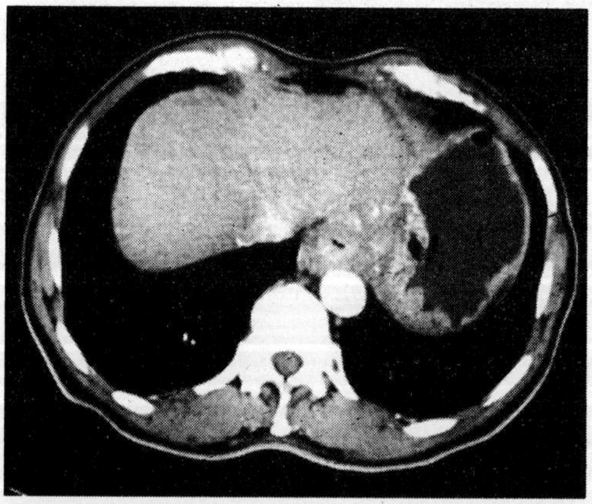

Fig. 65.3: Axial CT image shows mass at the gastroesophageal junction with spread along the fundus of the stomach

Pleural and Diaphragmatic Invasion

- Not accurately seen on CT because adhesions to these structures by tumor can easily occur without invasion.

Nodal Staging

- Nodal mets are very common as rich lymphatic network along oesophagus and lack of serosa allow early tumor spread.
- Endoscopic USG is most accurate for regional node mets. Regional L.N. extend from supraclavicular to celiac chain.
- MC nodes involved - Inferior periesophageal L.N. nodes near gastric cardia.
- Metastatic deposits may be +ve in nodes as small as 2-3 mm - central low attenuation is helpful but low sensitivity.
- Size threshold for supraclavicular nodes 5 mm
- Gastro hepatic ligaments nodes 8 mm.
- Other mediastinal and abdominal nodes 10 mm.

Distant Metastases

- Liver 32%.
- Lung (21%) – Present as single or multiple nodules ± pl. effusion.
- Adrenal: To differentiate between adrenal adenoma and mets.

Adenoma	**Metastases**
Homogeneous	Enlarged heterogeneous
Size <5 cm	gland with loss of normal shape

Attenuation value.

-5 to 10 HU.

PET: FDG is used.

For primary esophageal cancer – PET is as sensitive as CT.

For metastases – More sensitive than CT.

Disadvantages – Mediastinal invasion is not so well assessed.

Postoperative appearance and recurrence.

ESOPHAGO GASTRECTOMY

Early Postoperative Complications

- Anastomotic leak – mediastinitis, abscess.
- Lung parenchymal consolidation.
- Pleural effusion, empyema.
- Subphrenic abscess.

Table 65.4: Types of eosophago-gastrectomy

High esophagogastric anastomosis with gastric conduit ↓	Low anastomosis ↓
Both esophagogastric junction and stomach are located in right paravertebral area. Proximal esophagus about anastomosis may be dilated. In lower retrocardiac area, stomach passes from right to left directly anterior to descending aorta.	Esophagogastric junction and stomach lie in left paravertebral area.

Tumor recurrence – soft tissue mass; displacement of normal structures; distant metastases; L.N. enlargement.

LEIOMYOSARCOMA

- Seen in middle aged and older adults.
- Site: Middle and distal 1/3rd.
- Better prognosis than squamous cell carcinoma due to slow growth and late metastases.
- Growth pattern – polypoid or infiltrating.
- CT
  - Thickening of esophageal wall with large exophytic component.
  - Areas of central necrosis.
  - Extraluminally gas/oral contrast within tumor.

  Polypoid lesion is usually non obstructive.
- MR → Iso to muscle on T1W, hyper on T2W areas of signal void if air is present.

Malignant Spindle Cell Tumor

CT – Large intraluminal mass that expands oesophageal lumen without causing obstruction.
– Homogeneous soft tissue attenuation.
– Intense enhancement.

D/D – Malignant stromal tumor.
Malignant melanoma.

LYMPHOMA

- Associated with AIDS.
- Esophagus is least common site of involvement in cases with GI lymphoma.

Ba Swallow

- Irregular narrowing of distal esophagus due to contiguous spread of tumor from gastric function.
- Varicoid appearance may be seen in enlarged tortuous folds.
- CT – Marked diffuse thickening of esophageal wall; ulcerations; lymphadenopathy tend to be larger.
- D/D leukemic infiltrates.

Hematogenous Mets

- Kaposi's SA.
- Multiple stromal tumors.

PRIMARY MALIGNANT MELANOMA

- Very rare.
- **Barium swallow** – Bulky polypoid intraluminal mass that focally expands esophagus without obstruction.
- Grows intraluminally along long axis of esophagus.
- CT - Large oesophageal mass lymphadenopathy is less frequent.
- D/D - Spindle cell carcinoma.

METASTATIC DISEASE

Causes

CA breast – Most common cause distance site of origin of oesophageal metastases.
– Submucosal masses are common.

CA bronchus – May also infiltrate oesophagus directly.
– Fistula may develop between oesophagus and bronchus.

CA pancreas – Especially of tail region.

Melanoma

Bezoars

These are collections or concretions of indigestible foreign material that accumulate and coalesce in the G.I.T. usually the stomach and small intestine.

Can be classified into 4 types:

- Phytobezoar.
- Trichobezoar (Figure 66.1).
- Medication or pharmacobezoar.
- Lactobezoar or milk curd – secondary to an infantile formula.

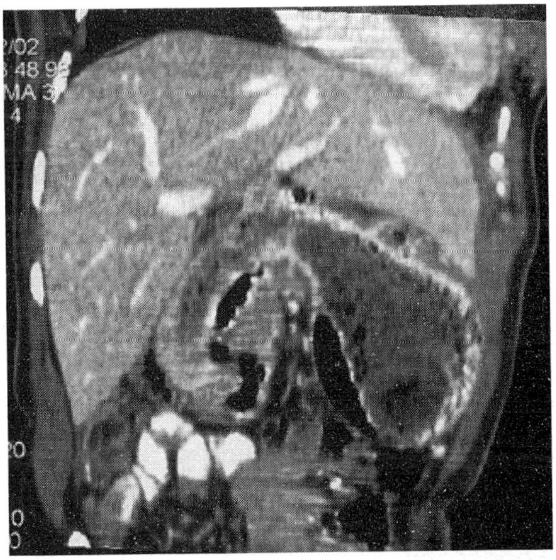

Fig. 66.1: Oblique MPR CT image shows a large trichobezoar in the stomach and proximal duodenum

Phytobezoar

- Most common.
- Commonly occur with food such as celery, pumpkins, grape, skin, raisins, leeks, beets, etc. These food contain large amount of non-digestible fibres, tannin in high concentration forms a coagulase when exposed to gastric acid.
- Although formed in stomach, most often migrate to the small bowel and become impacted in small bowel and may cause partial or complete small bowel obstruction in jejunum and proximal ileum.

Trichobezoar

- Most common in children and young adult females, there is increased association mentally retardation, psychiatric conditions.
- Usually confined to stomach.
- Results due to ingestion of large quantities of hair, carpet fibres, string or clothing.

Medication Bezoars

- Such medication includes antacid, fibre supplements enteric-coated aspirin and multivitamins.

PREDISPOSING FACTORS

- Most common – altered gastrointestinal anatomy from previous surgery – altered motility with delayed gastric emptying with reduction gastric mixing and peptic activity.
- Excessive consumption of foods with increased fibre content.
- Alteration in dentition and mastication.

SITE

- Stomach.
- Duodenum.
- Small intestine – bezoar may also seen in small bowel diverticulum.

Clinical Presentation

- Vague feeling of epigastric distress.
- Anorexia.
- Hemetemesis – Secondary to intermittent gastric outlet obstruction.
- Gastric ulceration – Secondary pressure necrosis in 1/4th of the part.
- Physical diagnosis – Palpable mass, abdominal distension, jaundice.

Radiological Features

Plain X-ray

- Mottled soft tissue opacity in the shape of the distended stomach or small bowel obstruction in case of small bowel bezoars.
- Soft tissue mass floating in the stomach at the air fluid level.
- A calcification rim may delineate the edge of bezoar, which may extend to the small intestine.

Upper GI Barium Study

- Bezoars on barium study appear as filling defect; barium is seen in the interstices of the bezoar giving a mottled appearance.
- Occasionally bezoars may be unusually smooth, simulating a large gas bubble, which is freely mobile with or without attachment to the gastric wall.
- Additional filling defects seen in distal small bowel may because of breakage of bezoars and lodging in small bowel.

Ultrasound

- Curvilinear bright echogenic band with posterior acoustic shadowing due to increased echogenicity of the hair/fibers as well as multiple acoustic interfaces created by food debris and air trapped within the highly compacted bezoar.

CT

- Large mesh like intraluminal mass of decreased attenuation. The mass can contain trapped air or contrast material and may demonstrate concentric rings.
- Orally administered contrast can be used to delineate the outer surface of the mass.
- Complication – Small bowel obstruction, perforation, peritonitis, abscess.
- Calcified bezoar – Lacks the mottled gas pattern and present as an olive stone on a golf ball.

M.R.I.

- Variable
  - ↓ SI on T1, T2 and fat supp. T2 air.
  - ↑ SI on T1 and T2 – due to H_2O and food trapped with in the bezoar.
  - ↑ On T1 and inversion recovery due to fat.
- Foci of inflammation due to gastritis or ulceration or perforation.

Endoscopy

- Radiograph with or without Ba may identify only 1/4th of bezoars.

- Definitive diagnosis of bezoar is established at endoscopy.

Differential Diagnosis

- Foreign bodies – Radiolucent filling defect in stomach and duodenum.
- Gastric neoplasm.
- Villous tumor/adenomatous polyps – in stomach and duodenum – predominantly villous element grossly appear as polypoid mass with numerous fronds like projection.
  - Site: Equally common in stomach and duodenum (papilla of Vater); risk of malignancy is proportional to the size of lesion.
  - Age > 50 years.
  - Clinical presentation: Signs and symptoms of upper GI.
  - Bleed – melena, guaiac +ve stool, iron deficiency anaemia and obstructive jaundice.
  - Malignant potential is increased.
  - Barium study – polypoid mass (2-9 cm). Reticular or soap bubble appearance with serrated feathery margins because of trapping of barium in multiple clefts between the fronds like projection of tumor.
  - Not mobile with change in patients position.
- Malignancy – Carcinoma, lymphoma, and leiomyosarcoma of stomach and duodenum may also manifest as bulky intraluminal mass, but these lesion rarely produce a soap bubble appearance.
- D/D features – In carcinoma thickening of gastric wall is 3 mm to 1 cm, there is distortion of normal rugal pattern with regional lymphadenopathy.
- G.I. lymphoma – NHL; most common pattern – sub mucosal spread; diffuse or localized gastric wall thickening with distortion of normal rugal fold pattern, luminal contrast material may extend into crevices between thickened gastric rugae. Contrast enhancement of thickened submucosal lymphatic tissue in minimal. Regional lymphadenopathy is seen.
- Leiomyosarcoma are of smooth muscle origin 50% intramural, 35% exogastric and 15% endogastric attachment with the wall. Ulceration and cavitation is common with metastases in liver and peritoneal cavity. Angiography shows a well-defined hyper-vascular mass with huge feeding artery and draining veins with intense tumor staining.

Gastric Carcinoma

- 95% of malignant gastric lesions.
- Most common – primary gastric malignancy (Adenocarcinoma).

Predisposing Factors

- Atrophic gastritis, H. pylori infection.
- Pernicious anemia.
- Adenomatous polyps.
- Partial gastrectomy.
- Intake of nitrates, smoked salty fish.
- Diet rich in vitamin C →↓ incidence.
- C/F loss of appetite, dyspepsia, weight loss, anemia.
- Ulcerating tumors → hemorrhage.
- Infiltrating tumors → early diagnosis.
- Tumors obstructing cardia → dysphasia.
- Gastric outlet obstruction → vomiting.

Early

Confined to mucosa and submucosa (irrespective and regional L.N. status).

Japanese Endoscopic Society

I. Elevated >5 mm.

II. Intermediate between I and III.

- 2A flat.
- 2B slightly elevated (<5 mm).
- 2C slightly depressed but do not extend through muscularis mucosa.

III. Ulcerating tumor, penetrating muscularis mucosa.

Advanced Penetrates beyond submucosa.

Bormann – four types:

1. Polypoidal mass.
2. Irregular ulcer with sharply circumscribed margins.
3. Ulcer with surrounding tumor infiltration.
4. Diffuse infiltration .
5. Linitus plastics.

Polypoidal Form (Figure 67.1)

Smooth submucosal filling defect of lobulated intraluminal mass with or without ulceration.

Ulcerative

- Usually in combination with polypoidal form.
- Rarely multiple ulcers without any surrounding mass.

Nodular

- Multiple submucosal nodules or masses.
- Ulcerated – Bull's eye lesion.

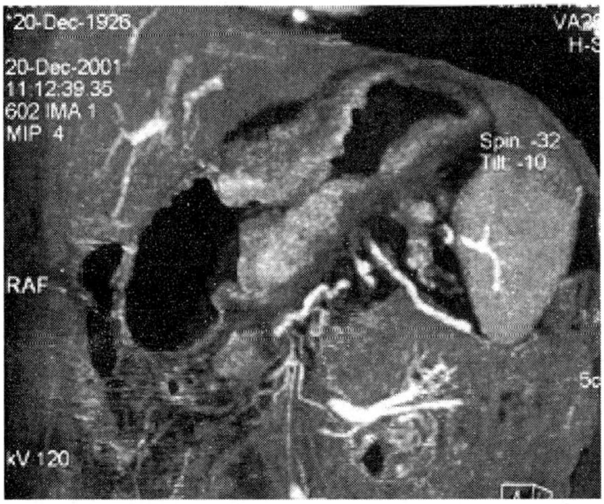

Fig. 67.1: Oblique MIP CT image show a gastric adenocarcinoma involving the body of the stomach

- A combination of above form.
- Transpyloric spread – 30-40%.
- Transcardiac spread – 10%.

CT Features suggestive of Lymphoma
(Figure 67.2)

Bulky homogenous tumor with pronounced thickening of gastric wall, preservation of perigastric fat plane, trans pyloric spread, multicentricity, widespread nodal disease, splenic enlargement.

CT Staging

1. Confined to bowel wall.

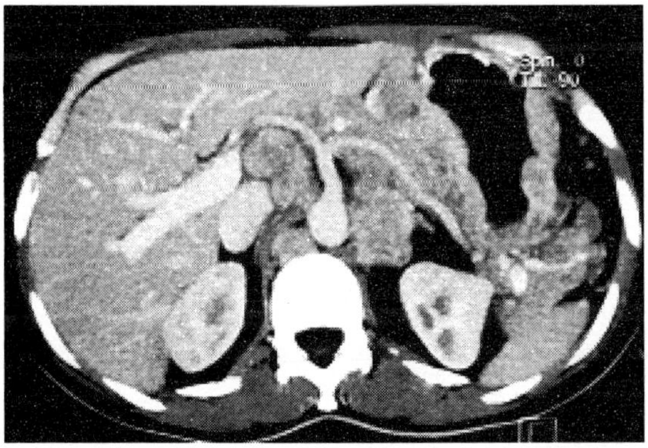

Fig. 67.2: Axial CT image shows gastric lymphoma with lymphadenopathy

2. Limited to regional nodes.
3. Widespread nodal disease (above and below diaphragm).
4. Disseminated to other bone marrow liver spleen – other organs.

TUMOR SPREAD

Lymphatic: Regional – L gastric, splenic celiac common Iliac.

Enlarged retro pancreatic and para aortic

distant metastasis

↓

CI Surgery

- Gastro hepatic and portal hepatis – 8 mm.
- Celiac axis to renal arteries – 10 mm.
- Renal arteries to aortic bifurcation – 12 mm.
- High attenuation (>100 HU), even if small.
- Well-defined, hypoechoic, spherical.
- Adjacent organ and diaphragm, pancreas, liver, transverse colon.
- Hematogenous – liver, lung, kidney, adrenal, brain.
- Peritoneal – ovarian – Krukenberg tumor – omental cake.

STAGING – CT, endoscopic, USG, laparoscopy.

CT Staging

I. Intraluminal mass, no wall thickening.
II. Wall thickness > 1cm.
III. Invasion of adjacent organs.
IV. Distant metastasis.

TNM T1 – Mucosa, submucosa.
T2 – Muscular is propria and subserosa.
T3 – Involvement of visceral peritoneum with or without invasion of adjacent organs.
T4 – Adj. organs.
No – Normal.
N1 – I-6 regional nodes (celiac, splenic, (b) gastric, common hepatic).

N2 – 7-15.

N3 > 15.

Mo – No mets.

M1 – Metastases.

Differential Diagnosis

Entire stomach	*Abdomen*
• Carcinoma	• Amyloidosis, sarcoidosis.
• Metastases from breast carcinoma	• Crohn's, TB, syphilis.
• Hodgkin's lymphoma	• Caustic ingestions, radiotherapy.
• Kaposi's sarcoma	• Eosinophilic gastroenteropathy.
• Neurofibromatosis (Figure 67.3)	• CMV gastritis.

Lymphoma

1.5% of all gastric malignancy.

51% stomach of GIT.

Lymphomas

- Primary – 10%.
- Secondary – 90%.

Dawson's Criteria of Primary GI Lymphoma

- No palpable L.N.
- Normal chest X-ray.
- Normal TLC, DLC.
- At laparotomy, alimentary lesions must predominate and L.N. involvement if any must be confined to draining area of the involved gut segment.
- No hepatosplenomegaly.

Table 67.1: Features differentiating lymphoma from carcinoma

	Lymphoma	Carcinoma
Age	Bimodal	Single peak
C/F	Abdominal pain Mass (lump)	Hepatomegaly, dysphagia, early satiety, vomiting
	Multicentric	Rare
Epicentre	Submucosa	Mucosa
Distensibility	Normal	Lost
Calibre	Normal or ↓	↓↓↓
Well thickness		
Mean	4 cm	1.8 cm
Range	1.1-7.7	1.1-3.2 cm
Enhancement	↑ (Mild)	↑↑↑
Invasion of adj. organs	(+)	(+++)
Perigastric fat plane	N	Lost
HSM	(+)	(-)
L.N.	(++) Both above and below renal hilum	(+)
Ext. to duodenum	(++)	(+)
Oesophagus contour	Regular	Irregular
Hemorrhage and Necrosis	(±)	(++)

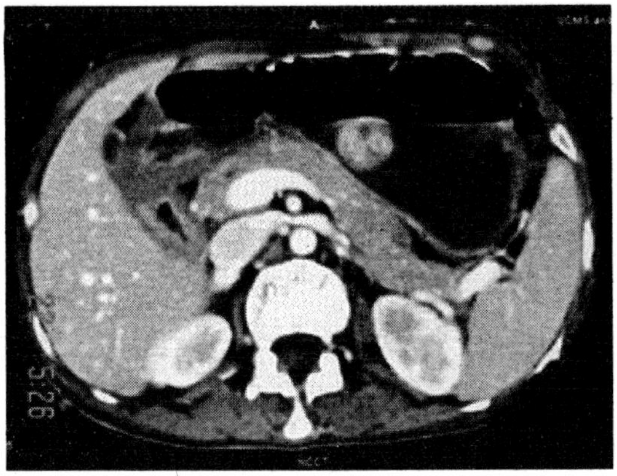

Fig. 67.3: Axial CT image shows gastric neurofibroma in a case of neurofibromatosis

Predisposing Disease

Celiac disease, Ulcerative colitis, AIDS, SLE, Crohn's, Immunocompromised states.

- Hodgkin's – 10%.
- NHL – More common – β cell – MALT (chronic H. pylori).

  (Lukes and Collins) T cell – celiac disease.

  Histiocytic.

C/F – Abdominal Pain, Most Common

Anorexia, weight loss with palpable abdominal mass:

- Initially submucosal, but soon progress to intraluminal fungating mass, or annular constricting lesions or ulcerations.

  Five types – infiltrative form: May be localised or diffuse.
- Diffuse enlargement of gastric folds.
- Large, serpiginous folds with nodular appearances, not effaced after buscopan.

D/D – Menetrier's disease

– Hypertrophic gastritis – involve the proximal half of stomach.

Gastrointestinal Stromal Tumors (GIST)

- 1% gastric malignancies.
- Fundus, body.
- M > F, middle aged and elderly.
- Large intramural tumors with central necrosis.
- Large exogastric component.
- May occasionally show dystrophic calcification.
- Metastases to:
  - Peritoneal cavity.
  - Hematogenous, liver, lung, bone.
  - Lymphatic – rare.
- Hypovascular.
- Difficult to differentiate between benign/malignant, event on histology.
- Benign, usually <10 cm homogeneous on CT, endoscopic US.

Kaposi's Sarcoma

- Tumor of blood vessel – in homosexuals, patients with AIDS.
- Multifocal submucosal tumors throughout GIT.
- Stomach, duodenum, small intestine – Most common site.
- Hemorrhagic patches on endoscopy.

On barium	Polypoidal mass.
	Submucosal nodules.
	Bull's eye lesions.
	Linitis plastica.
CT	Retroperitoneal nodes,
	splenomegaly.

Carcinoid

- Stomach – uncommon site (Antrum, lesser curvature).
- Slow growing submucosal nodule
  - Pedunculated.
  - Ulceration.
- Do not produce carcinoid syndrome.
- Hypervascular hepatic metastases.

Metastases

- Carcinoma breast.
- Melanoma.
- Carcinoma lung-nodules with central ulceration is the most common appearance.
- Lymphoma – Carcinoma breast can produce linitis plastica.

Crohn's Disease

The blending of antrum, pylorus and duodenal bulb into a single tubular or funnel shaped structure.

Pseudo Billroth I pattern.

Presence of residual pliability, distensibility and lack of nodularity.

At times mucosa may be shaggy and nodular cobblestone, fissures and fistulas.

Tuberculosis

- 10% of patients with gastric T.B. have associated duodenal involvement.
- 50% of gastric T.B. – antral.
- Mural nodularity, ulceration, short areas of narrowing.

Eosinophilic Gastroenteritis

- Mural narrowing and mucosal fold thickening.
- Transpyloric extension, peripheral eosinophilic, specific food allergies.

Duodenal Masses

DUODENAL MASSES

Benign	Malignant
Duodenal polyp	Villous tumors
Leiomyoma	Duodenal carcinoma
Ectopic pancreatic rests	Lymphoma
Brunner gland hyperplasia	Leiomyosarcoma
Duplication cyst	

DUODENAL POLYP

- Less common than gastric polyp.
- Hyperplastic polyps are rarely found in the duodenum.
- Most duodenal polyps are adenomatous.

Radiographic Findings

- Duodenal polyps usually appear on barium studies as smooth, small lesions in the first or second portion of the duodenum.
- They are usually less than 2 cm in size.

F/D

- Leiomyoma.
- Brunner gland hamartoma – Endoscopy.
- Antral mucosa (prolapsed) – It usually manifests as mushroom shaped defect at the base of the half.

Villous Tumors

- Adenomatous polyps in the duodenum that contain predominantly villous elements have been called balloon adenomas, papilloma or adenomatous papilloma.

C/F

- Seen in patients older than age 50.
- These present with signs or symptoms of upper GI bleeding such as melena, gives +ve stool or iron deficiency anaemia.
- Obstructive jaundice.

Radiographic Features

- These usually appear on barium studies as polypoid masses, ranging from 2 to 9 cm in size.
- These lesions often have a reticular or "soap" appearance with serrated, feathering margins because of trapping of barium in multiple clefs between the fronds like projection of tumor. The malignant degeneration may lead to the developments of annular lesions with shelf like overhanging margins.

- These tend to be located near the papilla of Vaters but occasionally lesions as far proximally as the duodenal bulb.
- Because these lesions are easily obscured by superimposed mucosal fold, they are best seen on double contrast studies with optimal distention of the duodenum.

Differential Diagnosis

- A large gastric bezoar – it is freely mobile.

LEIOMYOMAS

- These constitute about 90% of mesenchymal tumors and 40% of all benign tumors in the stomach and duodenum.

C/F

These usually occur with about equal frequency in men and women older than age 50.

- An epigastric pain or upper GI bleeding manifested by hematemesis, melena, gives +ve stool or Fe deficiency anemia.

Radiographic Findings

- These appear on barium studies as discrete submucosal masses.
- When viewed in profile, the lesions have a smooth surface that is etched in white on double contrast images and their borders form right angles or slightly obtuse angle with the adjacent duodenal walls.
- When viewed enface, the intraluminal surface of these tumors has abrupt, well-defined borders. The overlying mucosa is usually intact.
- These vary in size from tiny lesions of several mm to enormous masses that encroach significantly on the lumen.
- Tumor larger than 2 cm frequently contain area of ulceration manifested by a central barium filled crater within a smooth or slightly lobulated sub masses. Bull's eye or target lesions.

Differential Diagnosis

- Lipoma – These have tendency to change in size and shape on fluoroscopy.
- Duodenal ulcer – A leiomyoma usually has discrete borders whereas the oedematous mound surrounding duodenal ulcer tends to have more gradual transitions with the adjacent mucosa.

ECTOPIC PANCREATIC RESTS

- These are submucosal lesions.
- Usually discovered as incidental findings.

C/F

- Epigastric pain.
- Upper GI bleeding.

Radiographic Findings

- These usually appear on barium studies as smooth, broadbased submucosal masses.
- They almost always occur as solitary lesions, ranging from 1 to 3cm in size.
- Duodenal lesions are most frequently found in the proximal duodenum between the duodenal bulb and the papilloma of Vater.
- These often contain a central umblication or dimple representing the orifice of a primitive ductal system.
- This orifice is manifested by a central collection of barium ranging from 1 to 5 mm in diameter and 5 to 10 mm in depth.
- When viewed enface, these umbilicated lesions have typical "bulls eye" appearance.
- Rarely, barium may reflux into rudimentary ductal structures that terminate in tiny club shaped pouches.

6 Section

Differential Diagnosis

- Ectopic pancreatic rests – usually occur as solitary lesion.
- Metastatic disease lymphoma - Multiple lesions.
- Kaposi's sarcoma.

BRUNNER GLAND HYPERPLASIA/BRUNNER GLAND HAMARTOMA

- This occurs as a response to hypersecretion of acid in the stomach.

Radiographic Findings

- The diffuse form of Brunner gland hyperplasia is manifested on barium studies by multiple small rounded nodules in the proximal duodenum producing a characteristic cobble stone appearance.
- The nodules tend to be most abundant in the duodenal bulb with fewer nodules in the descending duodenum.
- Occasionally, central fleck of barium may be identified in the nodules.
- Brunner gland hamartoma may appear as one or more submucosal or sessile lesions, ranging from several millimetres to several centimetres in size.

DUPLICATION CYSTS

- These are hollow epithelium lined, spherical or tubular structures that are directly attached to GIT.
- They tend to occur on the mesenteric side of the bowel often sharing common blood supply and muscular coat with the adjacent bowel wall.
- These are usually spherical having no direct communication with the normal GIT.

C/F

- These have an approx equal sex distribution.
- Duodenal duplication cysts are discovered in patients older than age 20.
- Abdominal mass and bilious vomiting.

Radiographic Findings

- Abdominal plain films – presence of soft tissue mass indenting duodenal air shadows.
- Inferiorly displaced transverse colon.
- Barium studies – As smooth intramural or extrinsic masses involving the medial wall of the descending duodenum.
- They may considerably encroach on the lumen causing progressive obstruction.

USG

- These on USG usually appears as sonolucent masses with strong posterior wall echoes and then transmission.

CT

- Thin walled, fluid filled structures abetting the medial wall of the descending duodenum.
- Rarely there may be cyst wall calcification or enteroliths.

DUODENAL CARCINOMA

- It is a rare malignant tumor.
- These lesions are located in the post bulbar portion of the duodenum at or below the level of the ampulla of Vater.

C/F

- Nausea, vomiting, abdominal pain, weight loss, seizures or symptoms of upper GI bleeding.
- ↑ed incidence.
  - Gardner's syndrome.

- Celiac disease.
- Crohn's disease.
- Neurofibromatosis.

Barium Studies

- Polypoid, ulcerated on annular lesions at or more common distal to the ampulla of Vater.

USG

- A small hyperechoic mass is the head of the pancreas at the site of bile duct obstruction.

Cholangiography

- A polypoidal mass at the ampulla or abrupt termination of the common bile duct without mass.

CT

- A discrete mass or mass like thickening of the duodenal wall.
- T1W fat suppressed image – low signal intensity in the region of ampulla.
- Post gadolinium spin gradient echo images – areas of low signal intensity.

DUODENAL LYMPHOMA

- It usually results from contiguous spread of tumor from the distal stomach or proximal jejunum or from encasement of duodenum by a conglomerate mass of lymphomatous nodes in the retroperitoneum.
- CT – Nodular masses, cavitated lesions or long, infiltrated segment with mass like thickening of the duodenum.

LEIOMYOSARCOMA

- 10% of malignant tumor in the duodenum.
- Sex distribution equal.

C/F

- Upper GI bleeding.
- Weight loss.
- Abdominal pain.
- Palpable mass.
- Obstruction jaundice.
- 2nd or 3rd portion of duodenum.

Barium Studies

- Submucosal masses often containing areas of ulceration or cavitation.
- Rarely cause duodenal obstruction.

CT

- Exocentric lesions, which tend to project laterally from the 2nd portion of the duodenum.
- Often contain areas of low attenuation because of necrosis of the tumor.

Chronic Inflammatory Bowel Disease

This entity includes ulcerative colitis and Crohn's disease. Symptoms include abdominal pain weight loss diarrhea and the passage of bloody stools.

Epidemiology of Inflammatory Bowel Disease

Sonographic evidence of mural thickening of the bowel with a paucity of luminal content may be helpful in the detection of inflammatory bowel diseases (IBD). However the findings are non-specific and the differential diagnosis must be related to the specific segment of the bowel involved.

Table 69.1: Differentiating features between ulcerative colitis and Crohn's disease

Factor	Ulcerative colitis	Crohn's disease
Incidence (per 100,000)	2-10	1-6
Prevalence (per 100,000)	35-100	10-100
Racial incidence Ethnic incidence Sex	High in whites High in Jews Slight female preponderance	High in whites High in Jews Slight female preponderance

ULCERATIVE COLITIS (UC)

It is an inflammatory bowel disease of unknown origin. The prevalence of the disease is estimated at about 68 cases per 10,000 populations with an equal distribution between men and women and with a familial predilection (Table 69.1).

There is a possible genetic etiology but auto-immune mechanisms and psychological factors also play an etiological role.

Grossly a uniform and continuous inflammatory process with hemorrhages and ulcerations of colonic mucosa characterizes UC. The rectum is involved in the large majority of patients. The term backwash ileitis designates involvement of a 5-25 cm segment of the terminal ileum that may occur in patients with involvement of the entire colon. Fistulae and pericolic abscesses are rarely seen in patients with UC. During the chronic phase fibrosis with retraction and shortening of the colon causes Haustral loss and development of inflammatory pseudopolyposis without malignant potential. However the risk of associated carcinoma of the colon is markedly elevated for patients with long standing UC.

The clinical symptomatology of UC includes bloody diarrhoea with pus, low grade fever and weight loss. Extracolonic manifestations of UC include arthritis, skin changes and hepatobiliary disturbances. The clinical course of UC is characterized by periods of remissions and exacerbations. UC affecting the rectum has a different clinical presentation than classical UC. The disease is usually limited to the rectum without extension to the other colon segments, it may follow a hyperacute clinical course and the extracolonic manifestations are usually not prominent or may even be absent.

The most important complications of UC are colon perforation and toxic megacolon.

Radiological Diagnosis

The role of radiological study in patients with UC is:

- To confirm the endoscopic findings.
- To evaluate the extent and the severity of the mucosal lesions; and
- To demonstrate complications (Table 69.2) such as strictures, pseudopolyposis, toxic megacolon, perforation and malignancy.

On plain radiography of the abdomen the

Table 69.2: Complications and extraintestinal manifestations of IBD

	CD	UC
Local perianal disease		
• Anal fissures, rectovaginal fistulas, recto-vesical fistulas	+++	+
• Para rectal abscess	+++	+
• Rectal prolapse	++	+
Hemorrhage		
• Mild–may lead to anemia	+++	+
• Massive–may be life threatening	+	+++
Toxic megacolon perforation		
• Free with or without toxic megacolon	+	+++
• Walled-off	+++	-
Strictures		
• Fibrous-permanent	+++	-
• Muscularis mucosa hypertrophy reversible	+	+++
Cancer		
Systemic skin manifestations		
• Erythema nodosum	+++	+
• Aphthous ulcers of the mouth	+++	-
• Pyoderma gangrenosum	+	+++
Eye lesions		
• Conjunctivitis	+++	+
• Iritis, uveitis, episcleritis	+++	+
Arthritis		
• Peripheral joints – migratory non deforming, seronegative	+++	+
• Ankylosing spondylitis, sacroiliitis	+	+++
Hepatobiliary disease		
• Biliary		
– Pericholangitis	+	+
– Primary sclerosing cholangitis	+	+++
– Bile duct carcinoma	+	+
– Gall stones	+++	-
• Hepatocellular		
– Chronic active hepatitis	+	+
– Cirrhosis	-	+

diagnosis of UC is suggested by the striking absence of residue in the colon. Abnormally located free air collections may indicate free perforation in the peritoneal cavity. Air may also be detected within the wall of the colon indicating severe tissue necrosis.

Barium examination is the most appropriate technique to reveal the typical mucosal changes observed in UC. In patients with active disease the usual procedure for colon preparation cannot be applied because laxatives may cause an exacerbation of the inflammation and the examination itself should be conducted with great care in order to reduce the discomfort for the patient.

- During the early stage of the disease hyperemia and edema leads to a fine granular mucosal pattern composed of small dots of barium or to a coarser granular pattern composed of reticular or ring like structures.
- During the ulcerative phase of the disease, superficial and linear ulcerations become apparent, commonly located at the site of the attachment of the teniae. The ulcerations may also become deeper and extend over a short or longer distance in the submucosa.
- Polypoid lesions may first occur during the acute phase of the disease and are then composed of the remaining areas of normal mucosa or of islands of regenerative mucosa, which are dispersed among the numerous ulcerations.
- During the chronic phase of the disease or in patients with quiescent disease, another type of pseudopolypoid structure caused by chronic inflammation of the mucosa leading to marked tissue proliferation is commonly observed. These inflammatory pseudopolyposis may have a sessile, front like appearance or may be pedunculated.
- If the ileocecal valve is widely open or incompetent, it is likely that the disease process has extended to the terminal ileum: "back-wash ileitis". The involved ileal segment will show granular mucosal changes similar to those seen in the colon and a decreased peristaltic activity.
- The radiological features observed during the chronic phase of the disease are characterized by the definitive loss of mucosal folds, resulting in a marked "flat" appearance of the mucosa, shortening due to fibrosis of the hepatic and splenic flexures, which becomes less prominent. Finally areas of marked lumen reduction and constriction may become evident. These stenosing lesions characteristically extend over several cms and may be reversible.

The CT Findings in UC Consist of:

- Mild to moderate colonic wall thickening and increased pericolonic lipomatous tissue, growth with abnormally elevated attenuation of fibrolipomatous tissue in the perirectal space.
- On CECT scans and using water as endoluminal contrast medium three different layers may be visible within the thickened colonic wall the thickened muscularis mucosa and lamina propria have a high attenuation, a middle ring with low attenuation corresponds to the submucosal fat and the outer layer again has a higher attenuation due to the thickened muscularis propria. Although the CT features visible in UC are quite striking, they are not considered to be specific. Thus CT should not be recommended for the routine management of patients with UC, as its findings do not contribute to the diagnosis or to the differential diagnosis of Crohn's disease of the large bowel.

CROHN'S DISEASE

It is named after Burrill Bernard Crohn's an American physician. This is a chronic inflammatory condition of the gastrointestinal tract from unknown origin.

Anatomic Distribution of Crohn's Disease

Major site of involvement	*Percentage*
Small bowel only	30
Small bowel and colon	50
Colon only	20

From a pathological point of view, however, CD is characterized by chronic inflammation extending through all the layers of the intestinal wall and involving the mesenteric as well as the regional lymph nodes. In rare instances other segments of the alimentary tract (stomach, duodenum and oesophagus) may be affected by CD but this usually occurs in association with involvement of the distal ileum. Early pathological features of CD include hyperemia and edema of the bowel mucosa and of the mesentery associated with enlarged inflammatory lymph nodes. Another early typical gross pathological lesion of CD is a small superficial aphthous mucosal ulceration, commonly located over Peyer's patches in the small intestine and over the lymphoid aggregate in the colon.

Later during the course of the disease, the ulcerations tend to enlarge and to coalesce. Typically long linear longitudinal ulcerations develop along the long axis of the bowel. These multiple ulcers associated with the intervening remaining islands of submucosal wall thickening produce the so called typical "cobblestone" pattern. Fissures develop from the base of the ulcers destroying the full thickness of the bowel wall but will not result in free perforations because a fibrinous reaction of the serosa induced adherence of other intestinal loops into which the fissure ends. However the circumscribed inflammatory process commonly results in abscess formation and fistulisation. Extraluminal fistulous tracts may interconnect small bowel loops or a small bowel loop with a segment of the colon. It is not uncommon that fistulas may develop with adjacent non-intestinal pelvic organs such as the vagina and the bladder or with the skin. The fibrosing process, which develops in longstanding CD, results in narrowing of the lumen of the bowel and a generalized loss of flexibility of the bowel. The stenosing segments may be very long and extend over several cm. The fibrosing process also involves the mesentery, which becomes considerably thickened and tends to retract resulting in fixed loops of bowel.

In the large bowel skip areas of apparently normal bowel separate severely involved segments. Whereas in UC the rectum is almost always involved however, in patients with CD of the rectum is frequently spared (Table 69.3). Inflammatory pseudopolys may develop in long standing disease.

Radiological Features

During the early stage of CD minimal mucosal changes characterized by:

- The presence of very small nodular defects due to the focal granulomatous inflammation on barium studies. This pattern is very similar to that observed in lymphoid hyperplasia.
- The aphthous ulcers of CD are revealed radio graphically, as small central collections of barium surrounded by a radiolucent halo. This sign has been named "bull's eye" or "target" lesion.
- Other findings during the early phase of CD include changes in the thickness and anatomical orientation of the valvulae conniventes caused by inflammatory mucosal and submucosal thickening as well as lumen narrowing due to contractions and edema.

During a More Advanced Stage of the Disease

- The ulcerations become larger and confluent but the main feature is the narrowing of the lumen due to fibrosis.

Table 69.3: Differences between CD and UC

Factor	Crohn's Disease	Ulcerative Colitis
Distribution	Affects small bowel and large bowel	Affects large bowel only
Endoscopy findings	Rectum frequently spared inflammation not continuous (presence of skin lesions) Bowel wall is thickened and has a 'cobblestone' appearance due to deep ulcers and swelling of the tissue	Rectum always affected Inflammation is uniform Bowel wall is thin with loss of vascular pattern (blood vessels not visible)
Radiology	Strictures are common Deep fissures and fistulae are common Asymmetrical inflammation	Occur less commonly Occur less commonly Symmetrical inflammation
Histology	Presence of granuloma are almost diagnostic Inflammation extends through the mucosa and muscle of the bowel. The increase in white cells tend to be lymphocytes	Inflammation usually confined to mucosa The increase in white cells tends to be polymorphs
Diet	Remission achieved with enteral feed followed by exclusion/elimination diet.	Unaffected by diet
Clinical appearance	Patients often thin and may be malnourished due to intestinal malabsorption of nutrients Diarrhoea–Only sometimes with blood Abdominal mass common	Weight loss usually related to the severity of active disease Bloody diarrhea Rarely occurs
Smoking	Strongly associated with smoking Predicts a worse course of disease Increases risk of surgery and further surgery	Associated with non-smokers of ex-smokers Appears to protect against disease
Genetic factors	Susceptibility genes on chromosomes 12, 7, 3 and 2. Chromosome 16 strongly associated with Crohn's	Shares similar susceptibility genes HLA factors (like those that determine blood groups) appear to be important in predicting disease extent and behavior.

- The "string sign" is most frequently visible in the terminal ileum. It is caused by incomplete filling of a bowel segment due to irritability and spasm associated with marked ulceration.
- Displacement of intestinal loops may be due to abscess formation or to mesenteric fatty tissue increase and induration.
- The discontinuity of the ulcerations as well as the asymmetric involvement of the walls of the bowel with intervening areas of normal mucosa – called "skip" area – are typical features of CD.
- Pseudopolypoid lesions composed of islands of remnant inflamed tissue or of hypertrophic inflammatory tissue proliferations may lead to the appearance of filling defects of varying size and configuration.
- Internal fistulas are well demonstrated by barium study.
- Rectal involvement in CD is characterized by patchy discontinuous mucosal changes by collar-button ulcers and by sinus tracts.

The radiological differential diagnosis between UC and CD of the colon or granulomatous colitis is difficult and frequently impossible, particularly in chronic long-standing disease. Granular mucosa, diffuse rectal disease, continuous inflammation and a normal terminal ileum are in favor of UC. Patchy rectal involvements with collar-button ulcers on a background of normal mucosa, discontinuous involvement associated with lesions of the terminal ileum are features favoring CD.

In the acute phase of Crohn's disease, viral gastroenteritis, appendicitis Yersinia enterocolitis and Salmonella gastroenteritis must be excluded. If the Crohn's disease presents as a chronic recurrent illness then culture of the stools and rectal mucosa for giardiasis amebiasis intestinal tuberculosis, nongranulomatous ulcerative jejunoilitis, fungal infections and pseudomembranous enterocolitis must be done. If the inflammatory state is limited to the colon or rectum, ulcerative colitis, ischemic colitis, diverticulitis, and occasionally cancer of the colon may simulate Crohn's disease.

CT and MRI Features

The main contribution of CT in the evaluation of patients with Crohn's disease is its ability to display the degree of bowel wall thickening and the extraluminal bowel changes in the mesentery and the retroperitoneum. In patients with granulomatous colitis, the colon wall tends to be thicker and more homogeneous than in patients with UC.

Furthermore, CT demonstrates mesenteric or retroperitoneal abscess more appropriately than barium studies and displays its exact anatomic location and extent. In the chronic phase of the disease one can note an important proliferation of fibro fatty tissue representing a reaction to the chronic inflammation of the mesenteric fat. The "comb" sign is based on the prominence dilatation and tortuosity of the vasa recta coursing through proliferative mesenteric fat. This condition may cause displacement of the bowel loops as visualized on the barium study and the CT findings will be most helpful for detecting the cause of the bowel displacement.

CT can in some instances visualize fistulous tracts but in general MRI because of its multiplanar capabilities is better suited to display optimally the exact topographical course and the extent of these fistulas particularly in the perirectal fossa and the perineum.

Diverticular Disease of Colon

- It is a common abnormality in the elderly present in 1/3rd of patients >60 years.
- 2/3rd of patients > 80 years.
- Only 10% of patients have symptoms and 1% require surgery.
- Diverticular disease has two components:
  1. Muscular abnormality is sigmoid colon.
  2. Diverticula.

Diverticulosis–refers simply to the presence of diverticula.

Diverticulitis–refers to inflammatory changes within the diverticula which results in a muscular abnormality.

Primary change is 200% increase in elastin deposition in taeniae coli but not in circular layer.

↓

Shortening and pleating of sigmoid with formation of folds of mucosa and muscle layers.

↓

Diverticula arise from apices in between muscle clefts.

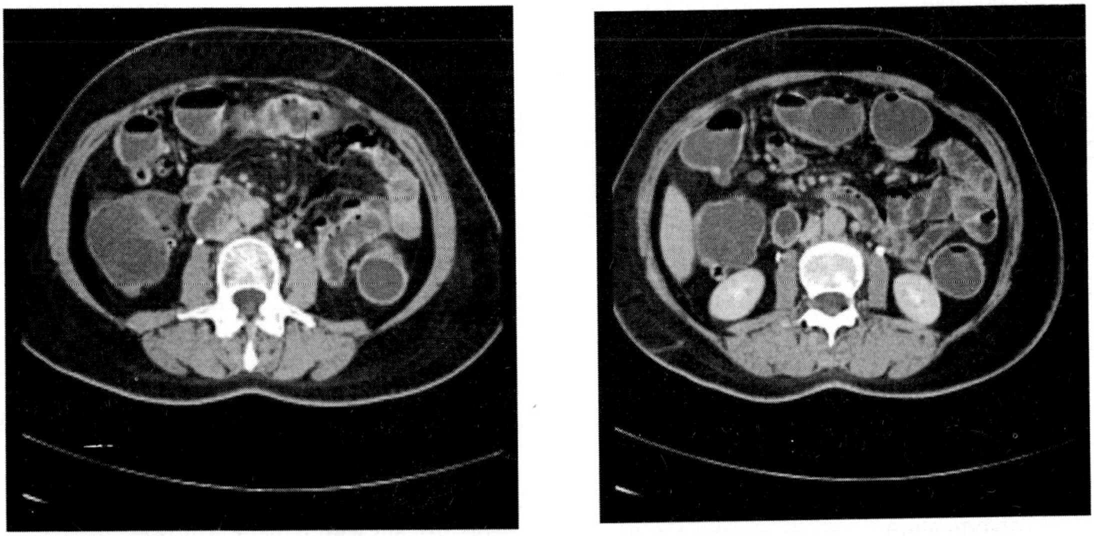

Fig. 70.1: Axial CT images show fluid and air filled diverticula arising from the right sided colon

Site: 80% in sigmoid (because it has high intra colonic pressure).

17% in entire colon.

4-12% isolated to calcium and ascending colon.

Diverticula

- Colonic diverticula are pulsion in type, secondary to high-pressure contractions during colonic segmentation.
- They are herniation of mucosa and submucosa through muscularis propria with wall layers of mucosa, submucosa and serosa.

Sites – Two types

1. Lateral diverticula – between mesenteric and antimesenteric – taeniae at points of weakness where branches of vasa recta penetrate muscle layer.
2. Intramural small diverticula on antimesenteric border.

RADIOLOGICAL INVESTIGATIONS ON BARIUM ENEMA

1. Muscle change
   a. Saw tooth sign: Concertina like or serrated appearance of affected area due to folds of mucosa and muscles.
   b. Persistent spasm during filling of barium, which is relieved by antispasmodics.
2. Diverticula: Appears as flask like or rounded outpouching from the bowel wall at apices between muscular clefts.

   En face

   a. Seen as ring shadows and sharp outer border fades centrally.
   b. Ba filled.
   c. Fluid level in crest or decubitus.
   d. Narrow neck seen as smaller eccentrically placed ring within larger circle of diverticulum.

Imaging in Diverticulitis and Its Complications

1. Plain X-ray Abdomen

a. Localised ileus.
b. Soft tissue mass due to collection.
c. Gas collection in abscess/fistula.
d. ± Pattern of small bowel obstruction.
e. Pneumoperitoneum (rare).

2. Barium Enema

a. Luminal contrast studies are unrewarding in the diagnosis of early diverticulitis.
b. Water soluble contrast enema may show tracking of contrast from a ruptured diverticulum to an abscess.
c. Focal area of eccentric luminal narrowing caused by pericolic/intramural inflammatory mass.
d. Marked thickening and distortion of mucosal folds.
e. Fistula to bladder, small bowel or vagina.

3. Ultrasound

a. Concentric, strikingly hypoechoic thickening of the bowel wall.
b. Inflamed diverticula seen as bright echogenic foci with ring down artefact or acoustic shadowing within or beyond the wall.
c. Inflammatory changes in pericolonic fat with a regionally - echogenicity with ± hypoechoic zones.
d. Abscess – seen as loculated collections.

4. CT-Scan

a. Circumferential bowel wall thickening >4 mm of homogenous density.
b. Presence of gas or contrast medium in the diverticula within the bowel wall.

c. Inflammation of pericolic fat seen as increase in attenuation, associated with fine stranding, small fluid collections and induration of sigmoid mesocolon.

d. Heterogenous pericolic collection of soft tissue density – phlegmon or abscess with air bubbles in a collection or an air fluid level.

e. Fistula may be seen or gas within the bladder associated with bladder wall thickening.

f. Pneumoperitoneum free fluid in peritoneal cavity.

g. Colonic or small bowel obstruction.

Differential Diagnosis

Colonic neoplasm.

Diverticulitis (Benign stricture)	Malignant stricture
Tapering ends	Irregular Shouldered ends
Long	Short
Intact mucosal pattern	Loss of mucosal folds with irregularity
Spikes of Ba filling the nodus of diverticula	Absentee of diverticulum

Ultrasound

1. Segmental concentric thickening of gut wall.
2. Diverticular may be seen as pockets of echogenic foci adjacent to gut wall with ring down artefact or acoustic shadowing.

CT Scan

1. Hypertrophic thickening of colonic circular muscle.
2. Diverticula are seen as intramural collections of air or contrast or as outpouching filled with air or contrast.

Complications of Diverticulosis

1. *Diverticulitis*

   Inflammatory changes in a diverticulum occur when inspissated faecal material abrades the mucosa.

   Common in sigmoid lesions, rare in caecal lesion to very rare in diverticular of transverse colon.

2. *Peri colic abscess*

   Inflamed diverticulum perforates at its apex and the abscess is discharged extramurally dissecting between the mesocolic fat and muscle or breakthrough the fat into the peritoneal cavity.

   Abscess are usually sealed off by omen turn and the sigmoid mesentery but may track to distant sites.

3. *Perforation*

   Free perforation with a considerable quantity of air intraperitoneally may be seen in elderly without much evidence of acute inflammation, severe generalised peritonitis may occur requiring urgent surgery.

4. *Fistula formation*

   Chronic inflammation creates adhesions, so that walled off collections cannot freely spread but result in formation of fistulous tract between adherent structures.

   Common colovesical fistula – pneumaturia or colovaginae.

5. *Obstruction*

   - Mild small bowel ileus due to inflammation.
   - Complete small bowel obstruction due to adherence of bowel to abscess with stricture formation.
   - Large bowel stricture may also occur.

6. *Hemorrhage*

   Bleeding from diverticula is profuse and

episodic. It is due to intimal thickening of the vasa recta over the apex of the diverticular with weakening of its wall and rupture.

7. *Giant cyst formation (pseudocyst)*

Large smooth walled air filled cavity with air fluid level in (L) iliac fossa may result due to expansion of a walled off sub serosal perforation.

CT might not be able to differentiate between diverticulitis and malignancy in 10% cases.

8. *Crohn's disease*

Small bowel commonly involved with skip lesions.

Ulcers, fistula formation abscess, fibrofatty proliferation within refractivity or attenuation of fat.

Colonic Duplication

The primitive foregut, midgut and hindgut develop during the fourth week in utero.

- The midgut lengthens, herniated out of the abdomen cavity and rotates 90° counter clockwise around the SMA during the 6th week in utero.
- By the 10th week, the midgut rotates an additional 180° as it returns to the abdominal cavity.
- The cecum descends to the right iliac fossa, where it becomes fixed*.

  (*The base of the small bowel mesentery, then runs from the ligament of Treitz in the left upper quadrant to the ileocecal valve in the right lower quadrant).
- Arterial supply.
- The cloacae is located at the distal end of the hindgut and at the end of the 6th week anorectal septum develops into a ventral urogenital sinus and a dorsal rectum.
- The anal membrane covering the cloacae ruptures at the end of the 8th week, forming the anal canal.

Duplication is rare congenital anomalies.

Causes

1. Failure of bowel to recanalize in utero.
2. Caudal twinning.
3. Incomplete separation of the notochord from the endoderm.

- The resultant structure may be tubular, communicating with the intestinal lumen, or more commonly closed cystic duplication.
- These cysts are lined by GI mucosa and contain a layer of smooth muscle within their wall.
- Duplication are usually found on the mesenteric side of the intestine.
- They frequently share a common wall and blood supply with the involved bowel.
- All regions of the gastrointestinal tract may be involved, however oesophagus and ileum are the most common site.
- Rectal duplication – are very rare.

Symptoms Vary From

- External fistula in perineum to fistulation in genitourinary tract – Most common form.
- Urinary retention and intestinal obstruction due to anorectal agenesis.
- Compression by a pelvic mass (of cystic duplication of rectum).
- Internal prolapse through the introitus.
- Most common form – mainly seen in tubular form of rectal duplication.

Association

- Often occur in association with other congenital abnormalities such as with large bowel duplication, exomphalos, meningocele, spinal, ureteral and urinary tract duplication.

Imaging

- Plain X-ray in case of obstruction – air fluid level and dilated bowel loops.
- USG – In cystic variety – an anechoic mass in the pelvis.
- Ba enema – show an extraluminal mass effect.
- Localized duplications occasionally communicated with the lumen and can fill with air on contrast material.
- CT / MRI but modality to show the duplication (Figure 71.1).
- Treatment – Resection is indicated for rectal duplication because of risk of neoplasia (adeno carcinoma).
- Surgical approach is dependent on the type of duplication. Post perineal and post sagittal approach seems to be the most common adopted route for excision of encysted form of rectal duplication.

Other approaches like transcoccygeal and abdomino-perineal procedures have also been adopted for the management.

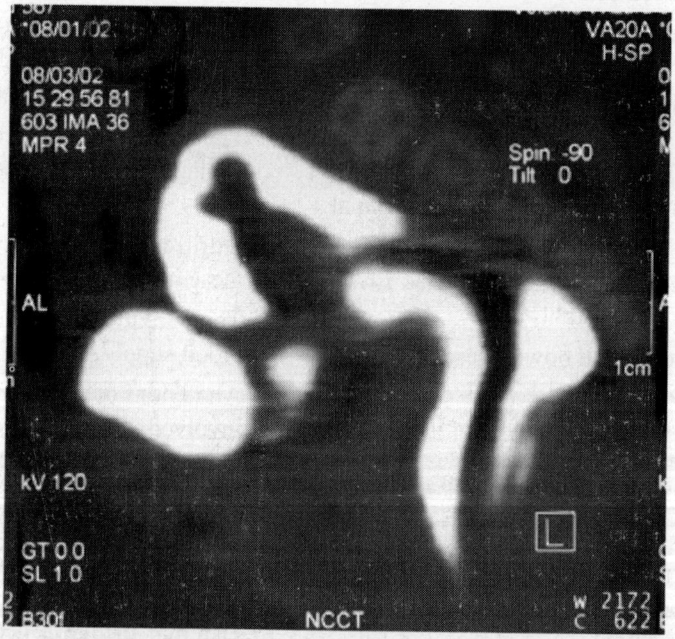

Fig. 71.1: Sagittal MPR CT image shows duplication of the rectum

Colonic Narrowing

CAUSES

1. Chronic Stage of Any Colitis

- *Inflammatory:* Ulcerative Colitis, Crohn's Colitis, Non-specific Benign Ulcer.
- *Infectious:* Amebiasis, Schistosomiasis, Bacillary Dysentery, TB, Fungal Disease, LGV, HZ, CMV, Strongyloides.
- Ischemic.
- **Traumatic: Radiation Injury, Caustic Colitis.**

2. Malignant Lesion

- *Primary*: Carcinoma, Lymphoma.
- *Metastatic*: From Prostate, Cervix, Uterus, Kidney, Stomach, Pancreas, Primary Intraperitoneal Sarcoma.

Colorectal Cancer

It accounts for two-thirds of all gastrointestinal malignant tumors. The large majority of colorectal carcinomas are adenocarcinomas. Its increasing frequency in the Western world and its rare occurrence in underdeveloped countries suggest etiological dietary factors such as fibre deficiency, increased fat intake and increased consumption of beef. The most common appearance of colon carcinoma is either polypoid or annular. Polypoid carcinomas are preferentially located in the caecum, the ascending colon and the rectum whereas annular and ulcerating lesions are more frequently seen in the transverse, descending and sigmoid colon. Most colon carcinomas are slow growing.

Radiological Diagnosis

On *plain films* of the abdomen, one may notice very rarely fine stippled calcifications either in the tumor itself or in liver and lymph node metastasis.

On *barium contrast studies* polypoid carcinomas are visible as a lobulated filling defect of variable size with a contour deformity along one margin of the bowel. On double contrast study, however, even large tumors may not be associated with a contour deformity because of marked adjacent lumen distension. Annular tumors show deformation of both margins with lumen narrowing. There is an abrupt transition between the tumor, where the mucosa is no longer visible and the normal aspect of the adjacent mucosa. This leads to a typical appearance of an "apple core" or an overhanging edge called the "tumor shoulder".

In case of obstruction due to intussusception, a not uncommon complication, one may observe the typical coiled-spring feature. In other patients with obstruction radiographic, features of colitis, characterized by narrowing and mucosal changes, is seen in the colon segment proximal to the obstructing lesion. CT will best display abscess formation secondary to perforation. Double contrast examination of the colon has a high sensitivity for detecting colorectal carcinoma if appropriate preparation of the colon is achieved. Transabdominal ultrasound, which is applied frequently as the initial study for examining patients with abdominal complaints, is able to visualize colorectal carcinoma in about 25% of cases as hypoechoic masses or wall thickening.

Similarly *CT* is able to display colon wall thickening as suggestive for colorectal carcinoma on routine abdominal scans but this method is mainly useful for staging of colorectal carcinoma. Recently, three-dimensional (3-D) visualization of the colon, also called virtual coloscopy, based on spiral CT or on MRI data, has become available. With this technique it is possible to identify changes of the colon mucosa and tumors originating from the mucosa.

Staging

The staging of colorectal carcinoma can be performed by endoluminal ultrasound (EUS), CT and MRI.

EUS is able to depict the degree of disruption of the muscular layers of the colon wall. Accuracy of EUS for T staging has been reported as around 80% and for N staging as ranging between 62% and 83%.

CT staging is based on an analysis of the thickness of the colon wall and the presence or the absence of tumor spread to adjacent or distant organs. CT has a low accuracy rate between 41% and 68%, which is largely due to its low sensitivity for detecting invasion of the different layers of the colon wall and lymph node metastasis.

MRI has the same limitations as CT for staging rectal tumors, although imaging in the coronal plane can be beneficial for evaluation of involvement of the musculus levator ani. Early experience with endorectal MRI suggests that this method may reach the same accuracy for staging of rectal adenocarcinoma as that achieved by EUS. Patients who have undergone resection of colon carcinoma with reanastomosis will show the same CT and MRI features for recurrent tumor as those of the primary tumor. In case of complete abdomino-perineal resection CT and MRI are the only modalities available for evaluating recurrent tumor. As neither CT nor MRI can reliably differentiate between recurrence and fibrosis or inflammation, it is advised to perform a baseline CT or MRI study 3-4 months after surgery with repeat examinations at regular intervals thereafter.

A criterion for CT staging of primary colorectal tumors is as follows:

- Stage I – Intraluminal mass without thickening of wall.
- Stage II – Thickened wall (> 0.6 cm) or pelvic mass, no invasion or extension to side walls.
- Stage IIIa – Thickened wall or pelvic mass with invasion of adjacent structures but not to pelvic side walls or abdominal wall.
- Stage IIIb – Thickened wall or pelvic mass with extension to pelvic side walls and / or abdominal wall without distant metastases.
- Stage IV – Distant metastases with or without local abnormality.

The above-mentioned criterion of CT staging correlates very well with the following surgico-pathologic staging system. A criterion of surgico-pathologic staging is as follows:

- Stage A – Limited to mucosa.
- Stage B1 – Extension into, but not through, the muscularis propria.
- Stage B2 – Extension through muscularis, no nodes.
- Stage C1 – Limited to bowel wall, positive nodes.
- Stage C2 – Extension through bowel wall, positive nodes.
- Stage D – Distant metastases.

[NOTE: This staging system represents the Astler-Coller version of the Duke's classification, as modified by Turnbull].

6

Section

CROHN'S DISEASE

CT and MRI Features

The main contribution of CT in the evaluation of patients with Crohn's disease is its ability to display the degree of bowel wall thickening and the extraluminal bowel changes in the mesentery and the retroperitoneum.

In patients with granulomatous colitis the colon wall tends to be thicker and more homogeneous than in patients with ulcerative colitis. Furthermore, CT demonstrates mesenteric or retroperitoneal abscess more appropriately than barium studies and displays its exact anatomic location and extent. In the chronic phase of the disease. One can note an important proliferation of fibro fatty tissue representing a reaction to the chronic inflammation of the mesenteric fat. The "comb" sign is based on the prominence, dilatation and tortuosity of the vasa recta coursing through proliferative mesenteric fat. This condition may cause displacement of the bowel loops as visualized on the barium study and the CT findings will be most helpful for detecting the cause of the bowel displacement. When the degree of liquefaction in an abscess is still limited minimal or no difference in attenuation value between an inflammatory phlegmonous, mass and an abscess will be noted and both conditions cannot be distinguished.

CT can in some instances visualize fistulous tracts but in general MRI, because of its multiplanar capabilities, is better suited to display optimally the exact topographical course and the extent of these fistulas, particularly in the perirectal fossa and the perineum.

Ulcerative Colitis

It is an inflammatory bowel disease of unknown cause affecting the colon.

Plain film findings are minimal unless toxic megacolon occurs. Bowel with active disease is collapsed and has minimal faecal content. A double contrast. Enema shows fine mucosal ulceration, evenly distributed circumferentially, with progressive disease, which starts at the rectum and extends proximally. While there is some overlap in the radiographic features of Crohn's disease and ulcerative colitis on barium enema, the typical finding in ulcerative colitis is that of mucosal granularity while in Crohn's, aphthous and fissure ulcers dominate, stricture formation occurs with both. Skip lesions, pseudodiverticula and fistula formation are features of Crohn's disease. A widened post-rectal space and reflux ileitis are seen in ulcerative colitis. With long standing disease the haustral pattern is lost and the colon becomes shortened and featureless. Complications include perforation and peritonitis. Backwash ileitis – involvement of the terminal ileum may occur in severe cases if there is an incompetent ileocaecal valve.

Infectious Colitis

Inflammation of the colon caused by various infectious agents. The diagnosis of infectious colitis is usually based on history, sigmoidoscopy and finally on examination of the stool for ova, parasites and bacteria. Barium study of the colon is not performed in most instances because clinically most cases will respond to medical therapy and the illness is of brief duration. In patients with persisting symptoms or unclear clinical and /or laboratory findings radiological examination may contribute to the diagnosis. However, the barium study findings are usually non-specific and may be similar to those seen in patients with either ulcerative colitis or Crohn's disease.

Ischemic Colitis

It is most commonly seen in patients subject to nonocclusive ischaemia, that is, patients with generalized atherosclerosis, hypovolaemia, hypotension and renal insufficiency. Ischaemic colitis has also been reported to occur in patients with vasculitis, obstructing colon carcinoma and with the use of vasoconstriction drugs.

Any segment of the colon may be affected, but the splenic flexure and rectosigmoid junction are most susceptible to injury. The left colon is more frequently involved, implicating that ischaemic colitis is most often a result of impaired perfusion in areas supplied by the inferior mesenteric artery.

Plain radiographs are often normal, or may show a picture of non-specific ileus and/or signs of submucosal bleeding and/or oedema. An early barium enema has wall oedema (thumb printing) as the most prominent finding. Ulcerations may also be present during the first 13 weeks after the onset of disease. Postischaemic strictures are easily visualized with barium enema. These strictures are usually smooth and tapered and sacculations may occur. CT often demonstrates localized thickening of the bowel wall and in cases with infarction, air in the wall.

Lymphoma

It appears most commonly in the caecal and rectosigmoid region. The tumor mass is often large, single, circumscribed and polypoid in the caecum. When the rectum is involved it is usually narrowed by a perirectal mass. Diffuse colonic lymphomatous polyposis may simulate benign nodular lymphoid hyperplasia or diffuse adenomatous polyposis and involves either long bowel segments or the entire colon. These lesions are often umbilicated due to aphthous ulcerations.

On barium examination primary colonic lymphomas usually appear as large ulcerated lesions or diffuse submucosal nodularity with or without aphthous ulceration.

Chapter 73

Colorectal Tumors

BENIGN TUMORS

1. Adenoma

- Most common benign neoplasm of colon.
- Incidence increased with age.
- Usually small (<1cm) larger in left colon.
- <1% of adenoma <1cm are malignant whereas >20% of adenoma >2 cm are malignant.

2. Lipoma and Teratoma

- Arise from submucosa.
- Complications – Intussusceptions.
- Ulceration of mucosa – hemorrhage.
- 70% of lesions are in right colon especially cecum.
- CT fatty attenuation (-60 to- 120 HU).

  Intusscepted lipoma – focal/diffuse soft tissue attenuation.

  D/D infarction or fat necrosis.

Diagnosis of teratoma is considered when a fatty mass contains soft tissue components and calcification.

D/D of lipoma – fatty infiltration of ileocaecal valve.

3. Hemangioma

- Affects young adults.
- Most common site – rectosigmoid.
- Most common clinical features – chronic rectal bleeding.
- There is an extensive network of vascular structures originating from submucosa with subsequent infiltration transmurally and in surrounding soft tissue.

  CT – Transmural thickening of involved segments.
  - Intramural and extrarectal phleboliths.
  - Vascular engorgement in the mesentery.

4. Cystic Lymphangioma

- Rare submucosal lesion.
- CT – Discrete well defined multilocular cystic mass with attenuation – 2 to 10 HU.
- D/D colitis cystica profounda.

MALIGNANT TUMORS

1. Colorectal Carcinoma (Figures 73.1, 73.2, 73.3 and 73.4)

- Age incidence > 55 years.

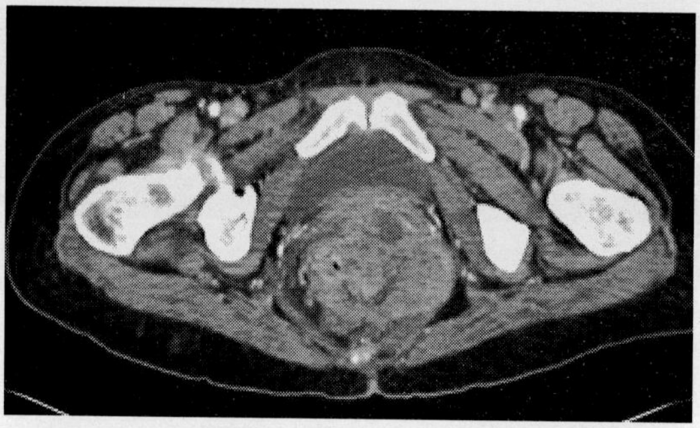

Fig. 73.1: Axial CT image shows a large rectal mass with perirectal invasion

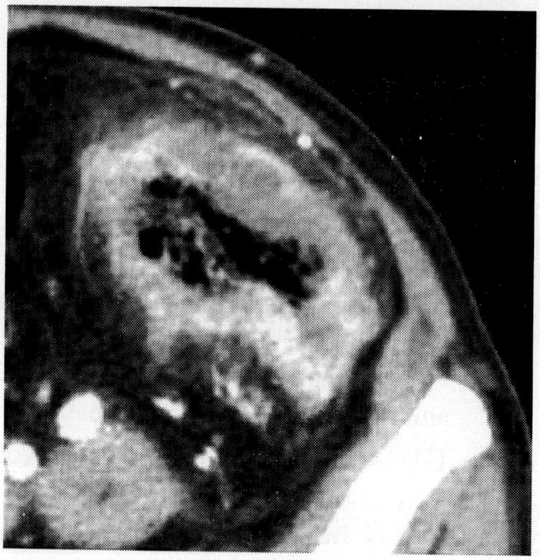

Fig. 73.2: Axial CT image shows mass in the left side colon with pericolonic invasion

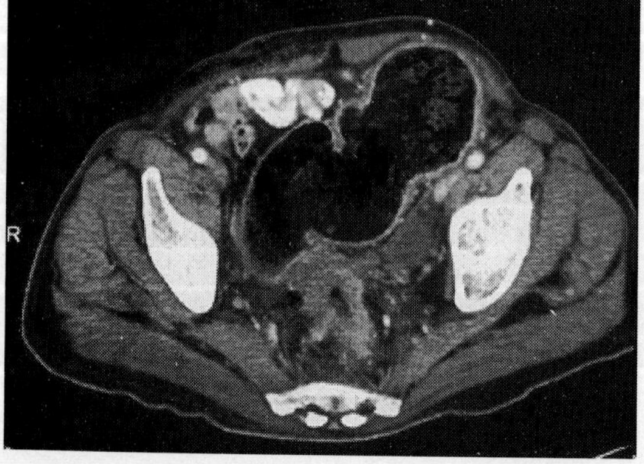

Fig. 73.3: Axial CT image shows a rectosigmoid

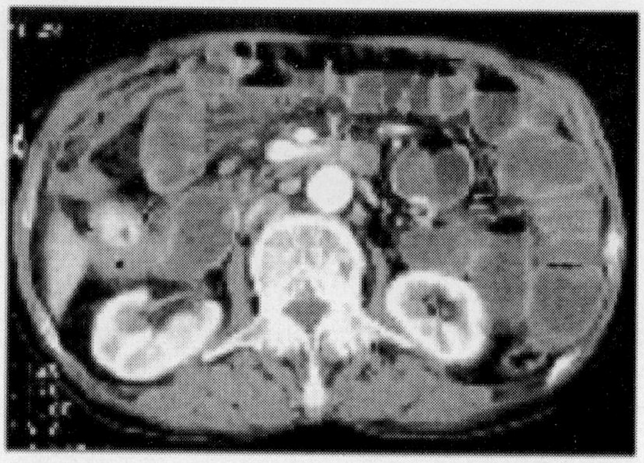

Fig. 73.4: Contrast-enhanced CT scan reveals colonic obstruction, with a well-enhanced concentric mass lesion visible in the hepatic flexure of the colon (arrows)

- Site 60% in rectosigmoid.
- Site 30% proximal to splenic flexure.
- Site 10% descending colon.
- Normal thickness of colorectal wall – 3 mm (when colon is distended with fluid).
  4-6 mm – suggests pathology.
  > 6 mm – definitely abnormal.

If pneumocolon is performed.

- Normal colon wall thickness = 2 mm.
- Normal rectal wall thickness = 3 mm.

DUKE'S CLASSIFICATION OF COLORECTAL CANCER

Stage	Description	% of operation	5 years % survival
A	Spread by direct continuity into submucosa or muscle only, No L.N. involvement	15	95
B	Spread beyond muscle layer into perirectal/ pericolic tissue. No L.N. involvement	35	70
C	Regional L.N. involved	50	30

Mucinous Adenocarcinoma

- As compared to non-mucinous tumors, these tumors have higher pathological stage at the time of diagnosis, greater tendency for mets and local recurrences. Unfavourable prognosis.
- CT – Low attenuation mass with intratumoral calcification.
- MR – Signal intensity is higher due to pressure of extracellular mucin.
- Peripheral or heterogeneous lace like enhancement pattern in characteristic.

Primary Signet Ring Cell Carcinoma

- Rare (0.1% to 2.4% of all CRC).
- Affects younger patients.
- Minimal mucosal alteration but permeates wall extensively causing narrowing so also known as linitis plastica type of carcinoma.
- Tends to spread to pelvic lymph nodes, ovaries and peritoneal surface with low incidence of hepatic metastases.
- CT shows
  - Long segment of concentric bowel wall thickening.
  - When rectum is involved extension to anal verge is common.
  - Target appearance may be seen with moderately enhancing inner wall due to fibrous tissue secondary to desmoplastic response.
- D/D includes metastatic linitis plastica (stomach, breast, gallbladder urinary bladder, prostate, lymphoma, inflammatory bowel disease, endometriosis and actinomycosis).

TNM CLASSIFICATION FOR COLORECTAL CANCER

T1 Tumor penetration to submucosa.

T2 Tumor penetration to mesenteric propria.

T3 Tumor penetration to perirectal fat/serosa.

T4 Tumor penetration to adjacent structures.

No –No Node.

N1 –1-3 peri rectal.

N2 >4 nodes.

N3 –Apical node or one along named vascular mark.

M0–No mets.

M1– Metastases present.

Early Carcinoma (T1)

- May present as a malignant polyp.
- Irregular lobulated surface and smooth in drawing of base, do not suggest malignancy.
- Irregularity of base – malignancy.
- Flat adenomas are more likely to have submucosal invasion.

Advanced Carcinoma

- May present as ulcerating or polypoid mass – broad irregular base.
- Circumferential growth – annular lesion with shouldered ends and irregular margins.
- Flat plaque like infiltration lesion – create abnormal mucosal lines (deformed/double line).
- Synchronous carcinoma is seen in 5% of patient and polyps in 23.4% patients.
- In lower rectum and anus, internal hemorrhoids should be distinguished from polypoid malignancy.

Tumor Spread

Extension of tumor beyond bowel wall. Mass with irregular outer border with soft tissue stranding in soft tissues. Stranding can also result from fibrosis – inflammation and congestive changes.

So criteria for confirming diagnosis on CT – tumor mass extending directly into adjacent muscles, obliterating the fat planes and enlarging the individual muscle or enveloping the neighbouring structures.

NODAL SPREAD

Left sided colonic and rectal tumors – mesocolic, left colic, inferior mesenteric L.N.

Right sided colonic tumors – L.N. at root of SMS – para-aortic and aortocaval L.N.

Hepatic flexure and proximal transverse colon – paracolic, gastro colic L.N.

Splenic flexure and distal transverse colon – middle colic L.N.

Low rectal and anal tumors – inguinal L.N.

* Any L.N. in perirectal fat should be considered malignant regardless of size.

DISTANT METASTASES

- Most common site – hepatic metastases.
- CT – Low attenuation lesion. Punctate or amorphous calcification is present if metastases are from mucinous adenocarcinoma.
- On dynamic helical CT scanning: Early phase – peripheral contrast enhancement; portovenous phase – lesion itself enhances with heterogeneous or target pattern; gradually lesion fills in with time becoming isoattenuating to liver.
- Liver resection for hepatic metastases is considered if CT shows.
- Metastases in only one lobe of liver not >4 in number.
- No other lesion present in normal appearing lobe.
- Lobe without lesion has normal function.
- No focal adenopathy is identified.
- No other distant mets is present.
- CTAP is a sensitive technique for detection of metastases.

COMPLICATIONS OF COLORECTAL CARCINOMA

1. Obstruction.
2. Perforation – Commonly due to bowel preparation, poor prognosis.
3. Pericolic abscess follows perforation, simulates diverticulitis.
4. Fistula formation – to small bowel, bladder, vagina.
5. Ischemic colitis – Develop in 1-7% patients.
   - Ba examination – Thumb printing with spasm or diffuse ulceration in colon proximal to carcinoma.
   - In contrast to irregular thickening in tumoral segment, ischemic colitis shows smooth regular thickening. Mean thickness 1 cm (tumoral 2cm).
   - Target sign with low attenuating central area is specific.
6. Intussusception.

Tumor Recurrence

Local recurrence is found in 50% patients during first 12 months and in 80% patients within 24 months. Features indicating tumor recurrence are:

- Invasion of surrounding structures (muscle, bladder).
- Enlarged local L.N.
- Soft tissue, mass increasing in size on follow up scans – commonly occur in pressured space and area of surgical bed.
- Pressure of ischiorectal fossa invasion.

GI Stromal Tumors

- Rare in large bowel. Rectum is a committee site than colon.
- Growth pattern:
  - Endocolic.

- Exocolic.
- Dumb-bell.

- CT – necrosis and cystic changes are more common with internal dystrophic calcification.
- Usually obstruction is absent or minimal despite large tumor.
- D/D of anterior rectal tumor – prostatic and gynaecological malignancies.
- D/D of retrorectal tumor – lymphoma, unusual sarcoma.

LYMPHOMA

- Most common site – caecum and rectum.

Four Forms

- Infiltrative – Long segment of concentric luminal narrowly.
- Polypoid – Difficult to distinguish from adeno-carcinoma lymphoma is greater possibility when:
  - Tumor extends to terminal ileum and shows deep fissuring and cavitation.
  - Associated diffuse mesenteric adenopathy.
  - Splenomegaly.
  - No evidence of invasion/obstruction of neighbouring viscera.
- Cavitary – Large tumor may excavate into mesentery producing a giant cavitated mass.
- Diffuse – Multiple nodules of small size: CT may not detect these but helps in staging.

TUMORS SECONDARILY INVOLVING COLORECTUM BY DISSEMINATION

1. Direct invasion from contiguous primary.

   Ovarian carcinoma – involves inferior border of sigmoid colon.

   Prostatic carcinoma – Anterior wall or circumferential involvement of proximal rectum.

   Renal carcinoma – right or left colon.

2. Direct invasion from non-contiguous primary.

   Gastric carcinoma – gastro colic ligament → inferior border of tracer colon.

   Pancreatic carcinoma – transverse mesocolon – sup. border of transverse colon.

3. Intraperitoneal seedling occurs in ovarian, gastric, pancreatic and colonic carcinoma. Tumor implantation in pelvis occurs.
   - Especially, anterior wall of rectum.
   - Small bowel loops in right iliac fossa.
   - Superior border of colon.
   - Right paracolic gutter.
   - Omental cakes of tumor especially at omental attachments with transverse colon.

4. Hematogenous spread – submucosal masses on antimesentric border of colon.

   These masses have smooth surface, polypoidal shape. Umbilicated metastases occur in carcinoma breast, lung, melanoma and lymphoma.

Application of Interventional Radiology in Malignant Colorectal Strictures

Metallic stenting for acute large bowel obstruction due to malignant strictures has impressive result as:

- It often avoids need for emergency surgery in elderly patient who are dehydrated and debilitated by metabolic disturbance produced by bowel obstruction and avoids need for two-stage surgery.
- If surgically incurable malignant stricture.
- Stenting provides non-surgical effective palliation without inconvenience of a colposcopy.
- Technical and clinical success rates of colorectal stenting are 78-100%.
- Specific colorectal stents are:
  - Schneider enteral stent.
  - Ultra flex stent.

Bowel Perforation

It is defined as full thickness disruption of the intestinal wall and with spillage of bowel contents into the peritoneal cavity with resultant peritonitis.

Upper bowel perforation → free when bowel contents spill freely into the abdominal cavity.

↓

Contained when a full thickness hole is created by an ulcer but free spillage is prevented because contiguous organs wall of the area e.g. duodenal ulcer penetrating into the pancreas. Large bowel perforation usually results in free intraperitoneal contamination.

Etiology

1. **Penetrating or Blunt Abdominal Trauma** In case of penetrating trauma the small bowel is the most commonly injured viscous because it is loaded and occupies most of the area of the peritoneal cavity. In addition it is highly mobile.
2. **Ingestion of NSAIDS, Aspirin and Steroids**.
3. **Presence of Predisposing Condition** – E.g. peptic ulcer disease – most common cause of duodenal perforation. Other predisposing conditions are acute appendicitis, diverticulitis and inflamed Meckel's diverticulum.
4. **Bacterial Infections** – E.g. typhoid fever may complicate by perforation in 5% cases.
5. Bowel injuries associated with endoscopy and laparoscopy.
6. Inflammatory bowel disease.
7. Perforation secondary to ischemia of ischemic colitis.
8. Intestinal malignancy.
9. Ingestion of caustic substances.
10. Foreign bodies.

Pathophysiology

Presence of bacteria in peritoneal cavity.

↓

Inflammatory response with localization of site by omentum or viscera.

↓

Phlegmon formation.

↓

Osmotic effects with shift of more fluids.

↓

Abscess formation.

↓

If untreated, bacteraemia, shock and multi organ failure ensues.

Clinical Signs and Symptoms

1. Severe abdominal pain and tenderness.

2. Vomiting.
3. Abdominal guarding.
4. Absent bowel sounds in generalised peritonitis.

Imaging Studies

Plain X-ray: Erect radiographs of the chest are recognized as the most appropriate first line investigation in bowel perforation for demonstration of free-air in peritoneal cavity.

A. Plain X-ray Findings in Pneumoperitoneum

1. *Erect Chest X-ray*

   Supine abdominal radiograph.

   Left lateral decubitus X-ray with horizontal beam, if patient cannot sit up.

   As the little at 1 ml free air can be seen.

   Patients should remain in position for 5-10 min before X-ray is taken:

   a. Erect X-ray shows free air under domes of diaphragm.
   b. Left lateral decubitus demonstrates gas between liver and abdominal wall.
   c. Supine radiograph may show collection of gas in right upper quadrant adjacent to liver in sub-hepatic space and Morrison's pouch.

- *Football sign*

  Large collection of intraperitoneal air seen as central radiolucency outlining the entire abdominal cavity along with visible falciform ligament surrounded by air.
- *Cupola sign*

  Gas entrapped under central tendon of diaphragm.
- *Rigler's sign*

  Visualisation of inner and outer walls of bowel loops caused by gas outside the bowel loop and normal intraluminal gas. Free air approx 1000 ml is required to elicit this sign.
- Free air may outline the ureters, lateral umbilical ligaments.
- Scrotal air may be seen in children.
- Gas within ligamentum teres seen as vertical slit about 2-4 cm right of spine between 11th and 12th ribs.

2. *Air Fluid Levels*

   Indicate the presence of hydropneumoperitoneium or pyopneumoperitoneum on erect X-rays.

B. Oral Contrast Studies

Not infrequently patients with acute abdomen and suspected perforation have no free gas on plain X-ray in which case oral contrast might prove whether or not bowel perforation is positive.

50 ml of water-soluble contrast in right lateral decubitus position.

C. Ultrasound

1. Intraperitoneal free fluid collection – internal echoes may be present due to faecal contamination.
2. Free air may be demonstrated
   - Total sound reflection at the soft tissue air interface.
   - High amplitude linear echoes with distal artificial reverberation echoes may be positive.
   - Gas foci may be seen in localized fluid collections.

     Site of bowel perforation may be detected by location of fluid and gas collection.
3. Bowel wall thickening, hypo peristalsis.

CT Scan is a valuable investigative tool providing differential morphologic information not obtainable with plain radiography or U/S. It is the standard criteria in assessment of pneumoperitoneum and can identify even small amount of gas present extraluminally.

- CT scans (Figure 74.1) may provide evidence of localised perforation e.g. perforated duodenal ulcer with leakage in area of gall-bladder and right flank.

- CT scans may show inflammatory changes in pericolonic soft tissues and focal abscess due to diverticulitis.

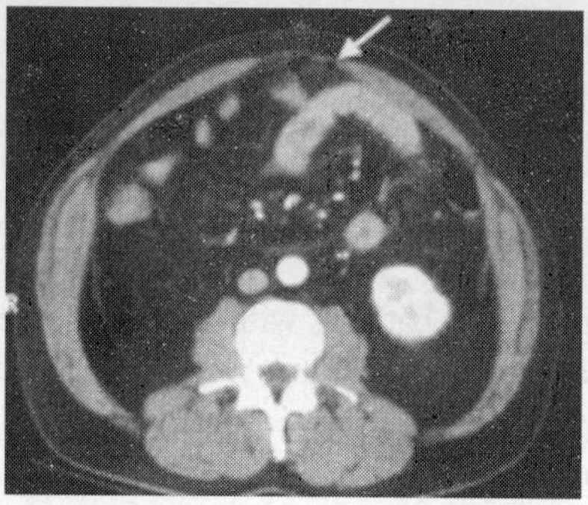

Fig. 74.1: CT Scan of abdomen shows free intraperitoneal air (*arrow*), suggesting intestinal perforation

- Cause of perforation may be diagnosed by CT scans.
- Extraluminal oral contrast material – given prior to CT exam is 100% specific for bowel perforation.
  - Bowel wall thickening may be positive which might show enhancement.
  - Mesenteric stranding can be associated with bowel perforation.

Limitation of Imaging Techniques

1. Free air may be missed on plain radiography because of inadequate technique.
2. Oral contrast material might not leak, if the perforation is too small or has sealed.

   It is sometimes difficult to opacify bowel in sick uncooperative patients.

   Oral contrast may obscure information such as appendicolith, and bowel hemorrhage.
3. Ultrasound is operator dependent and has limitations in obese and in those with large amount of intrabdominal gas.

Imaging in Acute Abdomen

- Patients with acute abdomen comprises the largest group of people presenting as surgical emergency.
- Following the history and the physical examination, the plain film radiographs have traditionally been on the first and most useful method of further investigation.

PLAIN ABDOMINAL RADIOGRAPHS

- In most of the acute abdominal conditions, the radiological diagnosis depends upon the gas pattern i.e. the distribution of gas in the dilated and non-dilated bowel and the presence of gas inside or outside the bowel lumen.
- In many cases a specific diagnosis can be made, however, not infrequently the appearance are nonspecific or even misleading and further investigation like USG, CT scan or radionucleide scan may be required.
- When the radiological diagnosis is specific or supports the clinical findings, surgery is often indicated without further investigation. However if there are clinical signs to indicate that, surgery should be performed, –ve or equivocal radiology should be ignored.
- It is often of value to view the radiographs initially in the absence of any clinical information. An objective evaluation of radiological signs can then be must and a full differential diagnosis considered without being based by clinical findings.
- However, to give a final opinion, full clinical history should be taken so that minor abnormalities are not overlooked.

Radiographic Techniques

- A supine abdomen and an erect CXR can be regarded as the basic standard radiographs.
- A horizontal ray abdominal radiograph either erects or left lateral decubitus is frequently taken to add more information and to demonstrate fluid levels.
- Patient should be in position for 10 min prior to the horizontal ray radiograph to allow free gas to rise to the highest point.
- The bladder should be emptied before supine radiograph is taken and the film should include the area from diaphragm to the hernial orifices.

CXR

- An essential radiograph in patients with acute abdomen because:
  - Best for showing small pneumoperitoneum. It is superior to the abdominal film as the X-rays penetrate almost

tangentially the top of the diaphragm (whereas in abd. film, the X -ray penetrates obliquely).

- A number of chest conditions presents with acute abdominal pain and mimic acute abdomen. These can be seen in CXR:
  - Pneumonia, particularly lower lobe.
  - MI.
  - Pulm. infarction.
  - CHF.
  - Pericarditis.
  - Pneumothorax.
  - Pleurisy.
  - Chest conditions e.g. pleural effusions in acute pancreatitis; aspiration pneumonia in patients with prolonged vomiting in internal obstruction may complicate acute abdominal condition.

Abdominal Radiograph

- A supine abdominal radiograph is probably the single most useful film.
- It allows visualizing distribution of gas, calibre of bowel, displacement of bowel, obliteration of fat lines etc.
- An exact abdominal radiograph is taken to both for fluid levels. However, the fluid levels do not contribute to diagnose of acute abdomen, as it usually does not distinguish between two most common causes of fluid levels like obstruction and paralytic illeus.
- However, 3 or more small bowel fluid level longer than 2.5 cm an abnormal and indicates dilated small bowel.
- (L) lateral decubitus abdominal radiograph is taken in patients who are unfit to stand erect.
- It is the projection of choice to see small pneumoperitoneum.
- In perforated antral/duodenal ulcer, air leaves in left lateral position instead of fluid. Also, air from perforated post gastric ulcer also remains in abdominal cavity instead of entry the lesser sac and hence detected easily. Gas altered dilated duodenal loop, which is the most common sign of pancreatitis, is best seen in the left lateral decubition projection.

PNEUMOPERITONEUM

- Detection of pneumoperitoneum in patients presenting with acute abdominal pain is important as in 90% of the cases, emergency surgery is required.
- With careful radiographic techniques, as little as 1 ml of free gas on chest Cx or (L) lateral decubitus can be detected with patient in position for at least 10 minutes before the film is taken.
- However, in cases in which erect/lateral decubitus film can't be taken, supine film is taken in which there are certain signs of pneumoperitoneum.
- 56% of patient with pneumoperitoneum have free gas detectable on supine radiograph.
- The signs are as follows:
  - An oval or linear collection of gas in the subhepatic space or hepatorenal fossa (Monson's pouch) (approx 50% of cases).
  - Gas on both sides of the wall of the bowel loop (Rigler's sign).

    (False +ves are seen when gas distended bowel loops are in contact, in which inner walls of the two loops are seen.
  - Small collection of gas between the bowel loops may sometimes be seen.
  - Visualization of falciform ligament, medial and lateral umbilical ligament when large amount of gas is present.
  - Large amount of gas accumulate beneath the diaphragm (Cupola sign).
  - Large amount of gas in the centre of the abdomen even the fluid collection (Football sign).

CT Scan

- It is the most sensitive method for detection of free peritoneal gas, which even the tiny bubbles of gas being visible.
- This requires reviewed images or wide window settings.
- No. of conditions are those, which stimulate free air, the punctured cavity on plain film (pseudo penumoperitoneum).

  There are:
  - *Chilaiditi syndrome*

    Distended bowel, usually hepatic plexure of colon between liver and diaphragm. This can be differentiated by visualization of the haustra/bowel wall.
  - *Subdiaphragmatic fat*

    Due to its constant position in lat decubitus views.
  - Other is:
    - Curvilinear film collapse.
    - Uneven diaphragm.
    - Distended viscus.
    - Omental fat.
    - Subprenic abscess.
    - Extramural gas in pneumatosis intestinals.
    - Apposition of distal gas filled loops.

Postoperative Puerperitoneum

- Seen in 60% of post laparotomy patients, however this is absorbed in few days.
- Any increase in volume of gas post operatively indicates anastomotic leak or further perforation.

Obstruction

- Diagnosis of int. obstruction depends on the demonstration of dilated bowel loops of bowel proximity with non-dilated/collapsed bowel distal to the pool of obstruction.

GASTRIC DILATATION

Causes

- Mechanised gastric outlet obstruction.
- Paralytic ileus.
- Gastric volvulus.
- Air swallowing, intubation.
- Secondary to intubation.
- Drugs.
- **Paralytic ileus** refers to an acute gastric dilatation often occur in old people (in association with fluid and elongated disturbance and has a high mortality.
- Mech. gastric outlet obstruction is caused by ulceration or carcinoma of the pylori antrum. A massive fluid fitted stomach with little gas present within the stomach which can be identified on horizontal X-ray film.
- Volvulus is the twisting of the stomach around the longitudinal or mesenteric axis. Contain both fluid and adequate air and is identified as a spherical viscus displaced upwards to the normal and is associated with raised normal hemi diaphragm.

Radiologically

- In volvulus gas filled stomach can be identified with greater curvature convex caudally and the pyloric antrum pointing cranially.

D/D Caecal volvulus: This can be seen by visualization as one or two haustra and the inferior part of the caecum pointing caudally (antrum pointing cranially).

SMALL AND LARGE BOWEL OBSTRUCTION

Small Bowel Obstruction

Causes are

- Postoperative adhesion in developed countries.

	Small bowel	Large bowel
Valvular conniventes	In jejunum	Absent
No. of loops	Many	Few
Distribution of loops	Central	Peripheral
Haustra	Absent	Present
Diameter	3-5 cm	5 cm +
Radium of curvature	Small	Large
Solid faeces	Absent	Present

- Strangulated hernias in underdeveloped countries.
- Complete obstruction leads to dilatated small bowel with accumulation of fluid and air with decreased calibre of large bowel.
- Plain film change usually appear after 3-5 hours and marked after 12 hours in cases of complete obstruction.
- With incomplete obstruction or film taken shortly after onset of symptom, plain films are normal and barium/USG may have to be one to established diagnosis.

Plain Film

- Dilated bowel loops in supine and multiple fluid levels in exact film establish the diagnosis.
- With bowel loops almost completely filled with fluid small bubbles of gas may be trapped in between rows of valvulae conventis or horizontal ray film. This is known as string of beads sign, which is virtually diagnostic of obstruction and is not seen in normal people.
- Repeated films are taken if interval film is normal.
- Still if the problem persists, barium or non-ionic contrast may be given. Inability of the barium contrast reaching the caecum at 4 hours implies to requirement of emergency surgery for small bowel obstruction.

USG

- Demonstrates dilated fluid loops of small bowel and an assessment of peristaltic activity can be made.

CT

- Demonstrates bowel calibre change and the level.
- The level of origin can be identified by carefully following the distended bowel loops, forward from D.J. junction backward from iliocaecal junction.
- CT scan shows adhesion, as adhesion can be suspected when bowel loops convulge to a point where there is the mass.
- Patients on conservative management can be followed radiologically to assess bowel diameter, thickening of bowel wall and valvulae conventis.

Strangulated Obstruction

- It's a mechanical/small bowel obstruction caused when two limbs of loop are incarcerated by a band/in a hernia with compromised blood supply.

Plain Film

- Soft tissue mass/pseudo tumor because of fluid in it.
- Thickened intestinal walls.
- If gangrene occurs, lines of gas may be seen in wall of small intestine.

CT

- More sensitive than plain film.
- A fluid filled closed loop is seen with mesenteric vessel converging towards the point of obstruction.
- If strangulation occurs, loop becomes thickened with venous congestion of the mesentery locally. If hemorrhage occurs, bowel wall is seen with increased attenuation. If necrosis occurs, gas may be seen in the bowel wall.

Volvulus

- Associated with incomplete rotation, malrotation or no rotation of gut and present in neonatal period or months or even years after birth.
- It is usually not possible to distinguish between simple obstruction, strangulated obstruction or volvulous obstruction on plain film alone.

Gall Stone Ileus

- It's a mechanical obstruction caused by gallstones impacted in the small intestine, usually terminal ileum but rarely in the duodenum or colon.
- Occurs in middle aged/elderly women.

Signs: Plain Film

- Gas within the bile ducts and/or the gallbladder.
- Complete or incomplete small bowel obstruction.
- Abnormal location of gall stones (if visualized).
- Change in position of gall stones (if visualized).

CT

- Dilated small bowel.
- Air in the biliary tree.
- Gallstone at the point of obstruction.

Intussusception

- Present as pain, vomiting and blood in stool and a palpable tumor.
- Plain film: Case of small bowel obstruction or as a soft tissue mass surrounded by a crescent of gas.
- Target sign has been described, comprising two concentric circles of fat density. This is due to the peritoneal fat surrounding and within the intussusception alternating with a layer of mucosa and muscle seen "end on".

USG

- Also shows similar target lesion with two concentric hyper echoic circles (Figure 75.1).

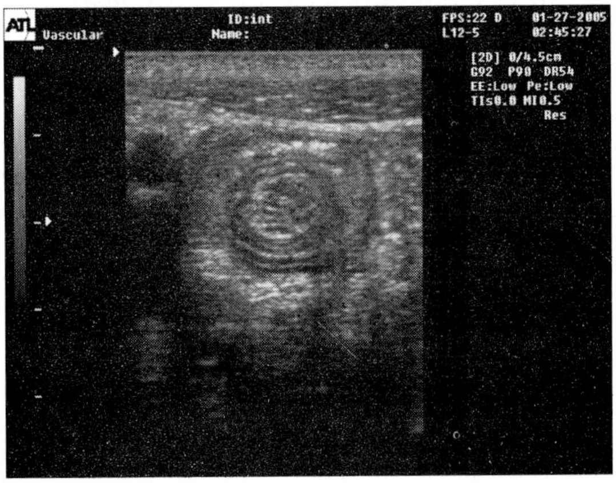

Fig. 75.1: US scan shows intussusception

CT

- Shows characteristic fat density centrally due to mesenteric fat being brought up between the intussuscipiens and intussuceptum (Figure 75.2).

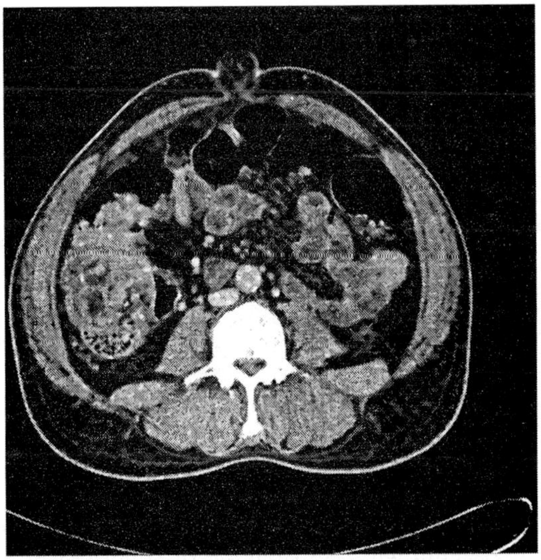

Fig. 75.2: Axial CT image shows ileocolic intussusception with an incidental umbilical hernia

Mesentric Thrombosis/Small Bowel Infarction

- Sudden onset abdominal pain with bloody diarrhoea in an elderly patient is suggestive of the condition.

Plain Film

- Gas filled, slightly dilated small bowel loops with multiple on fluid levels or fluid filled loops of small bowel may be seen.
- Wall may appear thickened due to submucosal hemorrhage or edema.
- Gas streak in bowel wall may be seen if there is gangrene and free gas may be seen if perforation has occurred.

CT

- Bowel wall thickening.
- Engorgement of mesenteric veins.
- ↑ed attenuation of mesenteric fat.
- Gas in the bowel wall.
- Gas in the mesenteric and portal vein (it is a bad prognostic sign).
- Non-enhancement of superior mesenteric artery and vein after contrast enhancement.

Large Bowel Obstruction

MC Causes

- Carcinoma (60% vs sigmoid colon).
- Diverticular disease.
- Volvulus.
- Radiological appearance depends upon the competence of IC valve if patterns are described.

  Type Ia: IC valve competent dilated colon and caecum with as distention of small bowel.

  Type Ib: Type IA proposes with small bowel dilatation.

  Type II: IC valve incompetent, colon and caecum not distended, instead small bowel dilated which simulate small bowel obstruction.
- When both small and large bowel dilatation is present in large bowel obstruction, the radiographic appearance is similar to paralytic ileus.

D/D: Lateral Radiograph

- Air in rectum – paralytic ileus.
- No air in rectum – obstruction.

Pseudo-Obstruction

- Mimics symptomatically, clinically and radiologically int obstruction associated with pneumonia, septicemia, drugs, DM, amyloidosis, collagen disorder. Most cases are idiopathic.

  Due to Ba enema, which rules out any organic obstruction.

Caecal Volvulus

- <2% case and adult intestinal obstruction.

Plain Films

- Occupies the right half or centre of the abdomen.
- One or two haustras are seen (distinguishes it from infected volvulus).
- Distended caecum with large gas/fluid filled viscus is seen.
- Identification of an attached gas filled appendix confirms the diagnosis.

Sigmoid Volvulus

- Seen in old, mentally subnormal patients.

Signs: Plain Film

- *Ahaustral margin*: Most important diagnostic point.

- *Liver overlap sign*: Overlapping of lower border of liver shadow.
- *Lower flank overlap sign*: Overlapping at haustrated and dilated descending colon.
- Often lies high in the abdomen, under the lateral hemidiaphragm at or above T10.
- Inferior two limbs converge.
- Air fluid ratio > 2:1.

Left flank overlap open above T10, superior convergence – are highly specific and sensitive sign.

Ba Enema

- Bird of prey sign: Smooth taper and narrowing at the point of torsion.
- Saw pattern of mucosa at the point of twist.
- Shouldering is seen at the site of torsion in chronic cases.

Acute Inflammatory Colitis

- The state of colonic mucosa, width of bowel lumen, the mucosal edge and the haustral pattern can be assessed by plain radiograph.
- Fury mucosal edges, widened clefts or absent haustratious indicative active disease.
- Course irregularity of mucosa is seen as ulceration when ulcerative colitis become extensive, mucosal islands/pseudopolyps may be seen.
- Bowel dilatation >5.5cm suggests the ulceration has penetrated the muscular layer and the patient needs urgent surgery.
- Follow up is done by daily plain radiograph to see change in colonic diameter, mega colon or a perforation.

Toxic Mega Colon

- Fulminant colitis with transmural inflammation with extensive deep ulceration.
- Perforation may occur; most common involvement is sigmoid colon.

Intra-Abdominal Abscess

- These can be subphrenic, subhepatic, right paracolic or left paracolic abscess.
- Plain film diagnosis require high index of suspicion. Small gas bubbles, which are usually unchanged in positive on consecutive film, displacement of organ and bowel and effacement of fat liver may be seen.
- Plain film combined with USG: Diagnostic in 90% of cases.

CT scan: Highly accurate in detecting intra-abdominal abscess. Pathological mass with attenuation of 15-35 HU with gas in it and showing ring enhancement after I/V contrast administration is characteristic.

- *Leucocytic scoring*: Leucocyte labelled with Iridium III is used. It has a sensitivity and specificity >90% in increasing int. abdominal sepsis.

False +ve: Other inflammation (lie IBD) non-infected thrombosis.

False –ve: Chronic abscess with low inflammatory response.

Appendicitis

- Most common acute surgical condition.

Plain Film

- Appendix calculus may be seen (0.5-6 cm).
- *Sentinal loop*: Dilated atonic ileum contained fluid level.
- Dilated caecum.
- Right lower quadrant mass due to fluid and edema.
- Scoliosis with concavity to the right side.
- Right lower quadrant non-indenting the caecum.
- Blurring of the right psoas outlie – unreliable sign.
- Gas in the appendix – unreliable sign.

USG Findings

- Blind ending tubular structure at the point of tenderness:
  - Non-compressible.
  - Diameter >7 mm.
  - No perstaltics.
- Appendicolitis casting PAS.
- High echogenecity, non-compressible surrounding fat.
- Surrounding fluid or abscess.
- Edema of caecal pole.

CT

- Appendix measuring >6 mm diameter.
- Failure of appendix to fill with oral contration or air upto its tip.
- Appendicolith seen.
- Enhancement of its wall with I/V contrast.
- Surrounding inflammatory changes like increased fat attenuation, fluid, phlegmonos, caecal thickening, abscess, extraluminal gas and LAP.

Acute Cholecystitis

- Acute inflammation of gallbladder, most commonly caused by obstruction of the duct by a stone.

Plain Film

- Gallstone in 20% cases.
- Duodenal ileus.
- Ileus or hepatic plexure of colon.
- (R) hypochondrial mass due to enlarged gallbladder.
- Gas within the biliary system.

USG Findings

- The positive sonographic Murphy's sign.
- Thickened echogenic gallbladder with hypoechoic margin.
- Indistinct gallbladder wall with pariechocystic fluid.
- Gallstone with PAS.
- Echogenic sediments caused by inspissated bile or pus.

Scintigraphy: Highly accurate in diagnosis of acute cholecystitis.

+ve scan: In a fasted patient, gallbladder not visualized but bile duct and duodenum are seen.

Empysematous choleocystitis is one type of cholecystitis in which gas is seen in the gallbladder wall or lumen. Cl. welchii sees this in diabetes due to infection.

Acute Pancreatitis

- Inflammation of the pancreas is known as pancreatitis.

Cause: Gallstones etc.

Plain Film

- Gas in the dilated duodenal loop with prone or (L) lateral position.
- Gas within pancreas (suggestive of an abscess).
- Dilated small bowel loop.
- Loss of left psoas outline.
- Opaque gallstones.
- Absent (L) psoas shadow.
- Elevated (L) hemidiaphragm.
- Renal halo sign, colonic dilatation.

USG

- Organ enlargement, indistinct boundaries, ↓ed echogenicity, duodenal atony may be seen.
- In necrotizing condition, liquid/semiliquid rather spreading beyond organ boundaries to the retroperitoneal and pararenal space.
- Pleural effusion/ascitis may be seen.

CT

- Demonstrate necrosis, hemorrhage and left behind parenchyma which enhances with intravenous contrast.

- Complication of pancreatitis, bile hemorrhage, abscess and pseudocyst can be seen.

Renal Colic

Plain film: Shows a ROS in the KUB region.

D/D phlebolitis: Are smooth in outline with radiolucent centre.

USG: Shows an edema shadow with a PAS.

NCCT: Usually not required.

IVP: To confirm the site and to simultaneously assess the renal function.

Acute Gynecological Disorders

Torsion of a cyst/ovarian, dermoid, salpingitis and ruptured ectopic presents as acute abdomen.

Torsion: Pelvic mass.

Dermoid: Diagnosed by its calcification, teeth or fat.

Salpingitis, present as ileus.

Ruptured ectopic: Pelvic mass, FF in the pelvis and paralytic ileus.

Leaking Abdominal Aortic Aneurysm

Plain Film

Central soft tissue mass, which may obscure psoas outline of (L) side. Freqeuently curvilinear calcification may be seen in AP view and is confirmed in lateral view.

USG will confirm the presence of aorta aneurysm but leak or a retroperitoneal hematoma requires CT scan.

Section 6—Alimentary Tract

Chapter 76

Blunt Abdominal Trauma

Evaluating patients who have sustained blunt abdominal trauma (BAT) remains one of the most challenging and resource-intensive aspects of acute trauma care.

BAT usually results from motor vehicle collisions, assaults, recreational accidents or falls. Men tend to be affected slightly more often than women. The most commonly injured organs are spleen, liver, retroperitoneum, small bowel, kidneys, bladder, colorectal, diaphragm and pancreas.

In 1990, approximately 5 million people died worldwide as a result of injury. Vehicular trauma is by far the leading cause of BAT in the civilian population.

Mechanisms

- Rapid deceleration causes differential movement among adjacent structures. As a result, shear forces are created and cause hollow solid, visceral organs, and vascular pedicles to tear, especially at relatively fixed points of attachment.
- When intra-abdominal contents are crushed between the anterior abdominal wall the vertebral column or posterior thoracic cage.
- External compression forces that result in a sudden and dramatic rise in intra-abdominal pressure and culminate in rupture of a hollow visceral organ.

The evaluation of a patient with BAT must be accomplished with all injuries prioritised accordingly. This implies that injuries involving the head, respiratory system, or cardiovascular system may take precedence over an abdominal injury.

Lab Studies

- Should include a CBC count, coagulation studies, blood type, and cross match. The presence of massive hemorrhage is usually obvious from hemodynamics parameters.
- Urine studies include urinalysis, urine toxicological screening, and serum or urine pregnancy tests in females of appropriate age.
- Serum electrolyte values, creatinine level, and glucose values are obtained.
- The serum lipase or amylase level is neither sensitive nor specific as a marker for major pancreatic or enteric injury. Normal levels do not exclude a major pancreatic injury. Elevated levels may be caused by injuries to the head and face or by an assortment of nontraumatic causes (e.g. alcohol, narcotics, and various other drugs). Amylase or lipase levels may be elevated because of pancreatic ischemia caused by the systemic hypotension that accompanies trauma. However, persistent hyperamylasemia or hyperlipasia should raise the suggestion of

significant intra abdominal injury and is an indication for aggressive radiographic and surgical investigation.

Imaging Studies

The important initial concern in the evaluation or a patient with BAT is an assessment of hemodynamics stability. In the hemodynamically unstable patient, a rapid evaluation must be made regarding the presence of hemoperitoneum. This can be accomplished using Diagnostic Peritoneal Lavage (DPL) or the FAST scan. Radiographic studies of the abdomen are indicated in stable patients when the physical examination findings are inconclusive.

Abdominal Trauma Radiograph Protocol

- AP supine and upright abdomen.
- Chest, upright view.
- If the patient cannot stand or sit, a left lateral decubitus (14 x 1-7) film of the abdomen should be done. The patient should lie with the right side up for 10 minutes before this film is taking. It is important to include the right hemidiaphragm to exclude free air.

Although the overall value of plain films in the evaluation of patients with BAT is limited, they can demonstrate numerous findings.

- The chest radiograph may aid in the diagnosis of abdominal injuries such as ruptured hemidiaphragm (e.g. a nasogastric tube seen in the chest) or pneumoperitoneum.
- The pelvic or chest radiograph can demonstrate fractures of the thoracolumbar spine.
- The presence or transverse fractures or the vertebral bodies, i.e., Chance fractures, suggests a higher likelihood or blunt injuries to the bowel.
- In addition, free intraperitoneal air, or trapped retroperitoneal air from duodenal perforation, may be seen.

Ultrasound

In many medical centres, the FAST (Focused Assessment with Sonography for Trauma) examination has virtually replaced DPL as the procedure of choice in the evaluation of hem dynamically unstable trauma patients.

- An examination is interpreted as positive if fluid is found in any of the 4 acoustic windows and is interpreted as negative if no fluid is seen. An examination is deemed indeterminate if any of the windows cannot be adequately assessed.
- The FAST examination is based on the assumption that all clinically significant abdominal injuries are associated with hemoperitoneum. However, detection of free intraperitoneal fluid is based on factors such as, the body habitus, injury location, presence of clotted blood, position of the patient, and amount of free fluid present.
- The minimum threshold for detecting hemoperitoneum is unknown and remains a subject of interest. Tiling *et al.* found that 30 mL is the minimum requirement for detection with ultrasound. They also concluded that a small, anechoic stripe in the Morison pouch represents approximately 250 mL of fluid, while 0.5 cm and 1 cm stripes represent approximately 500 mL and I L of free fluid, respectively.
- The current examination protocol consists of 4 acoustic windows with the patient supine. These windows are pericardia, perihepatic, perisplenic, and pelvic (known as the 4 Ps).
  - The **pericardial view** is obtained using a subcostal or transthoracic, window. It provides 4-chamber view of the heart and can detect the presence of hemopericardium, which is demonstrated by the separation of the visceral and parietal pericardial layers.
  - The perihepatic view images portions of the liver, diaphragm, and right kidney. It reveals fluid in the Morrison pouch, the subphrenic space, and the right pleural space.
- The perisplenic view provides view of the spleen and the left kidney and reveals fluid in

the splenorenal recess, the left pleural space, and the subphrenic space.

- The pelvic view uses the bladder as a sonographic window. This view is best accomplished while the patient has a full bladder. In males, free fluid is seen as an anechoic area (sonographically black) in the recto vesicular pouch or cephalad to the bladder. In females, fluid accumulates in the pouch of Douglas.

Reported sensitivities and negative predictive values for ultrasound in the detection of hemoperitoneum are 78-99% and 93-99%, respectively.

- Rozycki *et al.* studied 1540 patients and reported that ultrasound was the most sensitive and specific modality for the evaluation of hypotensive patients with BAT (sensitivity and specificity, 100%).
- Hemodynamically stable patients with positive FAST results may require a CT scan to better define the nature and extent of their injuries. Taking every patient with a positive FAST result to the operating room may result in an unacceptably high laparotomy rate.
- Hemodynamically stable patients with negative FAST results require close observation, serial abdominal examinations, and follow-up of FAST examination. However, strongly consider performing a CT scan especially if patient is intoxicated or has other associated injuries.

Abdominal Trauma Spiral CT Protocol (Upper Abdomen and Pelvis)

CT Technique

Most trauma centres use helical or multidetector CT to evaluate stable patients with significant injuries. Multidetector CT is used b/o Increase in speed (3 times greater than single slice helical CT) and increased anatomic coverage afforded by multidetector CT by the use of thinner collimation to improve spatial resolution.

Oral Contrast

If circumstances permit, administer 600 to 900 ml of water soluble oral contrast material 30 to 45 minutes before scanning, either orally or by nasogastric tube. An additional 300 ml of oral contrast material 15 minutes before scanning is helpful to opacify stomach and proximal small intestine.

Phase of Respiration	Suspended inspiration.
Slice of Thickness/Interval	7 mm.
Superior Extent	Diaphragm.
Inferior Extent	Symphysis pubis.

IV Contrast

- 150 cc at the rate of 2.5 cc/sec, with 60 second scan delay.
- Scan from the top of the liver to the iliac crest.
- Wait 2 minutes, then scan pelvis to symphysis pubis or lower if the proximal thighs need to be included as well.

CT Cystogram

- Contrast recipe 30 cc of 60% contrast added to 500 cc of sterile normal saline.
- Instil 100 cc of contrast through Foley catheters. Quick scan through bladder (spread three cuts over bladder, each cut 5 mm thick) and check images for extravasation.
- If initial scan is negative for rupture, continue with additional contrast with bottle hung 30 to 40 cm above table top until filling stops, and then spiral scan entire bladder at 7 mm to rule out intraperitoneal rupture.
- If initial scan is positive for extra-peritoneal rupture, continue with additional contrast, fill up to 300-400 cc total spiral scan bladder at 7 mm to rule out intraperitoneal rupture.

- Unclamp Foley catheters and proceed with abdominal/pelvis scan.

Others

- If NG present pull into oesophagus.
- If no ventilator, consider possibility of decreasing motion artefact by having respiratory therapy gate ventilator with scan acquisition.
- If there is evidence of severe renal trauma, consider delayed scans to evaluate extravasation of urine.

CT Diagnosis of Hemoperitoneum

Blood is unique as a biologic fluid due to its high protein content and high attenuation of the iron containing hemoglobin molecule. In patients without anaemia, CT attenuation values of blood are substantially greater than other fluid collections commonly encountered in the abdomen. Urine, bile, chyle and ascites fluid typically have attenuation values less than 15 HU.

Hemoperitoneum can be detected on CT with blood volume 100 ml. Blood reaches maximum attenuation at approximately 20 hours after injury and then stabilizes at a lower attenuation over the next 48 hours.

Free lysed blood within the peritoneal cavity only has attenuation values of 30 HU or more. Clotted blood has a higher attenuation and is on the order of 40-60 HU. Active arterial extravasation represents a unique contribution of CT in the diagnosis of abdominal trauma. The ability to visualize active bleeding cannot be demonstrated by any other modality short of arteriography.

Areas of active arterial extravasation appear as high attenuation density fluid collections that are isodense with adjacent major arterial structures, often on the order of 70-100 HU. There are invariably areas of hematoma formation around sites of active arterial extravasation.

Important CT Signs in Abdominal Trauma

- **The sentinel clot sign** refers to the fact that the attenuation of blood may be useful to identify the source of visceral injury. The attenuation of blood is highest in close proximity to sites of injury. Therefore clotted blood and active arterial extravasation due to parenchymal and vascular injuries will be of higher attenuation than free lysed blood elsewhere in the peritoneal cavity. Occasionally the sentinel clot sign may be useful to identify occult sources of injury.
- **The collapsed inferior vena cava sign** refers to the fact that patients who have undergone substantial blood loss may have decreased circulating venous return.
- The CT scan remains the criterion standard for the detection of solid organ injuries. In addition, a CT scan of the abdomen can reveal other associated injuries, notably vertebral and pelvic fractures and injuries in the thoracic cavity.
- CT scans, unlike DPL or FAST examinations, have the capability to determine the source of hemorrhage. In addition, many retroperitoneal injuries go unnoticed with DPL and FAST examinations.
- CT scans provide excellent imaging of the pancreas, duodenum, and genitourinary system.
- **Limitations of CT scans** include marginal sensitivity for diagnosing diaphragmatic, pancreatic, and hollow viscous injuries. Also, they are relatively expensive and time consuming and require oral or intravenous contrast, which may cause adverse reactions.

Diagnostic Peritoneal Lavage

Now known as abdominal paracentesis.

- DPL is indicated in blunt trauma. In:
  1. Patients with a spinal cord injury.
  2. Those with multiple injuries and unexplained shock.

3. Unstable patients with a possible abdominal injury.
4. Intoxicated patients in whom abdominal injury is suggested, and
5. Patients with potential intra-abdominal injury who will undergo prolonged anaesthesia for another procedure.

- The only absolute contraindication to DPL is the obvious need for laparotomy. Relative contraindications include morbid obesity, a history of multiple abdominal surgeries, and pregnancy.

With the availability of less, non-invasive, and better imaging modalities (e.g. FAST examination, CT scan), the role of DPC is now limited to the evaluation of unstable trauma patients in whom FAST results are negative or inconclusive.

Laparoscopy

- The most important limitation is its inability to reliably identify hollow viscous and retroperitoneal injuries, even in the hands of experienced laparoscopists.
- Diagnostic laparoscopy has been most useful in the evaluation of possible diaphragmatic injuries, especially in penetrating thoracoabdominal injuries on the left side.
- In blunt trauma, diagnostic laparoscopy offers no clear advantage over less invasive modalities such as DPL or CT scan and complications can occur from trocar misplacement.

Laparotomy

Indications for laparotomy in a patient with blunt abdominal injury include the following:

- Signs of peritonitis.
- Uncontrolled shock or hemorrhage.
- Clinical deterioration during observation.
- Hemoperitoneum findings after FAST or DPL examinations.

Finally, surgical intervention is indicated in patients with evidence of peritonitis based on physical examination findings.

Spleen

Most commonly injured abdominal organ. Injury to the spleen often leads to massive hemorrhage into the abdominal cavity. Because of its uniquely open circulation, it can bleed profusely with minimal injury.

Plain Radiography

Findings such as left lower rib fractures, pleural effusion, displacement of the gastric air bubble, or elevation of the left hemidiaphragm, can help in the diagnosis of splenic trauma. However, evidence of previous splenic trauma may be detected in the form of calcification from old hematomas.

USG can be very useful in the diagnosis of subcapsular and pericapsular hematomas of the spleen. If the capsule remains intact, it may be intraparenchymal or subcapsular hematoma. If the capsule ruptures, a focal or free intraperitoneal hematoma may result.

Fluid can be demonstrated in the LUQ surrounding the spleen. Immediately after the trauma the hematoma is liquid and can be easily differentiated from splenic parernchyma. After the blood clots, echogenicity of the perisplenic clot closely resemble the echogenicity of normal spleen.

This appearance may mimic that of an enlarged spleen (24-48 hours). Subsequently the blood liquefies and the diagnosis becomes easy. If the collection is crescentic and conforms to the splenic contour, the hematoma assumed to become subcapsular.

CT (Figure 76.1)

- Laceration – An irregular linear area of hypodensity on CECT.
- Intrasplenic hematoma – May appear hyperdense on NCCT. On CECT broader area of hypodense, nonperfused splenic parenchyma.
- Subcapsular hematoma – Crescentic collection of fluid that flattens or indents the underlying splenic parenchyma.

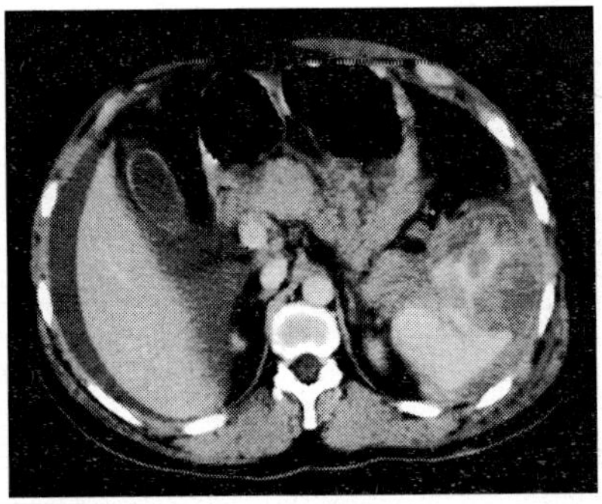

Fig. 76.1: Axial CT image shows splenic laceration and contusion

- Splenic infarcts – May occur following injury to the splenic vasculature and appear as wedge shaped area of non perfusion that extends up to the splenic capsule.

Nuclear scintigraphy with technetium sulphur colloid is also used to locate injury. Although not the diagnostic tool of choice, it may still have a role in the stable but uncooperative patient with local trauma to the LUQ. It may be especially useful in a patient with coexisting contrast allergy and skin injury, which would preclude both CT and ultrasound. Nuclear scintigraphy can also be used to follow return of splenic function. The resolution of this method, however, is significantly less than that of CT.

Angiography is also used to diagnose injury, but less invasive studies are more efficient and accurate.

MRI provides the best anatomical resolution but is contraindicated in an emergency setting.

Classification of Splenic Injury, Organ Injury Scaling Committee – 1987

The class I and a proportion of the less severe class II injuries can often be managed conservatively. The severe class II and the class III injuries have better outcomes with splenorrhaphy, and class IV injuries often require segmental splenectomy. The splenic artery divided into between 6 and 36 branches before entering the splenic parenchyma, providing segmental perfusion and allowing for partial resection in focal injury, class V splenic

Grade	Injury description.
I Hematoma	Subcapsular, non expanding, <10% surface area.
Laceration	Capsular tear, non bleeding <1cm parenchymal depth.
II Hematoma	Subcapsular, non expanding, 10-50% surface area or intraparenchymal, non-expanding <2 cm in diameter.
Laceration	Capsular tear, active bleeding or 1-3 cm parenchymal depth that does not involve a trabecular vessels.
III Hematoma	Subcapsular, either non-expanding >50% surface area of expanding.
Laceration	>3cm parenchymal depth or involving trabecular vessels.
IV Hematoma	Ruptured intraparenchymal hematoma with active bleeding.
Laceration	Laceration involving segmental or hilar vessels producing major devascularization (>25% of spleen).
V Laceration	Completely shattered spleen.
Vascular	Hilar vascular injury that devascularizes spleen.

injuries require splenectomy. Splenectomy is also favoured over splenorrhaphy for patients with lesser injuries but with medical contraindications to prolonged surgery.

Liver: 2nd most common predominant site of hepatic injury in blunt trauma is the right lobe, particularly, the posterior segment (Figure 76.2).

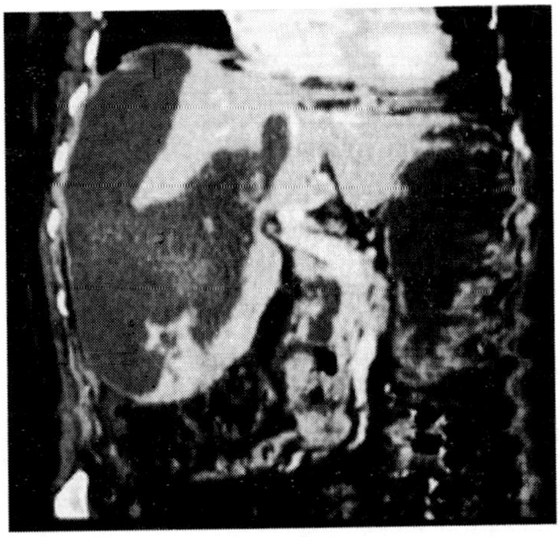

Fig. 76.2: Coronal CT image shows a large hepatic laceration

U.S.G.

Hepatic laceration – fresh hemorrhages or laceration appears echogenic (<24 hours). Laceration becomes more hypoechoic and distinct as a result of resorption of devitalised tissue, and ingress of intestinal fluid (within 1 week). 2-3 weeks later the laceration becomes increasingly indistinct as a result of resorption of fluid and filling of the spaces with granulation tissue.

C.E.C.T. Findings

- *Laceration:* Irregular linear, branching or rounded areas of low attenuation within the normal enhancing liver parenchyma. Commonly parallel with the hepatic or portal venous vasculature.
- *Bear Claw sign:* Parallel linear laceration on the surface of the liver of radiating out from the hilar region.
- Liver fracture (laceration extending between 2 visceral surfaces). Laceration extending into the perihilar region – increased incidence of bile duct injury and associated complication such as biloma and hemobilia.
- Intrahepatic hematoma is seen as poorly marginated confluent areas of low attenuation within the hepatic parenchyma. Often display a central area of high attenuation of clotted bld.
- Subcapsular hematoma is seen as peripheral, lenticular or crescent shaped fluid collections that flatten or indent the underlying liver. Most common site is inferolateral aspect of right lobe. Higher attenuation is seen early when clotted bld is present. Decreased in attenuation over time as clot lysis takes place.

Pancreas (Figure 76.3)

Pancreatic injuries from blunt trauma are relatively uncommon accounting for only 3-12% of all abdominal traumas.

Mechanism – Compression of pancreas between vertebral column and the anterior abdominal wall.

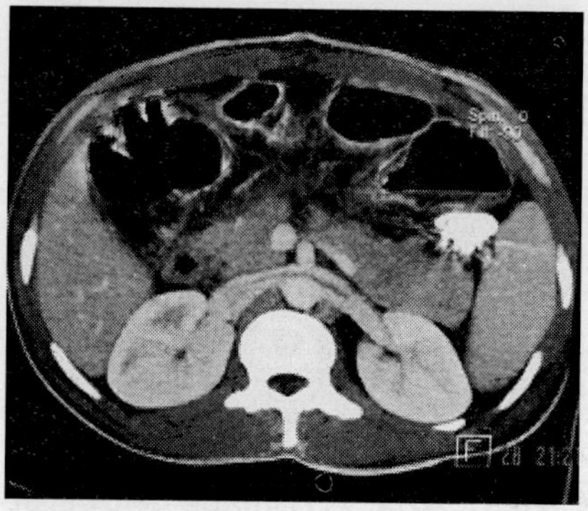

Fig. 76.3: CT MIP image shows laceration through the neck of the pancreas

USG can demonstrate the changes in the size, shape or consistency, large fluid collection surrounding the gland or pseudocyst. Limitation of USG in the region of body and tail below overlying bowel gases.

CT has been reported to diagnose pan injury in 67-85% of cases:

- Contusions – Focal low attenuation areas within the normal enhancing parenchyma.
- Laceration or fracture linear irregular areas of low attenuation often oriented perpendicular to the long axis of the pancreas. Fracture most commonly occurs at the neck or body of pancreas, where it overlies the spine.

Additional suggestive but non-specific signs of pancreatic injuries:

- Infiltration of the peripancreatic fat and mesentery.
- Thickening of the ant renal fascia.
- Tracking of fluid between the splenic vein and pancreas.
- Fluid in the anterior pararenal space or lesser sac.

Pancreatic laceration or fracture may be difficult to identify with CT within 12 hours of injury. As the time progresses, edema, inflammation, and auto digestion by exuded pancreatic enzymes often make the CT findings more apparent.

Thus if suspicion of pancreatic injury persists

despite initially NCT findings, repeat CT scans in 12-24 hours may be warranted.

Pancreatic Duct Injury: CT can't directly assess the integrity of the pancreatic duct; which is the principle determinant in the management of pancreatic injury.

Ductal disruption is likely to be present, if CT scans demonstrate a deep laceration or transaction of the pancreas.

In general ERCP or intraoperative evaluation is required for pan duct integrity.

Bowel and Mesentery

Occur in 3-5% of paitents sustaining bowel abdominal trauma.

Mechanism

1. Direct compression of the bowel between the vertebral column and the anterior abdominal wall.
2. Sudden marked increase in intraluminal pressure.
3. Shearing type injury at site of mesenteric fixation.

Most common site – Duodenum usually 2nd and 3rd part. Colonic injuries are less common after bowel abdominal trauma.

CT Signs of Bowel and Mesentery Injuries

Extraluminal air

- Extravasation of oral contrast material—very diagnostic but seen in very few cases.
- Free intra abdomonal air.
- Thickened and/or discontinuous bowel wall.
- High attenuation clot (sentinel clot) adjacent to the involved bowel loops.
- Streaky soft tissue infiltration of the mesenteric fat.

Free air in the IP or RP is a relatively specific sign of bowel perforation but seen only in 50% of cases.

Pneumoperitoneum is most commonly seen in the subdiaphragmatic area, along the ant peritoneal surface of the liver and spleen. Extraluminal air may also present between the leaves of mesentery or in the RP particularly in the ant pararenal space.

Intra abdominal fluid is very common but non-specific CT finding for bowel or mesentery. Fluid may be of low attenuation, representing extravasated, small bowel contents, or of intermediate to high attenuation from acute hemorrhage.

Intramural hemorrhage is seen on CT as circumferential or eccentric thickening of the bowel wall, often with intraluminal narrowing. Intense enhancement is also a sign of injury.

CLASSIFICATION OF RENAL INJURIES

In patients sustaining abdominal trauma, approximately10% will have an injury of the genitourinary tract. Of these injuries, half will be to the kidney. Blunt trauma (Constituting 80 -90%), occurring most commonly in falls, motor vehicle accidents and assaults.

Renal injury can be divided into 4 broad categories:

Grade 1 – Contusions and C-M laceration that do not communicate with the renal collecting system. Accounts for 75-85% of all renal injury. Treated non-operatively.

Grade 2 – Laceration that communicate with the renal collecting system. Accounts for 10% of the cases.

Grade 3 – Consists of shattered kidney and injuries to the renal vascular pedicle. Accounts for 5% of the total injuries.

Grade 4 – UPJ avulsion and laceration injuries require prompt surgery.

Renal injury must be presumed in every patient who is having gross or microscopic hematuria.

IVU is done with the double dose of contrast (100 ml non-ionic contrast medium for adults)

2 ml/kg for children. This should be performed as soon as possible to exclude a renal pedicle injury and to assess the contralateral kidney.

USG is best used in the follow up of the patients with known renal parenchymal traumatic injury.

Renal hematoma may be hypo, hyper or heterogeneous in appearance.

Subcapsular hematoma seen as perirenal fluid collection that flattens the underlying renal contour.

A shattered kidney will consist of multiple fragments of disorganized tissue with associated hematoma and urine collection in the renal bed.

Colour Doppler may help in the assessment of vascular pedicle injury.

R.N. imaging can be used to assess residual renal function after conservative treatment of renal injury.

ARTERIOGRAPHY for preoperative road mapping and therapeutic interventions such as embolisation of bleeding vessel and AVF.

MRI is not useful in acute situation.

CT (Figures 76.4 and 76.5) is the modality of choice. Renal contusion appears on NECT as focal swelling containing scattered foci of high density, fresh blood intermixed with normal homogenous soft tissue attenuation renal parenchyma.

CECT – The involved area often exhibits delayed and decreased enhancement.

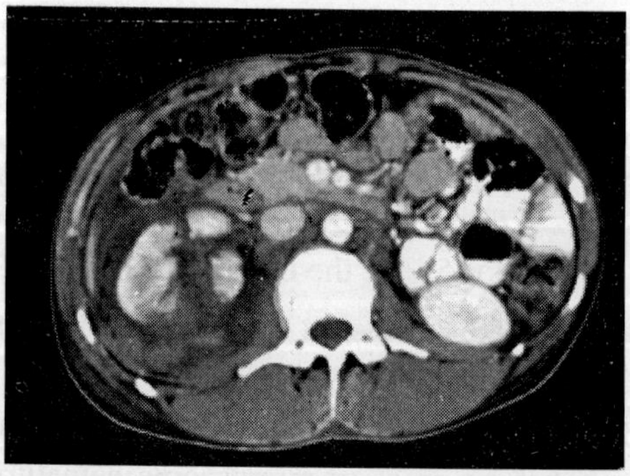

Fig. 76.4: Axial CT image shows a renal contusion and laceration with perinephric collection in the right kidney

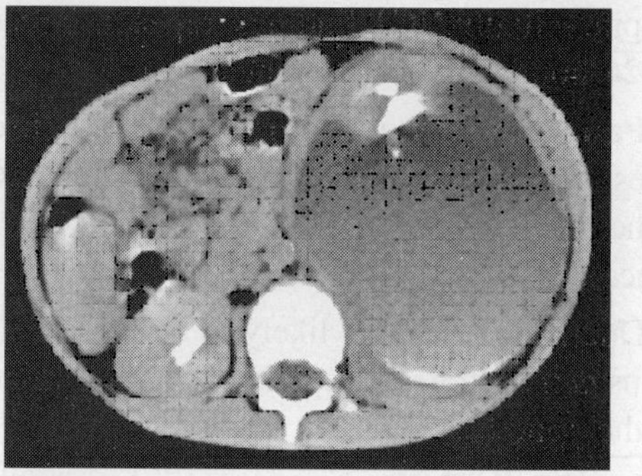

Fig. 76.5: Axial MIP CT image shows a large post-traumatic urinoma on left side with extravasation of contrast

A striated nephrogram resulting from stasis of urine in blood filled tubules has also been encountered.

Parenchymal laceration – Fig. 76.6 [a] appears as unenhanced areas disrupting the normal enhancing renal parenchyma.

Both contusions and laceration are usually associated with small subcapsular or perirenal hematoma (Fig. 76.6 [b]).

Subcapsular collection appears as lenticular collections that flatten the underlying renal contour while perirenal hematoma infiltrate or displace perirenal fat and may extend to the renal fascia.

Category 2 lesions on enhanced scans appear as parenchymal defects extending from the renal surface into the medulla where they may enter the collecting system and/or transect the kidney. Typically such renal fracture parallel intravascular tissue planes. Category 2 lesions are almost always associated with perirenal hematoma. Extravasation of opacified urine, into either renal parenchyma or the peri renal space, frequently occurs.

A shattered or pulverized kidney is recognized on CT as multiple fracture planes separating the enhancing or non-enhanced renal fragments fracture in this category usually shear across segmental renal blood vessel. A large perirenal hematoma is invariably present.

In renal pedicle injury, the occluded or avulsed main renal artery can be depicted on CECT. In

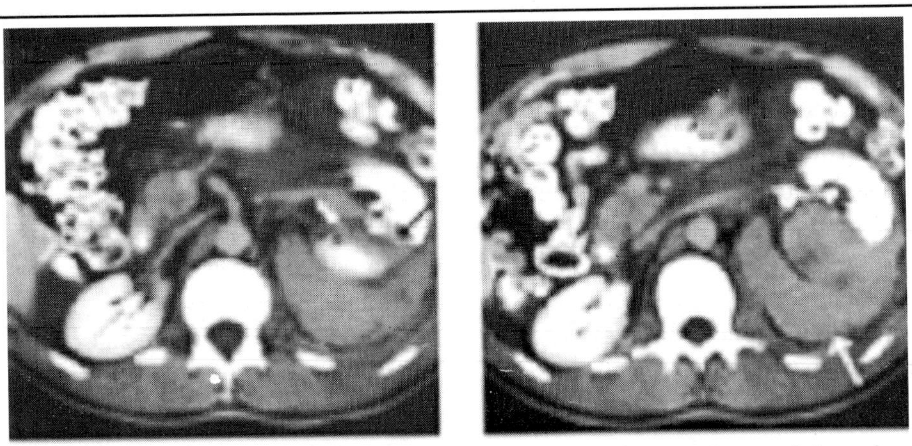

Fig. 76.6: Axial CT section showing grade 2 renal injury with (a) a deep posteromedial renal parenchymal laceration extending into the renal pelvis of the left kidney (arrow) and (b) a moderate perirenal hematoma (arrow) but no urine extravasation, indicating an intact collecting system

such injury, a normal sized, nonenhancing kidney is identified.

Subcapsular collateral vessels may normally perfuse a rim of cortical tissue.

Other associated findings include hematoma surrounding the renal hilum, abrupt cut-off of the contrast filled renal art, and retrograde filling of the renal vein. A wedge shaped infarct that is oriented with its base directed towards the renal capsule and its apex towards the real hilus.

Renal vein injury occurs in 20% of patients with solitary pedicle injury will produce an enlarged rather than normal sized kidney. Associated cortical rim enhancement is usually thicker than with arterial obstruction.

Demonstration of thrombus within a dilated renal vein on CT confirms the diagnosis.

CT findings of massive accumulation of extravasated urine in the medial, rather than dorsolateral aspect of perirenal space, absence of renal parenchymal injury and loss of ureteral opacification suggest ureteropelvic, junction disruption.

Ureteric Injury – It accounts for a relatively small no of ureteric injury. When present they commonly are associated with renal parenchymal art and venous injuries.

Most reported cases are hyperextension injuries sustained by children in motor vehicle accidents.

USG is not useful except to detect sizable fluid collection or hydronephrosis.

CT findings of isolated ureteral disruption in adults are non-visualization of the ureter distal to the point of disruption, intact renal parenchyma and confinement of extravasated urine to the medial perirenal space. In children however, the urine extravasation also expands into leaves of the renal fascia, anterior pararenal space, and the psoas compartment.

Urinary Bladder

Distended urinary bladder is more prone to injury then an empty one. Gross hematuria always accompanies bladder injury. Most patient with urinary bladder rupture complaint of suprapubic pain or tenderness. With an antero superior perforation, extravasation may be either intraperitoneal into the perivesical space (space of Retzius) or both.

With a postero superior tear, fluid can spread intraperitoneally. Retroperitoneally or both extravasations may also spread inferiorly into the perineum, the scrotum and the thigh if the urogenital diaphragm is disrupted.

Retrograde cystography is the preferred radiological procedure for evaluating patients with suspected urinary bladdar injury.

Properly performed CT is as sensitive for detecting urinary bladder injuries as conventional cystography.

CT scans of the pelvis should be obtained with the urinary bladder fully distended either by retrograde or antegrade means. Both delayed scans and repeat scanning of the pelvis after bladder drainage have been used to detect subtle bladder injury.

Angiography has no role in primary assessment of urinary bladder injury but may be of considerable value in the diagnosis and management of arterial bleeding associated with pelvic fracture.

Radionuclide scintigraphy can detect smaller amount of extravasation with great sensitivity but because of its inferior resolution compared to conventional radiography and CT, it is rarely used.

On CT bladder contusion or hematoma appears as focal or diffuse wall thickening without extravasation of contrast medium.

With intraperitoneal rupture of the urinary bladder extravasated urine, and contrast medium can be found surrounding the bladder or bowel and pooling in the paracolic gutters.

Extraperitoneal rupture results in extravasation of contrast medium and urine into the perivesical fat, anterior thigh, scrotum, and abdominal wall. Contrast medium can also extend cephalad to the perirenal and pararenal spaces.

Role of Intervention Radiology in GI Hemorrhage

ETIOLOGY OF GI HEMORRHAGE

UGI bleeding has many etiologies, including peptic ulcer, hemorrhagic gastritis, esophagitis, gastro-esophageal varices, neoplasm, and Mallory-Weiss tear. UGI endoscopy initially is performed to localize the source of bleeding and possibly to treat the cause of bleeding. However, endoscopy fails to find the source of bleeding in 10% of patients. Endoscopic treatment failures also can occur. With endoscopic diagnostic or treatment failure, angiographic evaluation and embolization are the next step. The results of endoscopy are important to the radiologist performing: Angiography, since the angiographic evaluation can be guided to a particular arterial distribution.

The two most common causes of LGI bleeding are diverticular disease and angiodysplasia. Less common causes include inflammatory bowel disease, neoplasia, and bowel ischemia. Endoscopy in the LGI tract is more problematic than in the UGI tract. When the colon is filled with blood and stool, the source of bleeding can be difficult to identify. As much as 40% of the colonoscopy is nondiagnostic regarding the source of bleeding. When endoscopy fails to identify the source of bleeding, a nuclear medicine study can help. Frequently, a nuclear medicine study can localize the source of bleeding to a particular arterial distribution, thus guiding the angiographic evaluation. The radionuclide scan can also help in determining the rate of bleeding, as arteriography is not helpful if bleeding has stopped.

- *Sclerotherapy*: Sclerotherapy is successful in controlling acute esophageal variceal bleeding in 80-90% of patients. Control should be obtained with 1-2 sessions. Patients continuing to bleed after two sessions, should be considered for alternative methods to control their bleeding.
- In the United States, sodium tetradecyl sulfate or sodium morrhuate generally has been used as a sclerosant. While polidocanol or ethanolamine has been more popular in Europe. Variations in the technique or the sclerosant used have not been shown to influence the outcome.
- Serious complications related to sclerotherapy have been reported in 15-20% of patients, with an associated mortality rate of 2%.
- Complications of sclerotherapy may include mucosal ulceration, bleeding, esophageal perforation, mediastinitis, and pulmonary complications. Long-term complications, such as esophageal stricture formation, also may occur.
- Endoscopic variceal ligation (banding):
  - Endoscopic variceal ligation is based on

the widely used technique of rubber-band ligation of hemorrhoids. The esophageal mucosa and the submucosa containing varices are. Ensnared, causing subsequent strangulation, sloughing, and eventual fibrosis, resulting in obliteration of the varices.

- Endoscopic ligation requires placement of an opaque cylinder over the end of the endoscope. This decreases the endoscopic field of view and may allow pooling of blood. Thus, in patients with active bleeding, visualization may be impaired more with ligation than with sclerotherapy.
- Recent trials have demonstrated that ligation and sclerotherapy achieved similar rates of initial hemostasis in patients whose varices were actively bleeding at the time of treatment.
- Local complications are less common with ligation compared to sclerotherapy. For example, esophageal strictures were found to be less common with ligation compared to sclerotherapy. Systemic complications, such as pulmonary infections and bacterial peritonitis, were not significantly different in the two groups. However, a trend was observed toward a decrease in these two complications in patients treated with ligation.

Transjugular Intrahepatic Portosystemic Shunt

- In 1994, the United States National Digestive Diseases Advisory Board established a set of clinical indications for TIPS placement (Shiffman, 1995). These accepted indications are as follows:
  - Acute variceal bleeding that cannot be successfully controlled with medical treatment, including sclerotherapy.
  - Recurrent and refractory variceal bleeding or recurrent variceal bleeding in patients who cannot tolerate conventional medical treatment, including sclerotherapy and pharmacologic therapy.
  - Unproven but promising indications include the following:
    - Therapy for refractory ascites.
    - Portal decompression in patients with hepatic venous outflow obstruction (Budd-Chiari syndrome), hepatic hydrothorax, or hepatorenal syndrome.
  - Absolute contraindications include the following:
    - Right-sided heart failure with increased central venous pressure.
    - Polycystic liver disease.
    - Severe hepatic failure.

Relative contraindications include the following:

- Active intrahepatic or systemic infection (Bacteria can colonize, the stent, causing persistent infection).
- Severe hepatic encephalopathy poorly controlled with medical therapy.
- Hypervascular hepatic tumors.
- PV thrombosis (Although PV thrombus may make the procedure more technically demanding, it is not an absolute contraindication to TIPS placement).

All patients undergoing TIPS placement should receive prophylactic broad-spectrum antibiotics. Appropriate resuscitation with fluid and blood products is indicated prior to the procedure. PV patency should be confirmed prior to attempts at TIPS placement.

All potential patients for TIPS placement undergo preoperative evaluation with duplex sonography to determine if the PV is patent. If the Doppler sonographic findings are inconclusive, arterial portography via the splenic or superior mesenteric arteries can be performed to evaluate PV anatomy and patency. In the presence of reversed intrahepatic portal flow, the PV may not fill during arterial portography. However, magnetic resonance venography may have a promising role in assessing PV patency prior to TIPS. An alternative approach in a patient with inconclusive sonograms can be wedged hepatic venography with CO_2 from the jugular vein.

Patients with cirrhosis often have coagulopathy, and severe coagulopathy should be addressed prior to an invasive procedure. Platelets are routinely administered when platelet counts are less than 50,000 mm^3, and fresh frozen plasma (FFP) is used with an international normalized ratio (INR) of greater than 2.0.

Most patients can safely undergo TIPS placement with intravenous conscious. Sedation involving short-acting benzodiazepines and opiates. Some institutions prefer general anesthesia during TIPS procedures because of the prolonged nature of the procedure and the degree of discomfort that many patients experience during the transvenous punctures. The technique is fairly standard and has been well described in the scientific literature, with some minor variations related to the interventionalist or the center at which the procedure is performed.

Commercially available sets that are specifically designed for TIPS placement are available in the United States:

- Colapinto transjugular and biopsy set (Cook, Bloomington, IN). This includes a 16-gauge colapinto puncture needle.
- Rosch-Uchida transjugular liver access set (Cook). This includes a 14-gauge needle with a trocar.
- Angiodynamics TIPS set (Angiodynamics, Queensbury, NY).
- Ring transjugular intrahepatic access set (Cook).
- Ring pediatric transjugular intrahepatic access set (Cook).

The right internal jugular vein is accessed, usually with ultrasonographic guidance. The left jugular vein may also be used if the right vein is unsuitable for any reason. Techniques involving a femoral venous approach have also been described, but these are used much less commonly, and they are technically more demanding (LaBerge, 1991).

With standard catheter exchange, a 5F catheter with a multipurpose curve is placed into the right hepatic vein. The catheter is wedged in a peripheral branch of the right hepatic vein. Wedged hepatic venography is then performed with carbon dioxide gas to opacify the portal venous system.

Typically, a 50-mL manual injection of CO_2 is used. This procedure usually demonstrates the location of the main PV, as well as that of the left and right branches. Frequently, more than one CO_2 injection is required to obtain a good portogram. If wedged injection fails to fill the PV, an occlusion balloon catheter may be used. Biplane CO_2 wedged hepatic venograms and biplane fluoroscopy can be used.

By using the wedged hepatic venogram images as a guide, the colapinto needle is advanced through the wall of the right hepatic vein and directed in an anteroinferior direction to access the right PV. Some have advocated injecting CO_2 as the needle is advanced through the liver to more definitively guide the puncture.

If a good wedged venogram cannot be obtained, selection of an appropriate site for puncture from the hepatic vein to PV is accomplished with a thorough understanding of the hepatic anatomy. The right hepatic vein lies superior and posterior to the PV bifurcation, and the right PV usually courses lateral to the T11 vertebral body. The portal bifurcation may be extrahepatic in a large percentage of patients. An extrahepatic puncture can lead to life-threatening hemorrhage, whereas puncture of a peripheral portal venous branch can create an angle that is too acute for successful TIPS placement.

From the right hepatic vein, the needle is usually aimed anteromedially and caudally, then advanced 3-4 cm within the liver. Several punctures may be necessary for success. Large volume paracentesis before TIPS in a patient with massive ascites can facilitate cannulation of the hepatic vein and puncture of the PV.

The needle is gently aspirated as it is withdrawn across the parenchymal tract. Once, portal venous blood is freely aspirated; contrast material is injected through the needle to verify the point of entry into the vessel. An intrahepatic access site with entry into the right PV at least 1 cm from the main PV bifurcation is desired. A guidewire and catheter are advanced into the PV, and portal venography is performed.

Pressure measurements are obtained in the PV as well as in the right atrium. The difference between the measured pressures yields the portosystemic gradient. If the pressure gradient is significantly elevated (>12 mm Hg), the TIPS are placed. If the gradient is not elevated, the presence of a competitive shunt, such as a spontaneous splenorenal shunt, must be evaluated. The spontaneous shunts can be used to lower the portosystemic gradient, but they are not true vessels and lack normal vascular integrity, which poses a risk for rupture.

The intrahepatic parenchymal tract is dilated with an 8- or 10-mm high-pressure balloon such as a Blue-Max balloon (Boston Scientific Vascular, Natick, MA). Images of the initial balloon waist are saved because they demonstrate the locations of the PV entry site and the hepatic vein exit site. A self-expanding metallic stent, such as the Wallstent (Boston Scientific Vascular), is then deployed across the tract and dilated to the desired diameter by using an angioplastic balloon.

Proper stent placement is crucial, especially if the patient is undergoing subsequent orthotopic liver transplantation. The stent should form a smooth and gentle curve and must extend adequately into the portal and hepatic veins. Overextension of a stent into the PV, hepatic vein, or inferior vena cava can be problematic for the transplant surgeon. The Wallstent significantly shortens as it is deployed, and the ability to predict and achieve appropriate final stent placement improves with experience. Self-expanding nitinol stents minimally shorten with deployment are also available from multiple manufacturers, and the use of one of these may be helpful for more predictable stent placement.

The stent may need to be dilated 8-12 mm, depending on the indication for TIPS and the stent used. Post placement venography is performed and pressures are measured to confirm adequate stent positioning, good flow through the TIPS, and reduction in the portosystemic gradient. If needed, additional stent placement or further balloon dilation can be performed to obtain a final portosystemic gradient of 8-12 mm Hg. Postplacement venography revealing persistent variceal filling indicates that insufficient decompression has been achieved with the stent. These varices can be selectively catheterized and embolized with coils.

Complications

A large number of complications can occur during and after placement of a TIPS (Freedman, 1993). Complications related to the puncture site include pneumothorax, vessel or tissue injury, and arteriovenous fistula formation. Ultrasonographic guidance for the jugular puncture can minimize these complications. Placement of the catheter in the right atrium can cause serious cardiac dysrhythmias. Cardiac monitoring should be continued throughout the TIPS procedure and during the initial post procedural period.

Complications can occur during the creation of the intrahepatic tract. The needle can, injure the hepatic artery or bile ducts. Capsular tears can result in life-threatening hemorrhage when they occur in association with a hepatic artery puncture. Portal venous puncture in an extrahepatic location can result in significant bleeding complications. Puncture of the right PV at least 1-2 cm distal to the PV bifurcation more often than not assures that an intrahepatic TIPS has been created.

A major concern of a newly placed TIPS is new-onset or worsened encephalopathy, which occurs in about 25% of treated patients. Patients often have hepatic encephalopathy immediately after shunt placement, and symptoms diminish as the shunt undergoes fibrous changes and resultant narrowing over time.

Aside from hepatic encephalopathy, the second most common complication associated with TIPS placement is shunt stenosis and occlusion.

Deterioration of the patient's hemodynamic status is also a concern after TIPS placement because acute increases in cardiac output and central venous and pulmonary wedge pressures can result in acute pulmonary edema and congestive heart failure (Quiroga, 1995). Patients should be closely monitored after the procedure until their hemodynamic status stabilizes.

Advanced TIPS Techniques

Various techniques to facilitate portal venous access, including ultrasound guidance, have been described. If standard portal venous access fails, the author prefers to percutaneously place a transhepatic Chiba (Cook) needle, which can be used as a target under fluoroscopy to advance the Colapinto needle. This approach adds an extra step to the procedure, and it is usually not appropriate in patients with large amounts of perihepatic ascites. Alternatively, puncture of a patent umbilical vein can provide access into the portal system. An approach for creating TIPS is by using a combination of transfemoral access to the hepatic vein with transmesenteric access to the portal system by means of minilaparotomy has also been described (Rozenblit, 1996).

If direct PV and right atrial pressures (measured to determine the portosystemic gradient) show a less-than-expected gradient, a competitive shunt (spontaneous splenorenal or large varices) should be excluded by advancing the catheter into the splenic or mesenteric vein and injecting bolus of contrast agent with digital imaging. Competitive shunts can be selectively embolized with coils, if necessary. Although the shunts may decrease the portosystemic gradient, they are thin walled and can spontaneously rupture, causing life-threatening hemorrhage. If no competitive shunt is found and if the gradient is less than 12 mm Hg, TIPS is not indicated, and alternate explanations for the bleeding should be sought. Upper GI bleeding may be related to a cause other than portal hypertension in as many as 25% of cases.

An 8 mm diameter stent is usually acceptable in patients with refractory ascites, whereas a 10-12 mm shunt may be needed in patients with life-threatening hemorrhage. Wallstents can be overdilated to about 10% larger than their nominal diameter to allow further gradient reduction. Nitinol stents cannot be overdilated in this way. In some cases, two parallel shunts are required to effectively lower the portosystemic gradient. Most commonly, TIPS result in complete reversal of intrahepatic PV flow and markedly reduce variceal blood flow.

SUPER SELECTIVE EMBOLIZATION

Super selective embolization of the mesenteric vessels is an alternative technique for treating massive lower GI bleeding. Rosch and colleagues first described this technique in 1972. Autologous clot, Gelfoam, polyvinyl alcohol, microcoils, ethanolamine, and oxidized cellulose can be used as embolic agents. Embolization involves superselective catheterization of the bleeding vessel to minimize necrosis, the most feared complication of ischemic colitis.

Rosenkrantz *et al.* reported three cases of colonic infarction. One patient, died following segmental colectomy, and the other patients revealed full-thickness bowel wall injury in the resected specimen. Intestinal ischemia and infarction have also been reported. In order to prevent this complication, perform embolization beyond the marginal artery as close as possible to the bleeding point in the terminal mural arteries.

Section 6—Alimentary Tract

Chapter 78

Hernia of the Abdominal Wall

ABDOMINAL WALL HERNIA (Figure 78.1)

A hernia is the protrusion of a viscous / part of a viscus through an abnormal opening in the wall of its containing cavity.

Table 78.1: Types of hernia

Abdominal	Pelvic
• Umbilical hernia (Figure 78.2)	• Inguinal – Direct – Indirect
• Ventral hernia	• Femoral hernia • Spigelian hernia • Obturator hernia
• Lumbar hernia	• Sciatic hernia
• Incisional	• Perineal hernia

Diagnosis of hernia is established clinically.

CT is the investigation of choice.

Differential diagnosis is between a hernia and a mass within the abdominal cavity or wall. In case of bowel herniation – complication like ischemia and obstruction.

Ventral Hernia

- Anterior and lateral aspect of abdominal wall.
- Majority through linea alba.

ANATOMY OF ABDOMINAL WALL

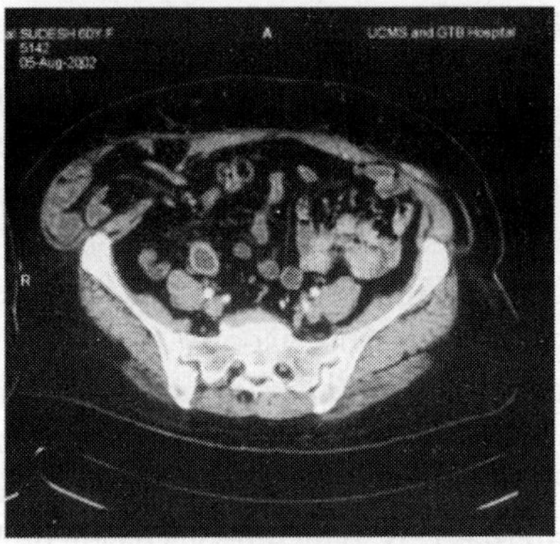

Fig. 78.1: Axial CT image shows hernia through the right anterior abdominal wall

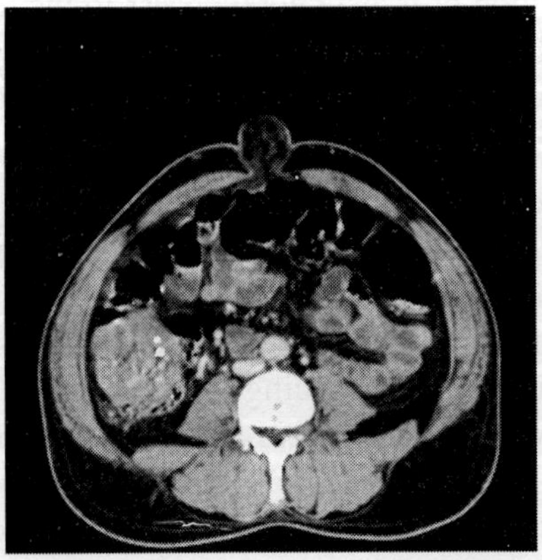

Fig. 78.2: Axial CT image shows umbilical hernia with fat as its content

- Above the umbilicus – epigastric hernia.
- Below the umbilicus – hypogastric hernia.
- *Contents:* Colon, properitoneal fat or bowel loops.
- Aperture – small – incarceration and strangulation.
- Common in manual labourers between 30-45 years.
- Sudden strain causes tearing of the interlacing fibres of the linea alba.
- Barium studies reveal distended bowel loops, proximal to a narrowing or obstruction in close relationship to a locally tender part of the abdominal wall.
- CT, MR, USG – reveal the actual defect and associated herniation in the ventral wall of the abdomen.

Incisional Hernia

- It is the herniation of peritoneal sac through an acquired scar in the abdominal wall, caused by a previous surgical operation (8%) or an accidental trauma.
- Tend to occur during the 1st 4 months after surgery.
- Most common site along midline and paramedian incision.
- Risk factors – Obesity, diabetes, malnutrition, etc.
- *Cause*: Division of motor nerves supplying the muscles around the wound. Inadequate hemostasis – wound hematoma, wound infection.
- *Contents*: Properitoneal fat, edge of colon, bowel loops.
- *Barium studies*: Profile view of old surgical scar while the patient strains on fluoroscopy will reveal the diagnosis.
- CT can show small defect in peritoneal and fascial layers of abdominal wall through which omentum or small portion of intestine protrudes in the subcutaneous fat. It can also detect ischemic changes caused by strangulated bowel loops.

Spigelian Hernia

- Variety of interparietal hernia, where hernial sac passes between the layers of the lower anterior lateral abdomen wall along the semilunar line.
- 2% of the anterior abdominal wall hernia.
- R: L = 1.6:1.
- Usually seen in male, mean age – 50 years.
- Congenital or acquired:
  - Previous operation.
  - Obesity.
  - Multiple pregnancy.
  - Prostatic increase.
  - Chronic pulmonary disease.
- Hernia can occur at any point along the semilunar line. 90% through spigelian fascia – broad and weak – region (because of Spigelian belt (S'belt)) is a 6 cm horizontal transverse zone located within a plane between the umbilicus and a line joining the both anterior iliac spines.
- Presentation – well localised constant abdominal pain with or without palpable lump.
- *Contents*: The defect and hernial sac usually small <2 cm, usually empty, but there may be small or large bowel, omentum or even part of stomach wall in the hernial sac.

  20%-25% of patients presents with strangulation.
- Imaging

  Plain X-ray/barium studies

  Bowel loops outside the confinement of the peritoneal cavity on tangential views.

  USG
  - Discontinuity of deepest layer of peritoneum and properitoneal fat on transverse scans.

– Hernial sac in interparietal plane – more prominent on valsalva manoeuvre.
– Sac contents like intestine or omentum and reducibility of content by probe compression.

Signs of Incarceration

- Free fluid in hernial sac.
- Bowel wall thickness in hernia (>4 mm) fluid within herniated bowel loops.
- Dilated bowel loops in abdomen.
- Absence of blood flow and peristalsis within hernia.
- Intramural gas and free gas in abdominal/hernial sac.
- CT – best to visualize the hernia defect and interstitial protrusion of the omentum or intestinal loops.

Adult Umbilical Hernia (Paraumbilical Hernia)

- Usually seen in females.
- *Contents*: Stomach, various segments of small or large bowel loops.
- *Incarcerated hernia*: X-ray distended bowel, loops and soft tissue density.
- Coned down lateral/cross table view of anterior abdominal wall with ↓ kVp – shows the omental fat on bowel loop.
- USG/CT: Bowel protruding through the umbilical defect.

Lumbar Hernia

- Two areas of weakness.
- Superior lumbar space bounded superiorly by 12th rib, anteriorly by internal oblique. Muscle and posteriorly by spinal muscle.
- Inferior lumbar triangle/Petit's triangle bounded inferiorly by iliac crest, anteriorly by external oblique muscle and posteriorly by latissimus dorsi muscle.
- Most are seen in larger superior lumbar space.
- *Contents*: Bowel loops, retroperitoneal fat, kidney or other viscera.
- Symptoms – Chronic low backache, intestinal obstruction.
- Bowel incarceration – 25%, strangulation in 10%.
- CT can best delineate the precise location and content of lumbar hernia.

Inguinal Hernia

Indirect – MC Type

- Peritoneal sac, containing bowel loops protrudes through the inguinal canal and emerges at its external ring.
- *Contents:* Small bowel loops, mobile colon loops.
- *Intestinal obstruction*: 15%.
- *X-ray supine*: Convergence of distended intestinal loops towards the inguinal region. Soft tissue density/gas containing mass overlying the ipsilateral obturator foramen.
- Ba studies show tapered narrowing or obstruction of intestinal segment as it enters the hernia orifice.
- CT/USG reveal the hernia contents and differentiate it from other masses.

Direct Inguinal Hernia–Less Common

- Mostly in males.
- Visceral protrusion directly through the lower abdominal wall in a weak area, medial to inferior epigastric vessels.
- Rarely becomes incarcerated.

Femoral Hernia

Predominantly in females.

- Herniation within the femoral canal.
- *Contents*: Retroperitoneal fat, edge of

omentum, small bowel can displace or narrow the femoral vessels and descend along saphenous vein.

- *Neck of hernia* – Always remains below are inguinal ligament and lateral to pubic tubercle.
- 8-12 times more prone to incarceration and strangulation than indirect inguinal hernia.

Obturator Hernia

- It occurs through the obturator canal in the superolateral aspect of the obturator foramen.
- 80-90% seen in elderly females.
- *Content*: (R>L) ileal loops.
- Contents are often incarcerated in the canal or in the space between the pectineus and obturator muscle.
- *Abdominal X-ray/Barium* – Bowel obstruction together with a fixed loop containing some gas or contrast in the obturator region.
- CT shows a soft tissue mass or opacified loop that protrudes through the obturator foramen and extends between the pectineus and obturator muscle.

Sciatic Hernia

- Rarest.
- Hernia exits the pelvis through greater or lesser sciatic foramen.
- *Contents* – Bowel, ureter, urinary bladder, ovary.
- Frequently complicated by incarceration, obstruction and strangulation.
- CT shows a hernial sac as a mass of thickened bowel and other pelvic contents protruding posterior to the ischial spine.

Section 7—Excretory System

Chapter 79

Embryological Development of Excretory System

1. DEVELOPMENT OF KIDNEYS AND URETERS

- Three sets of structures in urinary system appear during 5th – 7th week of intrauterine life called the:
  - Pronephros.
  - Mesonephros; and
  - Metanephros – responsible for permanent kidneys.
- Develops from two sources:
  1. Ureteric bud from mesonephric duct.
  2. Metonephrogenic cap from the intermediate cell mass of mesenchyme of lower lumbar and sacral region.

Table 79.1: Details of development

Ureteric bud	Metanephrogenic cap
Arises as an outgrowth of mesonephric duct. It forms	Condenses around ureteric bud and forms the glomerular capsules
1. Ureter	
2. Uretric pelvis	PCT
3. Major calyces	DCT
4. Minor calyces	The loops of Henle
5. Collecting tubules	

Migration of Kidneys (Figure 79.1)

The developing kidney is initially a pelvic organ and receives its blood supply from pelvic continuation of aorta, the middle sacral artery.

↓

- Later the kidneys ascend up the posterior abdominal wall. This so called absent is caused by growth of body in lumbar and sacral region and by straightening of its curvature. The ureters elongates as the ascent continues.

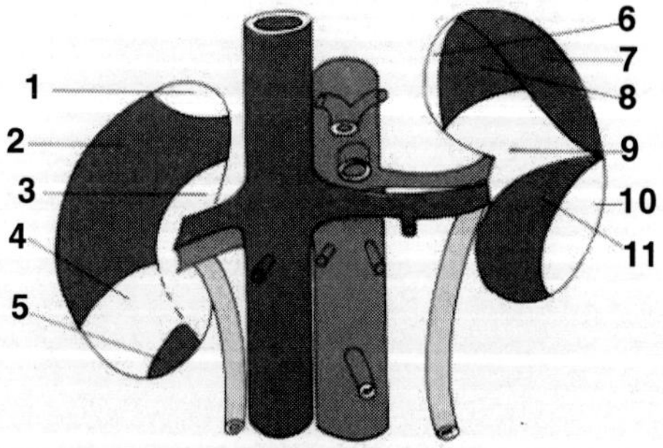

1. Suprarenal, 2. Liver, 3. Duodenum, 4. Colon, 5. Small Intestine, 6. Suprarenal, 7. Spleen, 8. Stomach, 9. Pancreas, 10. Colon, 11. Small Intestine

Fig. 79.1: Figure shows relationship of kidneys

2. DEVELOPMENT OF BLADDER

- In the seventh gestational week the rectal septum fuses with cloneal membrane dividing it into:

Ventral	Dorsal
Urogenital/sinus	Anorectal canal
Bladder	Rectum

Initially bladder is continued with atentosis, which eventually becomes a fibrous cord the cihous (known as median umbilical ligament in adults).

- As the bladder enlarges, the distal portion of mesonephric duct is incorporated as connective tissue into the bladder trigger. At the same time cultures comes to open separately into bladder.

  In infants/children – Abdominal organ often puberty – becomes a true pelvic structures.

DEVELOPMENT OF URETHRA

Males

Prostatic Urethra

1. Proximal part as far as opening of the ejaculatory ducts – Mesonephric ducts.

   Distal part — Urogenital sinus pelvic part.
2. Membranous urethra — Pelvic part of urogenital sinus.
3. Penile urethra — Phallic part of urogenital sinus.

Females

Upper two third–Mesonephric ducts.

Lower one third–Urogenital sinus.

RADIOLOGICAL ANATOMY

Plain Film of the Abdomen (X-ray KUB)

Outline of several structures can be seen on KUB including kidneys, psoas end bladder outlines. It also tells about the bowel gas pattern and the lung bases.

- The clarity of renal outline varies from person to person according to the amount of perinephric foli.
- Outlines were clearly viewed on oblique view owing to greater depth of renal tissue and fat when viewer in this position. The kidney appears as bear shaped structures with their concavity pointing medially.
- The renal hilum lies at the level of biventriculum.
- Upper pole lies at the level of T11 and lower pole opposite L3 vertebra.
- The right kidneys lies a variable distance lower than the left owing to presence of liver.
- The quiet respiration they move up and down .
- Principal use of KUB is in the assessment of urinary tract calculi.
- Apart from calyces the potential sites of impaction of stones are:
  1. Pelivuretric junction.
  2. When ureter kinks as it passes from pelvic brim to enter pelvis.
  3. Where ureter pierces bladder wall.

RELATIONS OF KIDNEYS

Anterior

- Right supra renal gland.
- Liver.
- Second part of duodenum.
- Hepatic flexure of colon and small intestine.

Out of above, the hepatic and intestinal surfaces are covered by peritoneum.

The lateral border of the right kidney is related to the right lobe of the liver and to the hepatic flexure of the colon.

Posterior

- The diaphragm.
- The costodiaphragmatic recesses of pleura.
- 11th/12th rib.
- The process quadratus lumbarum and transverse abdominal muscle.
- The subcostal, iliohypogastic and ilioinguinal nerves run downward and laterally.

COVERINGS OF KIDNEYS

1. *Fibrous capsule:* Surrounds the kidney and is closely applied to the outer surface.
2. *Perirenal fat:* Covers the fibrous capsule.
3. *Renal fascia:* Condensation of connective tissue that lies outside the pleurorenal fat and encloses the kidneys and suprarenal.
4. *Para renal fat:* External to renal fascia is a part of retroperitoneal fat.

EXCRETION UROGRAPHY

A. Parenchyma

- The renal parenchyma is bounded by surface of kidney outlined by perirenal fat and by the margins of calyceal system and the fat in renal sinus.
- The distance from the surface of the kidney to the ilio-psoas renal papillae judges the thickness of renal parenchyma.
- The renal parenchyma appears thicken at the poles than in the mid parrt of the kidney.
- On the right liver may flatten the upper and outer margin of the kidney and this is sometimes misinterpreted as localised loss of renal substance.
- Persistance of fetal lobulation into adult life cum produces characteristic notching of renal outline. Can be differentiated from other causes of irregularity by the symmetry and shape and by absence of any deformity of underlying calices.

B. Papillae and Calices

- The superior end of ureter expands to form the renal pelvis, which divides into 2-4 major calyces each of which divides into 2-4 minor calyces.
- Each calyx is indented by a papilla, which in the apex of medullary pyramid. The farnices extends around the convexity of the papilla.

3. ULTRASOUND

A. Parenchyma

- The low level echoes of renal parenchyma stands out clearly against the bright echoes of the surrounding perinephric fat and of the renal sinus fat.
- On good quality images cortex and medulla can be differentiated.
- The pyramids are seen as triangular structures of low reflectivity than the surrounding cortex.
- The arcuate arteries may be seen as bright dot at their bases.

B. Sinus

- The central cluster of bright sinus echoes is largely produced by renal sinus fat.
- The normal pelicalyceal system is not usually seen.

C. Ultrasound Gives Accurate Measurement of Renal Length

In a large study maximum length of normal

adult kidney was found to vary between 10-12.5cm.

- Renal length relates to body size and decreases with age.
- Measurement of renal length on USG is of order of 0.5 cm less than on IVU, which suffers from radiographic magnification.
- A difference of 2cm or more between two kidneys raises the possibility of unilateral disease. In young healthy adults cortical thickness is of index of 2.5-3cm at the poles and 1.5-2.0cm elsewhere. This may decrease substantially with age.
- The pelviuretric and vesico uretric junction may be seen on USG especially when discussed but otherwise normal ureter is not routinely demonstrated.

Bladder

- Routine examination requires it to be moderately full. The normal bladder has a triangular shape in the sagittal plane and that of a square with rounded off in transverse plane. The normal wall thickness is 2-8 mm when bladder is moderately full.

4. CT SCAN

- The normal renal parenchyma is of intermediate density (30-60 HU).
- The renal sinus and perinephric fat are low density around 10-50 HU.
- Following IV contrast the cortex enhances more rapidly than medulla appearing more dense from around 20-60 sec when there is maximum CMD. Around 60-110 sec, the renal parenchyma become homogenously high density around 80-120 HU.

5. M.R.I.

- On T1 weighted images the renal cortex is of similar signal intensity to liver. The medulla is slightly lower signal, similar to spleen.
- On T2 weighted images kidneys are diffusely high signal similar to spleen. The bladder is seen as a thin low signal of fat outside and urine inside the bladder.

Section 7—Excretory System

Chapter 80

Congenital Anomalies of Urinary Tract

EMBRYOLOGY

Development of urinary system from 3 stages:

1. Pronephron.
2. Mesonephros.
3. Metanephros.

Major events are:

- Emergence of ureteral band from each mesonephric duct.
- Development of each bud by mesoderm.
- Deviation of PCS and collecting ducts from bud.
- Development of nephrons from mesoderm.
- Confluence of lumen of DCT's with coll. duct.
- Ascent of kidney.
- Rotation of kidney.

Bladder and Urethra

Urogenital sinus → ant part of the cloacae

↓ Superior vesico urethral canal

↓ Inferior definitive bladder urogenital sinus

Mesonephric duct

Segment between mesonephric duct and ureter

↓

Trigone

Congenital Anomalies

Renal Anomalies

Abnormalities of number.

a. Unilateral renal agenesis.

Incidence 1/1000 to 1/1500.

Expected radiological findings in unilateral agenesis:

1. Absence of renal density on plain X-ray K.U.B.
2. On USG – Absence of Kidney in Renal Fosse, Absent Renal Artery when seen on Doppler.

Compensatory hypertrophy of contralaterals kidney.

3. On IVU, lack of excretion of contrast.
4. On cystoscopy, absence of ureteral meatus.
5. On cystoscopy, hemitrigone or blind ending ureter.
6. At aortography absent renal artery.
7. Evidence of compensatory hypertrophy.
8. Selective renal phlebography – demonstration of main renal vein – rules out agenesis.

Bilateral Renal Agenesis

- Uncommon.
- Incompatible with life–post natally.
- High incidence of pulmonary hypoplasia.
- Potter fascies.

Supernumerary Kidney

- Is an extra kidney, which is completely encapsulated and not fused.

  ↓

  Extreme degree of duplication.
- Lies cephalad, smaller with few calyces and single infundibulum.
- Can be U/L on B/L.

D/D – calculus.

- Inflammation.
- Hydronephrosis.
- Pyonephrosis.
- Radiologic findings include:
  1. At IVU, duplication of pelvis /ureter (Figure 80.1).
  2. Angio –separate renal arteries.
  3. Hydronephrosis +/-.

Abnormalities of Position

A. Malrotation of the Kidney

Findings include:

1. Upper pole of the kidney is located more laterally than the lower pole and thus the upper pole calyces are therefore lateral to lower pole calyces, pelvis usually placed more anterior.

   U/S – Abnormal axis of kidney detected with position of pelvis. Also rules out horseshoe kidneys however a 99mTcDMSA scan with anterior views are required to assess the fusion of the isthmus.

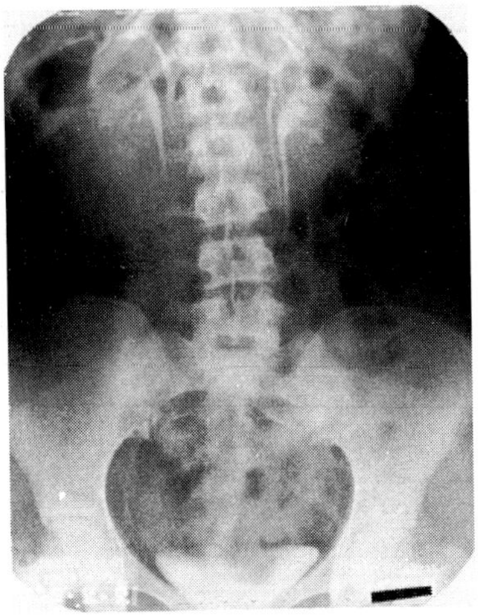

Fig. 80.1: Intravenous pyelography shows duplex pelvis with double proximal ureters on both sides

2. Ectopy (Figure 80.2)
   - USG – Extra small kidney seen cephalic to the normal kidneys. Smaller with few

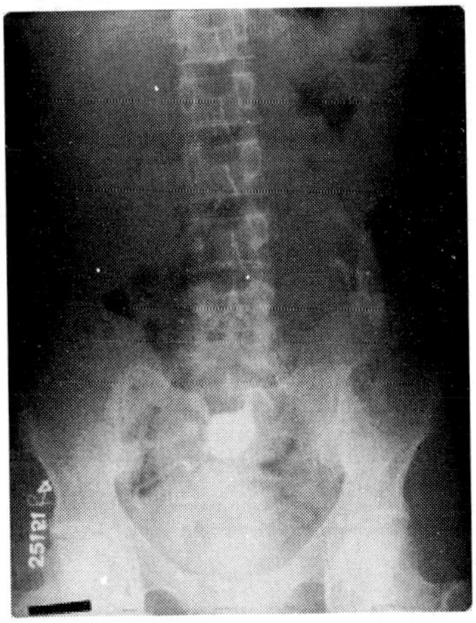

Fig. 80.2: Intravenous pyelography shows bilateral renal ectopia

calyces. On Doppler separate renal artery from aorta.

- Pelvic kidney is usually small or malrotated or present as pelvic mass or hydronephrosis.
- Supply – Common iliac, internal iliac.
- Thoracic ectopia – Lower thoracic aorta or upper aorta.

Abnormalities of Fusion

A. **Horseshoe kidney** (Figures 80.3 and 80.4) – Most common fusion anomaly.

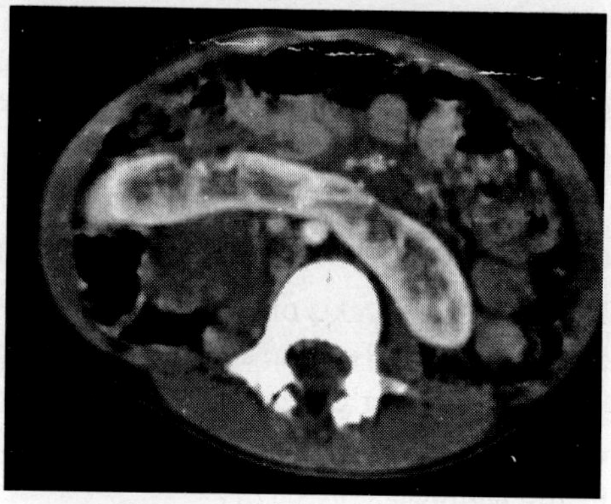

Fig. 80.3: Axial CT image shows a horseshoe kidney in a patient with a right retroperitoneal mass

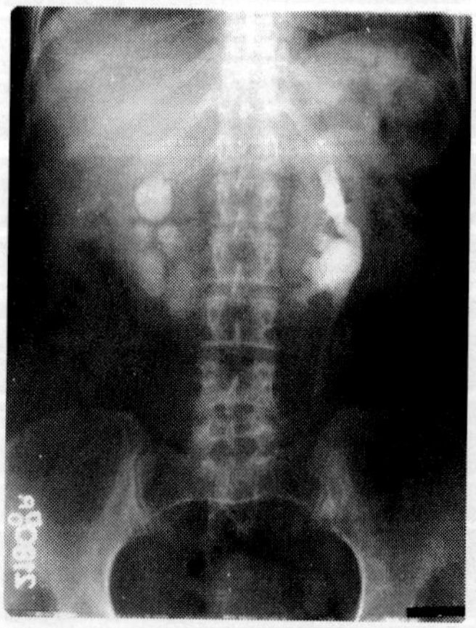

Fig. 80.4: Intravenous pyelography shows a horseshoe kidney with bilateral hydronephrosis, more prominent on right side

Fusion between 2 meta nephric blastomas.

95% ↓ Lower pole

5% ↓ Upper pole

- Joined by isthmus – Renal parenchyma
  Fibrosis tissue.

↓

Unable to ascents and rotate and located anterior to aorta and IVC.

Blood supply	Associated complications
IMA	prone to trauma
CIA	Obstruction
RIA	Calculus
IIA	Infections
	V.U.R.
	Carcinoma (Wilms).

Radiologic Findings are:

1. Plain X-ray – Kidney lie more vertically, near midline and at a lower level.
2. IVU – Lower poles more medial than the upper, isthmus may or may not be demonstrable.

   Ureters pass above the isthmus

   ↓

   And are more lateral than normal

   PUJ located anteriorly.
3. Aortography – Accessory renal vessels are common.

B. **Disk kidney**

- Single renal mass
  - Lump
  - Pancake
  - Doughnut
- S, C, L J shape.
- Usually two ureters opening normally.

C. **Crossed fused renal ectopia** (Figure 80.5)

- Ectopic kidney almost always lie caudal to the other.
- Malascent and malrotation.

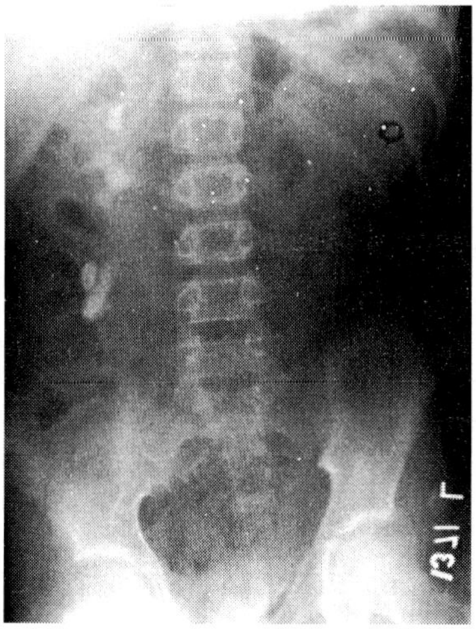

Fig. 80.5: Intravenous pyelography shows crossed renal ectopia on right side

Radiologic Findings are:

X-ray - Abnormal irregular renal mass on one side and the absence of renal mass on the other side.

IVU - Two complete PCS on one side usually one above the other.

Upper ureter is deviated as it crosses anteriorly across midline to its normal opening.

D. Abnormalities of form

Dysplasia	ARPD.
Multicystic kidney	ADPD.

Renal Dysplasia

Small.

US – Loss of normal CMD.

Small transonic areas (1-2 mm).

Smooth outline.

Focal dysplasia – USK – UPMARK kidney.

If B/L – CRF

↑ VUR

Syndromes associated are:

- Lawrence-Moon Biedl syndrome.
- Beckwith-Wiedemann syndrome.
- Meckel's syndrome.

Multicystic Dysplastic Kidney

- Large non-functioning with numerous cystic spaces.
- Ureteral atresia is always (+).

Polycystic Renal Diseases

ARPD	ADPD
Usually associated with liver fibrosis	Uncommon for it to present at infancy.
Caroli's disease	Ultrasound most sensitive
Enlarged kidneys	modality for diagnosis
Loss of CMD with bright medulla	

IVU – streaking of contrast.

↓

Best seen on delayed image.

RENAL PELVIC AND URETERIC ANOMALIES

A. Duplication/Ureteric Ectopia

- Results from the growth of two separate metanephric ducts with both buds reaching the blastoma.
- Seesaw peristalsis common lower ureter.

Development of distal ureteric insertion.

Radiologic Findings are:

1. Soft tissue mass at upper pole causing lateral displacement.
2. IVU delayed function upper dilated segment.

   "Drooping likely" sign.

   Dilated tortuous proximal ureter with distal insertion.

   Usually bilateral duplication.
3. Urethral triplication.

   Very rare anomaly classified into 4 types.

Type I	Complete with 3 separate orifices.
Type II	Double ureter with one being bifid – Two orifices.
Type III	Trifid ureter – One orifice.
Type IV	Double ureter with 3 orifices.

B. Blind Ending Ureter

From failure of metanephric duct to connect with the metanephric blastoma.

C. Ureteral Diverticulum

Due to persistent narrowing or obstruction, diverticulae appear which later on clinically manifest as incontinence of urine.

D. Congenital Ureteral Stenosis

Common sites - PUJ.

VUJ.

Findings – If distally— markedly dilated hydroureter

↓ Pressure defect of the filled blaster.

E. Ureteral Webs and Bands

- Very rare primarily.
- Are flap like leaflet or annular diaphragm with pin point opening.

↓

Obstruction

↓

Proximal hydrouretero nephrosis

F. Congenital Megaloureter

- Usually there is slight to moderate dilatation of the pelvic segment.

  Neurogenic/myogenic cause.

Retrocaval ureter.

Normal right ureter is anterior to IVC.

Normal deviation from supra cardinal veins.

↓

If there is persistent.

Subcardinal vein.

↓

Ureter lies behind IVC.

On IVU – Proximally dilated ureter with sharp medial deviation at L2-L3 level.

↓

Characteristically Reversed J Appearance.

G. Congenital Megacalicosis

- Marked caliceal dilatation with > 14 calices and very little dilatation of the renal pelvis.

H. Ectopic Ureterocele

Simple	Ectopic
↓	↓
Always non duplex	Always duplex moieties

Saccular dilatation of the intramural portion of a ureter as it passes through the bladder wall.

Cx. VUR

IVU – cobra head appearance.

BLADDER ANOMALIES

Exstrophy/Epispadias Male: Female = 3:1.

V

|

More benign	More severe	Genital stroma is normal.
Diastasis at pubic symphysis >25 mm.	Diastasis is 10+ few num only.	↑ adenoma/ adenocarcinoma incidence.

PRUNE BELLY SYNDROME

Ultrasound Diagnosis – Absent abdominal wall muscles.

+

Undescended testis

+

Renal dysplasia accompanied with grossly dilated PCS.

- Is a developmental abnormality due to mesenchymal arrest.
- Predominantly seen in males.
- Plain X-ray protuberant abdomen resulting from the lack of musculature.

Features of Renal Tract

- Small kidneys with abnormal calyces.
- Minimal dilatation of the PCs.
- Upper mildly dilated ureter with lower ureters showing marked tortuous disproportionate dilatation.
- UB thin walled, irregularly shaped, wide necked non-trabeculated bladder.
- Patent urachus/urachal diverticulum may be present.
- Post urethra is markedly dilated with conical narrowing.

Duplication of the Bladder

Two Types

Complete duplication	Diminution of lumen by long or transverse septum.

Urachal Anomalies

- Congenital patent urachus.
- Umbilical urachal sinus.
- Vesico urachal diverticulum.
- Urachal cyst.
- The alternating sinus.

URETHRAL ANOMALIES

Posterior urethral valves (Figure 80.6).

Bilateral hydronephrosis with distended urinary bladder on antenatal ultrasound with progressive oligohydramnios.

↓

Pulmonary Hypoplasia – Suspected post urethral valve.

Usually of ¾ types – Type-I is most common.

2 fold at the level of vern montanum with ventral central slit lit orifice.

Type III - Pin point eccentric orifice.

↓

Forward ballooning of the valve.

↓

"Wind in the sail appearance".

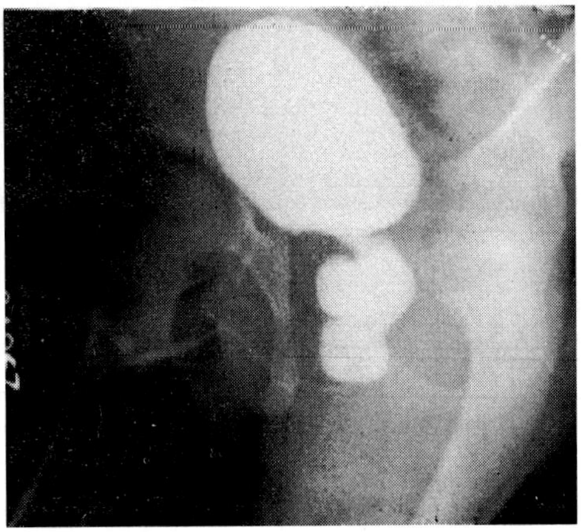

Fig. 80.6: Micturating cystourethrogram shows posterior urethral dilatation secondary to posterior urethral valves

Complications

- Urinoma.
- Urinary ascites.

Urethral atresia – Rare.

Rectourethral fistula – Usually accompanied with imperforate anus.

Urethral duplication – hypospadius.

Anterior urethral anomalies – valve, flap or diverticulum.

Section 7—Excretory System

Chapter 81

Radiology of Unilateral Enlarged Kidney with Dilated Pelvi-calyceal System

CAUSES

- Congenital mega calices.
- Mega cystic mega meter syndrome.
- Prime belly syndrome.
- Duplex kidney.
- PUJ obstruction.
- Pyonephrosis.
- Renal pelvic calculus.
- Benign polyp of renal pelvis.
- Multi locular cystic nephroma/Wilm's causing extrinsic obstruction.
- Ureteral filling defects (stone, blood clot, the papilloma, fungus ball).
- Ureteral valve, stricture.
- Retrocaval ureter.
- Primary on metastatic to invading or compressing ureters.
- Retroperitoneal fibrosis.
- Primary megaureter.
- Congenital ureterovesicle obstruction.
- Ectopic ureter.
- Ectopic ureterocele.
- Simple ureterocele.
- Bladder neoplasm obstructing UV given.

INVESTIGATIONS

1. **IVP:**

   Previously the imaging method of choice for pediatric kidney and collecting system has to a large extent supplemented by USG and nuclear scintigraphy.

   Commonly requested when an obstructing calculus or lesion is suspected.

2. **Retrograde Pyelography:**

   When more precise anatomic information is required. Test is valuable when IVP is contraindicated or causing poor renal function and inadequate contrast excretion.

3. **Antegrade Pyelography:**

   Prior to consideration of antegrade pyelography, clinical suspicion of obstruction should be high and previously confirmed by other examination – USG.

4. **Whitaker Test:**

   Generally used when a partial obstruction is identified but functional significance is uncertain. It explores the relationship between pressure and flow for a given partial obstruction. By using a constant flow rate (10 ml/min), the pressure generated to bypass the obstruction was obtained. After accounting for bladder pressure and intrinsic pressure of needle/tubing apparatus the resulting relative pressure is a quantitative measure of degree of obstruction. Higher pressures indicate greater likelihood of renal damage and parenchymal loss if no intervention undertaken. It is cited as gold standard for obstruction.

5. **USG:**
   - Non-invasive, quick, portable, inexpensive, requires neither CM nor ionizing radiation.
   - Provides anatomic information and may reveal level and cause of obstruction.
6. **Doppler ultrasound:**
   - Helps in distinguishing vessels from mildly dilatation (in some cases of what is termed mild HDN may in fact be prominent renal artery).
   - Evaluates ureteral patency by Doppler analysis of ureteral jets.

     With complete obstruction – no jet is detectable with partial obstruction – continuous low-level jet pattern i.e. asymmetric to other ureter.
   - Identifies functionally significant obstruction by detecting elevated intra renal arterial resistance.

     Obstruction can produce elevated RI, which includes dig (intrarenal arterial resistance – other obstruction):
     1. Elevation above threshold 0.7.
     2. Inter renal RI differentiation >0.6 to .1 with unilateral dilated.
     3. Abnormal RI response to diametis challenge.
7. **CT scan:**
   - NCCT is highly sensitive for detection of renal/ureteral calculi.
   - Once a potentially obstructed kidney is identified CT scan may aid determining the cause.
8. **MR:**

   MR urography has excellent diagnostic utility in patients of obstructive uropathy:
   - Is advantageous in children and pregnant women (therefore no radiation involved).
   - Can be performed even if renal function is impaired.
   - Demonstrates renal and surrounding anatomy.
   - Can assess function using I.V. Gadolinium.
   - Outlines dilated PCS; detects lower urinary calculi and depicts PVJ and extrinsic obstruction better than IVU.
   - Does not require bowel preparation and patient can be well hydrated.
9. **Nuclear renography:**

   It is very sensitive method to and renal parenchymal disease, renal function, cortical transit time and drainage phase. Also in study of renal hypertension. 99 m Tc mag-3, 99 m Tc DTPA, 99mTc GHA are the pharmaceuticals used in renal dynamic scintigraphy captopril renography is a method of choice for secondary hypertension.

CONGENITAL MEGACALICES

- It is the non-obstructive enlargement of calices accompanied by hypoplasia of medullary pyramid.
- This entity is important because it can be radiologically confused with obstructing or refluxing hydronephrosis.
- Renal pyramids are well defined; corticomedullary junction is distinct and cortical parenchyma is of normal thickness.

There is thinning of renal medullae. Papillae are flat or unapparent calix is therefore flat or converges outwards.

- It is a benign non-progressive condition.

IVU

- Caliceal dilatation of all or few of calices of one or both kidneys.
- Infundibular are short and broad, pelvis and ureters normal.
- No evidence of obstruction to ureter, bladder or urethra.
- Kidneys are larger than normal.
- Increase in number of calices.
- Prompt nephrographic phase, but opacification of pelvis and ureters may be delayed owing to large volume of contrast required to full calices.
- Associated nephrolithiasis.

USG

- Increased number of dilated calices.
- Normal thickness of cortex and thinning or attenuation of medulla.

PUJ OBSTRUCTION

- PUJ obstruction is by far the most common cause of neonatal hydronephrosis and a major cause of obstructive uropathy at all ages.
- Occurs most commonly in males than females.
- Most common on left side.
- Bilateral on 10-30%.
- Newborns and infants – palpable abdominal lump other children presents with abdominal pain; vomiting; hematuria; or UTI.
- PUJ obstruction may occur in duplex system where it affects the lower moiety.
- Malrotated kidney.
- Horse shoe and ectopic kidney (due to aberrant and multiple arterial vasculature).
- Associated with primary mega ureter and primary VUR.

Diagnostic Imaging

- In infants with known or suspected hydronephrosis from a prenatal ultrasound, a reevolution by abdominal ultrasound should be done soon after birth.

↓

- Diuretic hemogram.
- IVU at a later date, if indicated.
- Therein lies the challenge for clinician differentiating those who have asymptomatic hydronephrosis per se from those with obstruction, as obstruction needs surgical correction while non-obstructive hydronephrosis does not.

USG

- It provides the best evaluation of HDN both for screening and for follow up.
- The hydronephrotic kidney is enlarged, has a central cystic spaces, which is pelvis surrounded by multiple cystic areas which are dilated calyces.
- Ureter is not visualized.
- Differential Diagnosis multicystic dysplastic kidney – kidney is replaced by multiple cysts of variable sizes which do not communicate with each other, large one filterated at periphery.
- Renal length, A-P dia of renal pelvis, cortical thickness and echogenicity of cortex are important features noted on US.
- Progressive worsening of hydronephrosis were indicator of obstruction, whereas improvement in HDN suggests the opposite.

IVU

- Delayed opacification of collecting system.
- Marked pyelocaliectasis.

- Narrowing at PUJ.
- Incomplete visualization of a normal sized ureter.
- Retention of contrast material in collecting system on delayed films.
- In severe cases, nephrogram shows synergic, which is opaque rim of functioning parenchyma with multiple radio lucencies centrally placed.
- Contrast in compressed, realigned on dilated collecting tubules seen as curved bands (calyceal crescents) or dense dots (seen in E or B phase).
- Micturating cystourethrogram is indicated in all cases of neonatal hydronephrosis as VUR is found in upto 14% of children with suspected PVJ obst.
- Abdominal CT is requested in children presenting with a flank mass and shows hydronephrosis.
- When PUJ obstruction involves a horseshoe kidney, CT is best to assess isthmus anatomy. It is also used to determine level of obstruction in severely damaged kidneys.
- Following up of patients based on degree of hydronephrosis as measured by AP diameter and cortical thinning on US.
- Neonates with mild HDN (<12 mm) pre and postnatally require USG at 3 months and 1 year.
- If dilatation persists, CFB repeated at 2, 5 and 10 years of age.
- With moderate HDN (13-19 mm) and good function should undergo follow up US with nuclear renography at 3 months, 2, 5 and 10 years of age.
- Children with severe HDN (>20 mm) will have functional levels ranging from good to poor. After initial functional assessment, management should be conservative with follow up and nuclear renography at 3 months, 6 months, 1 year and yearly thereafter.
- Surgery is indicated if worsening HDN, deteriorating renal function, appearance of UTI, hematuria, pain or flank mass.
- Kidneys with dilatation >50 mm on AP dia should almost always have pyeloplasty by 6 months of age; kidneys with very poor function may warrant nephrectomy.

PYONEPHROSIS

- Infected debris with exudate or purulent material and in dilated and commonly obstructed urinary tracts.
- Proteus and E. coli.
- Hydronephrotic process caused by renal/ ureteric calculi.
- Clinically UTI with fever, flank pain, hematuria.

USG

- Echogenic material within dilated pelvicalyceal system, fluid debris is seen which changes with patients' position.

IVU

- Decreased renal function with poor visualization of kidney.

CT

- Hydronephrotic kidney with attenuation higher than that of uninfected urine fluid debris levels, renal stones and site of obstruction may be shown.

PRIMARY MEGAURETER

- Functional megaureter/ureteral achalasia.
- Juxtavesicular segment of ureter near the bladder is narrowed by increase in fibrous tissue or by circumferential tissue devoid of muscle.

IVU

- Dilated ureter tapers smoothly but abruptly just above ureterovesicle opening.
- Terminal aperistaltic segment is 0.5 to 4 cm in length.
- Mild forms are common – fusiform dilatation of lower ureter.
- It may cause severe obstructive HDN with parenchymal thinning and loss of renal function.
- In bilateral cases dilatation is assymetrical.

USG

- Hydronephrosis, hydroureter with narrow segment of distal ureter behind bladder.
- Increased persistalises with to and fro movements of urine may be seen in ureter.

MCU

- Should always be performed to make sure that VUR is not major cause of dilatated ureter. Clues to diagnose primary megaureter.
  1. Distal ureteral segment is normal in caliber.
  2. Opacity of refluxed contrast material in ureter is less than that in bladder (dilution by urine trapped above aperistalsis.
  3. Delayed drainage of contrast laden urine back its bladder.

ECTOPIC URETER

- An ectopic ureter is one that drains in an abnormal location either within bladder or extravesically.
- Intravesicle ectopia is not common.
- Ureter opens lateral/caudal to normal opening.
- Extravesicle ectopia is more common.
- Most common in girls.
- Associated with duplex system; upper pole ureter opens in ectopic position.
- Ectopic ureter opens in urethra, vestibule or vagina and clinically present incontinence of urine.
- In boys, opens in prostatic urethra, ejaculatory ducts, seminal vesicles, vas deferens or rectum.
- Incontinence is not +ve therefore opening is above external sphincter however, uretero-pyelocacectasis, inflammation prostatitis, or epididymitis most common complications.
- Ectopic ureter is usually unilateral.

IVU

- The termination of ectopic ureter may be demonstrated.
- A non-functioning upper renal mortality is present with corresponding PC system and ureter visualized only on delayed films.
- Lower pole moiety is displaced downwards and laterally giving appearance of drooping flower.

MCU

- Filling of ectopic ureter is possible if it terminates in urethra or by vaginography if in vagina.

USG

- Is helpful if anomalous ureter is dilated and can be followed down to and beyond bladder.
- Renal scan – demonstrate function.
- CECT or MR may demonstrate second ureter not demonstrated by other methods.

URETEROCELE

- Ureterocele is herniation of distal dilated end of ureter into bladder.
- Two types:
  - Intravesicle/simple ureterocele.
  - Ectopic ureterocele.

1. Intravesicle Ureterocele

- Most common in adults.
- <1 cm in diameters.
- Ureteral orifice is usually stenotic which is found on surface of ureterocele.
- Unilateral or bilateral seen in non-duplicated system.

MCU

- Radiolucent filling defect.
- S/E events and minimises diverticulum.

IVU

- Early films – round radio lucent defect in bladder.
- When contrast collects in its lumen – round/ oval density surrounded by radiolucent halo of ureterocele wall – cobra head appearance.

US

- Cystic mass with thin sharp wall protruding in lumen of bladder.
- It may be associated with hydroureter and hydronephrosis in severe cases.

2. Ectopic Ureterocele

Invariably associated with duplication, obstructs the ureter of upper pole moiety.

- Unilateral.
- Most common in males.
- Involved ureter is dilated and tortuous and renal moicty it drains is USG dysplastic.
- The distal dilated ectopic ureter terminates in a thin walled structure that balloons into bladder lumen and may extend through bladder neck into submucosal portions of proximal urethra.

  Ureter of lower pole renal moiety is usually associated and reflux and opens slightly superior and lateral to its normal position.

IVU

- 90% cases no function is seen in kidney/moiety drained by ureterocele bearing ureter.
- In duplex system, PC system of lower moiety is displaced downwards and laterally and its ureter is also displaced laterally by dilated upper pole moiety and its ureter – "drooping lily" appearance.
- Ureterocele is seen as rounded, eccentrically placed defect within specified bladder.
- Outline of ureterocele is clearly defined by contrast except for its margin, which is confluent with bladder base and neck.

  (Simple ureterocele is intravesicle and completely outlined).

USG

- Fluid filled mass in upper pole moiety of kidney with dilatation of ureter and fluid mass in bladder on same side.
- Ectopic ureterocele may show significant change in size and shape with ureteric peristalsis.

CT

Demonstatres hydronephrotic changes – dilated ureter.

Fluid filled mass on same side.

Section 7—Excretory System

Chapter 82

Renal Cell Carcinoma

- Most common primary malignant tumor of the kidney.
- M: F = 2.5:1.
- Mean age – 55 years originates from the cells of P.C.T. within the cortex.
- ↑ed incidence with WVHL and long term renal dialysis.

C/F Triad – Pain, Hematuria, Loin Mass

- 10% of RCC show calcification on plain film – if calcification with renal mass it is most likely malignant, especially if calcification is dense, central and amorphous.
- On IVP – primary large, unifocal, unilateral mass.
- Displacement, compression, distortion, stretching, invasion or amputation of calices and infundibulum.
  - Focal replacement of nephrogram with irregular margin.
- USG: Solitary mass, bulging the renal contours.
  - Usually iso to hypoechoic compared to normal kidney.
  - 10% hyperechoic, especially if small.
  - Calcification ±.
- CT – Method of choice for evaluation of suspected malignant renal neoplasm.
- Usually isodense or hypodense compared to normal renal tissue, occasionally hyperdense.
- Enhance variably but almost always less than normal renal tissue.
- 1/3rd show calcification.
- MRI: Intermediate signal intensity on TWI.
- Intermediate to high signal intensity on T2WI.

Indications for CT for Renal Neoplasms

- Urogram suspicious for renal mass (Figure 82.1).

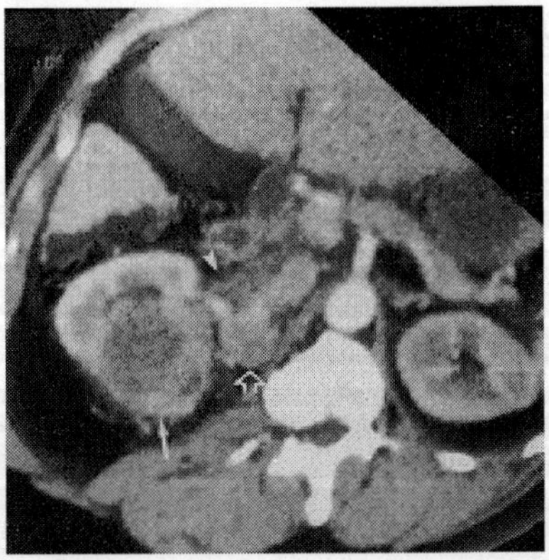

Fig. 82.1: CT scan obtained during the corticomedullary phase shows enhancing mass arising from the posterior portion of the right kidney (solid arrow). A low-attenuation filling defect is seen within the right renal vein and extends into the inferior vena cava (arrowhead). An enhancing node is seen near the renal hilum (open arrow)

- Sonogram suspicious for mass other than benign cyst.
- Normal urogram/sonogram but suspicious sign and symptoms of persistent hematuria.
- Metastases from unknown primary.
- Paraneoplastic syndromes.
- Syndromes associated with RCC – VHL, acquired cystic renal disease.
- Previous treatment for RCC.
- CT and MRI >90% accurate for most aspects of staging except for differentiation between I and II error rate – 50%, normal perinephric space (Figures 82.2 and 82.3).
- Primary sign bulky tumor in perinephric space.
- Secondary sign.
- Tumor extending to margin of kidney and ill defined peripheral outline.
  - Thickening of perinephric fascia.
  - Soft tissue strands in perinephric space.
- Treatment – I and II Radical nephrectomy.
- Nephron sparing surgery
- Also depend on being
  - I one functional kidney.
  - Small (<4 cm) tumor.
  - Possibility of benign tumor (e.g. Oncocytoma) able to pressure
  - Bilateral tumor independent blood supply.

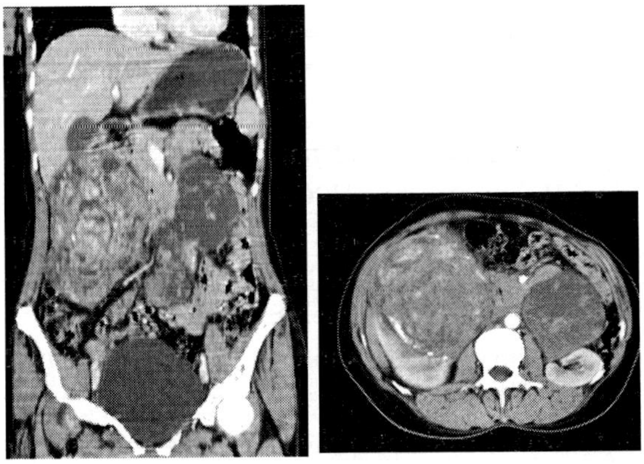

Fig. 82.2: Axial and coronal MPR CT images show large renal mass on right side with cystic retroperitoneal metastases

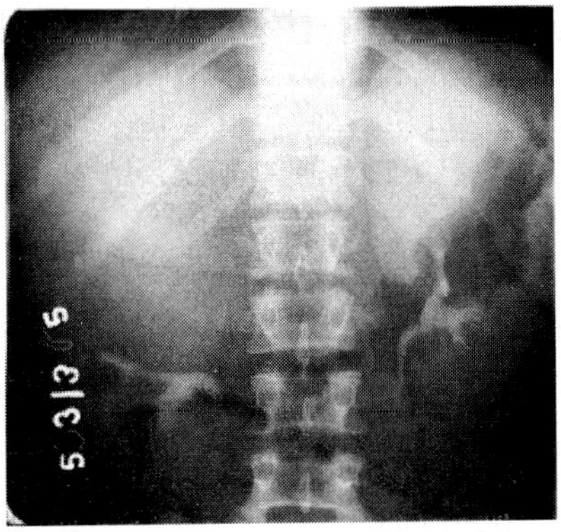

Fig. 82.3: Intravenous pyelography shows renal mass on right side

III– Radical nephrectomy with thrombectomy and/or lymphadenectomy.

IV– Palliative surgery ± radiotherapy ± chemotherapy ± embolisation.

Adenoma

- <3 cm in past.
- Size not relied criteria.
- <3 cm lesions can also metastasise.
- Needle biopsy not helpful heterogenous cell population – sampling error.

Oncocytoma

- Previously considered benign.
- Can metastasize.
- Any age, often asymptomatic.
- 1-20cm, usually solitary.
- Multiple 5%, bilateral 3%.

USG – Solid mass with internal echo's with hypoechoic centre.

CECT well defined solid enhancing mass with low attenuation central scar.

Angio – Characteristic rim and spoke wheel appearance.

TCC: Urothelial tumor, usually presents as filling defects within the renal pelvis or ureters.

But may present as a renal mass when its infiltration into renal substance.

Diagnosis based on recognition of altered renal contour, parenchyma of RCC on (T/MRI).

Collecting system and sinus fat, as well characteristics of mass lesion itself.

Diagnostic Criteria

- A mass that bulges renal contour:
  - Attenuating value/ SI different from normal renal parenchyma.
  - CT isodense, somewhat heterogenous 1/3rd calcification.
  - MRI – intermediate in SI-T1, somewhat hyper on T2.
- Enhancement different from normal renal parenchyma (usually less).
- Unsharp margins.
- If cystic-thick irregular wall, solicit enhancing component.
- Secondary sign – venous extension mats, LN adjacent organ invasion.

Staging

Table 82.1: TNM staging

Robson	Disease extent	TNM
I	Tumor confined to kidney (Small, intra renal, =7cm)	T1
	Tumor confined to kidney (large >7cm)	T2
II	Tumor spread to peri-nephric fat including Adrenal but within Gerotas' fascia	T3a
IIIa	Tumor spread to renal vein or IVc	T3b
IIIb	Spread to local LN	N1-N3
IIIc	Spread to local vessels and LN	T3b N1-N3
IVa	Tumor spread to adjacent organs (excluding, ipsilateral adrenal)	T4
IVb	Distant metastasis	M1

USG

Echo poor mass within the central hyperechoic area with or without dilated calyx or hydronephrosis.

CT

- Intraluminal soft tissue mass in the renal pelvis calices or ureter.
- Less vascular than RCC, enhances poorly with contrast.
- Obliteration of sinus fat.

Lymphoma

- Primary rare, usually secondary.
- Usually retroperitoneal lymphoma extends along lymphatics into renal sinus and perinephric space.
- Usually bilateral.
- Most common manifestation on IVU and ureteric displacement with variable hydronephrosis.
- On USG hypoechoic masses, rarely diffuse renal enlargement.
- CT well defined homogeneous into hypodense, enhance less than normal renal parenchyma.
- Hemorrhages, calcification, cystic areas – rare.
- Intermediate SI on T1.
- Intermediate to low SI on T2WI.

Angiomyolipoma

80% of patients with tuberous sclerosis have AML.

- 80% of AML occurs in patients without tuberous sclerosis.
- Documentation of fat.
- Hyperechoic on USG.

Metastases: Primary bronchogenic carcinoma, colorectal carcinoma, breast melanoma, testis, gynaecologic malignancies.

- Small (< 3 cm) multifocal (>50%) non-contour deforming.
- On CT isodense, enhance less than normal renal parenchyma.
- Associated with metastases elsewhere.
- Renal vein invasion rare.

Chapter 83

Renal Vein Thromboses

- Asymptomatic, often undiagnosed condition.
- Seen in neonates, infant.
- Incidence 0.26 to 0.7% in children.

Anatomic Consideration

- Venous system has no segmental distribution and has free anatomises.
- Small subcapsular vein – interlobular vein – interlobar vein.
- Venule rectae/Arcuate vein.
- Main renal vein at hilus–Left/Ureteral vein/ Gonadal vein/Supra renal vein.

  Right–Ureteral vein.

  Renal vein thromboses – subcapsular vein–perirenal vein.
- Systemic vein in para renal space.
- On (left) involves ureteral vein, gonadal vein etc.

Etiology

Intrinsic

- *Hypovolemia*: GI fluid loss, hemorrhage, dehydration (neonate of diabetes).
- *Primary renal diseases*: Glomerulonephritis, pyonephritis, amyloidosis, pan, sickle cell anaemia.
- *Trauma*: Blunt, surgical.
- *Neoplasms*: RCC, Wilm's tumor.
- *Hypercoagulable state*: Nephrotic syndrome systemic malignancy.

Extrinsic

- Pregnancy, Retroperitoneal tumors, abscess, lymphomas.

Functional

- CHF, tricuspid insufficiency, constrictive pericarditis.

Pathophysiology

1. Acute pulmonary occlusion:

- Tense swollen cyanotic kidney, renal vein pressure increased.

  Renal art flow – If increased swelling, renal artery perfusion arrested – destruction of kidney.
- If increased size in first 24 hours – peaks at 1 week – ↓ in subsequent 2 months – small atrophic kidney.

2. Acute partial occlusions:

- 80-90% occlusion – swelling and cyanosis – max ↑ at 1 week – ↓ to pre-thrombotic stage at 2 months – ultimate fate depend by formation of collaterals (starts as early as 24 hours after occlusion: max at 12 days to 1 month).

3. **Gradual occlusion:**

- Extensive collatererals. Kidney is normal → renal function with albuminuria.

C/F

- *Acute*: In infants and neonate's severe progressive lumbar or abdominal pain, kidney palpable and painful. Transient - in B.P. initial cross hematuria is followed by anuria or persistent microscopic hematuria.
- *Chronic*: Usually asymptomatic, may present like nephrotic syndrome; left varicocele, dilated superficial epigastric vein.

Lab Diagnosis

- Acute – Azotemia, acidosis, proteinuria, DIC like picture.
- Chronic – Pyuria, -ed FDP, glucosuria, RTA.

Radiographic Findings

Plain film: ↑ed in size in acute occlusion.

IVP: Can suggest but not confirmatory.

Acute Thrombosis

Enlarged oedematous renal mass.

Opacification of parenchyma, excretion in collecting system is poor to absent.

When seen calices – Pelvis are stretched, compressed excretion is often virtually occluded by surrounding parenchyma.

Gradual Occlusion

Normal opacification and excretion-anatomy in 1-2 weeks.

Normal IVP with notching of ureters or pelvis by dilated tortuous collaterals may be seen.

RGP

Helps to exclude obstruction in case of poor or absent function.

Splayed, distorted infundibulum seen as in IUP.

USG

- Gray scale finding are not pathognomic.

Reflects pathological changes of oedema and – hemorrhage in acute stage followed by collateral infiltration and fibrosis.

Immediate acute phase – Nephromegaly, with decreased cortical echogenicity due to edema.

Approx 2 weeks markedly ↑ed cortical echogenicity with preserved corticomedullary differentiation due to cellular infiltration with variable renal size.

Late ↓ed parenchymal echo which loss of LN differentiation due to fibrosis, ↓ed renal size.

There is loss of normal transmitted venous pulsation on affected side. Thrombus itself may be visualized.

Doppler may hold absent flow in main renal vein. If flow is seen it is steady with absence of any reflected pulsation from right atrium.

There is an internal arterial impedance, resulting in absent of reversal diastolic flow.

Arteriography

Renal arteriography, which focuses on venous phase, was initially favoured. Typical pattern is greatly enlarged kidney with delayed rate of flow with splaying ↓ in calibre with stretching of intralobular arteries.

Poor cortical opacification and nephrogram due to pruning of finer distal arterial branches.

Larger renal vein and site of obstruction may be seen in delayed venous phase.

In gradual obstruction – normal arterial study with venous collaterals in delayed phase.

Venography/Venocavography

- Venography with direct selective catheterisation is most definitive.
- Incomplete occlusion – radiolucent area.
- Complete occlusion – amputation of column.
- Collateral veins may be seen.
- Concurrent intra arterial, epinephrine facilitates evaluation of small vessels by diminishing flow.

However it is invasive and risk of dislodging the clot causing pulmonary embolism preferably preceded by IVC graphy which may show:

- Once of streaming effect on contrast column in IVC.
- Smooth wall appearance of IVC at level of renal vein.
- Retrograde reflux of contrast into main renal veins with subsequent propagation into intrarenal tributaries.

CT

- CT angio currently approaches the accuracy of conventional angiography in assessment of vascular anomalies.

  The renal veins can be depicted during early corticomedullary phase of enhancement hence different phases are recommended.

Acute stage – Hypoattenuating filling defect in an enlarged renal vein. Collateral vein may be seen later.

Secondary signs may be seen i.e. delay in renal cortical nephrogram. Renal enlargement.

MRI

Standard T1 weighted axial images and axial and sagittal gradient echo images can be taken.

Recently, MRA following gadolinium administration has shown encouraging results.

Radionuclide Renography

Useful in sequential assessment of renal perfusion in excessive oedema.

Scan indicating perfusion arrest warrants aggressive therapeutic approaches.

Section 7—Excretory System

Chapter 84

Renovascular Hypertension

Functional

- HT caused by renal hypoperfusion secondary to US changes in the kidney or from a lesion that impairs blood flows to a part or all, of one or both kidneys.

Operational

- HT that is shown to have remained cured or improved for at least 6 months after the revascularisation procedures.

Renovascular Disease

- Refers to disorders of the main renal artery and its branches; ± stimulation of RAAS. On angio—(+) of arterial abnormal whether the lesion is causing HT or not.

Renovascular HT

- Refers to arterial change kidney—↑ renin secretion—resultant HT.

Etiology

- 0.5-5% of all cases of HT. 3-10% of children ↓ RVH.

Common

- Renal arterial stenosis
  - AS.
  - FMD.
  - Neurofibromatosis.
  - William's syndrome.
  - Rubella syndrome.
  - Klippel trenaunay Weber syndrome.
  - Linear sebacious neuro syndrome.
  - Kawasaki disease.
  - Crohn's disease.

Less Common

- Trauma
  - RAT.
  - AVF.
- Renal artery emboli
  - Simple.
  - Mycotic.
- Renal artery compression
  - Band, mass, cyst, pheochromocytoma, neurogenic tumor, Wilm's tumor.
- Renal artery aneurysm/dissection.
- Arthritis
  - Takayasu's.
  - Syphilitic.

- Coarctation of aorta.
- Radiation damage to renal artery.
- Retroperitoneal fibrosis.
- Collagen muscular disease.
- Middle aortic syndrome.

Pathogenesis

- Hemodynamically significant RAS.
  ↓ Renal perfusion
  - Aberrent art. Baro receptors.
  - Macular densa of JGA (Na^+).
  - Postganglionic symp. Nerve ending at JGA.
- Incresed renin at JGA.
- Angiotensinogen → Ang. I.
  ↓ ACE.
  Ang. II.
- Vasoconstriction — Vasoconstriction
  - Adrenal aldosterone.
  - ↑Sodium reabsorption.
  - ↑ EBN.

  ↑ BP.

Clinical Clues that Suggest RVHT

A. High probability

1. Malignant or associated HT >180/100 mmHg and/or resistant to two or more drugs.
2. Unexplained azotemia – especially after receiving ACE (-) or angio-II antagonist.
3. Atrophic kidney or discrepancy in size between B>3.15 cms.
4. Epigastric bruit.
5. Unexplained pulmonary edema with or without LV systemic dysfunction.

B. Moderate probability

1. Abrupt onset of HT <30 or >55.
2. Patients with vascular disease.
3. Heavy or prolonged use of tobacco.
4. Low body mass index.

C. Low probability

1. Presentation typical of mild to moderate essential HT.

Diagnostic Modalities

1. Plain X-ray
   - Chest.
   - KUB.
2. Sonography.
3. IVU.
4. Doppler imaging (Figure 84.1)
   - Duplex.
   - CDI.

A

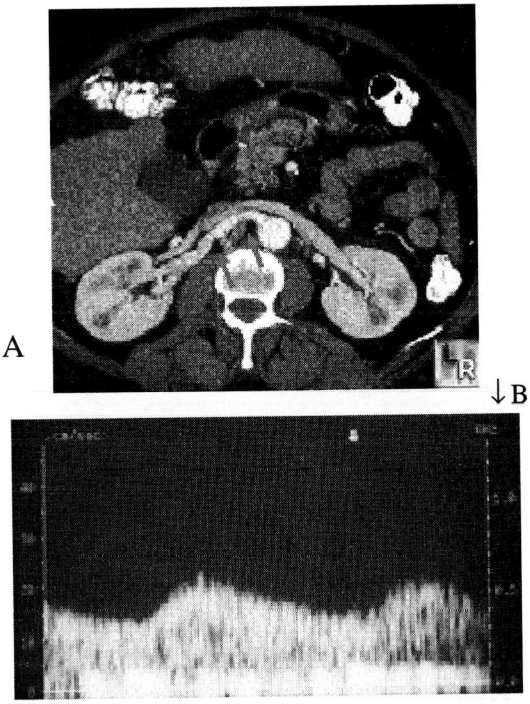

↓B

Fig. 84.1: A) Axial postcontrast CT section showing narrowed and beaded right renal artery suggestive of fibromuscular dysplasia. B) Doppler wave form in same patient showing parvus tardus flow

5. Arteriography
   - Conventional.
   - IVDSA.
   - IADSA.
6. Selective renal vein sampling for renin assays
   - Plasma renin activity.
   - Renal vein renin.
   - Renal vein renin ratio.
   - Renal to systemic renin index.
   - Post captopril renin measurement.
7. Radionuclide renography
   - Static.
   - Dynamic.
   - Captopril.
8. CTA.
9. MRA.

1. Plain X-ray

a. KUB

↓ Renal size.

Aneurysmal calcification.

Abnormal renal contour.

b. Chest

Suggestive of HT - LVt, aortic tortousity.

Rib notching.

Reverse 3 sign.

Mediastinum widening, osteopenia, vertebral. collapse.

↓

Features of Cushing's disease.

HT+ paravertebral mass – pheochromocytoma.

Clavicular erosions → Chr. Renal disease + secondary HPT.

2. USG

- Size discrepancy.
- S/o parenchymal disease.
- Aneurysms.

3. Urography

- Rapid sequence IVP or HT IVU.

  Scout – 90 ml of 50% Na diaurzoate → ½ mm, 1, 2, 3,4,5, 10 min – 20-30 min.

Findings

- U/L delay of a min or more in calyceal appearance of contrast.
- Disparity in size of 2 kidneys.
- Spidery pyelogram.
- Delayed hyperconcentration of contrast in PCS.
- Notching of PCS and upper ureter by art. collaterals.
- Focal parenchymal atrophys.

Status

- No role in evaluation of patients with RVHT.

4. Doppler Imaging

a. Duplex examination (renal artery).

Sites of examination:

- At astia/origin.
- Mid part.
- At renal hilum.
- Segmental art. at upper mid and lower poles.

Normal renal art signature

- Initial local ↑ in frequency during peak systole.
- Subsequently, prog. ↓ during rest of the cycle.
- Signal throughout is above baseline suggestive of low impedance flow with continuation forward diastolic flow.

Indices measured are:

Peak systolic velocity— 180 cms/sec.

R.A.R (PSV-renal a/PSV aorta)— > 3.5.

Findings in RAS

a. Proximal to stenosis PSV maintained with decreased diastolic flow.

b. At stenosis—PSV, RAR > 3.5.

c. Imm. distal to stenosis – turbulence.

d. Slightly function downstream. Classical tardu/ parvus pattern.

AT > 0.07 sec/700 ms.

AT <3m/sec/300 cm/sec.

Sensitivity – 87%; Specificity – 97%.

Location of stenosis.

Kidney size.

Non-nephrotoxic.

Non-dependant on anti HT.

Non-invasive and cheap.

5. Angiography Gold Standard for Diagnosis of RVH

a. Aortography for
   - Localizing renal artery.
   - To assess number of renal artery.
   - Localizing RAS.
   - Localizing prominent collateral artery.

b. Conventional selective renal arteriography

Selective catheter exchanged for aortography catheter over a flexible guide wire to the tip keeps just proximal to branching in the desired renal artery.

10-12 ml contrast injected 3-6 ml/sec.

Arterial phase.

Nephrographic phase.

Venous phase.

c. IVDSA.

Technique

- Pigtail catheter is passed through median cubital and satisfactory positioned in RA and is connected to injection plp. 40 ml of contrast (350 mg I/ml) 20ml/sec.

Images acquired at the rate of 2 fils/sec upto 10 sec.

Adv. over IVU

- Can detect U/L or B/L disease.
- RVR samples can be taken at same sitting allowing simultaneous evaluation of significance of detected stenosis.
- Outpatient procedure.
- Cost effective.

Adv. over IA DSA

- Avoids artery puncture.
- OPD procedure.
- Doesn't involve catheter manipulation in or near renal artery.
- More suitable for elderly.

Disadvantages

- Large dose of contrast used.
- Distal US and br. artery not adequately visualized.
- Image quality inferior to IADSA.
- Unsuitable in patients with low cardiac output.
- Over estimates stenosis in high grade aortic stenosis and under estimates in FMD.

d. IADSA
   - Adv. over conv. angio.
   - OPD basis as smaller size catheter is used.
   - Low dose of contrast.
   - Can be combined with PTRA, if desired.
   - Speedier, better resolution.

6. Angio Criteria for Determining Significance of Detected Stenosis

a. Severe stenosis with human diameter being <1.5 m or reduction by >75%.

b. Presence of post-stenotic dilatation in aortic stenosis lesion.

c. Presence of collaterals is virtually a reliable sign of stenosis being the cause of HT.

7. Selective Renal Vein Sampling

Specificity is high. Estimates clinical significance of RAS. Peripheral renin concentration in the normal range is used as an indication of no benefit from intervention. Not used as screening test.

1. **Plasma renin activity**

   Measures renin sample for peripheral diagnosis and has wide range of normal values.

   Disadvantage – Low sensitivity.

   - Errors in renin measurement.

2. **Renal vein renin ratio – RVR ratio**
   - Renal v. renin/IVC renin.
   - Normal RVR – 1.24.

     In stenosis – stenosed kidney RRVR > 1.5 (4 production).

     Normal kidney <1 (physio suppression).

3. **Renal to systemic renin index**

   RSRI – Renal vein renin-systemic renin/ systemic renin.

Radionuclide Renography

a. Conventional 123^{I}– OIH and ^{99}Jc DTPA used.

Further studies are suggestive if:

1. Asymmetry in the rate of rise in activity.
2. Time to peak activity (>5 min).
3. Delayed clearing of contrast uptake.

b. Captopril scintigraphy

Based on the principle that the renal function in an ischaemic kidney could abruptly be reduced further after a single dose of captopril and hence values in 2 kidneys could be measured and compared more easily with baseline renogram values.

Technique

- Active medical treatment and diuretics discontinued at least 2 days before the examination and patient is on salt restricted diet and fasting.
- Hydrated with water 10 ml/kg BW orally.
- Fixed with IV line.
- Baseline BP obtained. Radioisotope given IV and baseline renal scintigraphy performed.

↓

After 2 hours.

↓

50 mg captopril crushed and given orally with H_2O and BP taken every 15 min.

↓

After 1 hour.

Patient injected with 10 ml (370 Mbg) of ^{99m}Tc DTPA and Tc LAI T 3—after positioning the patient on gamma camera, 1 hour after oral captopril.

↓

Rapid sequence recording done for 1st/rim at the rate of 2 sec/frame.

↓

Next 30 min → sequential images taken at the rate of 1min/frame.

↓

Time activity curve, generated and scintigram obtained. Results analysed.

Positive results and indicated by

1. Split renal function >5% discrepancy is significant.
2. Time to reach peak activity >5 mm in affected kidney or < 2 min.
3. Delayed clearing of cortical uptake (i.e. renal cortical activity at 20 min >30% of peak renal activity).

   Sal – 90%, SP – 95%.

   There is good correlation between the appearance of captopril scintigrams and treatment results.

Disadvantages

1. Not suitable in patients with significant azotemia.

2. Does not pick up B/L RAS as it depends on lateralization to more diseased side.
3. Not helpful in solitary kidney.
4. 10-23% of patients with no response to captopril may benefit from revascularisation.

8. CT Angiography

Technique

- Continuous volumetric acquisition of patient data during a single breath used in the arterial phase of the contrast after injection enables subsequent 3D recovery.
- Initial scan obtained from L1 – L3.

  100-150 ml contrast injection at the rate of 8 ml/sec.

  Spiral scan obtained in a single breath hold time of 30 sec, beginning 30 sec. after the start of power injection using collimation—3mm pitch of 1 to 2.

  ↓ Post processing.

  Interpolation of spiral data into 2mm overlapping axial section.

  ↓

  3D rendering MIP.
  SSD.

  SN – 59-92%, SP – 82-98%.

9. MR Angiography

a. Time of flight—utilizes flow related enhancement to image the renal artery.

b. Phase contrast—utilises phase shift differences in measuring protons to display flow within renal or both can utilize 2D or 3D Fourier transformation for display.

   Based on the principle that most significant stenosis result in severe flow disturbance and subsequently signal loss in vs and there exists a convolution between length of signal used and degree of stensis which can be measured and hence the degree of stenosis assessed.

   <5 cm signal noise—60-70% narrowing.

   > 5 mm >75%.

   Signal noise extending—>95%.

   No flow detected > 99% or complete occlusion or artery missed.

Interventional Radiology

- PTRA.
- Endovascular stenting.

A. PTRA

- Should be the initial treatment of ostial lesions as well as less different lesions and that surgery should be reserved for technical failures and patients who restenose after 2 PTRA's.

Mechanism

- Fracturing of the atheroma.
- Tearing of intima and media.
- Dilating the adventitia.

Arterial access through transfemoral route and placement of catheter.

↓

Contrast run to show the morphology of stenosis in multiple projections.

↓

Pressure measured proximal to stenosis.

↓

Crossing the stenosis with a guidewire followed by passage of end hold catheter over the guidewire.

↓

Check ring to ascertain catheter position.

↓

Measure transstenotic pressure gradient.

>20 mmHg gradient is significant.

Exchange of catheter with an appropriate sized balloon catheter over guidewire.

↓

Balloon inflation across the entire length of stenosis.

↓

Mean pressure gradient followed by check angiography

↓

Removal of catheter, guidewire and sheath followed by hemostasis at preventive aortic.

Criteria for successful PTRA.

a. Luminal drain supports by 50%.
b. Residual stenosis <20%.
c. Transstenotic pressure gradient <20 mmHg and disappearance of collaterals.

B. Endovascular Stenting

Indication

- PTRA
  - Intimal flap.
  - Dissection.
  - Occlusion.
- Ostial stenosis.
- Restenosis after PTRA.
  - Inadequate primary angioplasty.

Radiology of the Abnormal Shape, Contour Capacity and Masses of Urinary Bladder

SHAPE AND CONTOUR ABNORMALITIES

1. Congenital

- Bladder hypoplasia/agenesis.
- Urachal anomalies.
- Diverticula (congenital).

2. Inflammatory

- Acute bacterial cystitis.
- Chronic cystitis.
- Emphysematous cystitis.
- Urine infections.
- Malakoplakia.
- Focal cystitis.
- T.B.
- Schistosomiasis.
- Hemorrhagic cystitis.
- Interstitial cystitis.

3. Mechanical

- Trabeculation.
- Diverticula.
- Cystocoele.
- Bladder herniation.
- Fistula.

4. Extrinsic Compression/Displacement.

5. Post Surgical.

CAPACITY

- Small capacity bladder.

1. Fibrotic/Thickened Bladder Wall

- Interstitial cystitis.
- Tubecular cystitis.
- Cystitis cystica.
- Schistosomiasis.
- Surgical resection, radiation therapy.

2. Neurogenic Bladder: Spastic Type

- Large capacity bladder.
- Prune belly syndrome.
- Neurogenic bladder, atonic type.

MASSES

Shape and Contour Abnormalities

Congenital Causes

Bladder hypoplasia/agenesis

- Rare congenital abnormalities.

Benign	Malignant
• Leiomyoma (HC)	• Urothelial carcinoma
• Hemangioma	• Urachal carcinoma
• Lipoma	• Lymphoma
• Fibrous tumor	• Rhabdomyosarcoma

- Sonographically bladder may be absent or very small.
- Associated with other congenital abnormality, incompatible with life.

Duplication

- Also rare anomaly associated with urethral duplication.
- On imaging, duplication is divided into 3 types:

Type I: A peritoneal folds, which may be complete or incomplete, separate two bladders.

Type II: An internal septum is present dividing the bladder. Septum may be complete/incomplete and may be distributed in a sagittal or coronal plane. There may be multiple septa.

Type III: There is a transverse band of muscles dividing the bladder into two useful quadrants.

Urachal Anomalies

- Fetal bladder tapers superiorly into urachus with communicates with allantois at the level of umbilicus. It closes around mid 2nd trimester becoming the median umbilical ligament but lies extraperitoneally.

Four types of anomalies are seen:

- Patent urachus (50%).
- Urachal cyst (30%).
- Urachal sinus (15%).
- Urachal diverticulum (5%).

Patent Urachus

- Presents at early age with micro leakage at umbilicus.
- Usually associated with maternal obstruction and hence serving as a protective mechanisms to allow normal fetal development.
- Can be easily demonstrated with sinography/cystography.
- CT/MRI/USG: A fluid filled structure extending from bladder to the umbilicus.

Urachal Cyst

- Forms with closure of umbilical end and bladder end of urachus with patent middle part.
- Often seen in the lower 1/3rd part.
- Increased incidence of adenocarcinoma is seen.
- USG/CT/MRI: There is characteristic appearance of cyst with some time, delicate peripheral calcification.
- Debris and increased echogenicities/densities may be seen inside the cyst with presence of infection and it is often associated with thickening of its wall.

Urachal Sinus

- Seen when the urachus closes at the bladder but remains at the periphery.
- Presents with infection and/or periodic discharge.
- Sinography: Shows a blind ending sinus.
- Cross-sectional imaging (USG/CT/MRI), it is seen as a fluid filled tubular structure.

Urachal Diverticulum

- Seen when urachus close at umbilicus and remains patent at the bladder.
- Incidentally seen.

- ↑ed risk of carcinoma and stone formation.
- CT/MR/USG: Diagnosed incidentally, with investigation along for some other purpose.
- Strongly associated with prune belly syndrome.
- Cystogram/MCU: Alone shows these congenital diverticula.

DIVERTICULA (CONGENITAL)

- Urachal diverticulum: Described above.
- Hutch diverticulum: Seen superior and lateral to the ureteric orifice.

INFLAMMATORY LESIONS

Acute Bacterial Cystitis

- Extremely common. Associated with gram negative organisms, E. coli, Klebsiella, and pseudomonas species.
- Most frequently seen in young and middle aged adults and may be associated with sexual activities.
- Commonly in old aged males when bladder outlet obstruction develops.
- No imaging features are seen unless infection is severe, when there may be thickening and irregularity of bladder wall.
- USG: There may be ↑ed echogenicities of the mucosa with presence of echogenic debris within the bladder lumen.
- CT: In extremely severe cases, mucosa appears of reduced density with irregularity of the luminal surface of bladder.

CHRONIC CYSTITITS

- In this, there may be gross wall thickening, reduction of bladder capacity and the development of VUR/ureteric dilatation.
- Due to inflammation, cluster of hyperplastic urothelial cells may develop in the submucosa, which are known as Brum's nests.

Brum's Nests

- Central portion degeneration aged resulting in → Cystitis cystica.
- Nests develop into glandular structure → cystitis glandularis.

USG: Chronic inflammatory changes are seen cysts are solid papillary mass may be seen.

D/D malignancy; can only be differentiated with cystoscopic biopsy.

Emphysematous Cystitis

- Rare condition associated with diabetes mellitus and is usually associated with E. coli.
- Both intraluminal and intramural gas is present.

USG: Echogenic foci with ring down artefacts or dirty shadowing within the bladder wall.

VIRAL INFARCTIONS

- Most often associated with adenovirus.
  - Quiet aggressive course, patients present with hematuria.

Imaging: Reduced bladder capacity with multiple small polypodial lesions of the mucosa seen on USG and CT examination.

MALAKOPLAKIA

- Rare granulomatous infection.
- Male: Female – 4:1, peak 6th decade.
- Associated with DM, acute liver disease, mycobacterium infection, sarcoidosis and following transplantation.

Imaging: Single or multiple mucosal-based masses ranging from 0.5-3.0 cm are seen manually at the bladder base and lower ureters, which may provoke stricturing.

Focal Cystitis

- May develop in response to classic irritation due to calculus, catheter, foreign body and associated paravesical disease particularly diverticulitis, pelvic abscess and Crohn's disease.

Imaging: Evidence of gross focal thickening with rest of the bladder normal.

CT/MRI: Will show the cause and delinate the exact anatomy.

TUBERCULOSIS

- Usually occurs due to hematogenous spread from two ways.
- Represents 10-20% of genitourinary TB and is virtually always associated with renal TB.
- Causes, bladder thickening, reduced bladder capacity, may obstruct urethra or may cause traction of ureteric orifice, which may lead to UVR.

Imaging: Shows, trabeculation with irregularity of bladder with decreased capacity. At late stages bladder appears thick walled and may calcify.

SCHISTOSOMIASIS

- Also called bilhariziasis.
- Caused by schistosoma hematobium.
- Female lays eggs in the bladder was which provoke edema and granuloma formation.

Imaging: When eggs provoke edema and granuloma formation there is evidence of focal polypodial swelling of cystography.

On USG: Normal in early or mild cases but often shows wall thickening and single/multiple polypodial lesions, which may be sessile or wavy and may protrude into the lumen. Metaplastic changes are most marked at bone and trigone.

- Late stage: Fibrosis and calcification.

Plain Radiograph: In late stage shows calcific opacities in regional bladder.

CT scan: Eggshell or linear calcification in the submucosa is seen in bladder and distal meter.

D/D: TB, differentiation by the fact that, in contrast of TB, in this, bladder capacity and contractility are surprisingly preserved.

- Schistosomiasis predisposes to carcinoma particularly squamous cell carcinoma.

HEMORRHAGIC CYSTITIS

- Develops following cyclophosphamide therapy.

Surgery: Evidence of nodular bladder with a large hematoma in bladder lumen. In late stages, there may be a contracted bladder.

INTERSTITIAL CYSTITIS

- Usually idiopathic, may be associated with atrophy.
- May be associated with autoimmune disease like PAN, SLE, RA.

Imaging: No imaging feature in the early stages but later bladder becomes contracted and may have a nodular wall.

MECHANICAL PROBLEMS

Trabeculations

- In this, the bladder wall appears thickened and its inner aspect shows an undulatory or ridged pattern which are very well seen by USG.
- Thickening of bladder wall may be normal in mild BOO however, it often rises with more severe chronic disease.
- Common causes of BOO in BHP: Other includes prostatic cancer, bladder wall stress, urethral stricture and calculi. On urologic studies high intravesical pressure, >15 cm of H_2O/Hg is seen.

DIVERTICULA

- In severe cases saculation and later diverticula develops.
- In early stages multiple, small outpouching of the bladder mucosae appear between trabecular known as saculation. When it is >2 cm, these are defined as diverticula.
- Produced due to focal herniation of the urothelium and submucosa though weak sites in the bladder wall.
- Acquired due to increased elevation of intravesical pressure associated with BOO or neurogenic bladder.
- Sacular/diverticula are formed so as to moderate the intravesical pressure by filling uretor during back emptying. This causes classical symptoms of double micturition.
- Cystogram/CT/MRI/USG will show a smooth thin walled diverticulum often associated with trabeculated bladder.
- Shows diverticula connected to the bladder by a narrow neck.
- Pre operative assessment by CT is required to delineate exact anatomy.

Complication: Calculus formation, infection and occasional malignancy.

CYSTOCELE

- Condition of abnormal descent with prolapse into the vagina.
- Degree of descent of bladder and duration cause stress incontinence.

Diagnosis

- Lateral standing cystogram: Decent of any part of the bladder that reaches below the inferior. Pubic ramus during straining indicates cystocele.

BLADDER HERNIATION

- Occur usually in inguinal/femoral canal with former roughly twice as often as latter.
- Usually small 2-3 cm, asymptomatic, however at risk of rupture during herniorrhaphy.
- May become large, act as a diverticulum and result in double micturition.

Contrast Examination: During IVP or cystogram may show the lesion.

FISTULAE

- Fistula between bladder and adjacent organs is not uncommon.
- Most frequently is colovesical and is due to diverticulitis.

Other causes:

- Carcinoma large bowel.
- Crohn's disease.
- Carcinoma UB (rare).

- Fistulae can be demonstrated by cystography, IVP or double contrast barium enema.
- USG, cystography will show focal bladder wall thickening and irregularity due to underlying cause. However, this can be missed in 40% cases.
- CT: will detect such missed cases and shows mass tumor, inflammatory tissue, focal wall thickness and air in bladder.

Vesicoureteric fistula: Associated usually with Crohn's disease.

Ba. MT demonstrates two fistulas.

VESICOVAGINAL FISTULA

- Usually due to surgery, mostly radical pelvic surgery for gynecological malignancy, rarely due to obstetric injury, TB, schistosomiasis.

  IVP/Cystography→ On lateral images usually easily makes the diagnosis.

EXTRINSIC COMPRESSION/DISPLACEMENT

- Under filled bladder often shows some distortion in shape by adjacent bowel loops when they are loaded with gas or fecal matter.
- Superior indentation by normal uterus is seen in females.
- USG will interpret it correctly.
- Pathologic lesion like enlarged uterus due to fibroid or an ovarian mass/cyst will cause extrinsic compression.
- **USG/CT scan/MRI** will delinate such lesions easily.
- Compression by urinoma/hematoma is seen following trauma or surgery. History suggests the diagnosis usually USG/CT/MRI will identify the cause easily.

PELVIC LIPOMATOSIS

- Rare condition, there is excess of adipose tissue within the true pelvis.
- Bladder appears pear shaped on contrast examination.
- Bladder base is elevated and capacity is reduced.
- There may be associated ureteric deviation and obstruction.
- The rectum and sigmoid colon appears elongated and narrowed.

CT: Is diagnostic and shows fat in the pelvis and rule out any mass lesion in the pelvis.

POST SURGICAL

Ileal Conduit

- Part of ileal coop is used to form new bladder and the ureters are implanted into it.
- Conduit predisposes to:
  - Bilateral reflux.
  - Chr. pyelonephritis—renal failure.
  - Calculi.
  - Stenosis at uretero ileal junction.
- Conduitogram/loopogram shows B/L reflux from a neobladder having typical small bowel mucosa.

BOARI FLAP

- Length of the flap of bladder is used depending upon the distal ureter deficit.

Imaging: Postoperative appearance range from subtle amputating of the superolateral aspect of the bladder on the affected side to an obvious tube of bladder extending superiorly.

MCU is diagnostic and shows reflux of contrast into the newly formed ureter as normal mechanism for prevention of reflux is lost.

CAPACITY

Small Capacity Bladder

- Interstitial cystitis.
- Tuberculous cystitis.
- Cystitis cystica.
- Surgical resection.
- Neurogenic bladder: Spastic type.

SPASTIC NEUROGENIC BLADDER

Causes

- Trauma.
- Parkinson's disease.
- Diabetes mellitus.
- Spina bifida.
- Multiple sclerosis.
- There is a low capacity high-pressure bladder that contracts involuntarily (detrusor instability) and results in incontinence.

- Radiological features include trabeculated thick walled bladder with sacculation and diverticulae and a typical cone shape referred to as "PINE CONE" bladder often with an open bladder neck due to sphincter dyssynergia. This may be associated with VUR.
- However, urodynamic studies are required to confirm and to plan diagnosis.

LARGE CAPACITY BLADDER

Autonomic Neurogenic Bladder

- In this, the bladder appears flaccid with high capacity.
- Seen in lower motor neuron lesions.
- **Imaging:** The bladder is thin walled smooth and enlarged, sometimes reaching upto the umbilicus.

PRUNE BELLY SYNDROME

- Also known as PBS triad syndrome, abdominal musculature deficiency syndrome.
- Consists of absent abdominal wall muscles, undescended testis and renal dysplasia associated with gross dilatation of the collecting system.
- Incidence is increasing as antenatal USG has permitted its early detection.

Aetiology

- Fetal urethral obstruction, which resolves in the latter stages of gestation but results in clinically apparent features of the syndrome at birth.
- Generalized developmental abnormality, which is possibly related to an early mesenchymal developmental arrest.
- Predominantly seen in males.

Triad

Deficient abdominal musculature, undescended testis and urinary tract dysplasia.

- Characteristic features of renal tract are:
  - Small kidneys and abnormal calyces, with minimal dilatation of the calyces and pelvis. Upper ureters are mildly dilated while lower ureters are shown disproportionate dilatation.
  - Bladder is thin, without trabeculation, has a large volume, is irregularly shaped and has a wide neck.
  - Patent urachus or a diverticulum may be present.
  - Post evacuation is markedly dilated proximally with a typical conical narrowing and this post stream in the distal urethra.

Imaging

- Plain X-ray abdomen shows a protuberant abdomen due to lack of abdominal musculature.

USG: Adding for demonstrating calyces and small lobulated kidneys.

IVU: Proximal dilated calyces with markedly dilated distal ureters.

MCU: Shows VUR in 2/3rd of the cases.

Post urethra is dilated in its proximal part.

MASSES

Benign

Leiomyoma

- Most common benign tumor of the urinary bladder.
- Surgery shows well-defined oval/spherical neural mass upto several centimetres diameter.

- Imaging cannot differentiate with benign from malignant, so biopsy is always required.

Hemangioma

May associate with:

- Additional hemangioma elsewhere in 30% cases.
- Klippel – trenaunay syndrome.
- Sturge-Weber syndrome.

Patient presents with recurrent episodes of gross hematuria.

Plain Radiograph: This may be identified, if there is presence of phleboliths.

USG: Solid predominantly hypoechoic mass with hypoechoic spaces within the thickened bladder wall.

IVP: Rounded/lobulated filling defect.

CT/MRI shows serpinigous vascular structures in the bladder wall.

MALIGNANT

MC is Transitional Cell Carcinoma (Figure 85.1)

- Tumors are classified into four growth pattern.
- In situ (non invasive).

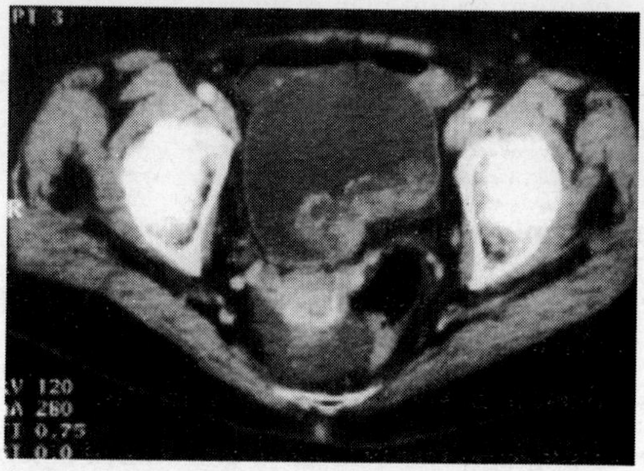

Fig. 85.1: A CT scan of the pelvis shows a large bladder tumor invading the base of bladder. The tumor appears to be musle invasive

TNM	Americal urological system	Histological description	CT criteria	MRI criteria
TIS	0	Ca in situ	NA	NA
T1	A	Superficial, limited to mucosa and submucosa	Stages→A→B_2 or T_1 and T_3a cannot be differentiated – tumor is detected	Stages→A→B_2 or T_1 and T_3a are diagnosed when the tumor is confined to the bladder wall with outer bladder being of low signal intensity of T2WI.
T2	B1	Superficial invasion of mucosa wall	–	–
T3a	B2	Deep invasion of muscular wall	–	–
T3b	C1	Perivesical fat invasion	Irregularity and soft tissue mass extending into perivesical fat	Interruption of low sigma/intensity bladder wall on T2WI and tumor extension to the perivesical fat on T2WI.
T4	C2	Invasion of adjacent organs	Direct tumor extension to adjacent organs or soft tissue mass extending from the tumor to obturator intense or pelvic node	Direct invasion of adjacent organ.
N	D1 (pelvic nodes)	Lymph node involvement	>10 mm	>10 mm
M	D2	Distant metastasis	Distant mets	Distant mets

- Papillary.
- Infiltrating.
- Combined papillary and infiltrating.

STAGING

- The diagnosis of bladder cancer is clinical and requires cystoscopy with biopsy.
- IV urogram/cystogram: Can diagnose tumor but small and the infiltrating tumors can remain undetected. Associated dense concentration of contrast material obscures intraluminal part of tumor.

USG: Sonographic detection is excellent and is = 95% appears as focal non mobile mass or of urothelial thickening, calcification in the papillary type may also be seen.

CT/MRI: Detection rate is higher than USG. Presently CT cystoscopy has been compared with fibreoptic cystoscopy. Reports have found that all tumor scan on conventional cystoscopy was also seen on CT cystoscopy. CT and MRI also help in staging its malignancy.

Staging USG: TAS has limited value. TRUS and transurethral USG allow better resolution; staging accuracy of 75-95% have been reported. However, with perivesical spread evaluation is limited and USG also does not allow LN assessment.

CT: Neoplasm appear sessile/pedunculated soft tissue, may have density similar to the bladder wall on CECT and occasionally intraluminal surface is entrusted with calcium.

- Lesions simulating bladder cancer is invasive carcinoma from prostate/ rectum, phaeochromocytoma, leiomyoma, lymphoma and malakoplakia.
- Major role of CT is to stage other than detect the primary neoplasm.
- CT cannot differentiate between the changes of bladder wall hence useful for detecting invasion of perivesical fat, LN and adjacent viscera.
- **LN metastasis:** CT is useful for LN assessment nodes >10 mm in short axis are considered malignant. Obturator and external iliac lymph nodes are involved 1st, followed by internal and common iliac nodes.
- Reported accuracy of CT to stage is 40-92%, for detection of perivesical extension is around 05-25% and LN detection varies from 65-97%.

MRI: MR staging also follow TNM classification.

- Papillary competent is best seen on T1WI, where it demonstrates higher signal intensity than the surrounding urine. On T2W1, both tumor and urine increases in intensity diminishing the tissue control.
- To evaluate infiltration, T2W and CE T1WI are needed. This spin action sequence demonstrates tumor with higher signal intensity, in contrast to lower signal of non-involved bladder wall.
- CE MRI has shown to aid in the differentiation of tumor from inflammatory post biopsy changes in the bladder wall or in perivesical fat.

Cancer shows	For LNs
earlier enhancement	
(6.5 sec after	Metastatic node show
contrast admn.)	early contrast
Which is 4 sec.	enhancement
faster than post	compared to
biopsy tissue	nonmetastatic LNs.

- Multi planar imaging facilitates clearly depicts direct tumor invasion into adjacent organs.
- Sagittal section imaging allows:
  - Assessment of uterine or vaginal imaging.
  - Assessment of seminal vesicles.
  - Invasion of prostate and rectum.

- LN assessment in similar to CT (i.e. >10 mm in short axis).
- The staging accuracy of MRI is slightly better than CT, but the improvement did not reach statistical significance. Published data shows:
  - Accuracy for CT around 40-92%.
  - Accuracy for MRI around 60-96%.
  - MRI better than CT for evaluation of tumors in differentiating between deep muscular (T3a) and perivesical tumor invasion (T3b).

URACHAL CARCINOMA

- Uncommon, <0.5% of bladder cancer.
- >90% are adenocarcinoma.
- Majority are in urachus immediately adjacent to the bladder wall and spreads towards the umbilicus in the perivesical space.
- Presents late and hence poor prognosis.
- Considerable extravesical component and position at the bladder wall suggests urachal origin rather than bladder carcinoma (bladder carcinoma is intravesical and involve posterolateral wall).

Imaging

- 2/3rd urachal carcinoma shows dystrophic calcification, which may be punctate or curvilinear. 3/5th have low-density cystic component.

USG: Lesions appear cystic with increased echogenicity because of high protein content.

CT: Demonstrate cystic and calcific components very well.

- Also demonstrates mass at the bladder wall and its characteristic extravesical spread.

PRIMARY LYMPHOMA

- Extremely rare (<1% of bladder malignancy).
- Usually non-Hodgkin.
- Present with marked hematuria, increased frequency.
- Radiologically, the appearance of the tumor is non-specific, shows large lobulated mass or focal wall thickening.
- Secondary involvement seen in advanced disease, found in upto 13% of post mortem examination in patients who die of lymphoma.

RHABDOMYOSARCOMA

- Most common pediatric bladder tumor.
- There is biphasic age distribution with peak at 2-6 years of age and 15-19 years of age.
- Tumor grows rapidly with primary invasion and lymphatic and hematogenesis spread.
- Presentation may be with bladder outlet obstruction or incontinence, hematuria infection or visible/palpable mass.

Imaging: Location at the bladder base and/or lying between lower urinary structure leading to difficulty in determining from which organ it has originated.

CT/MRI: Bladder rhabdomyosarcoma appears as a sessile or polypodial soft tissue mass that deforms the bladder base.

- Often project into the bladder lumen (botryoid or bunch of grapes appearance).
- Central necrosis and hemorrhage are other common findings.
- On MRI, it shows low signal intensity on TIWI and intermediate or high signal intensity on T2W1. Tumor enhances after intravenous administration of contrast.

Bladder Outflow Obstruction (BOO)

Approach to a Case of BOO

Most cases of BOO present in emergency with acute urinary retention. Pediatric population may present with distended abdomen and hydronephrotic kidneys. Difficulty in micturition, inability to micturate or post void dribbling is other presenting complaints. Pain due to distension of urinary system is another presenting feature and the patient may also present with hematuria.

Plain X-ray KUB: May reveal the presence of calculus, a soft tissue pelvic mass or bladder wall calcification.

IVP: It appreciates the anatomy of the urinary system and also crudely assesses the renal function and may reveal, or help in narrowing the differential diagnosis in depicting the cause of BOO.

USG: Now-a-days USG is probably the first investigation sought for in the patients with urinary complaints or abdominal masses. USG points to the diagnosis in most cases and further investigations are sought only for better characterization and staging of the pathology or for functional assessment. High frequency linear array probes produce excellent images of urethra, which has to be distended by instilling saline retrogradely.

MCU: The investigation details the anatomy of the bladder and the lower urinary tract especially the posterior urethra, some urodynamic information can be gained as well (Figure 86.1).

Urethrography: Ascending or retrograde urethrography details the anatomy of anterior urethra unto the distal sphincter mechanism.

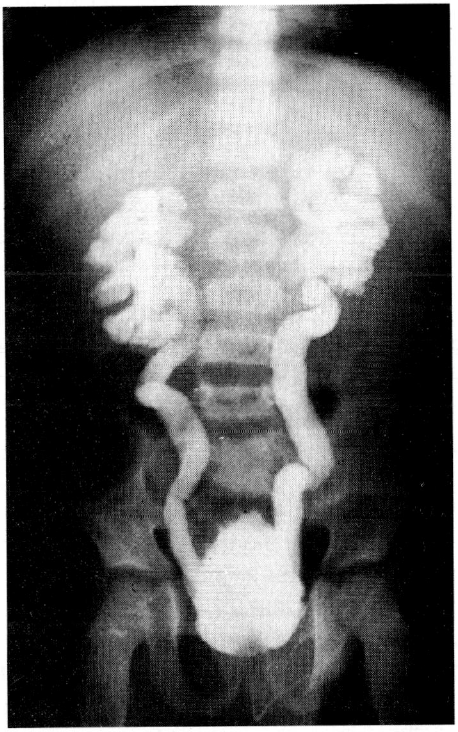

Fig. 86.1: Cystogram shows bladder outlet obstruction with severe vesicoureteric reflux

CT: CT is used to stage malignancy and in cases where diagnosis is in doubt and is also used in biopsy guidance where USG has failed.

MRI: Has the same indications as CT with having added advantage of better soft tissue contrast, multiplanar imaging and no radiation exposure.

Urodynamic Renal Tract Studies

- **Uroflowmetry:** The simplest and most widely applicable investigation is the measurement of urinary flow rate. It is by itself an adequate investigation for uncomplicated prostate related outflow obstruction in nearly 50% cases. The flow rate however is only of value if more than 200 ml is voided as the flow pattern is more important that the flow rate. It can be combined both with USG and IVP.
- **Ultrasound:** Cystodynamography this is the combination of USG with flow rate measurement. This is of value in patients who have had surgery and in those with compromised bladder function e.g. Detrusor failure and sphincter dysfunction.
- **Intravenous urodynamography:** After the 20-minutes' full-length film of an excretory urogram 20 mg of intravenous frusemide is given. When naturally full the patients voids in a flow meter and post micturition film taken.
- **Cystometry and videocystometrography (VCMG):** If a more detailed urodynamic investigation is necessary, measurement of detruso pressure during controlled filling and subsequent voiding, together with measurement of flow rate (filling and voiding CMG), are performed. The detrusor pressure is estimated by the automatic subtraction of rectal pressure (as an index of intra abdominal pressure) from the total bladder pressure. In addition to pressure and flow measurements, the initial bladder residual urine, the bladder volume at the time of patient's first sensation of filling, the tolerated bladder volume and the residual volume after voiding are measured. The VCMG combines pressure studies with imaging of the lower urinary tract.

CAUSES

Primary Bladder Causes

Congenital

- Bladder neck obstruction—Neurogenic.
- Ureterocele.

Acquired intrinsic defects

- Benign prostatic hyperplasia.
- Carcinoma prostate.
- Carcinoma bladder.
- Calculi.
- Diabetic neuropathies.
- Spinal cord disease.
- Anticholinergic drugs and alpha adrenergic antagonists.

Acquired extrinsic defects

- Carcinoma cervix, colon etc.
- Trauma.

Urethral Causes

Congenital

- Posterior urethral valves.
- Anterior urethral valves.
- Stricture.
- Meatal stenosis.
- Phimosis.

Acquired intrinsic defects

- Stricture.
- Tumor.
- Calculi.
- Trauma.
- Phimosis.

Acquired extrinsic defects

- Trauma.

Radiological Findings in BOO

- Bilateral hydroureteronephrosis with dilated tortuous ureters in later stages and sometimes ending up in caliceal rupture leading to urinoma formation or urinary ascites especially if BOO occurs during intrauterine life.
- Thick walled trabeculated bladder, with or without multiple diverticulae depending on the etiology of bladder outlet obstruction.
- Large or small capacity bladder.
- Dilatation of proximal urethra if urethral obstruction is the cause.
- Renal function impairment or loss in later stages.

Urodynamic Features: The urodynamic definition of BOO is a increased voiding detrusor pressure combined with decreased flow rate.

- Normal flow rate varies with age, sex and volume of urine voided.
- Normal male detrusor pressure—40-60 cm H_2O and of female is—20-40 cm H_2O.
- Most patients are diagnosed with a simple pressure studies but only problem cases require VCMG. It also shows anatomy.

Benign Prostatic Hyperplasia

- M.C.U. shows elevation of bladder base.
- Encroachment on the bladder neck by the enlarged median lobe.
- Stretching and narrowing of the prostatic urethra.
- On USG, transabdominal ultrasound shows an enlarged prostate with heterogeneous echotexture. Size estimation can be done reasonably well.
- Shows bladder changes—trabeculations/diverticulation.
- Backpressure changes in the kidneys can be assessed.
- Measurement of post void residuals urine more than 1/3rd of prevoid volume or absolute more than 50 ml is suggestive of significant obstruction.

Neurogenic Bladder

- Occurs as a result of neuropathy related with diabetes or spinal cord disease.
- Two types are known: atonic high capacity (LMN) bladder and spastic low capacity (UMN) bladder.
- Spastic low capacity bladder occurs because of a variety of causes including trauma, spina bifida, Parkinson's disease, multiple sclerosis and diabetes mellitis.
- There is a low capacity high-pressure bladder that contracts involuntarily (detrusor instability) and results in urge incontinence.
- Radiological features include trabeculated thick walled bladder with trabeculations and diverticula's and a typical cone shape referred to as pine cone bladder often with an open bladder neck due to sphincter dyssynergia. There may be associated VUR.
- The urodynamics assessment is necessary to plan treatment.
- Bladder neck dyssynergia is a congenital disease seen in younger age group. The VCMG findings are characteristics, when a normal person is asked to interrupt micturition, contrast agent is milked back into the bladder from the distal sphincter mechanism through the bladder neck "stop test". If there is obstruction at the level of bladder neck contrast agent will be trapped within the prostatic urethra "positive white side trapping sign".
- Flaccid high capacity bladder is seen in lower motor neuron lesions and the bladder is thin walled smooth and enlarged sometimes reaching upto the umbilicus.

Urethral Valves

- Posterior urethral valves are by far the most common and almost exclusively seen in male children.
- There are bilateral hydronephrotic kidneys with dilated ureters, thickened bladder wall with diverticula.
- MCU demonstrates dilated posterior urethra with shelf like PUV most commonly at the level of veru montanum.
- Three types are recognized:
  1. *Type I:* (Most common) are mucosal folds extending antero inferiorly from the caudal aspect of verumontanum.
  2. *Type II:* (Rare) mucosal folds extend antero superiorly from the verumontanum towards the bladder neck.
  3. *Type III:* Diaphragm like membrane located below the verumontanum.
- Vesico ureteric reflux is seen associated especially on the left side.

Role of Imaging in Vesical Mass

ANATOMY

UB when empty is a pelvic organ lying just behind pubic bone with a maximum capacity of 400-500 ml in adult.

- It is boat shaped when distended and has:
  - Superior surface which is covered with peritoneum over which lies intestine and is reflected over rectum to form recto-vesical pouch in males; and over uterus in females to form utero vesical fold.
  - 2 lateral surface related to pelvic bones.
  - Posterior surface/base.

Normal radiological appearance of a distended UB.

IVU: UB appears as centrally located oval or round structure having smooth outline. It often shows normal smooth indentation due to uterus/sigmoid colon on the superior surface of the bladder. After micturition it should be empty apart from little contrast trapped in mucosa.

USG: UB appears as a cystic structure with smooth outline. The wall should be sharply defined and barely perceptible (2-3 mm).

CT Scan: (Figure 87.1) Smooth outline contrasted against pelvic bone. It has thin wall and a uniform diameter. Contrast opacification of urine is variable depending on the amount of contrast reaching the bladder. As the contrast is heavier than urine dependent portion is more dense.

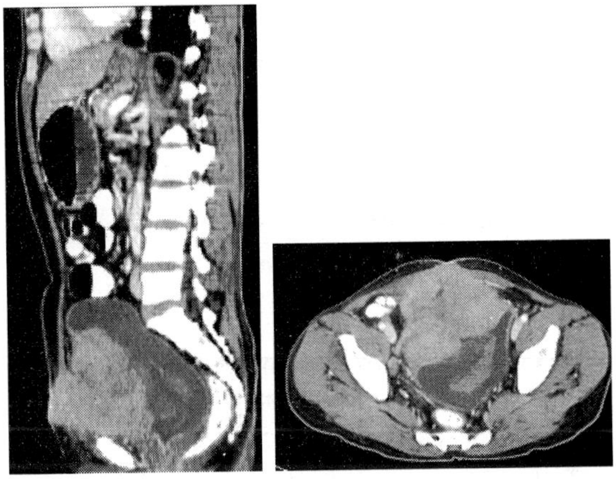

Fig. 87.1: Sagittal MPR and axial CT images show a vesical mass with spread to the abdominal wall

MRI: Bladder wall has low SI on T1W and T2W scans whereas urine because of its long T1 and T2 appears as low and high SI respectively. Urine and bladder wall has low signal intensity can be clearly distinguished. On T2W image: Bladder wall appear as low signal band contrasted with high signal urine and perivesical fat.

VESICAL MASS

Lesions included are:

1. Neoplasm.

2. Calculus.
3. Blood clot.
4. Cystitis.
5. Muscle hypertrophy in BOO.
6. Foreign bodies e.g. bulb of Foleys.

BLADDER TUMOR

- UB is the most common site of urothelial malignancy.
- Most common site:
  - Post wall.
  - Lateral wall (near UV junction).
- Common in males.
- HPE: 92% is TCC: Rest being:
  - SCC.
  - Adenocarcinoma.
- Predisposing factors
  - Smoking.
  - Exposure to
    - Aniline dye.
    - Rubber.
- Secondary tumor – Lymphoma, melanoma, CA rectum, CA prostate in male and Ca cervix in females, sarcomas in children.

"Role of imaging is to diagnose and stage the lesion". Crucial point is to identify the invasion of tumor into perivesical fat and adjacent viscera along with medial iliac and obturator nodes–as the presence of such a spread signifies in operable lesion.

TNM Classification

TIS: Carcinoma in situ.

T1: Tumor does not invade beyond lamina propria.

T2: Tumor invades superficial muscle layer.

T3a: Invades the deep muscle layer.

T3b: Tumor extends through bladder wall.

T4a: Tumor involves – prostate, uterus, vagina.

T4b: Tumor involves the pelvic side walls/ abdominal wall.

N0: No regional lymph node metastasis.

N1 Single, ipsilateral ext. or int. iliac LN.

N2 Contralateral, bilateral multiple LN.

N3 Fixed regional LN.

N4 Juxta regional LN.

M0: No distant metastasis.

M1: Distant metastasis.

IMAGING IN DIAGNOSIS AND STAGING

1. **EU:** Bladder mass appear as an irregular filling defect.
2. **USG:** Is most common screening modality now-a-days.
   - A high degree of accuracy has been reported for both endoscopic and transabdominal USG.
   - Endoscopic USG can identify all tumors except TIS.

T1: Appear as echo poor mass that cause no interruption of bladder wall.

T2: Infiltrate the echo dense bladder wall.

T3: Involves entire thickness of bladder wall.

On TA USG: Bladder mass may appear as hyper-hypoechoic lesion.

Multiple areas of calcification may be seen:

- Bladder wall oedema associated with chronic catheterisation/chronic cystitis; and hypertrophied bladder wall cannot be distinguished from a solid tumor.

3. **CT Scan:** Is unable to distinguish stages lower than T3a.

T1 and T2: Appear as localized/generalized thickness of bladder wall with clear definition of perivesical fat.

- Nodal staging by CT is dependent upon LN being enlarged, as CT is unable to detect tumor in normal sized nodes.

- Unenhanced scan may show calcification as 10% of tumor may calcify.
- Both CT and USG are useful in diagnosis of tumor in bladder diverticulum than could not be seen during cystoscopy.

4. **MRI** – Lesions >1-1.5 cm can be reliably detected on MRI.

   T1W: UB wall appears as medium SI higher than that of urine and lower than that of perivesical fat.

   - The tumor size/intravesical component/ extension into perivesical fat are best demonstrated on T1W or fat suppressed T2W scans.
   - The presence/absence of pelvic LN and ureteric obstruction can also be assessed in coronal or transverse plane.

   T2W: Tumor on heavily T2 weighted images particularly with fat suppression technique show an intermediate signal being lower than urine.

   - T2W image show extension through bladder wall and infiltration of adjacent organs, former being recognized by disruption of normal low signal band.

ADVANTAGES OF MRI OVER CT SCAN

- More precise delineation of tumor in bladder base and dome.
- Improved evaluation of local spread of tumor as MRI not only produces alteration in size and contour but also produce change in signal intensity.
- Demonstration of LN without IV contrast.
- In most cases it is able to differentiate stage T1/T2 from T3.
- Muscular hypertrophy in BOO there is no alteration in its normal low signal intensity, which can be differentiated from tumor causing altered signal intensity.

CALCULUS DISEASE

- A sharp echogenic lesion on USG casting a distal acoustic shadow and is mobile.
- If calculus is impacted, further evaluation by CT scan required as large calcification may obscure the underlying bladder pathology.

CYSTITIS

USG/CT: Appear as focal/diffuse wall thickening with post void residual urine.

MRI: There occur changes in signal intensity, so it cannot be differentiated from bladder tumor.

Blood Clot

- There is usually history of trauma or catheterisation.
- USG show an irregular echogenic lesion or bladder lumen, which is mobile, and with change in position its configuration changes and it can be well visualized on real time.
- However, solid tumor does not change its appearance.

MUSCLE HYPERTROPHY

- This produce bladder wall thickening and associated with BOO.
- **USG/CT:** Appears as thickened bladder wall with trabeculation sometimes associated with diverticulum.

Section 7—Excretory System

Chapter 88

Interventional Uroradiology of Upper Urinary Tract

With the advent of cross-sectional imaging including real time imaging by means of USG, the percutaneous approach to the collecting system of kidney has been adapted and modified to perform a variety of intrarenal and ureteric manipulations including:

1. Percutaneus nephrostomy.
2. Percutaneous nephrolithotomy.
3. Percutaneous endopyelotomy.
4. Percutaneous resection of urothelial tumors of renal pelvis.
5. Renal cyst puncture.
6. Aspiration cytology and biopsy of renal masses.
7. Pressure flow studies.
8. Percutaneous balloon dilatation of ureteric strictures.
9. Therapeutic ureteric occlusion.

Percutaneous Nephrostomy (PCN)

Indications

Emergency percutaneous nephrostomy

- Obstruction and infected urine.
- Obstruction and severe pain.
- Obstruction causing renal failure.

Elective percutaneous nephrostomy

- Obstruction with minor symptoms before treatment.
- Diversion of urine to heal urinary fistula.
- Pressure flow studies for equivocal upper tract obstruction.
- Percutaneous access for manipulations within kidney or ureter.

Technique

- Usually performed under LA with the patient in prone position, anxious patients may require intravenous sedation and young children always require GA. The puncture may be guided by fluoroscopy alone or preferably by real time USG. If renal function is adequate intravenous contrast medium given before the puncture will give additional fluoroscopic aid to the USG guided puncture.

Single or Double Puncture Technique

- If the kidney is functioning and the PCS is opacified, then it is easy to use 19 gauge sheathed needle for the caliceal puncture under fluoroscopic guidance so that a 0.35 guide-wire can be advanced into the renal pelvis.
- In poorly functioning kidney initial puncture with a fine needle allows opacification of the

PCS so that a calyx can be selected for the fluoroscopic guided sheathed needle puncture. An ultrasonic guided puncture is the best method of guidance for puncturing a posterior calyx.

Ultrasound Guidance

- When obstruction is severe, USG is required to localize the dilated collecting system. It can give good idea of angle and depth of the collecting system. With a small system and a difficult puncture it can be used to provide real time assistance during the procedure. The aim should always be puncture a posterior lower pole calyx passing through the least depth of parenchyma to reach the PCS, this puncture allows good access to pelvis and avoids interlobular vessels. A direct central puncture is more likely to cause vascular damage. The prone or prone oblique position of the patient is preferred.
- A large HDN can be drained using a combined needle and catheter system. The pigtail catheter is incorporated in the needle and a single puncture allows the introduction of the catheter.

Seldinger method uses a needle with a rigid or flexible 4F outer sheath, a flexible outer sheath is preferred as it allows respiratory movement of kidney and minimizes damage. A guidewire is introduced and the track dilated using Teflon fascial dilators and finally an 8F pigtail catheter is passed over the guidewire.

Complications

- Septicemia if infected, urine passes into the circulations.
- Hemorrhage is usually mild.
- AVM can occur if the puncture is made too centrally and are usually treated by selective embolization.

Percutaneous Nephrolithotomy (PCNL)

- PCNL can be done as a one-stage procedure for any type of stone without the kidney necessarily being obstructed. Patients with calculi greater than 2 cm are the best candidates for PCNL.

Technique

- Under GA, a retrograde catheter is passed up the ureter into the renal pelvis and a little methylene blue mixed with contrast media is injected and a PCN is performed. Track dilatation is then performed, either a rigid guidewire is used over which Teflon fascial dilators are passed or large balloon catheters can be used to dilate the track, alternatively metallic dilators can be used. After the track is dilated an amplatz Teflon sheath is advanced which is then used as an operative channel and to perform endoscopy. Nephroscopes are then used to remove calculi, small stones being extracted intact using grasping forceps. Large calculi require disintegration with either ultrasonic or hydraulic probes.

Percutaneous Endopyelotomy

Patients with PUJ obstruction can have an endoscopic treatment of the obstruction by this technique.

Technique

- Access is gained percutaneously in the same way as PCNL. A guidewire is passed into the renal pelvis via the ureteric catheter and brought out to the skin through the percutaneous endoscopic tract. The wire safeguards the PUJ and stabilizes it during treatment. Using an urethrotome the PUJ is cut open on the renal side of the pelvis. The resection is a full thickness cut through the retroperitoneal fat, which is extended 3 cm down the ureter. A tapered endopyelotomy stent is the introduced over the guidewire and is left in situ for 4-6 weeks to allow the PUJ to heal and surrounding fibrosis to form.

Percutaneous Resection of Urothelial Tumors of Pelvis

- This procedure is to be weighted against the possible seeding of tumor in the track and the introduction of tumor cells into the circulation thus only low grade well differentiated tumors can be treated in this way. The radiologist creates the percutaneous tract selecting the calyx that will easily lead to the tumor causing minimal vascular damage. The tumor is then resected using a resectoscope via an amplatz sheath thus inserted; a nephrostomy is left in situ to allow the track to heal.

Renal Cyst Puncture

- This is done only occasionally to drain large cysts that are symptomatic like parapelvic or intrarenal cysts causing pelvic obstruction. It is usually performed under real time USG guidance and if renal abscess is suspected a pigtail catheter can be left inside to allow drainage.

Aspiration Cytology and Biopsy of Renal Masses

The vast majority of renal tumors will require surgery and biopsy will not alter such surgical management. There are two situations when a tissue diagnosis will alter management as in cases suspected to be lymphomatous and in metastasis. FNAC reduces the risk of tumor seeding however the tissue obtained by core biopsy allows most accurate diagnosis.

USG guidance is usually sufficient and LA is all that is needed. Small centrally located lesions are better biopsied using CT.

Ureteric Manipulations

Ureteric Stones

Upper third calculi can be flushed back into the pelvis using a ureteric catheter; a PCNL can then be done. Alternatively a retrograde double J stent can be inserted to prevent the stone from dropping down the ureter and the patient can then be sent for ESWL. Impacted stones, which cannot be moved, can be fragmented and extracted through the kidney through the percutaneous tract using a nephroscope or an ureteroscope.

Middle third calculi present a major challenge and are removed using flexible ureteroscopes.

Lower third calculi can be extracted using rigid or flexible ureteroscopes and a basket catheter passed through the urethra.

Percutaneous Balloon Dilatation of Ureteric Strictures

Indications

- Postoperative strictures.
- Ligated ureters.
- PUJ obstruction.
- Malignant obstruction to facilitate stent placement.

Technique

This is mostly used for benign postoperative strictures. It can be done either in antegrade or retrograde fashion, but most commonly the antegrade technique is preferred after a PCN only difference is that a middle calyx is preferred after as it makes the access to ureter easier. A 7F angiography catheter and a 4-8 mm balloon are usually used.

Therapeutic Ureteric Occlusion

Indications

- Urinary fistulas.
- Severe dysuria and hematuria.
- Total urinary incontinence in inoperable patients.

- Total urinary incontinence or urinary fistulas leading to severe cutaneous infection.

Technique

After performing a nephrostomy and providing an external drainage the following can be used for occlusion:

- Synthetic tissue adhesive.
- Detachable or nondetachable balloon.
- Large bore occluding catheter.
- Silicon or nylon plugs.
- Gelatin sponge plug.
- Intraluminal electrocautery.
- Retroperitoneal ureteric clipping.

Section 7—Excretory System

Chapter 89

Role of Interventional Radiology in Lower Urinary Tract

The mainstay of interventional radiology in lower urinary tract is in:

1. Prostatic dilatation and stenting.
2. Transrectal USG guided biopsy of prostate.

PROSTATIC DILATATION AND STENTING

- Prostatic obstruction to urinary flow is very common age related disorder resulting in frequency, urgency, incontinence, dysuria and urea retention.
- Intermittent catheterization was for centuries the mainstay of treatment in this condition.

  In current urological practice, approx. 90% of patients undergoing surgical treatment have TURP. However, with longer follow up there is significant incidence of impotence, retrograde ejaculation and stricture formation and it is estimated that 12-15% of patients will require 2nd operation within 8 years.

  This suggest that symptomatic relief may be all that is required in many cases and it is in this that interventional radiology is playing role.
- 2 main radiological techniques are available:
  1. Balloon dilatation.
  2. Stent insertion.

Balloon Dilatation of Prostate

- This uses a low compliance fixed diameter balloon that is inserted transurethrally and dilated under fluoroscopic control.

  This technique is easier and less invasive. Procedure is carried out under IV sedation and analgesic and can be conducted as outpatient procedure. Dilatation of balloon reduces disruption of prostatic commissures and possibly stretching the prostate capsule.
- After prostatic dilatation, only small reduction in absolute prostatic volume occurs suggesting neither tissue necrosis nor atrophy is important factors.

  Dilatation with 35 mm balloon produce symptomatic relief in apprrox 70% of patients. The complication rate of balloon dilatation seems to be very low. Slight bleeding may occur after procedure but retrograde ejaculation, loss of patency and incontinence have not been reported.

Prostatic Stents

Metallic stents are used in the treatment of prostatic outflow obstruction and ureteric strictures.

- 2 types:
  - Temporary.
  - Permanent.

- Temporary stents are entirely intraluminal and become encrusted with phosphotic debris if they remain in contact with urine for long periods. This ultimately leads to infection.
- Urothelium covers permanent stents and this avoids the risk of encrustration, infection and stent migration.
- Stent offer better prospects of relief from the symptoms of obstruction and now seem to be reasonable alternative to surgery in elderly patients.

TRANSRECTAL USG GUIDED BIOPSY OF PROSTATE

- Ca prostate is the most common cancer in the world and its incidence is increasing. So diagnosis and management of ca prostate has become an important topic in recent years.
- A rise in serum PSA may be the 1st indication of prostatic pathology.
- The diagnosis is made by biopsy which is most accurately guided by TRUS.
- The normal anatomy of prostate is assessed 1st in axial and long planes.
- The peripheral zone (PZ) folds around the central zone (CZ) posteriorly.
- 80% of cancers originate in outer gland.
- 70% in PZ and remaining 20% in transition zone.
- 10% in CZ.
- The most obvious lesion representing cancer is the hypoechoic peripheral mass most oftenly seen posteriorly.

Biopsy

- An 18G needle is used. A transperineal approach is used. After cleaning the perineum LA 10-20 ml lignocaine is injected 1-2 cm and to anal sphincter and infiltrated into the apex of prostate using a spinal needle. This is all guided with transrectal ultrasound probe. Biopsies are taken with real time ultrasound control.

Patient Preparation

- Before biopsy 120 mg gentamycin is given I.V. At the time of USG 500 mg metrogyl suppository is inserted into the rectum. After biopsy ciprofloxacin 500 mg is taken twice daily for 5 days.

Complications

1. *Hematuria:* Most patients will experience mild hematuria for 2-3 days.

   If they are taking low dose aspirin, this should be stopped until hematoma has subsided.
2. Hematospermia.
3. *Infection:*

   The advantage of transperineal biopsy is a very low incidence of infection.

Section 7—Excretory System

Chapter 90

Lesions of the Urethra

NORMAL ANATOMY

- The urethral exit from the bladder neck to the external urethral meatus.
- In males, it spans a length of 15-20 cm and is divided into anterior and posterior urethra.
- Anterior urethra
  - Bulbar urethra.
  - Penile urethra.
- Posterior urethra
  - Prostatic urethra.
  - Membranous urethra.
- The prostatic urethra is 3-3.5 m in length and is lined by transitional epithelium, which is continuous with the mucosa of the urinary bladder.
- The posterior wall of the prostatic urethra is compared of a longitudinal ridge of smooth muscle and contains verumontanus (1cm), which tapers inferiorly becoming the urethral crests.
- The membranous urethra, 1-1.5 cm in length, is the posteral course then the congenital diaphragm and the site of change from transitional cell epithelium to stratified columnar epithelium.
- The urogenital diaphragm contains the Cowper's glands, which are situated on each side and posterior to urethra. These Cowper's gland secrete mucin during sexual stimulation which functions as a lubricant for the semen.
- The ducts of the Cowper's glands empty into the bulbar urethra.
- The bulbar urethra extends from the inferior urogenital diaphragm to the suspensory penile ligament superiorly and penoserotal junction inferiorly.
- The penile urethra extends from the suspensory penile ligament and penoserotal junction to external meatus, which is lined with stratified squamous epithelium.

RADIOLOGIC EVALUATION

- **Ureterography:** It is the most common investigation in the imaging or of the urethra and can be in antegrade or retrograde approach (Figure 90.1).
- **VC UG:** The bladder is filled with contrast via suprapubic or retrograde catheterisation and the urethra is assessed during voiding.
- **RGU:** The contrast is retrogradely injected with the urethral orifice occluded to prevent reflux of contrast. Urethral occlusion is usually achieved with either a Foley catheter with the

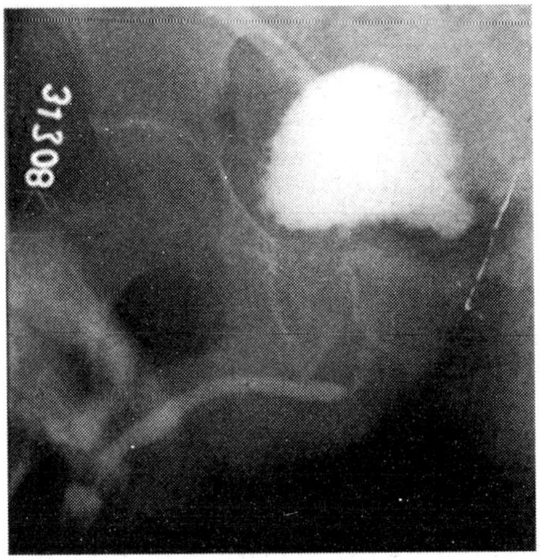

Fig. 90.1: Retrograde urethrogram and cystogram shows severe bladder outflow obstruction due to stricture of the posterior urethra

balloon inflated in the fossa navicularis or a catheter attached to a clamping device into the glans penis.

- **US:** It is able to assess both the urethral and periurethral tissues. The lumen of the urethra is anechoic when filled with saline (sono-urethrography) and the urethral wall is hyperechoic.
  - Abnormalities such as posterior urethral valves, ventricle cysts, urethral stones and stricture can be identified with US.
  - US can also assess associated periurethral abnormalities such as hematomas, abscesses and tumor invasion.
- **CT:** Urethra is seen as isodense to adjacent prostate and corporal tissues and therefore indistinguishable unless it is dilated, catheterized or contains stones.
- **MRI:** It provides excellent soft tissue contrast and despite the urethra and periurethral tissue to best advantage.
  - The urethra is isointense to muscles on T1W sequences.
  - The proximal prostatic urethra is rarely visualized on MR.
  - The verumontanum located in the mid to distal prostatic urethra, is high in signal intensity on T2W sequences.
  - The distal prostatic urethra has additional muscle layer, which demonstrates low signal on T2W.
  - The membranous urethra on T2W sequences demonstrates low signal representing the fibres of the external sphincter surrounding high signal epithelium.

Posterior Urethral Valves

- In this condition there is anomalous development of mucosal folds that obstruct the distal prostatic urethra in males.
- They manifest as bladder outflow obstruct of varying severity, the most extreme product are hydronephrosis, renal failure and Potter's syndrome.
- The milder forms present with lesser degree of outflow obstruction and poor urinary stream.
- MCU demonstrates dilatation of the prostatic urethra and a well defined linear filling defect obstructing the urine flow.

MULLERIAN DUCT REMNANTS

- The caudal part of the Mullerian duct in the male becomes obliterated (apart from caudal part, which persists as the verumontanum).
- Incomplete obliteration may give rise to cyst between the bladder and reaction.
- These may be asymptomatic or present with frequency, infertility, urinary obstructive symptoms or deep perineal pain on micturition or defecation.
- A cavity communicating with the posterior urethra derived from the caudal Mullerian duct may be seen (prostatic utricle) and is considered the male homologue of the uterus.

- Again this may be asymptomatic but is often associated with maldevelopment of the genitalia (hypospadias, crystorchidism, interest etc.) and may lead to urinary tract infection and calculi due to the presence of stagnant urine.
- These lesions may be demonstrated as cystic structure on CT, MRI and transrectal USG.
- Urethrography may demonstrate an extrinsic mass with a Mullerian cyst or a communicating narrow necked, often irregular cavity with a prostatic citricle.

HYPOSPADIAS

- In this congenital malformation the urethra terminates on the ventral surface of the penis, abnormally proximally.
- The meatus is found anywhere from just proximal to its normal site back as far as perineum in some cases.
- There is an association with other urinary tract anomalies and undescended testis.
- The anatomy is best demonstrated with urethrography but this may be difficult as the meatus is abnormal and usually narrowed, resulting in upstream urethral dilatation often with secondary infection.

COWPER'S GLANDS

- These paired glands are embedded in the urogenital in diaphragm and drain via ducts of variable length from a few mm to a few cm) and seen antero inferiorly onto the ventral surface of the perineal part of the bulbar urethra.
- They may be opacified during urethrography in the presence of stricture or inflammation.
- The ducts to the glands may be congenitally dilated (Cooper's duct syringocele), usually asymptomatically but on rare occasions associated with urethral obstruction.

OTHER CONGENITAL URETHRAL LESIONS

- The urethra is rarely duplicated congenitally, usually in the sagittal plane.
- The accessory urethra terminates along the shaft of the penis and is usually blind ending, although if it communicates with the bladder it is associated with continuous incontinence.
- Variable narrowing of urethra may occur, ranging from mild stenosis to complete atresia.
- The more severe forms are lethal, associated with obstructive renal failure and Potter's syndrome unless there is a persistent patent arachic or recto vesical fistula to decompress the system.

URETHRAL STRICTURES

Inflammatory

- Inflammatory urethral strictures may develop following urethritis.
- Classically it follows gonococcal urethritis but is occasionally seen following non-specific urethritis but is occasionally seen following non-specific urethritis with organisms such as chlamydia trachomatis.
- Urethrography should be avoided while there is active urethritis but on rare occasions the features of urethritis are observed on cystography and include contrast filling of the penile through glands and multiple small sessile filling defect due to polypoidal mucosal hyperplasia (urethritis cystia) especially with gonorrhoea.
- The stricture is typically situated in the anterior urethra, most commonly in the proximal bulbar urethra.
- Strictures may be multiplex and of any length.
- TB is a rare cause, being seen in the urethra in 2% or less of urinary tract TB. It almost always arises from a focus elsewhere in the urinary

tract, usually renal, sometimes as a result of direct extension of infection from the prostate or perineum.

- If severe, this may be associated with multiple urethra perineal fistulas.
- Rarely strictures may be seen following severe, usually chronic, urethritis from almost any cause including sero negative arthritides (Reiter's syndrome) and syphilic and chemical urethritis.
- This latter condition arises from therapeutic instillation of chemicals into the urethra (e.g. podophyllin or S- FU for treatment of condyloma acuminata).

TRAUMATIC

- This may follow iatrogenic or accidental trauma.
- Iatrogenic strictures most commonly follow catheterization (traumatic, failed or prolonged) and are usually at fixed narrowed areas, particularly the level of the membranous urethra and penoscrotal junction.
- They may also be seen following instrumentation and urethral surgery.
- They may be single or multiple and of variable length but are usually short.
- Accidental injuries to the posterior urethra are frequently associated with complete transition of the urethra. They are generally short (less than 2 cm long) and solitary.
- Strictures may be associated with pseudo diverticula and peri urethral absences developing upstream. Fistulas, inner urinary extravasation and false passages (exp. following iatrogenic trauma) may also occur.

URETHRAL TRAUMA

- It is almost entirely restricted to the more, being exceptionally rare in the female urethra under therein very major pelvic trauma.
- It should be suspected if pelvic trauma is associated with urinary retention or hematuria especially blood at the urethral meatus.
- Investigation is with careful ascending urethrography, which will demonstrate the presence and extent of the injury and allow classification into trauma to the posterior or anterior urethra.

Posterior Urethra

This is traumatised is around 10% for anterior pelvic fracture.

Male Posterior Urethral Injuries (Table 90.1)

- There may be some bladder filling on the retrograde urothrogram, allowing a diagnosis of partial or incomplete posterior urethral rupture to be made.

Table 90.1: Effects of trauma

Type	Membranous urethra	Bulbar urethra	Contrast extravasation	
			Perineum	Retroperitonic spare
I	Continuous or partial tear	Normal or stretched	No	No
II	Rupture above urogenital diaphragm	Normal or stretched	No	Yes
III	Rupture below urogenital diaphragm	Ruptured	Yes	No

- Complete rupture is associated with aborsence of bladder filling.
- While partial urethral tear usually heal uneventfully complete tear are much more likely to be associated with adverse sequelae such as urethral stricture (usually less than 1 cm or so in length) importance (upto around 10%) or incontinence (2%).

Anterior Urethra

- This is most commonly damaged during attempted catherizations or instrumentation, usually intragenically (occasionally self inflicted).
- In the community it is usually associated with blunt perineal trauma when the bulbar urethra and corpus spongionum are compressed against the inferior aspect of the anterior pelvic ring (straddle injury).
- The injury is not usually associated with a fracture.
- There may be urethral contusion only or some degree of rupture either partial or complete.
- In partial rupture the proximal urethra is demonstrated while in complete rupture there is an abrupt discontinent at the site of rupture.
- Extravasation is associated with both practical and complete rupture and contrast may enter the corpus spongiosum and veins.
- Even contusion alone may lead to subsequent stricture but this is more common with any degree of rupture especially complete.

URETHRAL TUMORS

Benign Tumors

- Fibroepithelial polyps are occasionally encountered, usually in children, sometimes in young adults.
- They appear as finger like processes 1-2 cm long originating near the verumontanum and present with intermittent outflow obstruction.
- Transitional and squamous cell papillomas are benign mesenchymal neoplasms lined with urothelium, which may be metaplastic.
- In the male they may be seen in the prostatic urethra (and may be associated with bladder papillomas) but are most often situated in the fossa navicularis and para meatal area.
- In the female they are usually found in the distal third of the urethra (urethral cannules).
- They usually present between 20 and 40 years of age with hematuria and/or discharge.
- They are seen as smooth solitary or multiple filling defects on urothrography.

Urethral Carcinoma

- This rare tumor is also unusual in being encountered more frequently in female than males.
- In the female it has peak incidence around 40-60 years and is usually associated with chronic inflammation and may be associated with fibrous polyps and caramels.
- It presents with blood appearing at urethral meatus and symptoms of irritation and obstruction.
- 75% of squamous cell carcinoma and most of the rest are TCC.
- Adenocarcinoma is occasionally encountered and arises from urethral diverticula, presumably reflecting the origin of the diverticulum from an infected paraurethral (Bartholin's) gland.
- Carcinomas appear as one or more serial irregular filling defects within the urethra on urethrography or as an irregular stricture.
- Lymph node metastases occur before blood borne spread, the distal third of the urethra metastasing to superficial and deep inguinal lymph nodes, the proximal two thirds to the external and internal iliac lymph nodes.

- In the males the peak incidence is above the age of 50. The commoner is carcinoma of the prostatic urethra usually TCC.
- It has a strong association with bladder TCC, especially with previous resection.
- Carcinoma in the remainder of the urethra (membraneous bulbar and penile) is strongly associated with chronic urethral inflammation (including STD) and strictures present in upto 75% of patients).
- As with carcinoma of the female urethra approximately 75% are SCC, most of the rest are TCC and adeno carcinoma is occasionally seen.
- Presentation is usually with insidious onset of poor urinary stream, hematuria and sero sanguinous discharge.
- On urethrography, carcinoma appears as well defined filling defect, it may be eccentric or circumferential and may be associated with irregular structuring.
- Metastatic spread is virtually always via the lymphatitis, the penile urethra metastasising to the deep inguinal and external iliac lymph nodes, the bulbar and posterior urethra to the internal iliac and obturator lymph nodes.
- MRI is the favored modality for staging urethral carcinoma in both sexes because of its better demonstration of the soft tissue anatomy of the perineum.

  T1 – Tumor invading subepithelial connective tissue.

  T2 – Tumor invading any of periurethral muscle, corpus spongiosum or prostate.

  T3 – Tumor invading any of the bladder neck, corpus cavernosum, anterior vagina.

  T4 – Tumor invading any of the other adjacent organs, including the bladder.

URETHRAL METASTASES

- Metastasis from distant primaries to the urothelium of the urethra is excessively rare.
- The urethra is more commonly involved by direct spread of tumor from adjacent organs, most often carcinoma of the bladder or rectum occasionally prostate vagina or cervix.

URETHRAL FILLING DEFECTS

- The most common urethral filling defects are calculi and tumors usually benign, occasionally, carcinoma and rarely metastasis).
- Other less common causes include the occasional urethral equivalent of inflammatory conditions seen elsewhere in the urinary tract (malcoplakia, urethritis cystica and the swollen mucosa of urethritis) and condyloma documinata.

CONDYLOMA ACUMINATA (VENEREAL WART)

- It is due to DNA papilloma virus and appears in a dermal wart on the genitalia and around on the conus.
- Condyloma may extend into the anterior urethra, where they appear as multiple sessile filling defects on urethrography.
- This procedure however may be associated with retrograde filling of the infecting agent into the bladder and is best avoided if the diagnosis is suspected in advance.
- There is an association with SCC of the vulva.

URETHRAL CALCULI

- Urethral calculi are uncommon and over 90% originate in the kidney and bladder.
- They may present with sudden obstruction of the urine flow or more chronic symptoms of urethritic dysuria and poor stream.
- A minority originate in the urethra in the association with a structural abnormality (usually structure or diverticula).
- They enlarge slowly and present with symptoms of prostate.
- In the female urethra they are usually seen in a mid urethral diverticulum. In the male they are generally found around the junction of the prostatic and membranous urethra.

STRUCTURAL LESIONS OF THE URETHRAL WALL

Urethral Diverticula

- These are rarely congenital, when they are classically saccular and situated in the midpenile urethra.
- They are associated with high grade obstruction in children and are difficult to distinguish from urethral valves.
- Acquired diverticula are strictly speaking pseudodiverticula, as they are lined with fibrous tissue or inflammatory cells rather than urothelium.
- They are inflammatory in origin and may develop from an abscess in the paraurethral glands or within the prostate gland.
- Mechanical causes play a part and they may develop immediately upstream of urethral stricture or following pressure necrosis with a long team urethral catheter usually on the inferior wall of the urethra at the panoserotal junction.
- Stasis of urine may lead to secondary infection and calculus development.
- If they become large enough, they may elevate the bladder base.
- They may be demonstrated on urethrography or ultrasound (transvaginally in the females).

URETHRAL FISTULAS AND SINUSES

- These form if there is an impediment to closure after urethral rupture or laceration.
- They may be secondary to rectal or gynaecological surgery, obstetric injury, radiotherapy and some inflammatory lesions (Crohn's disease, periurethral abscess, TB) or which stricture or carcinomas.
- They may end in the soft tissue of the perineum or continue onto the skin of the perineum or penis.
- Alternatively they may communicate with the rectum, colon, vagina or uterus.
- Conventionally diagnosis is with sonography or MW which will show an irregular track that may lead into an irregular cavity or into another viscera.
- MRI is also useful to show the fistulous track.

POSTERIOR URETHRAL VALVE (PUV)

- Most common congenital obstructive lesions of the urethra and most common cause of end stage renal disease in boys.
- These types of PUV have been recognized based on urethroscopic findings.

Type 1: Two fibro epithelial valve like fold originate from the lower pole of the verimontaneous and course obliquely to the most distal position of the prostatic urethra. Two folds fuse anteriorly leaving a cleft as the only passage for urine. This is the most common form of PUV.

Type 2: PUV related to superior urethral crest and its fine, is believed to be very rare or non-existent.

Type 3: This type of PUV is relatively less common as compared to type 1. In patients with this type of valve a transverse membrane is seen in the posterior urethra just below the verumontanum sometimes near the urogenital diaphragm.

- They manifest a bladder outflow obstruction of varying severity, the most extreme producing bilateral hygdronephrosis, renal failure and Potter's syndrome.
- The milder forms present with lesser degrees of outflow obstruction and poor urinary stream.
- Micturating cystourethrography demonstrates dilatation of the prostatic urethra and a well defined filling defect obstructing the urine flow.

Pneumoperitoneum

- One of the most significant sign in medicine.
- >90% of patients with pneumoperitoneum and acute abdominal pain require surgery.
- Erect CXR or left lateral decubitus X-ray can detect as little as 1 ml of air.
- CT (Figure 91.1) most sensitive – Wide window setting.
- It may not be possible to obtain erect or decubitus X-ray in every patient due to sick patient.
  - Horizontal shoot through.
  - Supine X-ray.

  Signs and pneumoperitoneum on supine X-ray.

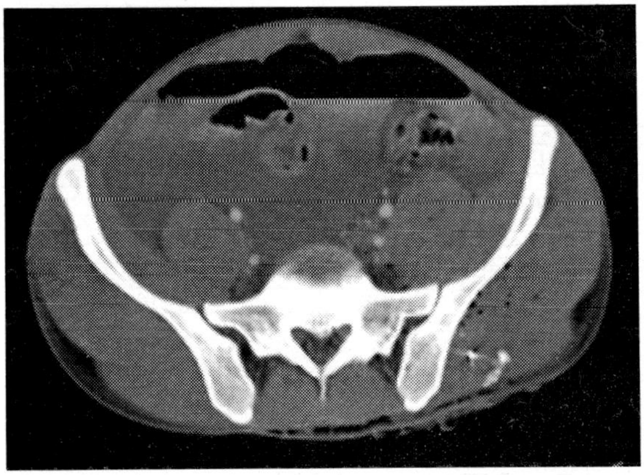

Fig. 91.1: Axial CT image shows hydropneumoperitoneum

- **Rigler sign:** Gas on both sides of the bowel, outlining the bowel wall.
- **Fallacy:** Overlapping loops of gas-distended bowel in mid abdomen can mimic this sign.
- **Triangle sign:** Air trapped between loops of bowel in a characteristic triangular configuration.
- ↑ed lucency in right upper quadrant due to air trapped between anterior aspect of liver and the abdominal wall.
- **Right upper quadrant sign:** Triangular or linear collection of air coming in inferolaterally to superomedially in right hypochondrium. Triangular collection in posterior right subhepatic space/hepato and fossa/Morrison's pouch. Linear collection—in anterior right subhepatic space.
- Visualization of falciform ligament.
- Inverted V sign in lower abdomen due to free gas outlining lateral umbilical ligaments, which courses inferolaterally from umbilicus on either side of midline.
- **Urachal sign:** Free air outlining urachus conical, widest inferiorly at its junction with urinary bladder, tapers superiorly.
- **Cupola sign:** Free intraperitoneal air beneath central tendon of diaphragm.

- **Football sign:** Usually in children with large amount of free air seen as generalized greater than normal radiolucency of the entire abdomen.

CAUSES

A. Perforated Viscous

- Most common cause of peritonitis with pneumoperitoneum—perforated peptic ulcer – Gastric/duodenal.
- In 30% perforations – No pneumoperitoneum.
- Colonic perforation (esp. cecal) give most abundant quantities of pneumoperitoneum:
  - Obstructing malignancy.
  - Toxic megacolon.
  - Diverticulitis—rarely.
  - Acute appendicitis—rarely.
  - Emphysematous—Cholecystitis/gastritis.
- Ulcerative/inflammatory bowel lesions:

Small bowel	–	Intestinal tuberculosis
	–	Typhoid fever
	–	Ulceration within Meckel's diverticulum
Large bowel	–	Chronic ulcerative colitis
	–	L.G.V.

- Infection – Peritonitis due to gas forming organism.
- Trauma – Penetrating injuries of abdominal wall with or without bowel injury.
- Blunt abdominal trauma with rupture of the hollow viscus.

B. Peritonitis

Iatrogenic→

Post laparotomy	–	X-ray – 60%
	–	CT – 83%

Patient supine – air along anterior abdominal wall.

Can be detectable upto 3 weeks – However, in obese children pneumo after 3 days may suggest the possibility of perforation.

↑ing air on serial radiographs – exclude breakdown of surgical anastomosis/perforation.

- Rarely following perforation during endoscopic procedures.
- Diagnostic pneumoperitoneum – obsolete.
- Peritoneal dialysis – Intra abdominal therapeutic embolisation.
- Abdominal causes.
- Pneumatosis intestinalis – can lead to pneumoperitoneum.
- Incomplete perforation of the peptic ulcer – valve are like flap that permits the escape of gas only.
- Similar mechanism may explain leakage from gastric carcinoma.
- Crohn's disease.
- Rarely gas can traverse the intact bowel wall of a distended viscus.
- Line from stomach – aerophagy, gastroscopy, excessive intake of oral sodium, bicarbonate, misplaced oxygen tube.
- Jejunal pneumatosis.
- Gynaecological course.
- Rubin test (obsolete).
- Vaginal douching.
- Water sports.
- Knee chest exercise.
- Pelvic examinations in the postpartum period.
- Post MTP.
- Intrathoracic causes – severe pulmonary

disease – COPD, asthma, cavitary pneumonia, rupture of an emphysematous bleb, positive pressure ventilation.

- Silent perforation.
- Steroid therapy/chemotherapy/antibiotic therapy.
- In elderly/comatose patients, in patients with other serious medical conditions.

PSEUDO PNEUMOPERITONEUM

- Chilaiditis syndrome – distended bowel, usually hepatic flexure interposed between the line of the diaphragm. Look for bowel folds.
- Subdiaphragmatic fat – lucent crescent under diaphragm.
- Extension of posterior para renal fat.
- Decubitus view.
- **Curvilinear pulmonary collapse:** Parallel to a just above the diaphragm may simulate a pneumoperitoneum.
- Subphrenic abscess – raised dome with splinting of dome of diaphragm.
- Associated basal atelectasis, pleural effusion.
- **Subpulmonary pneumothorax:** Decubitus view.
- Apposition of gas distended bowel loops mimicking Rigler sign.
- Intramuscular gas in pneumatosis intestinalis.
- Uneven diaphragm and interposed omental fat between the liver and the diaphragm may also simulate free gas.

Section 8—Peritoneum, Mesentery and Retroperitoneum

Chapter 92

Mesenteric Lesions

NORMAL ANATOMY

SMALL BOWEL MESENTERY

It is a broad fan shaped fold of peritoneum that connects the jejunum and ileum to posterior abdominal wall.

- Extends from duodenojejunal junction on left of spine obliquely to ileocecal junction on the right.

Contents

- Superior mesenteric artery and vein.
- Lymphatics.
- Lymph nodes.
- Nerves.
- Fat.

CT shows fat containing area central to small bowel loops in which jejunal and ileal vessels appear as round or curvilinear densities.

Normal mesenteric fat attenuation -100 to -160 Hounsfield unit.

LARGE BOWEL MESENTERY

Transverse Mesocolon

Extends from anterior surface of pancreas to transverse colon. Contains middle colic arteries and vein.

Sigmoid Mesocolon

Extends from posterior pelvic wall and contains sigmoid and hemorrhoidal vessels.

On Ultrasound

- Increased echogenicity of mesenteric fat is suggestive of oedema, inflammation with mass lesions can be evaluated for size, location, internal architecture and vascularity. Mesenteric thickening may be appreciated.

CT Features of Mesenteric Pathology

1. Increase in attenuation of mesenteric fat known as Misty Mesentery.
2. Distortion of architecture.
3. Loss of definition of mesenteric vessels.
4. ± Thickening of peritoneal lining.

D/D of Mesenteric Lesions

1. Mesenteric edema.
2. Lymphedema – Inflammation, neoplasm, surgery, radiation therapy.

3. Inflammation:
    - Pancreatitis.
    - Crohn's disease.
    - Appendicitis.
        - Diverticulitis.
        - Tuberculoma.
        - Mesenteric panniculitis.
4. Hemorrhage.
5. Mesenteric neoplasms.
    - Primary.
    - Secondary.
6. Mesenteric venous thrombosis.
7. Mesenteric cysts.
8. Miscellaneous:
    - Pseudo tumoral lipomatosis.
    - Systemic amyloidosis.
    - Endometriosis.

Diffuse Mesenteric Edema

Can occur due to hypoalbuminemia, mesenteric ischemia and lymphatic or venous obstruction.

CT

- Increased density of mesenteric fat.
- Poor definition of mesenteric vessels.
- Relative sparing of retroperitoneal fat.
- Associated subcutaneous edema and bowel wall thickening.

Inflammatory Conditions

1. Pancreatitis

Most commonly affects transverse mesocolon and less often the small bowel mesentery.

There is streaky or confluent increased density of mesenteric fat. There is dissection of mesenteric fat. There is dissection of fluid along mesenteric leaves with formation of abscesses, pseudocyst and enteric fistulae.

2. Crohn's Disease

It is a granulomatous disease of the alimentary tract.

a. Fibro-fatty proliferation of mesentery.
    - ↑ Density of fat (-70 to -90 HU).
    - Separation of bowel loops.
    - Lack of soft tissue mass or fluid collection in affected region.

b. Diffuse inflammatory reaction of mesentery:
    - Ill defined ↑ in density.

c. Abscess seen as water density mass.

d. Communication of mass/collection with bowel seen as leak of air or oral contrast.

e. Vascular dilatation and tortuosity as well as wide spacing and prominence of vase recta – comb sign.

f. Associated bowel wall thickening and mesenteric adenopathy.

Diverticulitis

Inflammation of pericolonic fat characterized by poorly defined soft tissue density and strands. Associated CT findings include colon wall thickening. Intramural sinus tracts, mural or extramural abscesses, fistulae and peritonitis.

Tuberculous Peritonitis

- Mesenteric lymphadenopathy.
- High-density ascites (20-45 HU).
- Thickening and nodularity of peritoneal surfaces, mesentery and omentum.

Bacterial Peritonitis

Thickening of peritoneum and mesentery with increased density of mesenteric fat and ascites.

Mesenteric Panniculitis

It is a non neoplastic inflammatory process involving the adipose tissue of the mesentery.

- Has a 2-8:1 male predilection.
- Age >50 years, rare in children.
- Cause of the disease is unknown.

Predisposing Factors

- Recent surgery – 17%.
- Undercurrent disease like cholelithiasis, aortic aneurysm, peptic ulcer, gastric carcinoma – 25%.
- Prior abdominal trauma, drug use, autoimmune disease, retained suture.

Stages

1. **Mesenteric lipodystrophy:** Fatty degeneration of mesentery. Histologically foamy macrophages and lymphocytic infiltration is present replacing mesenteric fat.
   - Involvement of gastrointestinal vessels and chylous ascites may be present.
   - Signs of inflammation are minimal – Asymptomatic.
2. **Mesenteric Panniculitis:**
   - Inflammatory changes in mesenteric adipose tissue.
   - Infiltration of plasma cells, foreign body giant cells and foamy macrophages.
   - Puckering of mesentery with adherent masses.
   - Abdominal pain, nausea, fever, weight loss.
   - Blood tests are usually normal.
3. **Retractile Mesenteritis – Final stage.**

   Histologically collagen deposition, fibrosis and inflammation with scarring and retraction of mesentery.
   - Formation of abdominal masses.
   - Intestinal obstruction.
   - Jejunal mesentery is more commonly affected.
   - Criteria for diagnosis involve absence of pancreatitis and inflammatory bowel disease.
   - Definitive diagnosis is by biopsy.

Barium Study

May reveal displacement of bowel loops. Bowel loops may be dilated, fixed or narrowed.

U/S

Shows ill defined heterogeneous mass in the mesentery with mesenteric thickening.

CT Features

1. Well defined soft tissue masses (Figures 92.1, 92.2, 92.3 and 92.4) with areas of interspersed fat with higher attenuation than retroperitoneal fat.
2. Cystic components in the mass due to dilated lymphatic due to obstruction.
3. Maximum transverse diameter of mass is 7-15cm and mass is directed towards left abdomen due to greater predilection for jejunal mesentery.
4. A hyper attenuating stripe surrounds the mass in 60% cases.
5. Scattered small soft tissue nodules may be present. Enhancement is positive because of inflammation.
6. Hypodense fatty halo surrounding nodules and mesenteric vessels.

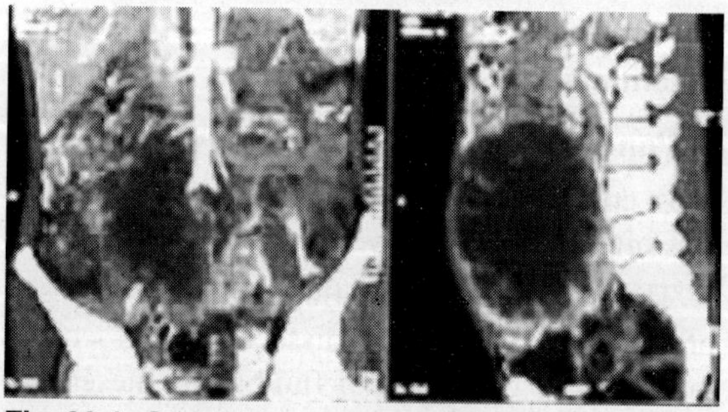

Fig. 92.1: Coronal and sagittal MPR CT images show a large mesenteric sarcoma

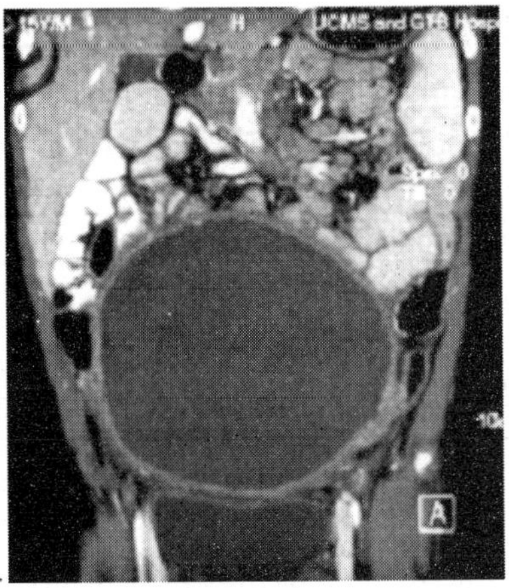

Fig. 92.2: Coronal MPR CT image shows a large mesenteric cyst

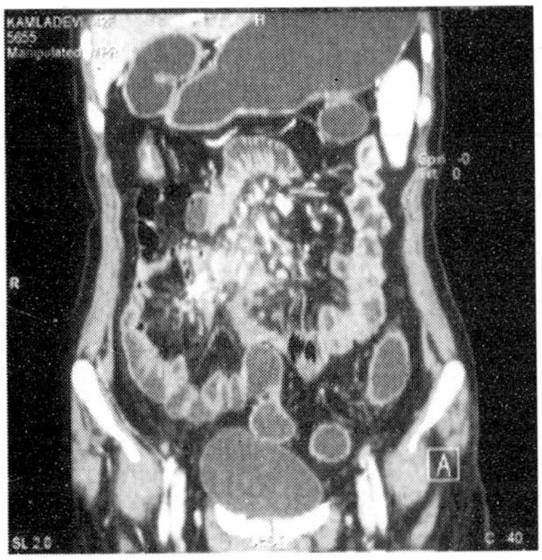

Fig. 92.3: Coronal MPR CT image shows a large retractile mesenteric mass

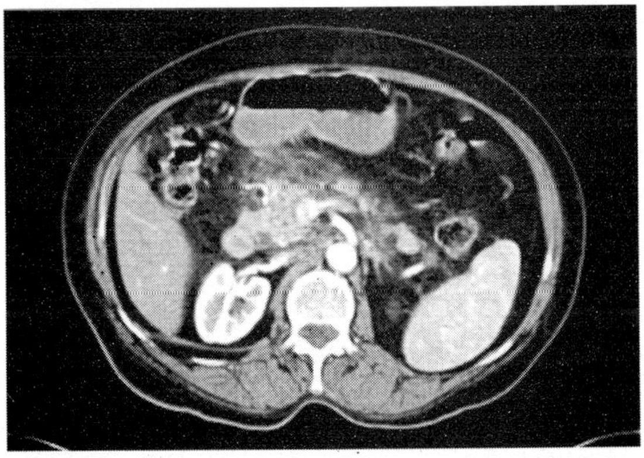

Fig. 92.4: Axial CT image shows mesenteric inflammation in a case of acute pancreatitis

7. Inflammatory mass tend to surround vessels rather than displacing them (D/D from tumors).
8. In later stages fibrosis predominates with increased attenuation of masses.
9. Calcifications are common.

MRI: Fluid or inflammation – low on T1, to high on T2.

Fat – high on T1 and T2.

Fibrosis – Low on T1 and T2.

D/D: 1. Pyogenic peritonitis.

2. Tumors.
   - Lymphoma.
   - Lymphosarcoma.
   - Desmoid tumor.
   - Metastatic carcinoma

Mesenteric Venous Thrombosis

Cause – Portal hypertension, intra abdominal inflammation, obstruction hyper coagulation and tumor thrombus.

U/S shows ↑ echoes in veins.

Doppler is the modality of choice for diagnosis and establishing the cause of increased internal echoes. Doppler shows absence of colour within these vessels with little or absent flow on pulse doppler.

CT – SMV is involved in 95% cases.

Chronic thrombus – Enlarged vein with central hypodensity surrounded by hyper vascular wall.

In acute cases – thrombus is hyperdense.

There is associated mesenteric edema.

Mesenteric Cysts

Lymphangiomas, pseudopancreatic cysts, enteric duplication cysts.

Appear as unilocular or multilocular cystic masses.

Mesenteric Hemorrhage

Associated with blunt abdominal trauma, rupture of aneurysm, excessive anticoagulation or thrombocytopenia.

Acute hemorrhage produces localised hyper attenuating soft tissue masses adjacent to bowel loops (50-60 HU) approaching water density with time.

Mesenteric Neoplasm

Primary

1. Mesenteric desmoid tumor

Locally invasive fibromatosis lesions, occurring more commonly in females and predominantly in patients with Gardner's syndrome.

On CT – Soft tissue mass with well defined irregular margins, displacing adjacent visceral structures.

40-60 HU with no enhancement.

MRI—Low signal on both T1 and T2 due to fibrous tissue.

2. Lipomatous tumor

Benign lipomas consist of a fat density mass liposarcomas – mixed fat and muscle density.

3. Malignant mesothelioma

- Peritoneal thickening irregular or nodular with mesenteric and omental thickening.
- Multilocular cystic mass.
- Ascites.
- Thickening of perivascular bundles by tumor.

Secondary Neoplasms

- **Metastatic carcinoma** from stomach, colon or ovary by direct spread along ligamentous attachments.
- Intraperitoneal seedling.
- Lymphatic and hematogenous disseminated.
- Direct spread - Causes stranding of mesentery with or without masses/nodules.
  Involvement by carcinoid produces characteristic features evident on CT scan.
- CT picture - Triad of calcification within mesenteric mass.
  Radiating soft tissue strands.
  Mural thickening of adjacent small bowel loop.
- Rounded cake like masses – mainly lymphoma.
- Ill-defined masses – ovarian carcinoma, lymphoma, metastases.
- Cystic—Ovarian carcinoma.
- Stellate pattern – radiating pattern of mesenteric leaves by ovarian, breast, colonic, pancreatic carcinoma.
- Pseudomyxoma peritonei—low attenuation mucinous masses may be capsulated, or diffuse with septations.
- Lymphatic dissemination – causes mesenteric adenopathy lymphedema.
- Hematogenous emboli – nodules seen.

Mesenteric Ischemia

CLASSIFICATION

Acute Mesenteric

- Occlusive.
  - Arterial
    - Embolic.
    - Thrombosis.
    - Dissection.
- Venous secondary to abdominal surgery, infection and hypovolemic status.
- Non occlusive hypo perfusion secondary to hypovolumic shock, low cardiac failure.
- Chronic **mesenteric**
  - Intestinal angina.
  - Mesenteric.

Chronic arterial disease resulting from:

- Atherosclerosis.
- Tumors.
- Fibro muscular dysphasia.

SMA more than IMA including smaller colic more frequently than celiac.

Rare Causes:

- Small bowel hernia.
- Adhesions.
- Intussusceptions.
- Antiphospholipid antibody syndrome (APS).

PATHOPHYSIOLOGY

Acute ischemia

↓

Submucosa, edema, congestion, thrombi, hemorrhage (sec to anoxia)

↓

Necrosis of mucosa

↓

Membrane formation (patchy)-patients experiences malabsorption, diarrhea and rectal bleeding

↓

If severe

↓

Bacterial invasion and granulation tissue

↓

If extends to serosa

↓

Dense adhesions

↓

Perforation – acidosis shock and hyperemia.

Mortality and Morbidity: The major cause of mortality is bowel necrosis with morbidity as high as 70% in such cases.

CLINICAL SYMPTOMS/SIGNS—ACUTE

- Abdominal pain—Initially with dull pain.
- Diarrhea.
- Rectal bleeding.
- Peritoneal sign sec. to infection.

Emergency Angiography

Emboli, arterial and venous occlusion and arterial mesenteric vasoconstriction.

Patients of **chronic ischemia**—post prandial abdominal pain, typically several minutes after meal, hence are reluctant to eat—weight loss—chronic diarrhea.

Rare Causes

- Small bowel hernias.
- Adhesions.
- Intussusceptions.
- Antiphospholipid antibody syndrome (APS) with hypercoagulable state secondary to circulatory immunoglobulins without interacting with phospholipids in all membranes.

VASCULAR OCCLUSION

Acute mesenteric thrombosis.

SMS occlusion	Embolus. Blunt trauma. Iatrogenic during repair.
Embolic occlusion. Usually lodged at bifurcations.	Near origin of middle colica.

- Seen as reversed meniscus sign or intraluminal filling defect on angio.
- Stacked coin appearance.

VASOSPASTIC MESENTERIC ARTERIES

Due to poor perfusion secondary to poor LVF, volume loss, shock.

Angio

- Patent vessels with fusiform narrowing at the origin of branch of SMA.
- Irregularities and spasm of the arcades.
- Incomplete filling of vasa recta.

Venous Thrombosis

- Is an infrequent cause of intestinal infarction.
- Cirrhosis with pulmonary hypertension.
- Tumor thrombosis.
- Trauma.
- Inflammatory.

CHRONIC INTESTINAL ISCHEMIA

- Intestinal angina due to insufficient blood flow.
- Visceral pain and/or absorption and motility disturbances.
- Biplane aortography.
- Occlusion/high grade stenosis with impaired collateral flow.

ACUTE MESENTERIC ISCHEMIA – ISCHEMIC COLITIS

- Pain, diarrhea, blood loss.
- On X-rays

↑ Bowel gas	
Thickened bowel wall	Also detects association of obstruction, free gas
Thumb	Intussusception,

printing or volvulus.
Featureless
colon
Intramural gas

- On barium study
  - Thumb printing
  - Transverse ridging
  - Thickened mucosal folds
  - Ulceration
    - Deep
    - Collar-button
  - Scarring and stenosis.
- USG—Shows wall thickening and oedema.
  - Doppler can assess vessel status of proximal vessels.
  - Associated liver, portal and other pathology assessed.
  - Angiography not of much help.

In Emergency setting—Modalities—Plain X-ray and than CT Scan. However at the later date barium studies, US and Doppler and if required angiography.

MESENTERIC INFARCTION

- Acute is more dramatic and lethal SMA affected

  On X-ray Diffuse dilatation
  Segmental bowel wall thickening
  ↓
  - "Pinky prints"
  - Intramural gas
  - Portal venous gas

  On CT Wall thickening
  - Intramural gas
  - Intraportal gas
  - Hypercoagulable states more common
    Polycythemia Vera
    Splenectomy
    OC's

  Idiopathic.
- On Angio
  - Normal large veins with only hyperemia and thickening of the bowel wall

    Veins fail to opacify
  - Prolonged arterial phase
  - Intense bowel wall opacification.
- Differential Diagnosis
  - Appendicitis.
  - Bowel trauma.
  - Colitis, Pseudomembrane.
  - Diverticulitis.
  - Crohn's disease.
  - Nacrotising colitis.
  - Pneumatosis intestinalis.
  - Typhilitis.
  - Ulcerative colitis.

Section 8—Peritoneum, Mesentery and Retroperitoneum

Chapter 94

Retroperitoneum Masses

RETROPERITONEUM MASSES

- **Lymph node mass**
  - **Malignant**
    - Lymphoma
    - Testicular tumors
    - Prostate carcinoma
    - Colonic carcinoma
    - RCC
    - Bladder carcinoma
    - Endometrial and cervical carcinoma
    - Ovarian
    - Melanoma
  - **Benign**
    - HIV inflammation
    - Cirrhosis
    - Sarcoidosis
    - Castlemann's disease
    - Amyloidosis
    - Lymphangio-leiomyomatosis
- **Primary retro-peritoneal tumor**
  - **Malignant**
    - Liposarcoma
    - Leiomyoma
    - MPH
    - Hemangiopericytoma
    - Primary extragondal GCT
    - Fibrosarcoma
    - Neurofibrosarcoma
    - Ganglioneuroblastoma
    - Rhabdomyosarcoma
  - **Benign**
    - Paraganglioma
    - Neurofibroma
    - Neurilemmoma
    - Teratoma
    - Lipoma
    - Hemangioma
    - Lymphangioma
    - Dermoid
- **RPF**
- **Others**
  - **–Hemorrhage**
  - **–Infectious process**

1. LYMPH NODES

- Normal size
  - Retrocrural <6 mm
  - Gastro hepatic <8 mm
  - Celiac
  - Int. iliac <7 mm
  - Obturator <8 mm
  - Mesenteric < 10 mm
  - Para-aortic
  - Pericaval.
- Few specific L.N. patterns on CT
  1. In Whipple's disease – L.N. attenuation is +10 to +80 HU due to deposition of fat and fatty acids.

2. Enlarged low density L.N. are also seen in:
   - M. tuberculosis and MAI.
   - Histoplasmosis.
   - Testicular malignancies esp. terato carcinoma.
   - Epidermoid carcinoma of genitourinary tract.
   - Lymphomas.
3. Calcified L.N. seen in:
   - Post-inflammatory conditions.
   - Mucinous carcinoma.
   - Sarcoma.
   - Treated lymphomas.
4. L.N. with low attenuation centre and rim enhancement M. tuberculosis.
   - MRI.

     In upper abdomen T1W sequence. Are useful (L.N. signal < fat signal).

     In lower abdomen and pelvis T2W sequence are useful (L.N. signal > muscle signal).

     Melanoma L.N. mets have high signal even on T1W.
   - M.R. contrast agent – iron oxide is useful to detect L.N. mets.

     Iron oxide phagacytosed and taken up in lymphatic system.

Normal L.N. accumulate iron oxide.	Malignant L.N. do not accumulate iron oxide.
↓	↓
Low signal on T2 and T2*W SE MRI	L.N. signal not ↓ or on hetero-geneously ↓.

- Ga^{67} SPECT F18 FDG or C11 methionin PET are also useful.

Important causes of retroperitoneal lymphadenopathy.

2. LYMPHOMA

a. Most patients with NHL have abdominal involvement	<50% of HL have abdominal involvement
b. Bulky paraaortic L.N. enlargement is common	Bulky L.N. masses are less common
c. Mesenteric disease seen in >50% patients	In <5% patients

In majority post contrast enhancement is similar to muscle but may be dramatic (more than 60 HU) in few cases.

In treated lymphomatous L.N.:

- Attenuation decreases.
- Size decreases.
- Mesenteric stranding increases.
- Dystrophic calcification.

3. TESTICULAR MALIGNANCIES

- Lymphatic drain near renal hilum.
- Mats from right testis – Tend to be midline.

  Right suprahilar L.N. are not involved without involvement of right hilar L.N.

4. HIV INFECTION

Specific CT characteristics:

a. L.N. of homogenous soft tissue attenuation – MAI, NHL.
b. Disproportionately large mesenteric L.N. with retroperitoneal adenopathy.
   - M. tuberculosis.
c. Post contrast enhancement—muscle – Kaposi SA.
d. Calcification in L.N.—extra pulmonary P.

Chapter 94

carinii also multiple focal low attenuation – splenic lesions, liver lesions.

Pleural and peritoneal free fluid.

e. Massive lymph node enlargement (>3 cm) – lymphoma.

5. LIPOSARCOMA (Figure 94.1)

- Inhomogeneous poorly marginated or infiltrative masses that may contain fat attenuation.
- Fat in liposarcoma can be seen as:
  - Low attenuation on CT (mean—10 HU).
  - High T1W signal intensity on SE MRI.
  - High T2W signal intensity on SE MRI.

  Signal loss on fat saturated T1W MRI.
  - 3 distinct CT patterns of liposarcoma.

  1. Solid pattern — CT unit >20 HU.
  2. Mixed pattern—Discrete fatty areas <-20 HU and other areas > + 20HU.
  3. Pseudocystic pattern – homogenous density between 20 to +20 HU.

  May simulate cystic lymphangioma.

HISTOLOGIC VARIANTS

Well differentiated (lipogenic) liposarcoma—

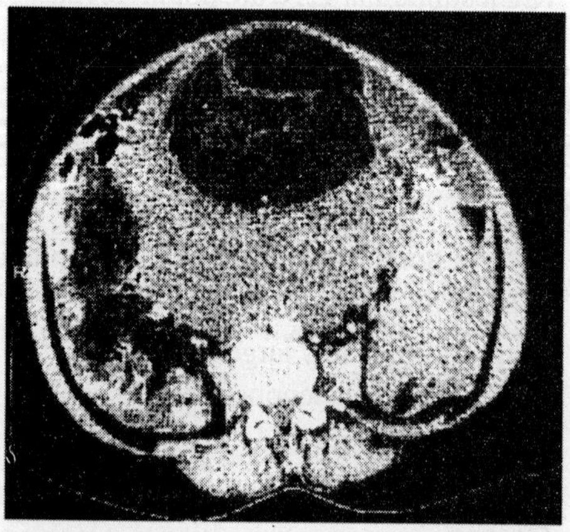

Fig. 94.1: Axial CT image shows a large heterogeneous liposarcoma

usually has mixed pattern with abundance mature fat.

Poorly differentiated liposarcoma – little fat.

Liposarcoma with round cell/pleomorphic histology—solid pattern.

Differentiating features between lipogenic liposarcoma and nature lipoma.

- Soft tissue septa >2 mm thick.
- Septal irregularity and bulging.
- Obvious enhancement.

LEIOMYOSARCOMA

- Large heterogeneous mass with low attenuation or high T2W signal intensity components (that represent necrosis) without presence of fat or Ca^{++}.
- Mimics lymphoma but leiomyosarcoma is more heterogeneous.

Malignant Fibrous Histiocytoma

- High grade tumor.
- Large heterogeneous soft tissue attenuation mass containing areas that show low attenuation or high T2W signal intensity representing necrosis.
- 25% tumor contains dystrophic calcification.

HEMANGIOPERICYTOMA

- Originate from blood vessel wall.
- Very vascular and show brisk enhancement on CT/MRI.
- May contain calcification in few cases.

PRIMARY EXTRAGONADAL GCT

- Only 5-10% of GCT originate outside gonads and most of them occur in mediastinum.
- Affect young adults.
- Heterogeneous mass with soft tissue attenuation.

- If teratomatous—may contain fluid density, fat-fluid level and Ca^{++}.

BENIGN NEOPLASMS

1. Paraganglioma

- Most common site for extra adrenal pheochromocytoma i.e. paraganglioma is the para aortic region from the level of adrenal gland to aortic bifurcation.
- CF if that are:
  - Episodic headache.
  - Palpitation.
  - Diaphoresis.
  - Hypertension.
- Seen as well defined soft tissue mass in the immediate para aortic location.
- Small – homogenous.
- Large – heterogeneous with necrosis and hemorrhage.
- May contain calcifications.
- Enhance briskly following contrast (a blockers should precede contrast).
- MRI – extremely high signal on T2W ± low signal rim due to hemosiderin deposition.

2. NEUROFIBROMA

- Usually in-patient with NF nerves courses through the tumor.
- CT – well defined sharply marginated homogenous soft tissue mass with near water attenuation.
- Usually located adjacent to vertebral column or deep psoas muscles.
- Neural foramina may be eroded.

If mass is heterogeneous – malignant degeneration.

3. NEURILEMMOMA

- Encapsulated tumor arising from peripheral nerve sheath nerve fibre confined to capsule of tumor.
- Usually seen in young to middle aged adults.
- Most common site – soft tissue of head and neck and extremities.
- CT/MRI
  - Heterogeneous soft tissue masses.
  - May contain cystic areas.
  - Iso intense on T1W MRI.
  - Very hyper intense on T2W MRI.

4. TERATOMA

Contain components of all 3 germ layers.

CT/MRI – Fat attenuation component +ve ± fat fluid level.

Calcification/Ossification

Dermoid Plug

Malignant degeneration occurs in <1% cases and is more common in post menopausal patients teratoma with dermoid plugs.

5. LIPOMA

- Well-defined homogeneous fat density lesions with thin capsule.
- Fine septa should be seen traversing through these.

6. HEMANGIOMA

- Soft tissue attenuation on CT with brisk post contrast enhancement.
- May contain calcification.

RETROPERITONEAL FIBROSIS (Figures 94.2, 94.3 and 94.4)

- Rare inflammatory and fibrotic process most

94 Chapter

frequently involving caudal aspect of retroperitoneum.

- Usually affects middle aged to elderly men.
- Associated disease:
  - Reidel's thyroiditis.
  - Fibrosing mediastinitis.

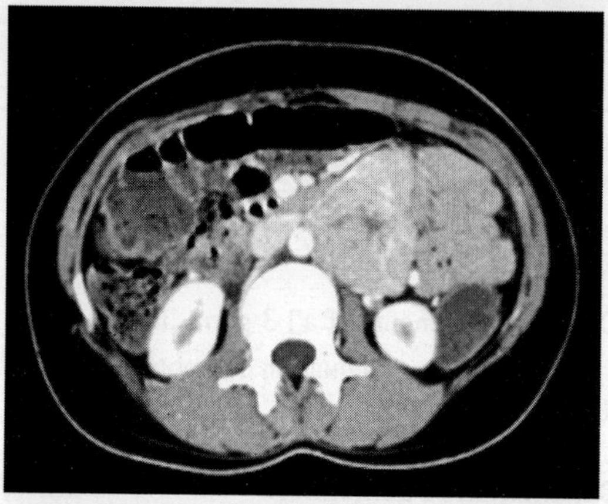

Fig. 94.2: Axial CT image shows a large vascular mass in the left retroperitoneum

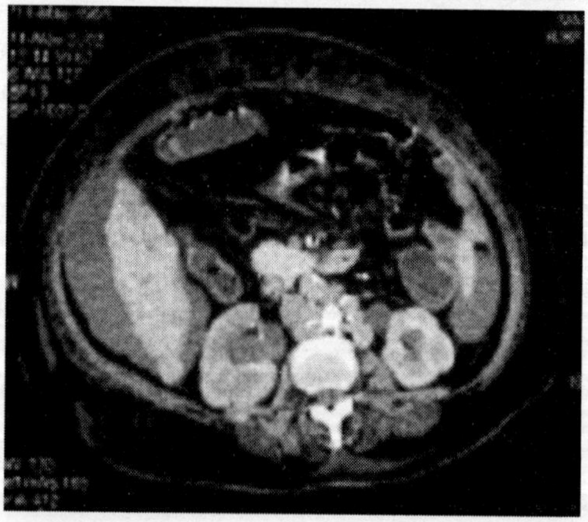

Fig. 94.3: Axial CT image shows malignant retroperitoneal fibrosis with nodular liver, ascites and hydrouteronephrosis on right side

  - Mesenteric fibrosis.
  - Rheumatoid arthritis.

CAUSES

1. Idiopathic (70%): Immune response to ceroid and oxidized LDL.

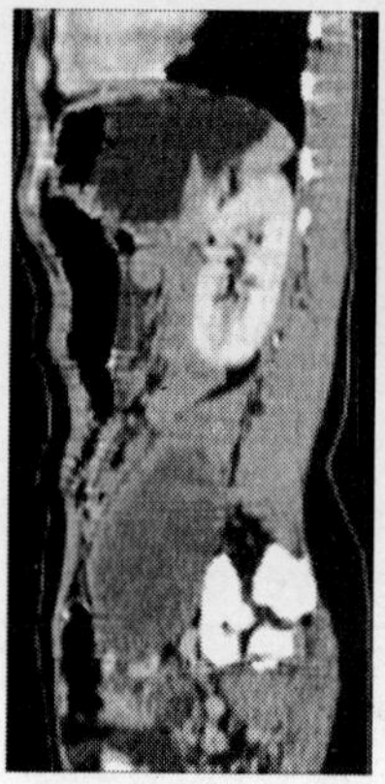

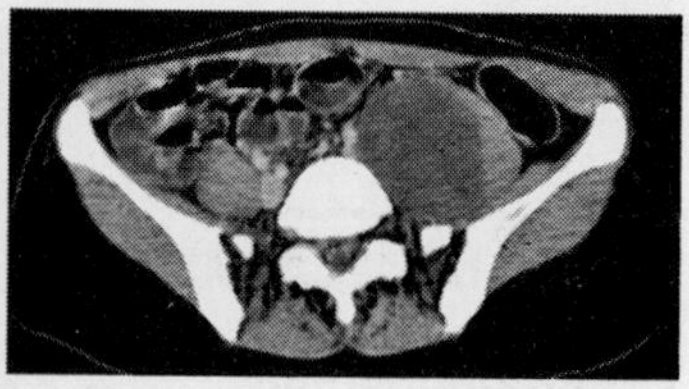

Fig. 94.4: Axial and sagittal MPR CT images show psoas abscess in the left retroperitoneum

2. Drugs: Methyserzide, β blockers, methyl dosage, hydralazine, antibiotics and few analgesics.
3. Systemic infections of TB, syphilis, actinomycosis, brucellosis, fungal infections.
4. Ford inflammatory or infectious conditions e.g. diverticulosis, appendicitis, extravasation from urinary tract.
5. Previous surgery or radiation treatment.
6. Trauma.
7. Retroperitoneal hemorrhage.
8. Marfan's disease.
9. Inflammatory bowel disease.
10. Malignant process – primary or mets esp.
    - Carcinoid.
    - Stomach carcinoma.
    - Breast carcinoma.
    - Ovarian carcinoma.
    - Prostate carcinoma.

- CT findings range from minimal periureteral stranding to large lobulated masses obliterating fat planes between aorta and IVC.
- RPF typically shows obvious post contrast enhancement.
- MRI – low signal on both T1W and T2W SE MRI.

Malignant/active RPF—high and heterogeneous T2W signal.

Differential Diagnosis

1. Metastatic L.N. Mass

Table 94.1: Features differentiating metastasis from retroperitoneal fibrosis

Metastases	RPF
Mass like configuration	Plaque like and infiltrative rather than nodular
Can occur anywhere	Tends to be centred as L4 level
Displaces aorta, IVC and ureters Can cause anterior displacement of great vessels.	Surrounds rather than displaces the anterolateral aspect of grade vessels; may displace ureters medially

2. Lymphoma

Enlarged L.N. are often centred more cranially in retroperitoneum and may be bulkiest at the level of renal hilum.

3. Malignancies Infectious Process

May invade/destroy adjacent bones and organs.

4. Neoplasms

Grow more quickly than RPF on sequential scans.

5. Hemorrhage

Acute life has high attenuation and infiltration between fascial planes.

Section 9—Reproductive System

Chapter 95

Embryological Development of Male Reproductive System

DEVELOPMENT OF TESTIS

- On each side of the embryo a primitive gonad arises from the genital ridge a condensation of tissue near the adrenal gland.

The primitive gonad develops a cortex and medullae. Until the 6th week of development these structures are identical in both sexes.

In genetic males (XY).

Primitive gonad starts developing into testis as early as 7th week with the formation of primitive seminiferous cords in medulla and the cortex regresses (Figure 95.1).

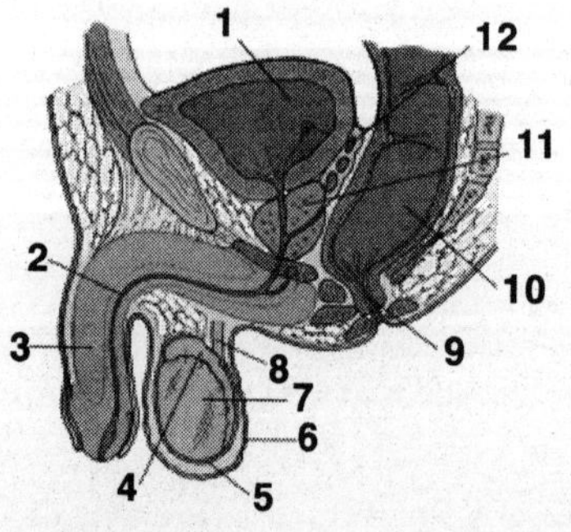

1. Bladder, 2. Urethra, 3. Penis, 4. Epididymis, 5. Tunica vaginalis, 6. Scrotum, 7. Testis, 8. Vas deferens, 9. Anus, 10. Rectum, 11. Prostate, 12. Seminal vesicles

Fig. 95.1: Male reproductive tract

DEVELOPMENT OF EPIDIDYMIS VAS DEFERENS, SEMINAL VESICLES

- At the 8th week of developments, the embryo has both male and female primordial genital ducts.

  Male—Wolfian duct (Mesonephric duct).

  Female—Mullerian duct (Paromesonephric duct).

These ducts are present as paired structures.

In genetic males.

↓

The developing testes secrete hormones.

Leydig cells	Sertoli cells
	↓ ↓
Testosterone	Mullerian inhibiting substance MIS
Promotes development and differentiation of Wolfian duct	Causes regression of Mullerian ducts by apoptosis

1. Duct of epididymis.
2. Vas deferens.
3. Ejaculatory ducts.

A small diverticulum arises which form the seminal vesicles.

- The testosterone metabolite, dehydroxy testosterone induces the formation of male external genitalia by 5th month.

TESTICULAR DESCENT

- The developing testis lies in the retroperitoneum below the developing kidneys. During the 10th week of intrauterine life the precursor of gubenaculum develops as a fold of peritoneum, which can be traced from its attachment between the vas and epidedymis to the region of developing phallus. Progressive contraction of peritoneal folds leads to testicular descent.
- The processus vaginalis start as an outpouching of peritoneum about the 10th week and recedes the testis in its journey through the abdominal wall down to the scrotum.

3rd month	→	Iliac fossa.
7th month	→	Deep inguinal ring.
Later part of 7th month	→	Travelling down the inguinal canal.
8th month	→	Superficial inguinal ring.
Shortly before/ at birth	→	Scrotum.

RADIOLOGICAL ANATOMY

1. USG/USG Doppler

The adult testes are ovoid structures measuring:

- 3-5 cm—Length.
- 2-10 cm—Width.
- 3 cm—Anteroposterior diameter.

Testicular size and weight decrease with age. A dense white fibrous capsule, the tune albugineu, surrounds the testes. Multiple thin saptations arises from innermost aspect of tunica albuginea and converge posteriorly to form mediastinum testis. The mediastinum testis support for entering and exiting testicular vessels and ducts.

- Normal testis has a homogenous grannular echotexture composed of uniformly distributed intermediate level echoes. Similar to that of the thyroid.
- The septa testis may be seen as linear echogenic or hypoechoic structured.
- The mediastinum testis is sometimes seen as linear echogenic band extending arochiocaudally within the testis.
- The tunica albuginea is not normally visualized and a separate structure.

EPIDIDYMIS

- The epididymis normally is echogenic or slightly more echogenic than the testis and its texture may be coarser.
- The head of epididymis lies lateral to the superior pole of testicle appears slightly more echogenic than the remainder of the epididymitis and has a maximum diameter of 8-15 mm.
- The epididymis tapers down through the body to the tail, which has a maximum diameter of 1-3 mm.
- The appendix testis, a remanant of the upper end of paramesonephric duct, is a small ovoid structured located most commonly on superior pole of testis. The appendix testis is visualized sonographically in 80% of testes and is more readily visible when hydrocele is present.
- The scrotal skin and subcutaneous tissues is severe as hyperechoic structure 5-7 mm thick.
- The velocity waveform of the normal capsular and intratesticular arteries—show high level of antegrade diastolic flow through the cardiac

cycle reflecting the low vascular resistance of testis.

- Supratesticular arterial waveform is of high resistance type—affecting high vascular resistance of the extratesticular masses.

PROSTATE

- The normal prostate is roughly bean shaped, the concavity of bean facing posteriorly.
- The central zone and transitional zone have same intermediate echogenicity and are inseparable on USG. They can be referred as central gland and in size and heterogeneity with age as benign prostatic hyperplasia develops in transitional zone.
- The peripheral zone is seen as an echogenic layer lying posteriorly. It is the site of most prostatic tumors, which generally appears as relatively echopoor areas.

Table 95.1: Transabdominal USG vs transrectal USG for prostatic evaluation

Transabdominal USG	Transrectal USG
Rough estimate of size normal prostatic dimension in adult male are approximately 4 cm in craniocaudal and transverse plane and 3 cm in anteroposterior plane; with maximum volume of 20-25 ml	Used in investigation of: 1. Suspected prostatic cancer 2. To assess prostate and stromal vesicles in infertility 3. Prostatitis

SEMINAL VESICLES

- The seminal vesicles appear as paired lobulated echo structures, which often contain multiple small echofree areas.

CT

- The seminal vesicles appear as tubular structures related to the superior aspect of prostate, posterior to lower bladder and anterior to rectum.
- There is a fat plane between the seminal vesicles and the bladder.
- The prostate is usually of homogenous soft tissue density but often show multiple foci of calcification increasingly from adulthood onwards.

MRI

- On T1 weighted images; the prostate appears as intermediate signal mass without visible zonal anatomy.
- The prostate zonal anatomy is often seen from about the age of years, before which there is insufficient central gland for contrast. The peripheral gland shows high signal on T2 weighted sequences compared to the intermediate signal of central gland. The capsule is seen at thin high signal line on T2 weighted sequences. BPH produces nodularity and heterogenicity on all sequences, especially T2 weighted sequences.

  The seminal vesicles appear multicystic and high signal on T2 weighted sequences and intermediate signal on T1 weighted sequences.
- The testis is homogeneous high signal on T2 weighted sequence with the low right at the mediastinum and somewhat heterogenous high signal within the epidedymis.

On T1 weighted sequences the testis and epididymis are homogenous and intermediate similar to muscle.

Testis—Anatomy and Pathologic Lesions

ANATOMY

- Scrotum divided by midline septum, with each half containing testis and associated structures.
- Tunica vaginalis–lines scrotal sac and envelops the structures. Closely applied to tunica albuginea but less closely to epididymis with an invagination on both sides between testis and epididymis–epididymal sinus.

Testis

- An ovoid organ.

Size at birth	1.5 cm in length.
	1 cm in width.
Before 12 years	1-2 cm^3
Post puberty	Average $5 \times 3.5 \times 3$ cm.

Tunica Albuginea

- Covers the testis, projects into the interior of testis to form mediastinum testis. Septae arise from mediastinum.

Epididymis

- Head, body and tail.

  Head – globules major, consists of 8-12 ducts converging into a single layer duct in body.

  Vas – continuation of the epididymis, runs upwards parallel to the epididymis.

- Four testicular appendages – appendix testis, the appendix, epididymis, the vas deferens and the paradidymis – remnants of embryonic ducts. Appendix testis – attached at upper pole in the glove between testis and epididymis.

Blood Supply

- Testicular arteries – directly from abdominal cortex, through inguinal canal.
- A network of capsular branches is formed over the testis, breaching pre T. albuginea and forming a network of centripetal and fugal arterion.

Pampiniform plexus of veins – found around the upper pole of testis usually on same side as the epididymis and vas.

(R) Testicular vein	-	IVC.
(L) Testicular vein	-	(L) renal vein.

ULTRASONOGRAPHY

- Supine position, scrotum supported with towel.
- 7-10 MHz high frequency, linear array transducer.
- The colour Doppler and Doppler parameters are optimized to display low flow velocities.
- Power Doppler US – may be used.

US Anatomy

- Prepubertal testis – low to medium echogenicity.
- Pubertal and post pubertal – medium homogenous echogenic reflecting the development of germ cell elements and tubular maturation.

Mediastinum Testis

- Echogenic band in cranio caudal direction.

Rete Testis

- (Normal) seen in 18% patients.
- Hypoechoic area with striated configuration near med. testis.

Tunica Vaginalis

- Space between two layers contain small amount of fluid seen as echofree area adjacent to head of epididymis.

Epididymis

- Best seen in oblique view.

Head – Pyramidal structure, 5-12 mm in maximum length.

Isoechoic to testis, echotexture coarser than testis.

Body – 2-4 mm in diameter normally indistinguishable from peri testicular tissue.

Tail – 2-5 mm in diameter, curved structure at lower pole.

- The otherwise normal appendix testis and appendix epididymis are typically seen only when a hydrocele is present.
- The appendix testis – ovoid structure, 5 mm in length.
  - Groove between testis and epididymis.
  - Isoechoic to testis occassionaly cystic.

MRI – Should be performed with a surface coil.

- Patient supine towel is placed under the scrotum to raise it from between the thighs.
- In patients with cryptorchidis, the abdomen and pelvis may also need to be evaluated.
- Although not generally needed, gadolinium contrast material can be administered to help characterized undeterminate masses.
- Normal testis has homogenous intermediate signal intensity on T1W1 and high signal intensity (slightly less than third) on T2WI.
- T. albuginea – thin low signal intensity band surrounding the testis.
- Internal architecture is better seem on T2WI.
- Thin low signal intensity septa – sean radiating back to mediastinum.
- Epididymis – Iso or slightly hypointense relative to testis on T1WI and hypointense on T2WI.
- In general testicular tumors.

  Isointense relative to testis – T1WI.

  Hypointense relative to testis – T2WI.

  Or may be heterogenous.

PATHOLOGIC LESIONS

Inflammatory

- Epididymo – orchitis.
- Acute orchitis.
- Syphilis.
- Chronic epididymo orchitis.
- Atrophy.
- Tuberculosis.
- Spermatocele.
- Varicocele.
- Sperm granuloma.

Focal Intratesticular Lesions

- Cysts.
- Calcified foci – microlithiasis.
- Macrocalcifications.

Trauma

- Testicular torsion.
- Testicular trauma.
- Heratocele.

Tumors

- Benign testicular lesions.
- Malignancy
  - Germ cell tumors.
  - Sex cord stromal tumor.
  - Lymphoproliferative metastatis.

Tumor Scar

- Myeloma/plasmocytoma.

Epididym Orchitis

- This is a common cause of acute scrotal pain in adolescent boys and adults.
- On examination, in early disease epididymis palpated as an enlarged tender structure separate from the testis.
- Prehn sign.
- Scrotal pain relieved when the testis are deviated over the symphysis pubis.
- To differentiate from testicular torsion.
- Adolescents.

  Sex transmitted disease – N. gonorrhoea and ch. trochomatis.

  Prepubertal ad >35 years – E. coli and P. microbilis.

US: An enlarged hypoechoic or hyperechoic (presumably due to hemorrhage) epididymis.

- Indirect signs – reactive hydrocele or pyocele, scrotal wall thickening, seen in most cases.
- Epididymis is the organ primarily involved with orchitis developing 20-40% due to direct spread of inflammation.
- Diffuse testicular involvement is confirmed by testicular enlargement and heterogenous echotexture.
- Gray scale US – Findings non-specific but acute epididymo orchitis is the most common disorder with these findings.
- Orchitis – characterized by oedema of testis contained within a rigid T. albuginea resulting in heterogeneous echo the process may be seen as a diffuse or focal involvement.
- Heterogenous echotexture – not always indicate orchitis. Leukemia and lymphoma – similar appearance, but are bilateral, infection in unilateral.

Color Doppler and Power Doppler

- Hallmark of scrotal infection is hyperemia of the epididymis, testis or both.
- Sensitivity of CD US imaging in detecting scrotal inflammation is nearly 100%.
- In

20% epididymitis	Hyperemia on CDFI.
40% orchitis	Gray scale US – normal.

- In acute epididymitis – Increased number of and concentration of identifiable vessels with hyperemia resulting in high flow low resistance pattern.
- RI measurement not a standard US proceeding but may provide useful information.
- RI normal rarely <0.5 but > half patients with epididymo orchitis <0.5.
- PSV— >15 cm – diagnostic accuracy of 90% or ratio >1.7.
- Reversal of flow during diastole in acute epididymis orchitis—Suggestive of venous infarction.

Acute Orchitis

- Inflammation of testis – whether infective or due to other etiology like acute ischemia produce oedema in testicular tissue.

US: Demonstrate swollen, poorly reflective

testicular tissue which may be generalized or focal in distribution.

If focal – usually multifocal.

Important feature – testicular tissue pattern appears normal and homogenous with no evidence of disorganization.

- Normal epididymis – separates inflammation secondary to epididymitis.
- Clinical presentation and other features are important as similar appearances may be seen in cases of epididymo orchitis, primary orchitis, ischemia, trauma, lymphoproliferative infiltration.

Syphilis

- Now extremely rare.
- Epididymis is seldom involved.
- Testis involved in two form:
  1. Diffuse orchitis – widespread interstitial fibrosis, painless, seldom presents for USG.
  2. Gumma formation – focal poorly reflective intratesticular lesions.

Chronic Epididymo Orchitis/Periorchitis

- These two terms – denote chronic inflammation in the scrotum.
- Chronic inflammation, commonly repeated episodes of epididymis, produces a patchy, inhomogenous increase in reflecting of epididymis.
- Tunica layers – thickened, particularly T. albuginea.
- Calcification may form on tunica layers.
- Fibrous strands – in tunica sac.
- Testis may be atrophic.

Atrophy

- May result from a wide range of causes – like chronic inflammation, ischemia and trauma.
- Frequently seen in cryptorchidism with late descent of the testis into scrotum or following orchipexy may be natural phenomenon of ageing.
- Size of testis is very variable – Unilateral easy to appearance.
- The testis is globally reduced in volume and reflectivity and this too is more early appreciated if unilateral.
- If both are affected – somewhat subjective.
- A greater contrast between testicular substance and the mediastinum and associated stromal strands can usually be demonstrated.

Tuberculosis

- Epididymis – main site in scrotum.
- Infection is almost always by retrograde spread from focus of infection higher in urinary tract.
- Infection usually starts in the lower pole of epididymis.
- Epididymis – enlarges, commonly abscess formation occur.
- Liqufection may occur leading to echofree collections on USG.
- Testicular involvement – swelling with reduced reflectivity and focal intra testicular abscesses.
- Adjacent scrotal wall is commonly involved with sinus formation and cause thickening of the tunica vaginalis.
- Involvement of contralateral epididymis may occur.
- Resolution may lease large extra testicular masses often with large areas of calcification.

Sperm Granuloma

- Extravasation of sperm into epididymal tissues causes granuloma formation and eventually fibrosis.
- Despite small size – frequently symptomatic.
- They can be extremely difficult to localize with US and palpation technique is often valuable (Figure 96.1).

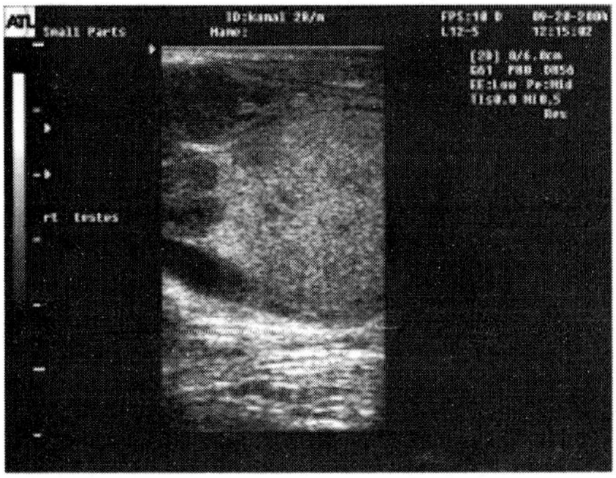

Fig. 96.1: US scan shows granuloma in the testicular parenchyma

- US demonstrates small (<1cm) focal lesions in epididymis that may be of or ↓ed reflectivity depending upon the degree of fibrosis present.

Intratesticular Spermatocele

- It is a cystic intraparenchymal lesion attached to the mediastinum in the area of rete testis.
- Communicates with seminiferous tubules unlike simple ectasia of rete testis.
- Cystic contain spermatozoa and can be septated.

Intratesticular Varicocele

- Newly defined condition, pathogenesis and clinical implications are not yet well established.
- Can occur in association with extra testicular varicocele but more commonly found alone.
- Patients may have pain, related to passive congestion of the testis.
- Ultrasound is similar to extra testicular varicocele including anechoic, serpinginous tubular structures of varying sizes.
- CDFI demonstrate the venous flow pattern with a characteristic venous spatial waveform that increases during a valsalva manoeuvre.

Cysts

- Benign cysts – occur in upto 10% of male population.
- Frequently located close to rete testis or peripherally abutting the tunica capsule of the testis.
- Occasionally related to previous trauma, may be with calcification.
- USG clearly demarcated echo free lesion with no disorganization of surrounding testicular substance.
- As some testicular neoplasms may be predominantly cystic, if some doubt, repeat scanning at short intervals.

CALCIFICATION

Microlithiasis

- Uncommon condition, discovered incidentally at ultrasound.
- Characterized by intratubular calcifications, within a multilayered envelope containing organelles, vesicles and collagen fibres.
- Ultrasound multiple echogenic foci with no posterior acoustic shadowing due to structure or small size.
- Although minor calcification within the testis is normal, typical ultrasound appearance of TM is of multiple non shadowing echogenic areas measuring 2-3 mm and randomly scattered throughout the testicular parenchyma.
- 5 or more foci per transducer field abnormal.
- TM is associated with cryptorchidism, pseudohermaphroditism, testicular atrophy and subfertility as well as Down's syndrome and Klinefelter syndromes.

  It appears to have an associated with testicular cancer.
- TM has a potential link with intratubular germ cell neoplasia (IGCN). IGCN is likely to be the precursor of GCT. It is found adjacent to most tumors and is seen in contralateral testis in upto 5% of cases.
- Recent studies – suggest a frequency occurrence and tumor development—15-27%.

Microcalcification

- Coarse calcification (above 3 mm diameter) that are relatively few in number, are seen within some malignant testicular tumors, particularly non-seminomatous GCT.
- A solitary substantial focus may be associated with the so-called burnt out primary tumor.
- Infection, trauma or infarct may also produce dystrophic calcific areas. Usually solitary or few in number.

Testicular Torsion

- Most common scrotal disorder in children.

Etiology

- "Bell and Clapper" deformity – high insertion of tunica vaginalis or spermatic cord.
- Abnormally loose mesordium between testis and epididymis.

Peak Age

- First year of life or adolescence.
- Sudden severe pain, -ve urine analysis, history of similar episode, nausea and vomiting, swelling and tenderness.

Salvage Rate

- Onset of pain and surgery.
  <6 hours—80-100%.
  6-12 hours—76%.
  12-24 hours—20%.
  > 24 hours—near 0%.

US in Acute Stage

- Testicular and epididymal enlargement with ↓ed echogenicity.
- ↑ Size of spermatic cord.
- Scrotal skin thickening.
- Hydrocele (occasionally).
- Loss of spermatic cord doppler signal.
  - Sensitivity—44%.
  - Specificity 67%.

Nuclear Imaging

- Decreased perfusion/occasionally normal.
- Nubbin sign – bump of activity extending medially from iliac ant denoting reactive -ed blood flow in spermatic cord with abrupt termination.
- Rounded cold area replacing testis surrounded by rim ↑ed activity indicating hyper perfusion.

Testicular Trauma

- Main consideration is the continuity of the capsule.
- In severe trauma, there may be rupture of the testis with the testicular substance fragmented into several parts and this may be difficult to differentiate from associated hematoma.
- Less severe trauma Low reflectivity area – infarction.
  High reflectivity area – hematologic.
- Hematocele.

Benign Testicular Lesion

- Derived from the stromal elements of the testis.
- Small impalpable tumors may present with secondary hormonal effects.
- US – demonstrates, small, poorly reflective or even cyanotic lesions.
- Tissue within the lesion is disorganized to a varying degree and the lesions may or may not be clearly demarcated.
- Some cases may show better demarcation and less tissue disorganization.

Epidermoid Tumors

- Well-defined, avascular rounded lesions on USG.

- Solitary, multiple or bilateral.
- Calcification patterns – multiple foci, curvilinear along the wall or a target pattern of concentric circles.
- Otherwise usually diffusely echo poor.
- If typical features, partial orchidectomy.

Cryptorchidism

- In majority of prepubertal males the testis may normally be retractile, however, if the testicle can never be located within scrotum—undescended.
- Most commonly lies in the inguinal canal (72%) followed by presacral (20%) and abdominal (8%), in abdomen – anywhere from deep inguinal ring to renal hilum.
- Failure of descent by the age of 2-3 years is associated with abnormal development of the testicle.
- May be atrophic with poor spermatogenesis.
- Undescended testis (esp. abdominal) if >5 years – ↑ ed incidence of malignant neoplasia (40 times).
- There is also an increased risk in contralateral, normally descended testicle.

USG

- Can be regarded first line of investigation to locate the testis – quick and able to locate at its most common sites.
- Helpful first to examine the normal descend testis.
- Undescended testis – oval, homogenous hypoechoic structure.
- High-resolution real time ultrasound can reliably detect a testis located in inguinal canal between extensive inguinal ring and scrotal neck.
- If it is not found there, suprapubic perineal and femoral areas should be scanned.
- If above internal inguinal ring difficult to detect by USG due to bowel gases.

Problems on US

- In groin – inguinal hernia.
- Pars infravaginalis of gubernaculums testis.
- Hypoechoic and nodular in appearance.

MRI

- If testicle not found on US a more extensive search may be performed with MRI.
- The diagnosis of under testis can be made when elliptical mass is seen in pathway of testicle descent round – abdomen.
- Abdominal testis – when located close to internal inguinal – ring can be seen lateral to the bladder or adjacent to the iliac vessels or psoas muscle.
- Inguinal canal – distinguish from L.N.
- Sporadic cord structures – helpful landmarks.
- The ductus deferens and testicular vessels – often traced. Ductus is rarely seen caudal to under testis.
- Another important landmark – PIG (pars infra vaginalis gubernadum) the distal bulbous termination of the gubernaculums, always caudal to under testis.
- Usually atrophies remains if undescended as a fibrotic remnant, may be misdiagnosed as undescended testis.
- MR on signal intensity and from media testis.

CT

- Oval soft tissue mass along pre expected path.
- Abdominal testis difficult to detect.
- Possibly of malignant degeneration should be considered when >2 cm in longest dimension on CT images or has heterogeneous enhancement.

Venography

- Three distinct patterns.

- Demonstration of barbinitorn plexus.
- Testicular parenchyma.
- Blind ending testicular vein.

Testicular Cancer

- Although uncommon, it is the most common malignant in males between 20-40 years of age.

95%	-	Germ cell origin.
04%	-	Lymphomas.
01%	-	Rare tumors such as metastasis, leydig cell and sertoli cell tumors.

Germ Cell Tumors (GCT)

- 50% seminoma (Figure 96.2), less aggressive, older age group (30-45 years).
- Remaining 50%
  - Non-seminomatous GCT younger age (15-30 years).
  - Majority produce biochem marker.
  - Teratoma – yolk sac tumors.

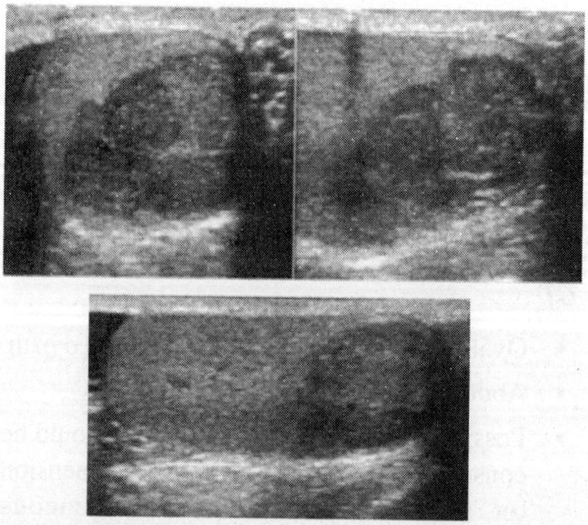

Fig. 96.2: USG images of the left testis demonstrate a heterogeneously hypoechoic intratesticular lesion consistent with a tumor in the lower pole of the left testis with a small hydrocele also visible. A seminoma was diagnosed at surgery

Risk Factor

- Undescended testis.
- Testicular atrophy.
- Microlithiasis.
- Previous testicular malignancy.
- Infantile hernia.
- Low birth weight.
- Maternal DES.

C/F

- Painless scrotal mass inseparable from testicle.
- Occasionally widespread pulmonary and abdominal mets.
- Leydig and sertoli cell T.—visualization or gynaecomastia.

USG

- Investigation of choice:
  - Sensitivity approaching 100%.

Table 96.1: Royal marsden staging system

Stage	I	No effect of metastasis
	I M	Rising serum tumor markers
Stage	II	Abdominal lymph node mets
	A	2 cm dia or less
	B	Between 2 and 5 cm dia
	C	5 cm dia or above
Stage	III	Supradiaph nodal mets
	M	Mediastinal
	N	Cervical or axillary
	O	Without abdominal L.N. mets
	ABC	Relates to size as in stage II
Stage	IV	Extralymphatic mets
	Lung	
	L1	3 mets or less
	L2	>3 mets, all 2 cm dia or less
	L3	>3 mets, at least one > 2 cm in dia
	H	Liver mets
	Br	Cerebral mets
	Bo	Bone mets

- Tumors seen as lesions with replacement of the normal architectural pattern by material of low echogenicity.
- Small tumors without mass effect.
- Occasionally hydrocele.
- Histology can't be predicted from the USG appearance. Classically seminoma – well defined, uniformly echo poor.

- Large tumors (>1.5 cm) – ↑ vascularity on CDFI. Smaller over – often hypovascular.
- D/D – focal or diffuse acute orchitis, abscess, infarct and hemorrhage.
- If an intra testicular lesion is not showing progressive resolution within a short time – orchidectomy would be recommended.
- Lymph node metastasis L.N. along IVC and aorta in lumbar region at L2 level. Almost always stenting on effected side.
- Bilateral involvement is uncommon – primary left sided.

  Bilateral more commonly seen when right sided.
- Following initial lymphadenopathy, disease may spread cranially or caudally.
- Iliac and and inguinal L.N. involved by retrograde spread or if tumor is grossly invasive within the scrotum.
- Hematogenous spread is rare before lymphatic except for choriocarcinoma.
- Royal Masden staging – more widely used, not only describes the site of metastasis but also volume of tumor.
- CT – conventional staging method.

  L.N. > 1cm usually involved (spec. 87%).

  > 1.5 cm – almost always (spec. 98%).

  Most nodes < 1 cm are uninvolved but 25-30% of untreated stage I disease develop subsequent mets. So a visible mode of <1 cm in diameter is best regarded as equivocal especially if above 8 mm and the scan should be repeated in 3 months.
- Metastatic mass – seminoma – usually homogenic NSGCT – heterogeneous, central necrosis.

MRI

Still controversial. L.N. criteria – same as CT.

Inferior to CT for detecting lung metastases.

Better soft tissue contrast – assist differentiation of potential tumor deposits from native structures or areas of solid tumor from fibrosis or cystic degeneration.

- Follow up scans – performed relatively frequently.
- Sometimes a small patient presents with widespread mets.
- Confirmed histopath – malign teratoma.
- In small proportion – small prim lesion with (echo poor USG appearance).

  Rarely – A small echogenic area within testicle.

  Suggestive of a scar of burnt out primary described with seminoma and NSGCT.

Testicular Lymphoma

- Most common testicular tumor in male > 60 years.
- Bilateral in 25% and in assoc with extranodal disease.
- Virtually always NHL.

USG

Well defined mass of low echogenicity expanding the testicle.

It often extends to involve the epididymis and spermatic cord.

Metastases:

- USG mixed, often predominantly reduced echogenicity, indistinguishable from primary malignant.
- From urinary tract – prostatic carcinoma, carcinoma bronchus or malignant melanoma.

Cryptorchidism

- It is the complete or partial failure of the testes to descend from the intra-abdominal position to the scrotum during gestation. The exact etiology is not known.
- Incidence in premature male infants is 9.2-30%. In full-term infants, the incidence is 3.3 to 5.8%, and in infants aged 1 year it is 0.8%.
- It is bilateral in approximately one to two-thirds of patients. A palpable testis within the inguinal canal may not require any imaging before proceeding with surgical correction. Despite the fact that completely undescended, intra-abdominal testes are usually not amenable to sonographic imaging. Ultrasound should be the initial imaging study for cryptorchidism when a testicle is not palpable in the inguinal canal.
- **Embryology:** The testis develops from the elongated embryonic gonad in the celomic cavity lying ventral to the mesonephric ridge. It migrates from its intra-abdominal position to the scrotal sac beginning at 36 weeks, guided by the contractile cord like structure termed the gubernaculums testis. The distal bulbous portion of the gubernaculums testis is termed the pars infravaginalis gubernaculi. After complete descent into the scrotum, the gubernaculums testis atrophies; however, it persists if the descent is not complete. Interruption of this normal migratory process results in ectopic positioning of the testis.
- The most common location of the cryptorchid testis is in the inguinal canal (72%), followed by prescrotal (20%) and abdominal (8%).
- Testicular malignancies occur in 10% of men with cryptorchid testis. Seminoma is the most common reported malignancy. Because malignant neoplasms occur 12-40 times more commonly in the undescended than-in-the descended-testis, it is widely agreed that orchiopexy be performed in patients younger than 10 years of age and orchidectomy in those who are seen after puberty. Orchiopexy does not alter the risk of malignant degeneration. The incidence of malignant transformation also is increased in the unaffected testis.
- Preoperative localization of a nonpalpable testis by radiological methods often helps in planning the surgical approach and shortens the anesthesia time. US, CT, MRI, arteriography/venography laparoscopy is used for diagnosis.
- US is the first modality to be used in preoperative localization of an undescended testis. If US cannot identify the testis, MRI and CT are the subsequent modalities of choice. Both can detect an abdominal testis. Angiography is used if CT/MRI fails.

Laparoscopy is performed if none of the radiological modality is able to give an unequivocal diagnosis, but it is expensive as well as invasive.

- Other conditions to be considered:
  - Testicular ectopia (normal descent but abnormal location, such as perineum, femoral supra-pubic regions; in nonpalpable testis in the scrotum search these areas to exclude ectopia, which is rare in the contralateral hemiscrotum).
  - Retractile testes (often bilateral, normal condition; commonly seen in prepubertal boys; absent in adults).
  - Congenital absence (anorchia; rare 4% of patients who clinically have an undescended testis, actually have unilateral absence).
  - Atrophic testis (usually secondary to torsion; no colour flow Doppler or contrast enhancement seen).
  - Lymph node (fatty hilum, characteristic location adjacent to vessels helps identification).
  - Pars infravaginalis gubernaculi (Occasionally mistaken for testis).
  - Hypospadias and inguinal hernia (associated conditions).

ULTRASOUND

- US is the first imaging modality performed on a cryptorchid testis. As 72% of cryptorchid testes are in the inguinal canal therefore, they are easily accessible to US examination.

  With grey-scale sonography, the undescended testis is oval and homogeneous in character but is smaller and slightly less echogenic than the contralateral, descended testis. Rarely, a thin white line or bright echogenic band representing the mediastinum testis can be seen. This can help differentiate, the testis from all inguinal lymph node.

False Positives:

- Rarely, an undescended testis can be confused with inguinal hernia; real time peristalsis confirms the presence of bowel.
- Persistence of pars infravaginalis gubernaculi has been mistaken for the testis. The presence of an echogenic band (mediastinum testis) identifies the maldescended testis.

- **Limitations:** US cannot detect an intra-abdominal testis.

COMPUTED TOMOGRAPHY

- It is the procedure of choice in the localization of the nonpalpable testis.
- Five different CT patterns have been encountered in patients with undescended testis spermatic cord absent, testis absent; spermatic cord in the inguinal canal, testis in the abdomen; spermatic cord not seen.
- Cryptorchid testis is seen as an oval soft-tissue mass along the expected course of testicular descent. Uniform enhancement is seen with intravenous (IV) radiographic contrast.
- When the undescended testis is unusually large or contains areas of low attenuation, it may be either because of malignant degeneration or epididymitis.
- CT is almost as accurate as US in detecting an undescended testis in the inguinal region. CT is much better than US in detecting an undescended testis that is located abdominally. In one study evaluating undescended testis, CT and US accuracy were 96% and 91%, respectively.
- **False Positives:** A lymph node can be differentiated readily by the presence of fatty hilum and its characteristic location. Limitation CT uses radiation.

MAGNETIC RESONANCE IMAGING

- Perform MRI from the level of the kidneys to the level of the pelvic outlet.

- The pulse sequences used are TI, T2, and post-gadolinium T1-weighted images in the axial and coronal planes.
- An oval mass that appears as low signal on T1-weighted images and high signal on T2-weighted images is characteristic of an undescended testis. Identification of the mediastinum testis is helpful.
- An undescended testis is hypointense to the contralateral normal testis.
- MRI detects the malignant degeneration in cryptorchid testis well.
- MRl has better soft-tissue contrast and multiplanar capability.

  False Positives: When the testis is higher in the abdomen, bowel loops and lymph nodes can mimic the undescended testis.
- CT is much better at differentiating the undescended testis from the bowel loop. Oral contrast agents are used to facilitate the identification of bowel loops on MR.
- Gadolinium infusion MR venography is an alternative, non-invasive method of evaluating the undescended testis, especially the vanishing testis. It is superior to MR imaging alone.
- MRI is preferred as the modality of choice at some centres where the equipment is readily available and where the radiation exposure is the major concern.

ANGIOGR APHY

- Testicular arteriography is not only technically difficult but also painful.
- Testicular venography is less traumatic than arteriography, but it is also associated with a high radiation-dose and some morbidity, although the false negative rate is low. It has fallen out of favor because of the availability of non-invasive test.
- The following findings are diagnostic:
  - Demonstrated presence of the pampiniform plexus.
  - Visualization of testicular parenchyma.
  - A blind ending testicular vein (usually indicates absent testis).
- Angiography is accurate but invasive, thus is not preferred.

Congenital Uterine Anomalies

Mullerian duct anomalies are an uncommon but often treatable cause of infertility. Patients with Mullerian duct anomalies are known to have a higher incidence of:

- Infertility.
- Repeated First Trimester Spontaneous Abortions.
- Fetal Intrauterine Growth Retardation.
- Fetal Malpositions.
- Preterm Labor, and
- Retained Placenta.

The role of imaging is to help detect, diagnose, and distinguish surgically correctable forms of Mullerian duct anomalies from inoperable forms.

Embryology (Figure 98.1)

Two paired Mullerian ducts ultimately develop into the structures of the female reproductive tract. The structures include the fallopian tubes, uterus, cervix, and the upper two thirds of the vagina. The ovaries and lower one third of the vagina have separate embryological origins not derived from the Mullerian system.

Complete formation and differentiation of the Mullerian ducts into the segments of the female reproductive tract depend on completion of 3 phases of development as follows:

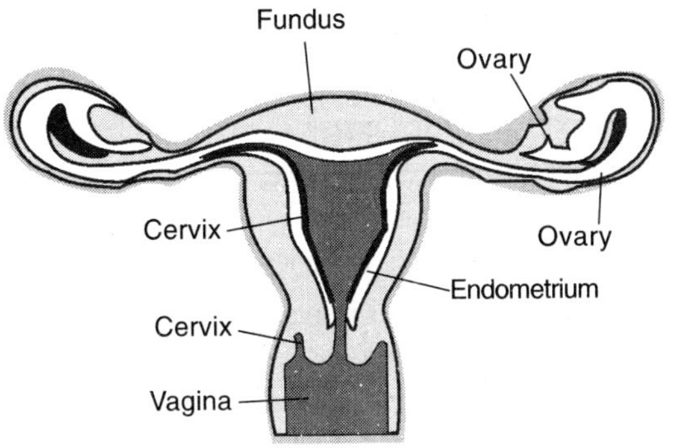

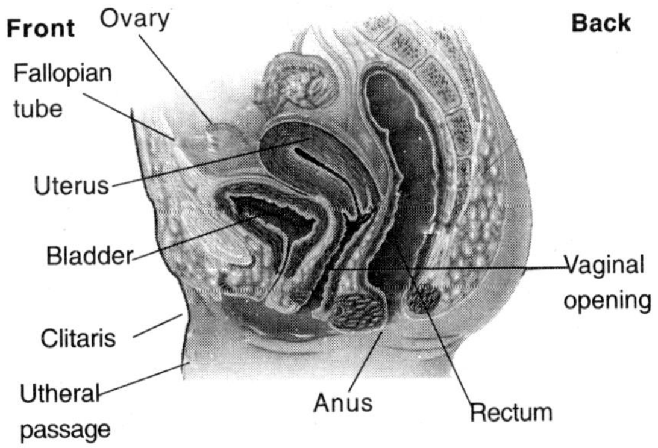

Fig. 98.1: Female reproductive system

- **Organogenesis:** One or both Mullerian ducts may not develop fully, resulting in abnormalities such as uterine agenesis-or-hypoplasia (bilateral) or unicornuate uterus (unilateral).

- **Fusion:** The process during which the lower segments of the paired Mullerian duct fuse to form the uterus, cervix and upper vagina is termed lateral fusion. Failure of fusion results in anomalies such as bicornuate or didelphys uterus. The term vertical fusion occasionally is used to refer to fusion of the ascending sinovaginal bulb with the descending Mullerian system (i.e., fusion of the lower one third and upper two thirds of the vagina). Complete vertical fusion forms a normal patent vagina, while incomplete vertical fusion results in an imperforate hymen.
- **Septal Resorption:** After the lower Mullerian ducts fuse, a central septum is present, which subsequently must be resorbed to form a single uterine cavity and cervix. Failure of resorption is the cause of septate uterus.

In the US, Mullerian duct anomalies are estimated to occur in 0.1-0.5% of women. The true prevalence is unknown because the anomalies usually are discovered in patients presenting with infertility. Full term pregnancies have occurred in patients with forms of bicornuate, septate or didelphys uteri; therefore, true prevalence may be slightly higher than currently estimated. Simon *et al.* found that in the healthy fertile population, Mullerian duct anomalies have a prevalence of 3.2%.

Certain types of the anomaly can increase morbidity, such as in patients with obstructed or partially obstructed Mullerian systems who present with hematosalpinx, hematocolpos, retrograde menses, and endometriosis. In addition, a fairly high association exists between Mullerian duct anomalies and renal anomalies such as unilateral agenesis. Often, the anomalies are found only when dedicated renal imaging is performed after the Mullerian abnormality is discovered however. These patients most commonly present for medical attention because of infertility and repeated pregnancy loss.

Anomalies may be diagnosed in infancy, adolescence, or young adulthood. Female patients may present with a mass resulting from an obstructed Mullerian system as infants (mucocolpos) with primary amenorrhea, mass (hematocolpos), or delayed onset of menarche as adolescents or with problems of fertility and/or carrying pregnancy to term as adults.

Mullerian duct anomalies are categorized most commonly into 7 classes according to the American Fertility Society (AFS) Classification Scheme (1988) as follows (Figure 98.2):

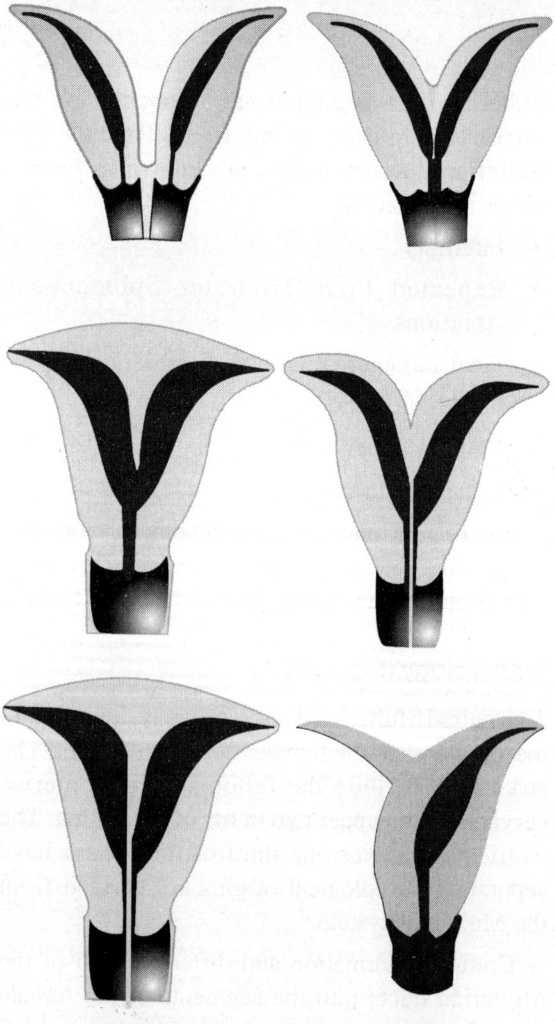

Fig. 98.2: Uterine anomlies

- **Class I (Hypoplasia/Agenesis):** This class includes entities such as uterine cervical agenesis or hypoplasia. The most common form is the Mayer-Rokitansky-Kuster-Hauser syndrome, which is combined agenesis of the uterus, cervix, and upper portion of the vagina. Patients have no reproductive potential aside from medical intervention in the form of in vitro fertilization of harvested ova and implantation in a host uterus.
- **Class II (Unicornuate Uterus):** A unicornuate uterus is the result of complete, or almost completes, arrest of development of Mullerian duct. If the arrest is incomplete, as in 90% of patients, a rudimentary horn with or without functioning endometrium is present. If the rudimentary horn is obstructed, it may come to surgical attention when presenting as an enlarging pelvic mass. If the contralateral healthy horn is almost fully developed, a full-term pregnancy is believed to be possible.
- **Class III (Didelphys Uterus):** This anomaly results from complete nonfusion of both Mullerian ducts. The individual horns are fully developed and almost normal in size. Two cervices are inevitably present. A longitudinal or transverse vaginal septum may be noted as well. Didelphys uteri have the highest association with transverse vaginal septa but septa also may be observed in other anomalies. Metroplasty can be considered however, since each horn is almost a fully developed uterus, patients have been known to carry pregnancies to full term.
- **Class IV (Bicornuate Uterus):** A bicornuate uterus results from partial nonfusion of the Mullerian ducts. The central myometrium may extent to the level of the internal cervical os (bicornuate unicollis) or external cervical os (bicornuate bicollis). The latter is distinguished from didelphys uterus because it demonstrates some degree of fusion between the two horns, while in classic didelphys uterus, the two horns and cervices are separated completely. In addition, the horns of the bicornuate uteri are not fully developed typically; they are smaller than those of didelphys uteri. Some patients are surgical candidates for metroplasty.
- **Class V (Septate Uterus):** A septate uterus results from failure of resorption of the septum between the two uterine horns. The septum can be partial or complete, in which case it extends to the internal cervical os. Histologically, the septum may be composed of myometrium or fibrous tissue. The uterine fundus is typically convex but may be flat or slightly concave (< 1 cm fundal cleft). Women with septate uterus have the highest incidence of reproductive complications. Differentiation between a septate and a bicornuate uterus is important because septate uteri are treated using endovaginal hysteroscopic resection of the septum, while if surgery is possible and/or indicated for the bicornuate uterus, an abdominal approach is required to perform metroplasty.
- **Class VI (Arcuate Uterus):** An arcuate uterus has a single uterine cavity with a convex or flat uterine fundus, the endometrial cavity, which demonstrates a small fundal cleft or impression (= 1.5 cm). The outer contour of the uterus is convex, or flat. This form is often considered a normal variant since it is not significantly associated with the increased risks of pregnancy loss and the other complications found in other subtypes.
- **Class VII (Diethylstilbestrol-related Anomaly):** The uterine anomaly is seen in the female offspring of as many 15% of women exposed to DES during pregnancy. Female fetuses that are affected have a variety of abnormal findings that include uterine hypoplasia and a T-shaped uterine cavity. Patients also may have abnormal transverse ridges, hoods, stenoses of the cervix, and adenosis of the vagina with increased risk of vaginal clear ceil carcinoma. Imaging findings are pathognomonic for this anomaly.

Once a Mullerian anomaly is suggested based on evidence from the patient history and physical examination, the clinician may opt for additional imaging workup. Imaging criteria for distinguishing forms of uterine anomalies are based on the configuration of the endometrial cavity and (primarily) on the configuration of the uterine fundus.

Typically, the first examination ordered is a pelvic ultrasound (U3) with transabdominal and, if feasible, endovaginal imaging. Mullerian duct anomalies may be suggested on endovaginal 2-dimensional (2D) sonographic imaging but may not be excluded on the basis of negative US findings. Newer 3-dimensional (3D)/4D sonographic techniques offer relatively higher sensitivity and specificity.

Hysterosalpingography (HSG): Performed under fluoroscopy, allows evaluation of the uterine cavity and tubal patency. Anomalies may be suggested but positive findings often are nonspecific for precise diagnosis.

MRI is considered the criterion standard for imaging uterine anomalies. MRI provides high-resolution images of the uterine body, fundus, and internal structure. In addition, it can help evaluate the urinary tract for concomitant anomalies. In the past, intravenous urography was used for this purpose. Most types of uterine anomalies can be diagnosed confidently using pelvic MRI.

Limitations of Techniques: Although US is often the first imaging modality chosen because of its availability, short scan time, and low cost, several limitations are encountered during imaging. Image quality from transabdominal and endovaginal examinations is operator dependent. Overlying bowel gas can hamper transabdominal imaging. Endovaginal imaging, although superior to the transabdominal approach, may not always be possible, as in patients with vaginal septa. Image resolution is a limiting factor.

HSG probably is the only imaging modality providing high-resolution imaging of the uterine cavity and fallopian tubes, but it is limited to imaging only the endoluminal contour therefore, characterization of Mullerian anomalies can be difficult. For example, visualization of 2 uterine cavities on HSG does not aid the radiologist in distinguishing septate, didelphys, and bicornuate uteri, which are 3 entities with radically different treatments. Since HSG uses ionizing radiation, ensure that the patient is not pregnant at the time of the examination. In patients who are not pregnant, ovaries receive a small dose of radiation and the risk to the unfertilized ova is unknown.

MRI provides high-resolution images of the uterine cavity, the configuration of the uterus (body and fundus) and the ovaries. MRI is limited by motion artifact (patient movement, bowel peristalsis) and other features that degrade image quality (e.g., metal prostheses, clips and filters) and cannot be performed in some patients (e.g., patients who are claustrophobic, have pacemakers, or are obese).

Other Problems to be Considered

Congenital renal anomalies, amenorrhea (primary and secondary forms diagnosed using endocrinological workup.

RADIOLOGICAL FINDINGS

HYSTEROSALPINGOGRAPHY (Figure 98.3)**:** Typically, the question of Mullerian duct anomaly arises during HSG examination if the typical trigone configuration of the cavity is not demonstrated.

A common finding is separation of the uterine cavity into right and left compartments. A divided uterine cavity can result from septate, bicornuate, or didelphys uterus. Certain criteria are used to increase confidence in diagnosing of the 3 entities.

- **Intercornual Distance** (distance between the distal ends of the horns i.e. ends that are continuous with fallopian tubes).
  - If <2 cm, the likelihood of septate uterus is increased.
  - If > 4 cm, the likelihood of didelphys uterus is increased.

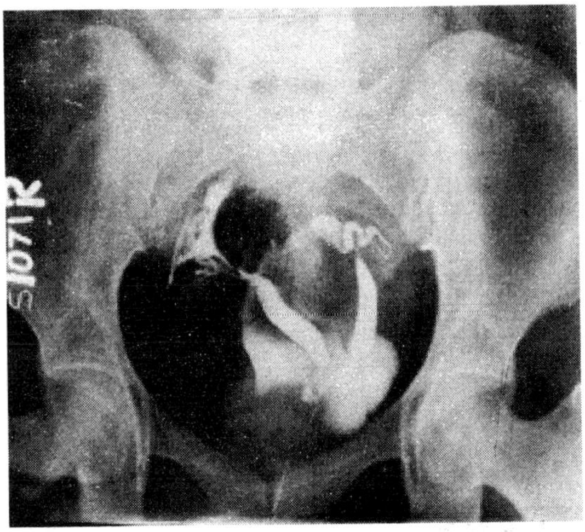

Fig. 98.3: Hysterosalpingogram shows bicornis bicollis uterus

- Measurements of 2-4 cm (typical distance in a normal uterus) were indeterminate in an abnormal cavity configuration.

- **Intercornual Angle** (The angle formed by the most medial aspects of the two uterine hemi cavities).
  - If the angle is less than 60°, septate uterus is more likely.
  - For larger angles, the anomaly is more likely to be a bicornuate uterus.
- **T-shaped Cavity:** A hypoplastic, irregular, T-shaped uterine cavity is pathognomonic for in utero DES exposure. The uterus typically is much smaller than average and many forms of cavity appearance exist with varying, but usually symmetric, regions of narrowing or dilatation in the segments of the T. MRI and US examinations typically demonstrate uterine hypoplasia only.

Degree of Confidence: A large overlap exists between the subtypes when comparing uterine cavitary configuration, intercornual distance, and intercornual angle. In several studies, HSG had significantly less accuracy for diagnostic precision compared to MRI or US. In the studies, much of the final pathology was based on laparoscopic or surgical findings primarily of the appearance of the uterine fundus, which HSG was not able to assess.

Currently, HSG has been all but abandoned as a primary modality for workup of potential congenital uterine anomalies. Anomalies incidentally discovered on HSG are referred for further evaluation using MRI or US.

The only anomaly in which HSG plays a significant role in diagnosis is DFS uterus (AFS class VII). The abnormal uterine cavity can be depicted clearly on HSG but often is visualized as only uterine hypoplasia on MRI or US.

PELVIC ULTRASOUND

Most commonly, 20 EVS is used to help evaluate uterine anatomy. Transabdominal 2D imaging may be performed, ideally through a distended bladder, but offers reduced sensitivity and specificity because of increased distance from the uterus and, often, intervening bowel. Preliminary studies indicate that 3D techniques in sonography may offer improved sensitivity and specificity for detection of uterine anomalies.

US appearance of Mullerian anomalies (AFS classification system).

- **Class I (Hypoplasia/Agenesis):** Findings of agenesis include:
  - Absence of the cervix and/or uterus with a blind-ending vagina. In uterine agenesis, no identifiable uterine tissue is present.
  - In uterine hypoplasia, the endometrial cavity is small with a reduced intercornual distance (<2 cm).
- **Class II (Unicornuate Uterus)** (Figure 98.4)
  - The unicornuate uterus appears banana shaped without the usual rounded fundal contour and triangular appearance of the fundal cavity.
  - Uterine zonal anatomy is normal.
  - If present, a rudimentary horn can be observed as a soft tissue mass with similar echogenicity to myometrium.

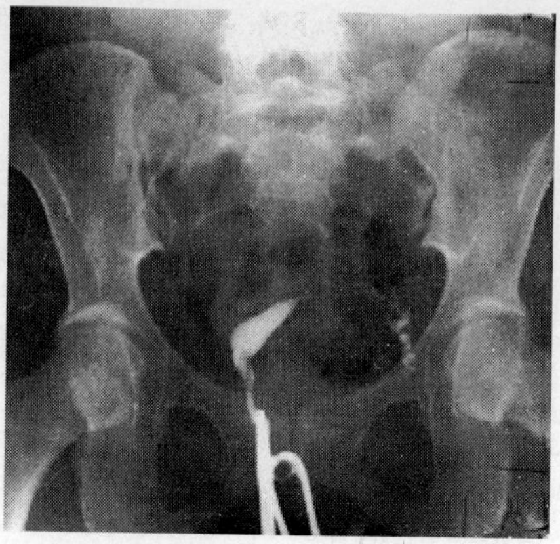

Fig. 98.4: Hysterosalpingogram shows a unicornuate uterus

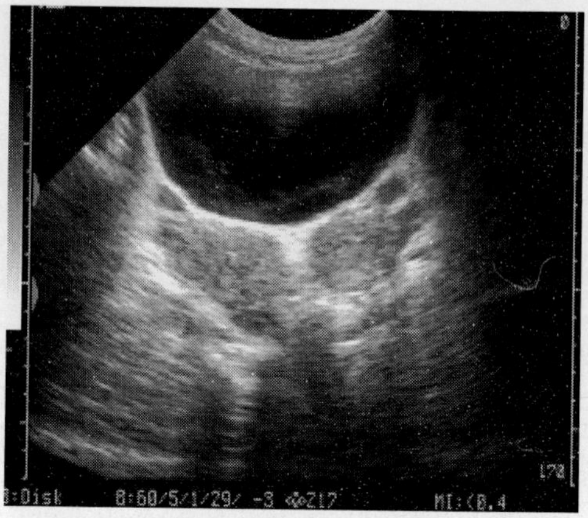

Fig. 98.5: US scan shows a bicornuate uterus

- If obstructed, a rudimentary horn with functioning endometrium may present as a complex hemorrhagic cystic structure.

- **Class III (Didelphys Uterus)**
  - Two separate normal-sized uteri and cervices are observed.
  - A vaginal septum may be difficult to visualize.
  - The two uterine horns are usually widely splayed, and endometrial and myometrial zonal widths are preserved.
- **Class IV (Bicornuate Uterus)** (Figure 98.5)
  - US may demonstrate two uterine cavities with normal endometrium.
  - The most important imaging finding is a concave fundus with a fundal cleft greater than 1 cm. This has been shown to be a reliable means of distinguishing bicornuate from septate, uteri.
  - 3D US may play a useful role in making this diagnosis. An increased intercornual distance (>4 cm) may be observed. The cleft is visualized best on oblique coronal images in the plane of the long axis of the uterus. The septum separating the two horn demonstrates echogenicity identical to myometrium.
- **Class V (Septate Uterus)**
  - US may demonstrate a convex or flattened fundal contour.
  - The intercornual distance usually is normal or decreased <4 cm), and each uterine cavity usually is small.
  - The septum may be composed of muscle or fibrous tissue and is not a reliable means of distinguishing septate from bicornuate uteri.
  - A more reliable means to differentiate the two involves examining the fundal contour (see Class IV). Confirm ambiguous US findings using MRI.
- **Class VI (Arcuate Uterus)**
  - US may detect the abnormality but, typically, it is not clinically significant because arcuate uterus has no significant negative effects on pregnancy outcome.
- **Class VII (DES related)**
  - US may detect the abnormality as uterine hypoplasia typically, DES-related uterus is diagnosed confidently using HSG.

Degree of Confidence: Some preliminary studies find that 3D US is highly sensitive (upto 100%) and specific (upto 100%) in diagnosing major Mullerian anomalies. Studies also have found 2D endovaginal sonography to be a highly effective means of diagnosis, with 75-100% sensitivity and upto 95% specificity. Positive predictive value was higher with 3D scanning compared to 2D scanning (100% vs 50%, respectively).

It has been found that transabdominal 2D US failed to visualize the uterine cavity adequately in as many as 35% of patients although it adequately imaged the uterine fundus in 90% of patients.

MAGNETIC RESONANCE IMAGING

MRI of the uterus is performed following administration of 1.0 mg IM of glucagon to decrease motion artifacts associated with bowel peristalsis. For the diagnosis of most anomalies, 5 main sequences are sufficient:

- Coronal single-shot fast spin-echo (FSE) images of the kidneys, ureters, and pelvis provide well localized and survey views of kidneys and ureters. This sequence is important because of the high incidence of associated renal anomalies (upto 5000), including agenesis, kidney duplication or pelvic kidney.
- Axial Tl spin-echo (without fat-saturation pulse) images: Fat signal is useful to delineate pelvic structures. An anterior saturation band is used to attenuate ghosting artifact from respiration.
- Sagittal T2 FSE (without fat-saturation pulse) image: Fat signal is useful to delineate pelvic structures. An anterior saturation band is recommended. This sequence is useful for determining anterior versus retroverted uterus and to set up subsequent oblique scans along the long and short axes of the uterine fundus.
- Oblique long-axis T2 SE (without fat-saturation pulse) images are similar to sagittal T2 FSE sequences but obtained along the long axis of the uterus (perpendicular to the sagittal plane, usually a slightly oblique coronal). This plane is ideal for visualization of the uterine cavity and uterine fundal contour.
- Oblique short-axis T2 FSE (without fat-saturation pulse) images are perpendicular to the long axis and sagittal planes (usually oblique axial), providing short-axis (target) views of the uterine cavity useful for visualizing a transverse-septum if present.

MRI Appearance of Mullerian Anomalies (AFS Classification System)

- **Class I (Hypoplasia/Agenesis)**
  - Findings are similar to US.
  - When uterine hypoplasia is associated with hormonal dysfunction (infantile uterus), not only is the uterus small, but the zonal anatomy is differentiated poorly on T2-weighted images.
- **Class II (Unicornuate Uterus):** Findings are similar to US.
- **Class III (Didelphys Uterus):** Findings are similar to US.
- **Class IV (Bicornuate Uterus):**
  - Findings are similar to US.
  - The cleft is visualized best on oblique coronal images in the plane of the long axis of the uterus. The tissue separating the two horns demonstrates signal intensity identical to myometrium on all pulse sequences. The inferior portion of the septum may be fibrous, with low T1 and T2 signal intensity.
- **Class V (Septate Uterus):** Findings are similar to US.
- **Class VI (Arcuate Uterus):** Findings are similar to US.
- **Class VII (DES related):** MRI may detect this abnormality as a hypoplastic uterus.

Degree of Confidence: MRI has consistently demonstrated high sensitivity and specificity (almost 100%) for evaluation of uterine anomalies.

MRI had the added advantage of detecting other incidental abnormalities, including a dermoid and submucosal leiomyoma, found on EVS to be indeterminate and no visualized, respectively.

Section 9—Reproductive System

Chapter 99

Lesions of Female Reproductive Tract

Müllerian Duct Anomalies

- Congenital anomalies of female reproductive tract occur in 1-15% of women.
- Embryologically the uterus, upper 1/3rd of vagina and fallopian tubes derived from paired müllerian ducts. At 10 weeks following conception the ducts migrate caudally and undergo fusion and subsequent canalisation. The process may be interrupted at any time leading to various types of congenital anomalies.
- Patient with congenital uterine anomalies may be completely asymptomatic or may present as infertility or spontaneous abortions or menstrual disorders.
- Müllerian duct anomalies are frequently associated with renal anomalies especially renal agenesis or ectopia.
- HSG (Figures 99.1 and 99.2) and USG have been the primary imaging modalities but each has its own limitations. HSG permits the contour of the endometrial cavity to be defined but its relationship to the myometrium cannot be defined. Hence HSG cannot differentiate between septate and bicornuate uterus.
- MRI has proved to be accurate and non-invasive means of evaluating patient with congenital anomalies, allowing precise classification.

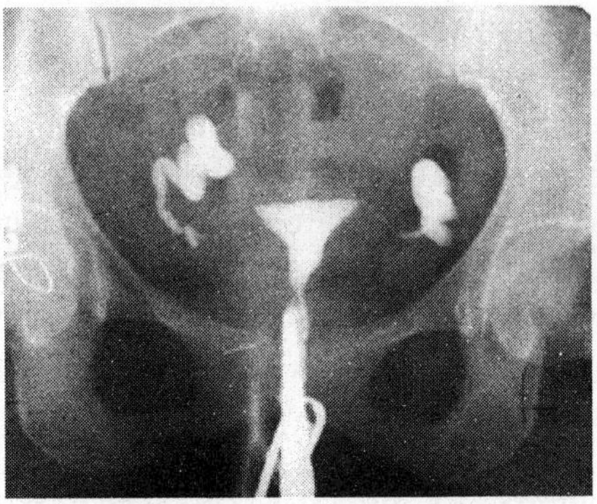

Fig. 99.1: Hysterosalpingogram shows bilateral blocked fallopian tubes with hydrosalpinx

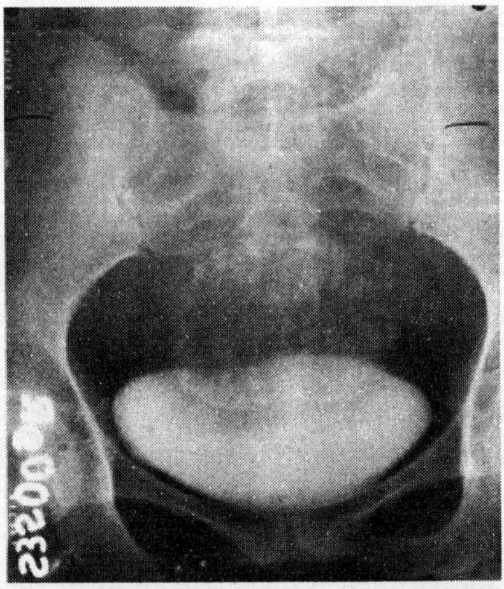

Fig. 99.2: Cystogram phase of the intravenous urography shows a large calcified fibroid producing an indentation on the fundus of the bladder

- The introduction of 3-D ultrasound allows identification of congenital anomalies, thus replacing the use of MRI in this field.
- USG with IVP are other important investigations to be seen associated with renal anomalies.
- The clinical classification of müllerian duct anomalies follows the guidelines proposed by Buttrams and and Gibbons. These can be classified as:

Class I

- Müllerian agenesis or hypoplasia. Non-development of rudimentary development of the müllerian ducts results in uterine aplasia or hypoplasia.
- USG or HSG shows absence of uterine or small uterus.
- T2W sagittal images are most useful for identifying the presence of a uterus. Uterus hypoplasia can be diagnosed when uterus is small in size and the myometrium is of lower than normal signal intensity.

Class II

- Unicornuate uterus results from non-development or rudimentary development of one müllerian duct. There are 3 sub-type of this anomaly.
  1. Presence or absence of rudimentary horn.
  2. Whether or not the rudimentary horn contains the endometrium.
  3. Whether or not the rudimentary horn communicates with the main uterine cavity.
- Patient with rudimentary horn communicating the uterine cavity might be benefited from surgical removal of the rudimentary horn.
- MRI shows characteristic banana shaped uterine cavity with normal dimensions of endometrium and myometrium.
- If the rudimentary horn is present the MRI can usually distinguish it from an adnexal mass suspected on USG, as well as determined if there is endometrium contained with it.

Class III – Uterus Didelphis

- Results from nonfusion of the two müllerian ducts.
- Two separate normal size uteri and cervices are demonstrated on imaging with septum extended upto the upper vagina. The uteri are widely separated with preservation of the endometrium and myometrial widths.

Class IV – Bicornuate Uterus

- Partial fusion of müllerian ducts produces the bicornuate icterus. In this anomaly the dividing septum is composed of myometrium.
- Depending upon extent of nonfusion it can be divided as:
  - Bicornuate bucollis – here the myometrial septum extends upto the external OS.
  - Bicornuate unicolic – here the myometrial septum extends upto the internal OS.
  - Partial bicornuate.
  - Arcuate.
  - It is very difficult to differentiate the bicornuate uterus from septate uterus on HSG. USG and/or MRI are essential to distinguish between these entities.

Class V – Septate Uterus

- Results because of incomplete resorption of final fibrous septum between two müllerian ducts.
- The subseptate uterus occurs more frequently than the completely septate uterus.
- The fundal contour is normal and the uterine septum is of low signal intensity on both T1 and T2W images in contrast to medium to high signal intensity myometrium separating the two-endometrial cavity in bicornuate uterus.

- The differentiation between septate and bicornuate weight is clinically significant as different surgical procedure are needed for their treatment.
- 3D ultrasound may also document an outward concavity in bicornuate uterus as opposed to the convexity seen in septate or normal uterus.

Class VI – Diethylstilbestrol Related

- Uterine anomalies have also seen in patients who had in utero exposure of DES. Imaging demonstrates a diffuse decrease in size of uterus and an irregular T-shaped uterine cavity.

Congenital Anomalies of Vagina

1. **Absent or hypoplastic vagina**
   - Absent vagina with absence of uterine and fallopian tube indicate total failure of müllerian ducts development.
   - In MRKH syndrome (Mayer Rokintansky Kuster Hauser) there is vaginal agenesis or hypoplasia with intact ovaries and fallopian tubes and variable anomalies of uterus, urinary tract and skeletal system.
2. **Transverse vaginal septum or imperforate ligaments**
   - These patients present as teenagers with cyclic abdominal pain. USG shows distended uterus filled with blood or pus.
3. **Vaginal duplication**
   - These patients often present with the incidental findings of vaginal septum that is usually asymptomatic.

ACQUIRED LESIONS

Uterus and Cervix

- Benign conditions.

1. Leiomyoma

- These are the most common uterine tumors and consist of predominantly smooth muscle with varying amount of fibrous and connective tissue.
- 25% of white and 50% of black women older than 30 years have at least one leiomyoma.
- Leiomyoma may be:
  – Intramural – Most common type.
  – Submucosal – Only 5-10% but most symptomatic.
  – Sub serosal.

USG Appearance of leiomyoma depends on size, site and age of tumor.

- The myomatous uterus is typically enlarged and its outline may be irregular or lobular.
- The most common appearance of LM is well marginated, hypoechoic rounded or oval mass within uterine body.
- When the muscular component predominates, the lesion is hypoechoic solid mass with poor sound through transmission.
- Increased echogenicity is suggestive of fibrous degeneration as tiny cystic area act as echogenic foci and allowing more pronounced through transmission.
- With further ageing, the LM may undergo cystic degeneration presenting as anechoic mass with acoustic enhancement.
- Area of calcification may be present, usually in older women. These calcification may be seen on plain radiography.
- Distortion of endometrial cavity echo is helpful in identifying submucosal LM, submucosal leiomyoma may mimic endometrial lesions and sonosalpingography may aid in making diagnosis.

- Special care should be taken when evaluating a pregnancy within a leiomyomatous uterus as multiple fibroids increase the frequency of malposition, retained placenta and premature uterine contractions.

HSG Submucosal LM are especially likely to cause distortion of the uterine cavity. While subserosal and small intramural leiomyoma are often associated with normal HSG findings.

- Single LM causes a smooth and rounded filling defect on the uterine contour.
- Multiple LMs are associated with separate filling defects and sometimes gross distortion of uterine cavity.
- Large leiomyoma may cause a cresentric or spindle shaped elongation of uterine cavity.
- LM may cause cornual distortion or obstruction to tubal filling.
- LM arising from cervix may elongate and distort its outline.
- Subserosal LM sometimes are large enough to deform the uterine cavity or compress or deviate a fallopian tube.

CT The characteristic feature of uterine LM is an enlarge uterus with solid enhancing mass having lobulated. Contour with speckled, streaked, or curvilinear calcification. The presence of dystrophic calcification is most specific sign of LM. However, it is seen only in 10% cases. In absence of carcinoma myoma cannot be distinguished from carcinoma on the basis of attenuation value.

- In absence of calcification both USG and MRI are superior to CT for demonstrating the myoma.

MRI is most sensitive imaging for LM being able to diagnose lesions as small as 3 mm. MRI is indicated when the USG examination is indeterminate or limited as in uteroflexed uterus.

- MRI facilitates differentiation of pedunculated myoma from adnexal mass on the basis of typical signal intensity.
- LM is typically seen as sharply marginated homogenous areas of very low signal intensity of T2WI and isointense to myometrium on T1WI.
- The appearance of myoma after administration of gadolinium is variable.
- Degenerative fibroid may have moderately high signal intensity on T2WI.
- The definitive diagnosis can be made by showing the 'claw sign' the stretching of myometrium around the base of the lesion.

2. Adenomyosis

- Is characterised histologically by the presence of endometrial tissue and stroma within the myometrium.
- The most common consequence of invasion of myometrium by endometrial cells is simply diffuse enlargement with no alteration in echo texture or uterine contour.
- Although, some time focal, the adenomyosis is more generally diffuse involving particularly the post uterine wall.

HSG It is difficult to diagnose this condition on HSG. Irregular endometrium may be the only finding but penetration of contrast material into myometrium, which give, speculated appearance may raise the suspicion of the diagnosis.

USG TVS shows an enlarged uterus with focal or diffuse change in texture. While the diagnosis of diffuse adenomyosis can be suggested on US the findings of focal adenomyosis are hard to distinguish from LM.

MRI is useful in diagnosis of adenomyosis. Present on T2W images as focal, ill defined, oval or elongate lesions within the junctional zone or diffuse widening of JN zone. Adenomyosis generally depicts low signal intensity in all pulse sequences but may contain areas of high signal intensity suggestive of hemorrhage.

- Contrast enhancement is similar to myometrium.

Endometrial Polyp

- Is localized overgrowth of endometrial glands and stroma covered by endometrial epithelium.
- This may be sessile or pedunculated.
- They usually arise in fundus.
- They are multiple in 20% cases.
- They are usually asymptomatic. If symptomatic present as vaginal discharge or bleeding.

HSG It is seen as irregularities in the outline of the uterine cavity or as filling defects.

USG Features include – non-specific thickened endometrium a focal echogenic area in the endometrium or occasionally an endo-cavitory mass surrounded by fluid.

- The submucosal fibroid may mimic on endometrial polyp but may be differentiated by a broader base and more irregular contour.

MRI Endometrial polyps are seen as low/intermediate signal masses within endometrial cavity. Contrast enhanced MRI has improves the sensitivity of detection.

Endometrial Hyperplasia

- Is the most common cause of vaginal bleeding in the both pre and post menopausal women.

USG Shows endometrial thickening, which is difficult to differentiate from polyps and carcinoma even on TVS.

- HSG can be helpful to differentiate it from polyp.
- Confirmed diagnosis is made by endometrial biopsy.

MRI Shows diffuse thickening of endometrial strike on T2WI which is isointense or slightly hypointense relative to normal endometrium.

- But these findings are non-specific and can also be seen with carcinoma endometrium.

AV Malformation

- Uterine AVM may appear on gray scale imaging as subtle myometrial in homogenecity, tubular space in myometrium, intramural uterine mass, and endometrial mass or prominent parametrial vessel.
- Doppler ultrasound shows low resistance blood flow PI (0.3 to 0.6) with high peak systolic velocities. Spectral analysis of the venous flow also shows high flow velocities and systolic velocity peak similar to arterial pattern, which suggest AV shunting.
- The Doppler parameter may be similar in gestational trophoblastic disease but the two can be differentiated with serum BHCG test which is negative with AVM.

MRI AVM appears as a focal uterine mass or as disruption of the junctional zones with serpinginous flow related signal voids and prominent parametrial vessels.

MALIGNANT LESIONS OF UTERUS AND CERVIX

Endometrial Carcinoma (EC)

- This is the most common malignant of female reproductive tract in developed countries.

- This present as postmenopausal bleeding with peak incidence between age of 55 to 65.
- Risk factors include unopposed oestrogen intake nulliparity, obesity, diabetes and stein-luventhal syndrome.
- Upto 90% of endometrial cancers are adeno-carcinoma. Rest include sarcoma, mixed tumors and metastasis.
- Endometrial carcinoma arises from body of uterus. Early growth is exophytic in endometrial cavity followed by progressive invasion of myometrium causing uterine enlargement.
- Tumor spread caudally into vagina and axially to involve adnexa, parametrium and other pelvic organs. Lymphatic spread is complex and any group of pelvic nodes or retroperitoneal para aortic LN may be involved.
- Hematogenous spread to lungs, liver, bone and brain can occur late.
- The endometrial carcinoma are staged according to FIGO staging system:

Stage I	Tumor confined to the body of uterus.
Stage II	Tumor involving body of uterus and cervix.
Stage III	Tumor extending outside the uterus but not outside the true pelvis.
Stage IV	Tumor extending outside the true pelvis or involving mucosa of bladder/rectum or distant metastases.

Conventional Radiography

- Chest radiography are routinely done in all patients diagnosed to have endometrial carcinoma.
- Skeletal radiography or scintigraphy can be performed if bone metastases are suspected.
- IVU or barium studies are obsolete in evaluation of endometrial carcinoma.

USG

- Is an important modality for diagnosing as well as staging the EC TVS is more accurate than TAS.
- Early EC typically appear as widening of endo-layer double layer thickness of >5mm in postmenopausal women as considered abnormal. But in women on estrogen therapy upto 7 mm is considered as normal.
- On sonohysterosalpingography EC is seen as intra cavitatory polyp or as asymmetrical thickening of endometrial lining.
- Obliteration of endometrial halo is suggestive of myometrial invasion. Larger tumor causes enlargement and distortion of the uterus.
- USG is less accurate in detecting LN mets.

Benign vs. Malignant Disease of Uterus on USG

- In women presenting with postmenopausal bleeding. It is important to distinguish benign condition as cystic atrophy, cystic or adeno-matous hyperplasia or endometrial polyps from malignant ones.
- Many studies say that malignant uterine tumors are more likely to have:
  - Thickened echogenic endometriums are retroverted.
  - Lack as sub endometrial halo.
- Cystic changes are present in 76% of benign conditions manifesting with endometrial thickening but in 24% of endometrial malignancy.
- Most endometrial tumors at least in part were echogenic. But in 10% cases they were isoechoic so difficult to detect.
- No difference in Doppler parameter has been found between malignant and benign uterine disease.
- So neither the TVS nor Doppler imaging can accurately distinguish benign lesion from malignant.

- In contrast enhanced CT EC is seen as a hypo dense mass relative to normal myometrium.
- Irregularity of uterine outline and stranding of parametrium in suggestive of extrauterine spread.
- CT can demonstrate LN enlargement and distent mets.
- Myometrial invasion is difficult to access on CT.

MRI

- Is the investigation of choice for evaluation of EC and staging it.
- On non-enhanced MRI EC is isointense with the normal endometrium.
- EC shows enhancement after intravenous gadolinium and it is particularly helpful in detection of small tumor even if they are confined to endometrium.
- Obliteration of junctional zone on MRI is suggestive of myometrial invasion.

Other Uterine Malignancy

- Sarcoma of uterus is highly malignant. They are rare (2/100000).
- Sarcomatous change in leiomyoma is extremely rare. Their USG appearance is identical to that of benign tumor. The only diagnostic clue of leiomyosarcoma is relatively rapid growth in postmenopausal women.
- Other systemic malignancies such as lymphoma or metastases are very uncommon in the uterus. When they are present the USG appearance is non-specific.

Gestational Trophoblastic Disease

- Includes:
  - Hydatiform mole (Figure 99.3).
  - Invasive mole.
  - Choriocarcinoma.
- They arise from the foetal tissue within the maternal host. This tumor has a unique and

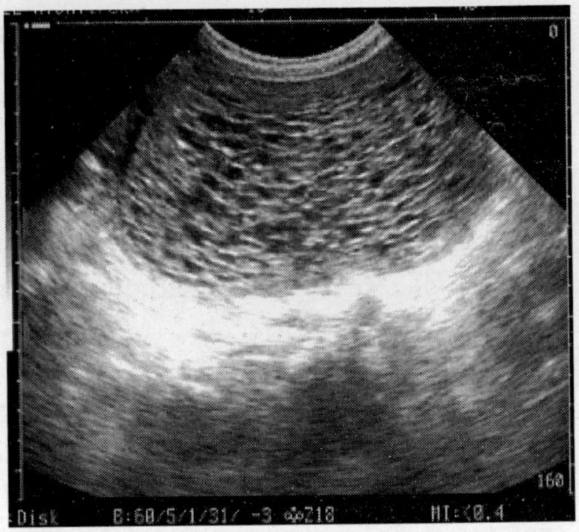

Fig. 99.3: US scan shows hydatiform mole

characteristic tumor marker HCG.

- The role of imaging in this disease is to document metastatic disease or to evaluate persistent disease.
- There is no specific imaging finding that allow differentiation of complete mole from invasive mole or choriocarcinoma.

USG

- Show soft tissue mass distending the endometrial cavity with multiple small cystic spaces. These findings are nonspecific.

CT

- Shows enlarged uterus. On CECT the uterine enhancement is heterogenous. Extrauterine manifestations are seen as bilateral ovarian enlargements by multilocular thecalestein cyst. Regional spread is checked by enhancing soft tissue density in parametrium or obliteration of pelvic fat or muscular plane.

MRI

- T2WI shows heterogenous increased signal intensity mass that obliterates normal uterine zonal anatomy.
- T1WI show iso to hyper intense mass on post contrast images tumors show enhancement.

Carcinoma Cervix

- It is the most common malignancy of female reproductive tract. It is the second most common site of malignancy after breast in female body.
- Patients usually present with post coital bleeding or vaginal discharge.

USG

- Early CA cervix is difficult to detect with USG either TAS or TVS. More advanced cancer is seen as enlarged cervix or irregular, hypo echoic mass that may mimic a cervical myoma. If tumor obstruct the endocervical canal hydro or hematometra seen.

CT

Shows enlargement of cervix. On CECT low attenuation area may be seen with the tumor. These areas may be due to necrosis or ulceration.

MRI

MRI is superior to USG or CT for delineation of the primary site and extent. T2WI shows intermediate signal intensity mass, which is greater than normal low signal intensity of cervix. T1WI tumors are usually isointense with normal cervix and may not be visible. Contrast enhancement is used in estimation of tumor necrosis and in suspected advanced disease involving rectum and bladder.

Conventional Radiography

- Chest X-ray is always done to detect pulmonary metastasis. They appear as multiple pulmonary nodules, which frequently cavitates. Mediastinal lymphadenopathy may also be seen in advanced disease.
- IVU, barium enema to see the invasion of uterus, rectum and sigmoid colon cross sectional imaging as US, CT and MRI are preferred now.

Staging

- Invasive cervical cancers are staged accordingly to FIGO staging system into 4 stages:

Stage 0:	Carcinoma in situ.
Stage I	Invasive tumor confined to cervix. IA – Preclinical. IB – Clinically detectable.
Stage II	Spread beyond uterus. IIA – Involvement of upper third of vagina. IIB – Involvement of paramet-rium not extending to side wall.
Stage III	Extension to the pelvic side wall/ lower third of vagina/hydro nephrosis. IIIA – Involvement of lower third of vagina. IIIB – Involvement of pelvic sidewall and/or hydronephrosis.
Stage IV	Pelvic visceral involvement or distant metastases. IVA – Involvement of bladder or rectum. IVB – Distant metastases.

OVARIAN LESIONS

Benign

1. Physiological cysts:
   - Follicle cyst – size 3-5 cm.
   - Lutein cyst:
     - Corpus luteum.
     - Theca lutein cyst.
   - The corpus lutein cyst tends to be larger than follicular cyst and has thicker wall.
   - These cysts may show hemorrhage. Bleeding is more common with corpus lutein cysts.

- These lutein cysts are associated with polycystic ovarian disease, hydatiform mole, choriocarcinoma, chronic gonadotropin or cloniphan therapy.

CT

On CT a simple ovarian cyst is homogenous, unilocular water density mass with smooth thin walls and no internal contents.

MRI

Simple ovarian cyst is a well-circumscribed homogenous mass with a smooth interface, are peripherally located and having smooth and almost imperceptible wall. The cyst contents are low signal intensity γ on TW1 and very high signal intensity γ on T2WI.

2. Para ovarian cyst:
   - Per ovarian cyst arises in broad paratubal cyst.
   - Ligament between the ovary and the fallopian tubes.
   - These cysts are not physiological hence its dimensions remain constant throughout menstrual cycle.
   - Specific diagnosis is not possible unless a normal ovary is seen separately from the cyst.
   - On sonography a complicated paraovarian cyst may resemble an endometrioma, serous cystadenoma or a hemorrhagic cyst.

Endometriosis

- This is the most prevalent cause of chronic pelvic pain occurring in upto 65% of women with pelvic pain. Endometrial tissue is present outside the uterus in the pouch of Douglas, the ovaries, covering the peritoneum of the bowel and bladder.
- Some patients are symptomatic, while other present clinically with dysmenorrhea, dysparunia, abdominal pain, dysfunctional uterine bleeding and infertility.
- Two forms have been described diffuse and localised (endometrioma). The diffuse form is more common or chocolatic cyst). The diffuse form is rarely diagnosed by USG because the implants are too small to be imaged.

Ultrasonography (USG)

The characteristic sonographic appearance of endometrioma is a well defined unilocular or multilocular predominantly cystic mass containing diffuse homogenous, low level, internal echoes. Occasionally a fluid-fluid level can be seen.

- The appearance may be similar to a hemorrhagic ovarian cyst. However, a hemorrhagic cyst more frequently demonstrate a reticular internal pattern and is more frequently associated with free fluid in cul-de-sac.
- A hemorrhagic cyst will resolve or show significant decrease in size over the next few menstrual cycles whereas endometriomas tend to show little change in size and internal echopattern.
- Endometriomas may be confused with an ovarian neoplasm or tubo ovarian abscess.

MRI

Endometriomas appear hyperintense on T1WI and heterogeneously hyperintense on T2WI. The use of fat suppression increases the detection rate.

Table 99.1: Ultrasonographic criteria

Technique	US features	Criteria indicative of PCO
TAS	• Ovarian volume • No. of follicles (4-10 mm)	>15cm^3 >10
TVS	• Ovarian volume • No. of follicles (2-5 mm) • Increased echogenicity of ovarian stroma	>17.6 cm^3 >15 Present
TVS	• Ovarian volume • No. of follicles (2-8 mm) • Increase echogenicity of ovarian stroma	>9 cm^3 >10 Present

Imaging of small implant (<1cm) is difficult even with MRI.

POLYCYSTIC OVARIAN DISEASE

- Is characterized by bilaterally enlarged polycystic ovaries, secondary amenorrhea or oligomenorrhea and infertility. About 50% of patients are hirsute and many are obese.
- TVS is the gold standard for diagnosing PCOD.
- Various ultrasonographic criteria have been laid for the diagnosis of PCOD.
- The most consistent feature of PCO, which is not seen in normal cyclic ovary, is the presence of small follicles around an echodense ovarian stroma.
- The presence of a very prominent thick endometrial echo is suggestive of PCO especially if other vs. clinical and endocrinologic findings point to this diagnosis.

Ovarian Torsion

- It is an acute condition requiring prompt surgical intervention caused by partial or complete rotation of the ovarian pedicle on its long axis.
- It is mostly associated with an adnexal mass usually a dermoid cyst but may also occur spontaneously.

USG

Shows unilateral ovarian enlargement which is oedematous with multiple small cystic structure at the periphery.

Table 99.2: Types of ovarian neoplasms

Type	Incidence	Example
1. Surface epithelial stromal tumors	65% to 75%	• Serous cystadenoma • Serous cystadeno carcinoma • Mucinous cystadenoma • Mucinous cystadeno carcinoma • Endometrioid carcinoma • Clear cell carcinoma • Transitional cell carcinoma • Brenner
2. Serum cell tumors	15-20%	• Teratoma • Dermoid • Immature teratoma • Dysgerminoma • Yolk sac tumor
3. Sex cordstromal tumors	5-10%	• Granulosa cell tumor • Thecoma and fibroma • Sertoli Laydig cell tumor
4. Metastic tumors	5-10%	• Genital primary – Uterus • Extragenital primary – Stomach – Colon – Breast • Lymphoma

- Small amount of free fluid may be seen in the cul-de-sac secondary to obstructed veins and lymphatus.

Color Doppler

- Demonstrate lack or severe restriction of arterial flow.
- The ovary has dual blood supply and torsion may affect one arterial blood supply more than the other resulting in partial arterial flow on CDS.
- The arterial waveform may exhibit a lack of diastolic flow with a spike configuration of the systolic peak.
- Arterial flow may be present even in a non-viable ovaries absent venous flow may be sensitive of non-viability.

Ovarian Neoplasm

- It is the 3rd most common gynecological malignancy; it has the highest mortality rate as a result of late diagnosis.
- Increasing age, multiparity, a history of breast, endometrial or colon cancer, or a family history of ovarian cancer has been associated with a higher risk of developing ovarian cancer.

SONOGRAPHIC FINDINGS

- Ovarian cancer usually present as an adnexal mass. Sonography shows the gross morphological condition of the tumor but not histology.
- It is difficult to distinguish benign from malignant ovarian tumor by sonography.
- Well-defined anechoic lesions are more likely to be benign, whereas lesions with irregular walls, thick irregular septations, mural module and solid echogenic elements favour malignancy.

Serous Cystadenoma

- Zoographically they are usually large, thin walled unilocular cystic masses that may contain thin septations.

Serous Cystadenoma Carcinoma

- Quite large, multilocular cystic masses containing multiple papillary projections arising from the cyst walls and septal echogenic solid material may be seen within loculation. Ascites is frequently present.

Mucinoma Cystadenoma

- Huge cystic mass upto 15-30 cm multiple thin septae are present and low level echoes caused by mucinous material may be seen in dependent part. Papillary projections are less frequently seen than serous counterpart 5% or bilateral.

Mucinoma Cystadenocarcinoma

- Large multi loculated cystic mass containing papillary projections and echogenic material. Penetration of tumor capsule or rupture may lead to intra peritoneal spread of mucin secreting cells that fill the peritoneal cavity with gelatinous material known as pseudomyoma peritonei. Sonographically it is similar to ascites or may contain multiple septations in the fluid that fill much of pelvis abdomen.
- A ruptured mucocele of the appendix and metastatic colon can also lead to pseudomyoma peritonitis 15-20% of bilateral.

Endometroid Carcinoma

- Cystic mass containing papillary projections. Some time it may present as solid mass that contain area of hemorrhage and necrosis. 20-30% are bilateral.

Clean Cell Tumor

- 20% are bilateral. Usually present as non-specific complex, predominantly cystic mass.

Transitional Cell Ca (Thinner)

- Uncommon (1-2% of all ovarian tumor). 6-7% are bilateral. They are hypoechoic solid mass. Calcification may occur in the outer wall.

Germ Cell Tumor

- 95% are benign cystic teratoma. These tumors are more commonly seen in active reproductive years.
- Cystic teratoma has a variable appearance ranging from completely anechoic to completely hyper echoic. Certain features are considered specific. These include a predominantly cystic mass with an echogenic mural nodule "the dermoid plug". The dermoid plug usually contains hair, teeth or fat and frequently cast acoustic shadow. An echogenic dermoid may appear similar to bowel gas and may be overlooked.

Struma Ovarii

- Is a teratoma that is composed entirely or predominantly of thyroid tissue.

Immature Teratoma

- <1% of all teratoma and contain immature tissue from all three germ cell layers. Sonographically these present as solid masses. Those mostly occur in first two decades of life.

Dysgerminoma

- This tumor occur predominantly in women <30 years and is bilateral in 15% of cases.
- Dysgerminoma and serous cystadenoma are the two most common ovarian neoplasm seen in pregnancy.
- Sonographically they are solid mass predominantly echogenic but may contain small an echoic area caused by hemorrhagic or necrosis.

Yolk Sac Tumor

- Occurs in female <20 years.
- Almost always unilateral.

Table 99.3: Differentiating features between benign and malignant disease

Sonographic characteristics	Benign disease	Malignant disease
1. Size	Small <5 cm	• Large >10 cm
2. External contour	Thin wall	
	Well defined	• Thick wall
	borders	• Ill defined or irregular borders
3. Internal consistency	Purely cystic	• Solid or complex
	Thin septations	• Thick or irregular septations
		• Papillary projections
		• Echogenic solid nodule
4. Doppler	High resistance	• Low resistance flow
	No flow	
	Avascular nodules	• Vascular nodules
5. Associated findings		• Ascites
		• Peritoneal implant

- Increased level of serum alpha feto protein may be seen in association with this tumor. Sonographic appearance is similar to that of dysgerminoma.

Sex Cord Stromal Tumors

- Granulose cell tumor: Occur in postmenopausal part.
- Nearly all are unilateral
- Estrogenically active ovarian tumor and 10-15% of patient eventually developed endometrial carcinoma.
- Sonographically they vary from very small to large masses. Small masses are predominantly solid having an echogenicity similar to uterine fibroid. The larger masses are multiloculated and cystic having the appearance similar to cystadenomas.

Sertoli Cycling Cell Tumor (Androblastoma)

- Rare (0.5% of ovarian neoplasm).
- Occurs in <30 years of age.
- Almost all unilateral.
- Signs and symptoms of mascularization may occur.
- Appearance similar to granulosa cell tumor.

Thecoma and Fibroma

- 70% occur in postmenopausal female.
- Unilateral.
- Thecoma frequently show clinical sign of estrogen production. Fibroma is rarely associated with estrogen production therefore asymptomatic despite reaching a large size.
- Ascites is seen in half patient with fibroma larger than 5 cm in diameter.

Meig's Syndrome

- Occur in 1-3% patients of ovarian fibroma (associated ascites and pleural effusion).
- Sonographically these tumors are hypoechoic mass with marked posterior attenuation of the band beam.
- The main D/D is – Brenner tumor.
- Pedunculated uterine fibroid.

Metastatic Ovarian Tumor

- 15% of ovarian malignancies are metastatic in nature.
- Common primary sites are stomach, colon and breast. Uncommon sites are lung, gall bladder, pancreas.
- Kurkenberg tumor is the term used for specific histological pattern of mucin secreting signet cells with sarcomatous stroma usually from a gastric primary.
- On imaging ovarian metastasis are usually bilateral large and lobulated. These are often indistinguishable from primary ovarian carcinoma. Ascites, peritoneal nodules and omental deposits are seen in both primary and metastatic ovarian tumors.
- Hematogenous spread to liver is rare with primary ovarian carcinoma but common with metastatic ovarian disease.
- Ovarian lymphoma is usually a part of disseminated non-Hodgkin's lymphoma.
- Ovary is the most common organ of female genital tract to be involved in leukemia.

Section 9—Reproductive System

Chapter 100

Uterine Masses

Imaging Appearance of Uterus

- The uterus lies in the true pelvis between the urinary bladder anteriorly and the rectosigmoid posteriorly.
- Uterine position is variable depending on the varying degree of bladder and rectal distension.
- The cervix is relatively fixed in the midline.
- Flexion refers to the axis of the cervix relative to the vagina.
- Version refers to the axis of the cervix relative to the vagina.

USG

- Myometrium consists of three layers distinguished by sonography.
- The intermediate layer is the thickest and has a uniform homogenous echotexture of low to moderate echogenicity.
- The inner layer is thin compact and relatively hypoechoic and surround the echogenic endometrium and referred to as "sub-endometrial halo".
- The thin outer layer is less echogenic than the intermediate layer and is separated from it by arcuate vessels.
- The endometrial cavity is seen as a thin echogenic line as a result of specular reflection from the interface between the opposing surfaces.

CT

Uterus appears as a pear shaped organ between the bladder anteriorly and rectum posteriorly and appears as homogenous in density. CT cannot differentiate the zonal anatomy of the uterus as USG and MRI.

MRI

- T2 weighted scans displays the characteristic zonal anatomy, with three distinct areas in uterine body.
- Hyperintense central zone representing the endometrium combined with secretions in the endometrial canal.
- Outer area of intermediate signal due to myometrium and a low signal junctional zone between a layer of compressed myometrium.
- Changes in size and signal intensity of the three zones in uterus occur during the menstrual cycle with an increase in the volume and signal of the myometrium in the secretory phase.
- Following I/V gadolinium chelate the endometrium and myometrium enhance, with the junctional zone remaining of low signal intensity.

Differential Diagnosis of Uterine Masses

Benign

- Uterine fibroids (99%).
- Pyometra.
- Hemato/hydrocolpos.
- Transient uterine contraction during pregnancy.
- Bicornuate uterus.
- Adenomyosis.
- Intrauterine pregnancy.
- Lipoleiomyoma (<50 cases in world literature).

Malignant

- Cervical carcinoma.
- Endometrial carcinoma.
- Leiomyosarcoma.
- Invasive trophoblastic disease.

Uterine Fibroids (Leiomyoma)

- Benign overgrowth of smooth muscles and connective tissue and is the most common cause of uterine enlargement second only to pregnancy.
- Fibroids are hormonal dependent and an increase in growth occurs in 15-32% of cases within the first trimester and not during the remainder of pregnancy. Shrinkage occurs in puerperium and after menopause.
- It is asymptomatic in 70-75 % of cases but may present as hypermenorrhea, palpable mass or as pain due to pressure effects, torsion, infarction or degeneration.
- Mostly seen at fundus and corpus, around 3% are seen in cervix.
- They may be intramural (within the confines of uterine outline), subserosal or exophytic which may secondarily become broad ligament fibroids or may become parasitic secondary to development of a separate blood supply from the omental or mesenteric vasculature, submucosal fibroids are also called as fibroid polyps and they may be pedunculated and may extrude out of cervical canal partially or completely.

USG

Especially TVS has 60% sensitivity and 99% specificity and 87% accuracy in diagnosing fibroids.

- Most commonly they present as hypoechoic masses but may also be uniformly echogenic, isoechoic presenting as focal bulge of uterine contour or may have mixed attenuation secondary to calcifications especially in postmenopausal age groups.
- They may also show anechoic regions secondary to internal degeneration: atrophic, hyaline, myxomatous, lipomatous, calcareous, necrobiotic and hemorrhagic.

CT: They present as hypo, iso or hyperdense to mixed attenuation masses with solid areas showing some contrast enhancement.

MRI: (86-92% sensitivity, 100% specificity, 97% accuracy).

- They present as sharply marginated homogenous focal area of intermediate signal intensity on both T-1 and T-2 weighted scans.
- Occasionally inhomogeneous high signal intensity on T2W scans may result from hemorrhage, hyaline degeneration or when it is a highly cellular leiomyoma.
- Hyperintense rim is seen in 33% cases due to dilated lymphatics, veins or edema.
- In post enhanced scans 65% are hypointense, 23% isointense, 12% hyperintense relative to myometrium.

Adenomyosis (Endometriosis Interna) (Figure 100.1)

Focal or diffuse benign invasion of myometrium by endometrium.

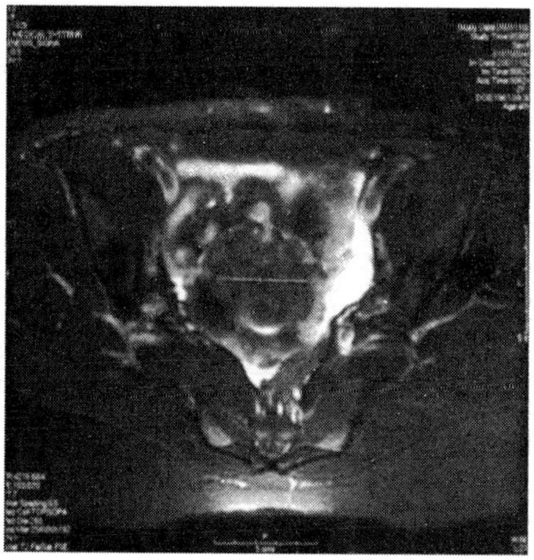

Fig. 100.1: MRI axial image showing multiple uterine masses

- Asymptomatic in 5-70% of cases most common presenting complaint is menorrhagia.
- Focal adenomyosis also known as adenomyoma presents as oval mass of ill-defined margins with a contiguity to the junctional zone.
- Diffuse adenomyosis there is smooth uterine enlargement.

USG

- Poorly defined hypoechoic heterogeneous areas are seen in the myometrium.
- 1-3 small myometrial cysts are seen occasionally with Swiss cheese appearance of myometrium.

MRI

- Myometrial mass with indistinct margins primarily of low signal intensity on all sequences.
- Diffuse or focal widening of junctional zone> 12 mm.
- Central high density spot on T1 and T2 W scans.
- Enhancement always less than the adjacent myometrium.

Cervical Cancer

- 6th most common cause of cancer death in women and is the 3rd most common gynecological malignancy.
- Peak age 45-55 years.

USG

- Bulky enlargement of cervix may be seen or in early cases only heterogeneity of cervix may be seen (Figures 100.2 and 100.3).
- Fluid filled uterus secondary to obstruction.
- Signs of parametrial invasion > mm soft tissue strands extending from cervix to the parametrial soft tissue masses in parametrium eccentric parametrial enlargement obliteration of fat planes.

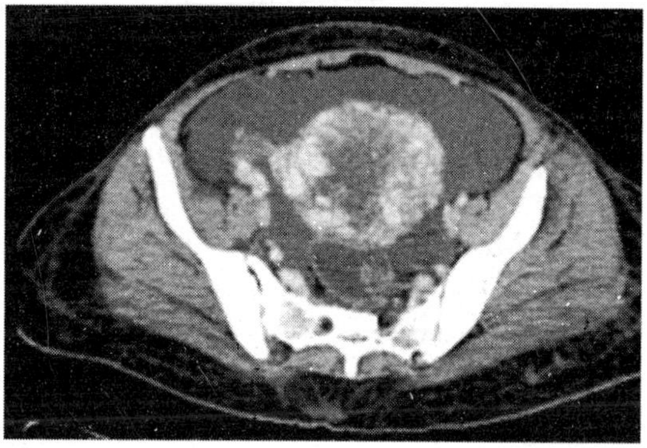

Fig. 100.2: Axial CT image shows cavernous hemangioma of the uterus

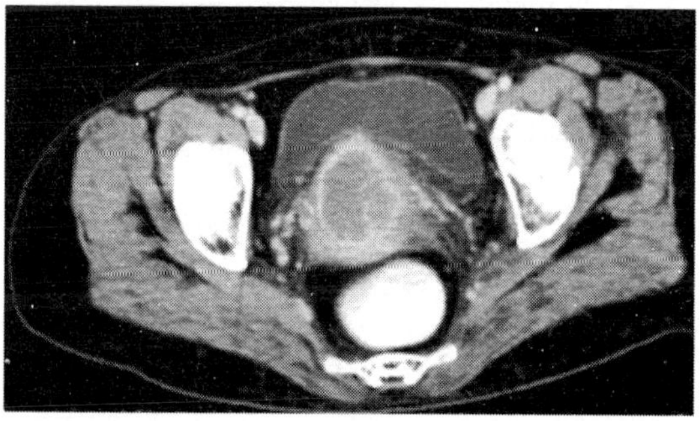

Fig. 100.3: Axial CT image shows a large cervical mass

MRI

- Isointense mass on T1W images.
- Hyperintense focal bulge/mass on T2W.
- Blurring and widening of junctional zone secondary to obstruction of cervical os.

Staging (FIGO)

0. Carcinoma in situ.
I. Confined to cervix.
   - Ia Microinvasion of stroma.
   - Ib Invasion confined to cervix.

II. Extension beyond the cervix but not to pelvic walls/lower third vagina.
   - IIa Vaginal invasion excluding lower third.
   - IIb Parametrial involvement except pelvic sidewalls.

III. Extension to pelvic walls and lower third of vagina.
   - IIIa Invasion of lower third of vagina.
   - IIIb Parametrial involvement till pelvic sidewalls.
   - IVa Mucosal involvement of bladder, rectum.
   - IVb Spread to distant organs including nodal metastasis.

Endometrial Cancer

- Most common invasive gynecological malignancy.
- Peak age 55-62 years.

USG

- Normal size or enlarged uterus.
- Echogenic thickened endometrium.
- Inhomogeneous endometrial echotexture with irregular hypoechoic areas.
- Pulsatility index of < 1.5.

MRI

- Slightly lower signal intensity than endometrium but higher than myometrium on T2W scans.
- Endometrial thickness abnormal if > 3 mm in postmenopausal and > 10 mm in patients on HRT.
- Disruption or absence of junctional zone.
- Hyperintense areas penetrating into myometrium.

FIGO staging

0 In situ.
Ia Limited to endometrium.
Ib Invasion to less than half of myometrium.
Ic Invasion to more than half of myometrium.
   - Iia Endocervical glandular involvement only.
   - Iib Cervical stromal invasion.

IIIa Invasion of serosal adnexal/peritoneal metastasis.
IIIb Vaginal metastasis.
IIIc Metastasis to pelvic/para aortic lymph nodes.
IVa Invasion of bladder/bowel mucosa.
IVb Distant metastasis.

Ovarian Tumors

- 25% of all gynaecological malignancy.
- Risk factors.

HISTOLOGIC CLASSIFICATION OF OVARIAN NEOPLASM

1. **Serous cystadenoma carcinoma**

MC – 30% of all ovarian malignancy ↑

Table 101.1: Types of tumor

Type	INC	Ex.
1. Surface epithelial stromal Tumor	65-75%	S. cystadenoma. M. cystadenoma. Endometrial. Clear cell ca. Transitional cell ca.
2. Germ cell Tumor	15-20%	Teratoma. – Dermoid. – Immature. Dysgerminoma. Yolk sac tumor.
3. Sex cord stromal Tumor	5-10%	Granulosa cell tumor. Sertoli leydig cell tumor. Thecoma and fibrous.
4. Metastatic ↑	5-10%	Uterus, stomach, colon, breast lymphoma.

50 - 70%—benign.

Adenoma-4th-5th D CO – perimenopausal/ Post menopausal.

20% - 50% of bilateral.

USG large thin walled unilocular cystic masses with thin replication and papillary projection.

Carcinoma large, multilocular cystic mass, containing multiple papillary projection.

Echogenic solid material within the loculation.

2. **Mucinous CA and CC 25% of all OVT**

85% - Benign.

Less freq. bilateral.

USG – huge cystic mass (15-30 cm); multiple thin septal, low-level internal echoes.

Papillary projections are less frequent.

Pseudomyxoma peritoni may be seen.

3. **Endometrioid Tumor–**Nearly all malignant.

25-30%—Bilateral.

Cystic mass with papillary projections. OR

Solid mass with areas of hemorrhage and necrosis.

4. **Transitional cell (Brenner) Tumor–**1 to 2%.

Nearly always benign.

6-7% are bilateral.

Hypoechoic solid mass.

Calcification in outer wall.

Cystic area – unusual – when present.

Coexistent cystadenoma may be present.

5. **Germ Cell Tumor**

Derived from primitive germ cells.

95% benign cystic teratoma.

Most common ovarian malignancy in children and young adults.

Cystic Teratoma

15-25% of ovarian tumor.

Variable from complete anechoic to hyperechoic dermoid plug i.e. tip of the iceberg sign. A mixture of mesh of hair, sebum gives rise to a dermoid mesh.

Fat fluid/hair fluid level may be seen.

Postmenopausal Female Unilateral

Small masses – Solid, larger masses, multiloculated and cystic.

Thecoma/Fibroma

Hypoechoic mass with marked post-accentuation of sound beam.

Meig's syndrome with ascites and pleural effusion seen in 1-3% of ovarian fibromas.

Metastatic Tumor

5% to 10% of ovarian tumor.

Most common primary sites – Breast and GIT.

Bilateral solid masses, may have necrosis.

Ascites may be seen – either primary or mets T.

lymphomas – diffuse, disseminated form, bilateral.

CT and MRI

- Do not play a primary role in initial evaluation.
- To determine tumor extent.
- Sensitivity of CT and MRI in detecting small intra peritoneal implants (<1cm) is low.

CT Feature of Ovarian Carcinoma

- Multiloculated cyst with thick septations of solid component.
- A thick walled cysts/a combined solid and cystic mass (Figure 101.1).
- Uniformly solid mass (Figures 101.2 and 101.3).

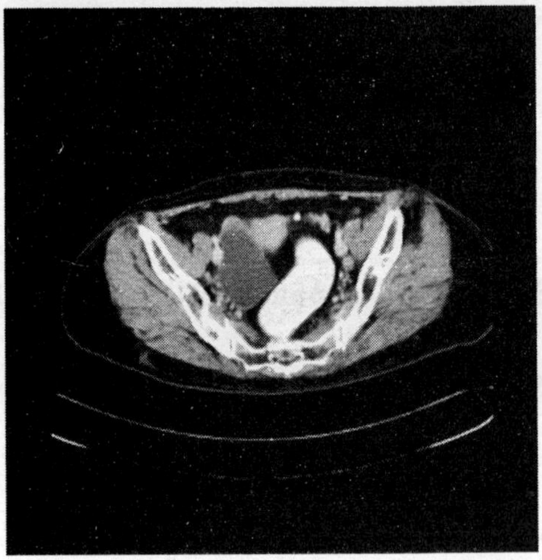

Fig. 101.1: Axial CT image shows a right ovarian cyst

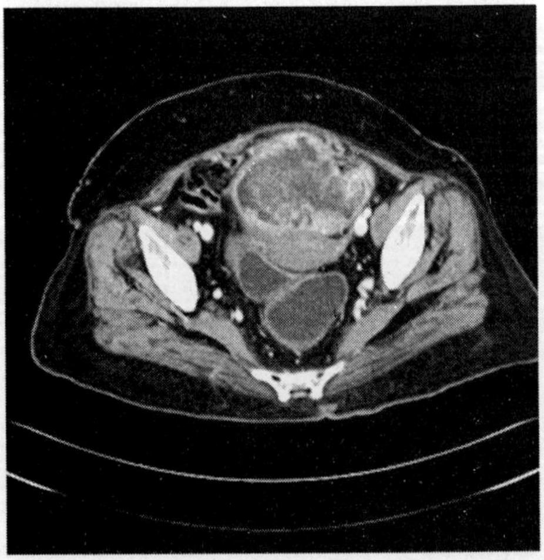

Fig. 101.2: Axial CT image shows a large heteogeneous left ovarian mass

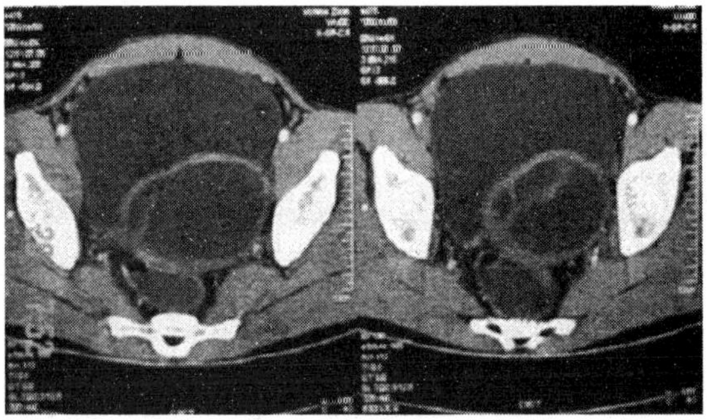

Fig. 101.3: Axial CT images show cystic and septated ovarian mass

- Calcification and contrast enhancement is absent.
- Useful in detecting tumor involvement of adjacent bowel loop and encasement of ureters, HDN spreads to the peritoneum, mesentery and greater omentum, liver, spleen, pelvic and para-aortic LN ascites and pseudomyxoma peritonii.

CT is most commonly used to detect persistent or recurrent ovarian cancer and document tumor response to subsequent therapy.

Staging Classification for Ovarian Carcinoma

Stage I

Growth limited to the ovaries:

IA One ovary, no ascites.

IB Both ovaries, no ascites.

IC One or both ovarian ascites present (malignant cells in the fluid).

Stage II

Involving one or both ovaries with pelvic extension.

IIA Extension of met to the uterus or tubes only.

IIB Extension of met to other pelvic viscera.

Stage III

Growth involving one or both ovaries with wide-spread intra peritoneal mets (omentum, small intestine, and its mesentry) limited to the abdomen.

Stage IV

Growth involving one or both ovaries with distant metastasis outside the peritoneal cavity.

Chapter 102

Localized Hyperostosis of Skull

Causes Include

1. Hyperostosis Frontalis Interna.
2. Fibrous Dysplasia.
3. Meningioma.
4. Osteoma.
5. Ossifying Fibroma.
6. Hemiatrophy.

HYPEROSTOSIS FRONTALIS INTERNA

- Hyperostosis Frontalis Interna is characterized by excessive growth or thickening of the frontal bone of the skull. It is a common abnormality found in as many as 12 percent of the female population exclusively in post menopausal women.
- It affects females 9 times more often than males.
- It is found in multiple generations suggesting that the disorder may be inherited as a dominant trait.
- The disorder appears to be hormone related, as it is associated with a variety of conditions such as seizures, headaches, obesity, diabetes insipidus, excessive hair growth and sex gland disturbances.
- On X-ray and CT it is characterised by irregular nodular thickening of inner table of skull vault.
- Lesions are bilateral symmetrical and spare midline.

MENINGIOMA

- Commonly invade the bony skull and produce localized hyperostosis.
- Radiological diagnosis is suggested by classical site e.g. Parasagittal or sphenoidal ridge and also by enlarged vascular markings leading to the lesion or signs of raised ICT.
- 75% of meningiomas occur in women with average age of onset is 50 years.
- Hyperostosis is confined to inner table but later it may grow through the diploic and outer table and even present as palpable lump. It may show sunray spicules when protruding externally.
- Meningiomas of anterior skull base constitute 40% of intracranial meningiomas. Of these 50% occur in sphenoid wing and 50% in tuberculum.
- Sphenoid wing meningiomas may be associated with hyperostosis of the sphenoid ridge and may be very invasive, spreading to

the dura of the frontal, temporal, orbital and sphenoidal regions.

- Meningiomas of the tuberculum sella may extend into both optic canals resulting in painless proptosis. About 15% of the olfactory groove meningiomas grow into the ethmoid sinuses.

OSTEOMA

- Arise principally from skull PNS and mandible.
- Benign slow growing tumor consisting entirely of well differentiated bone with broad base and well defined margins.
- Size usually not more than 1 cm, however large osteomas may be 2.5 cm.

Two Types

- Dense variety or Ivory osteoma.
- Spongy variety commonly occurring in cranial vault and is shown to contain moderate fibrous tissue (variant of FD).
- Usually asymptomatic but growth from inner table can produce raised ICT. Growth in PNS may cause mucocele especially involving the frontal sinus.
- Large osteomas may perforate through sinus and cause pneumocephalus. Large osteoma in frontal and ethmoid sinus may cause proptosis due to orbital invasion.

PAGET'S DISEASE

- Paget disease of the bone (osteitis deformans) is a metabolic disorder characterized by abnormal osseous remodeling.
- The final or cold stage demonstrates less evidence of continual osseous remodeling due to progression of osteoblastic activity and decline of elastic activity so that disorganized new bone of increased density replaces lytic bone so that previously laid woven bone is converted to dense lamellar bone.
- Paget disease typically is seen in older individuals and is uncommon before age 45 years. Onset of disease may occur earlier in men than women. Male-to-female ratio is approximately 1.8: 1.
- The radiographic findings of Paget disease include trabecular coarsening and distortion and cortical thickening observed in the sclerotic phase, typically involving the axial skeleton.
- In the skull, the sclerosis of inner table is pronounced and later the diploic spaces and outer table become thickened resulting in classic widespread cotton wool appearance.

HEMIATROPHY

- Hemiatrophy of one cerebral hemisphere is not frequently encountered. When this develops early in life (during the first two years) and is supposed to be caused by intrauterine and perinatal carotid artery infarction leading to cerebral hemiatrophy and is known as Dyke Davidoff Masson syndrome.
- The classical clinical presentation includes seizures, facial asymmetry, contralateral hemiplegia or hemiparesis and mental retardation.
- CT of head shows atrophy of the entire right hemisphere with compensatory ipsilateral skull thickening and paranasal and mastoid sinus enlargement along with widening of diploic space.
- There is ipsilateral midline structural shift, ventricular dilatation and sulcal enlargement. The compensatory cranial changes occur to take up the relative vacuum created by the hypoplastic cerebrum.

FIBROUS DYSPLASIA

- Fibrous dysplasia is a skeletal developmental

anomaly of the bone-forming mesenchyme that manifests as a defect in osteoblastic differentiation and maturation. Virtually any bone in the body can be affected.

- It is a non-hereditary disorder of unknown cause.

PATHOPHYSIOLOGY

- In fibrous dysplasia, the medullary bone is replaced by fibrous tissue, which appears radiolucent on radiographs, with the classically described ground-glass appearance.
- Trabeculae of woven bone contain fluid-filled cysts that are embedded largely in collagenous fibrous matrix, which contributes to the generalized hazy appearance of the bone.
- **Sex:** The incidence is equal in males and females.
- **Age:** The initial manifestations of fibrous dysplasia are most commonly found in persons aged 3-15 years.
- The following 4 disease patterns are recognized:
  1. Monostotic form.
  2. Polyostotic form.
  3. Craniofacial form; and
  4. Cherubism.

MONOSTOTIC FORM

- Approximately 70-80% of fibrous dysplasias are monostotic.
- This form most frequently occurs in the rib (28%), femur (23%), tibia, craniofacial bones 10-25%, and humerus, in decreasing order of frequency.
- This form most frequently occurs in those aged 10-30 years.
- The degree of bone deformity is relatively less severe as compared to polyostotic form.

POLYOSTOTIC FORM

- Approximately 20-30% of fibrous dysplasias are polyostotic. The common sites of involvement are the femur (91%), tibia (81%), pelvis (78%), ribs, skull and facial bones (50%), in decreasing order of frequency.
- The dysplasia may be unilateral or bilateral, and it may affect several bones of a single limb or both limbs with or without axial skeleton involvement.
- Two thirds of patients are symptomatic before they are 10 years of age.
- Often, the inital symptom is pain in the involved limb associated with a limp, spontaneous fracture, or both.
- Leg-length discrepancy of varying degrees occurs in about 70% of patient's involvement. The structural integrity of the bone is weakened, and the weight-bearing bones become bowed.
- The curvature of the femoral neck and proximal shaft of the femur markedly increase because a femoral lesion commonly causes severe coxa vara abnormality, Shepherds-Crook deformity, which is a characteristic sign of the disease.

CRANIOFACIAL FORM

- This pattern of the disease occurs in 10-25% of patients with the monostotic form and in 50% with the polyostotic form. It also occurs in an isolated craniofacial form.
- Sites of involvement most commonly include the frontal, sphenoid, maxillary, and ethmoidal bones. The occipital and temporal bones are less commonly affected.
- Hypertelorism, cranial asymmetry, facial deformity (i.e., leontiasis ossea), visual impairment, exophthalmos, and blindness may

occur because of involvement of orbital and periorbital bones.

- Involvement of the sphenoid wing and temporal bones may result in vestibular dysfunction, tinnitus, and hearing loss.

CHERUBISM

- This special variant of fibrous dysplasia is an autosomal-dominant.
- Disorder of variable penetrance. It occurs in children and is more severe in boys. Regression may occur after adolescence.
- The jaw is broad and protruding. Involvement of maxilla and mandible is symmetric.

Other Features

- Fibrous dysplasia may be associated with endocrinopathies in 2-3% of cases.
- These include precocious puberty in girls, hyperthyroidism, hyperparathyroidism, acromegaly, diabetes mellitus and Cushing syndrome.

McCune-Albright Syndrome

- Sexual precocity in girls, with polyostotic fibrous dysplasia and cutaneous pigmentation, constitutes McCune-Albright syndrome.
- It may be associated with hyperthyroidism and, hence, exophthalmos.
- Cutaneous pigmentation is the most common extraskeletal manifestation in fibrous dysplasia.
- It occurs in more than 50% of cases of the polyostotic form and is ipsilateral to the side of bony lesions, a feature that differentiates this disease from pigmentation in neurofibromatosis.
- The pigmented macules or *cafe-au-lait* spots are related to increased amounts of melanin in the basal cells of the epidermis.
- They tend to be arranged in a linear or segmental pattern near the midline of the body, usually overlying the lower lumbar spine, sacrum, buttocks, upper back, neck and shoulders. Similar lesions may occur on the lips and oral mucosa.

X-ray

- Common locations for lesions are the ribs, craniofacial bones, femoral neck, tibia, and pelvis.

Radiographic Findings include:

- Long and short tubular bones.
- The usual appearance of fibrous dysplasia includes a lucent lesion in the diaphysis or metaphysis, with endosteal scalloping and with or without bone expansion and the absence of periosteal reaction.
- Usually, the matrix of the lucency is smooth and relatively homogeneous classically described as a ground-glass appearance. Irregular areas of sclerosis may be present with or without calcification. The lucent lesion has a thick sclerotic border and is called the ring sign.
- The lesion may extend into the epiphysis only after fusion. Premature fusion of the ossification centers may occur, resulting in adult dwarfism.

Skull and Facial Bones

- The frontal bone is involved more frequently than the sphenoid, with obliteration of the sphenoid and frontal sinuses. The skull base may be sclerotic.
- Single or multiple, symmetric or asymmetric, radiolucent or sclerotic lesions in the skull or facial bones may be present.
- The external occipital protuberance may be prominent however; these features are less

common in Paget disease, neurofibromatosis and meningioma.

- Most commonly, maxillary and mandibular involvement has a mixed radiolucent and radiopaque pattern, with displacement of the teeth and distortion of the nasal cavities.
- The diploic space is widened, with displacement of the outer table. The inner table of the skull is spared in fibrous dysplasia, unlike Paget disease.

Pelvis and Ribs

- These bones have lucencies, with a diffuse ground-glass appearance and ring lesions. Cystic lesions are common. Protrusio acetabuli is a feature on the pelvic radiograph.

Spine

- Spinal involvement is common in polyostotic disease and rare in monostotic disease. Well-defined, expansile, radiolucent lesions with multiple internal septa or striations involve the vertebral body and, occasionally, the pedicles and arches.
- Paraspinal soft tissue extension and vertebral collapse are rare. Kyphotic deformity and spinal cord compression may occur.

CT Scan

- CT findings complement plain radiographic findings.
- CT demonstrates the nature of the lesion better by characterizing the matrix of the lesion. It also depicts expansion of the effected bone and its subtle mineral contents.
- It can demonstrate subtle nondisplaced pathological fractures.
- CT is extremely useful in evaluating the extent of disease in complex locations such as the facial bones, pelvis, chest wall and spine.
- Usually, attenuation is in the range of 70-130 HU.
- In the skull, the outer table always expands outward. Therefore, the lesion is invariably convex both tables are intact, although they are thinner.
- In the spine, CT can demonstrate the extent of bony disease and compromise of the spinal canal space.
- Paraspinal soft-tissue extension can be demonstrated at CT.

MRI

- Useful in assessing malignant change and demonstrating extension of the tumor into the surrounding soft tissues.
- On T1-weighted MRIs, the lesion has low-to-intermediate signal intensity equal to that of muscle. T2-weighted images also show low signal intensity owing to the high content of collagen and bone.
- In children, T2-Weighted images show hyperintense signal greater than that of subcutaneous fat this finding is characteristic of fibrous dysplasia.
- As fluid-fluid levels are reported in fibrous dysplasia, on short-inversion time inversion-recovery (STIR) images, the signal intensity of the lesion may be very high.
- For postoperative follow-up, gadolinium-enhanced MRI is useful in demonstrating the proliferation of fibrocellular tissue.

Malignant Degeneration

- The estimated frequency is 0.4-1%.
- The interval from the diagnosis to the development of malignancy varies and is usually years or decades.
- Most often, skull and facial bones undergo malignant change in monostotic disease, whereas femoral and facial bones undergo malignant change in polyostotic disease.

- Osteosarcoma and fibrosarcoma are the most common tumors.
- Radiographic features suggestive of malignant degeneration include a rapid increase in the size of the lesion and a change from a previously mineralized bony lesion to a lytic lesion.
- Clinical findings of increasing pain and an enlarging soft tissue mass suggest malignant change.

Metabolic Changes

- Hypophosphatemic rickets and osteomalacia have been noted in patients with fibrous dysplasia.

OSSIFYING FIBROMA

- Considered as localized form of FD and differs by the presence of osteoid.
- Relatively rare in skull usually effecting young people.
- Most frequently commence in PNS particularly in antrum.
- Unlike FD lesion is discrete, circumscribed, round and oval in shape confined to a part of the bone and frequently appears encapsulated.

Skull Lesions

SKULL

- Complex structure > 20 bones.
- Through survey as a routine procedure – not cost effective.

Four Standard Projections

1. *Lateral view*

   Suspected side near film.

   - 2.5 cm anterior to EA meatus and 1 cm above OM line.
2. *PA view*
   - OM line – vertical.
   - CR – Tilted 20° caudally.
   - Centring on the inion.
3. *Towne's view*
   - Supine.
   - CR – 30° caudally.
4. *Basal view*
   - Hanging head position.
   - OM line – horizontal.
   - Centring between angle of mandible.

Normal Appearance

Sutures

- Readily recognized on films of adult.

Skull

- Outer sarated, inner linear.

Infants

- Radiolucent linear bands.

Vascular Markings

- Meningeal markings recognized by the constant position and course.
- Increase gradually in size from above downwards.
- External surface – supra orbital and middle temporal arteries.
- Diploic vascular markings – Extreme variable in size, number and position.
- Most prominent in parietal region.
- Short course, widening and narrowing.

Pituitary Fossa

- Length 11-16 mm.
- Depth 8-12 mm.
- Breadth 9-19 mm.
- Usually small pituitary fossa – no particular significance – myotonia congenital, hypo pituitarism, radiotherapy as child.
- J. shaped sella – elongated sella, exaggeration of normal slight impression of sulcus chiasmaticus.

- Normal.
- Optic chiasm glioma.
- MPS.
- NF.
- Chronic hydrocephalus.

SKULL VAULT

- Pacchonian impressions.

Inner Table by Pacchonian Bodies

- Host numerous in parasagittal location.

NORMAL INTRACRANIAL CALCIFICATION

- Pineal – rarely in children, most adult skulls 3-5 mm diameter.
- Habenular commissure – lies directly anterior to the pineal at the back end of 3rd ventricles.
- C shaped calcification, open part facing posteriorly.

Choroid Plexus

- Frequently calcified.
- Punctate foci to 1 cm dense calcification.
- Usually bilateral and symmetric.

Dural Calcification

- Middle aged and elderly.
- Most easily recognized in falx or tentorium.

Petroclinoid Ligaments

- On a lateral film as a linear calcification between tip of the dorsum and petrous apex, interclinoid ligament may also calcify.

Pacchonian Bodies

- Difficult to identify.

Basal ganglia and dentate nuclei – often idiopathic.

SKULL IN NEONATES AND INFANTS

- May appear elongated and sometimes show overlapping of bones, change too normal within a week.
- Vault is thin, no different into inner or outer lobe, no vascular or convolution makings.
- Wormian bones occasionally seen in suture unite with vault as growth proceeds.
- Anterior and middle fossa are short, slope downward more than adult.

Suture -	< 1 month	1.5-10 mm.
	> 3 months	< 3 mm.

- Supraoccipital and exoccipital regions – occipital.
- Mendosal suture – occipital bone.
- Metopic suture – disappears by 9 months.
- Posterior fontanel – closes by 4-6 months.
- Anterior fontanel – at 15-18 months.

ABNORMAL SKULL

Congenital Lesions

- Abnormal shapes of skull.
- Dolicocephaly – abnormally long in relation to transverse diameter.
- Brachycephaly – Broad in relation to length.

Craniosynostosis (Figure 103.1)

- Due to premature fusion of skull suture.

Trigonocephaly (Triangular Head)

- Is due to premature fusion of metapic suture. Frontal bones appear wedge shaped.

Scaphocephaly (Boat Shaped Skull)

- Premature fusion of sagittal suture. Narrow Dolicocephalic skull – most common form of craniosyntosis.

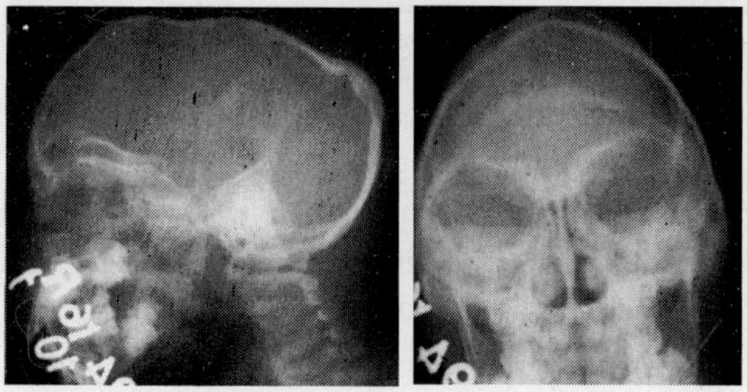

Fig. 103.1: Radiographs of the skull show craniostenosis

Plagiocephaly (Slanting Skull)

- Unilateral premature fusion of coronal and labdard suture.

Microcephaly

- Generalized premature fusion.
- Small brain, mental retardation.

Oxycephaly, Acrocephaly and Turicephaly

- Brachycephalic skull resulting from premature fusion of coronal and lambdoid suture.
- Same cases – Compression of optic nerves, mental handicap and other neurological lesions.
- Apert's syndrome–Syndactyly.
- Carpenter's syndrome – Polydactyly.
- Crouzon's disease – Acrocephaly with facial hypoplasia, hypertelorism, oxophthalamos, parrot beak nose, pragmatism.

Lacunar Skull

- Round oval or finger shaped pointing on the inner surface of infant skull.

  Usually associated with anomalies of CNS, most common myelomeningocele and encephalocele, hydrocephalus.
- High mortality in children.
- Disappear by 4-6 months, if survives.

Cranial Meningocele and Encephalocele

- Above defect beneath a scalp swelling should always raise the possibility of encephalocele.
- Basal encephalocele usually presents in infants with nasal obstruction. Basal view of skull – defect in the sphenoid or sphenoethmoid region.

Platybasia

- Flattening of base of skull.
- Basal angle – angle between plane of the clivus and the floor of the anterior fossa (125°-142°).

Basilar Impression

- Indicates an elevation of floor of the posterior fossa, which occurs as a congenital anomalies often in association with atlanto-occipital fusion or klippel – Feil syndrome.

Basilar Invagination

- Acquired condition from disease causing bone softening.
- Rickets, osteomalacia, Paget's disease, scurvy and hyper parathyroidism.
- Usually symptomless, may cause pressure on and distortion of the brain stem and obstruction of CSF.
- Chamberlin's line – more than half of odontoid peg.
- Cleidocranial dystosis – persistence of metopic suture and anterior fontanelle and failure of fusion of the lower labdoid sutures.

Congenital Parietal Foramina

- Symmetric bilateral large ovoid defects in posterior parietal region.
- Symptomless – may be familial.

Sinus Pericranii

- Due to small emissary vein, causes a midline defect in the frontal bone which the vein traverses.

Hypertelorism

- Distance measured between the medial walls at junction of medial angular process of the frontal bone with the maxillary and lacrimal bones.

  Adult: Women – 25 mm.

  Men – 28 mm.
- Associated with Sprengel's shoulder, failure of segmentation of sternum, congenital heart disease.
- Secondary hyperterlorism – frontal encephalocele or mucocele of the ethmoids, fibrous dysplasia, OI.

Raised ICP

Radiological signs are:

1. Suture diastasis.
2. Sellar erosion.
3. Pineal displacement.
4. Increased convolutional markings.

Infants and Children

- Sutural diastasis is the first and most prominent result of ↑ ICP.
  - Coronal and sagittal – markedly effects.
  - May show carniolacunae, if with meningocele.

  Older children and adolescents – suture appear abnormal with excessive interdigitation.
- Sellar erosion is a late sign and implies long standing—ICP.
- Incidental convolutional markings – nor necessarily pathological.

Adults

- Erosion of the dorsum sella is cardinal sign in adults, no sutural diastasis.
- Commences as slight porosis of anterior cortex of dorsum sellae.

Pinceal Displacement

- Another important sign in adults lies within 3 mm of midline on PA projection.

INTRACRANIAL CALCIFICATION

Tumors

Gliomas – In over 5% calcification seen

oligodechdogliomas – 50%, serpinginous calcification.

Craniopharyngiomas – Calcification in 75%, few punctate foci to densely calcified mass.

- Position – Midline just above the sella.
- Shape of sella – Bent forward as if pressed from above.

Meningiomas – Calcification on plain film in about 10% of cases.

Calcification – Ball like and amorphous, parasagittal.

Hyperostosis of the vault, increased vascular markings leading upto the site of attachment.

Dermoids – Most common in the post fossa, base of skull – arc like calcification.

- Associated with small central defect in occipital bone.

Epidermoid – Occasionally show arc like calcium.

Teratomas – Pineal and suprasellar region calcification.

Pineal Tumors

Lipoma – Usually occurs in relation to corpus callosum – characteristic marginal calcification

CPP, chondromas, metastasis (bracket sign).

Vascular lesions (Figures 103.2 and 103.3).

Aneurysms

- Arc like calcification in region of circle of Willis.
- Mostly <1 cm in diameter.

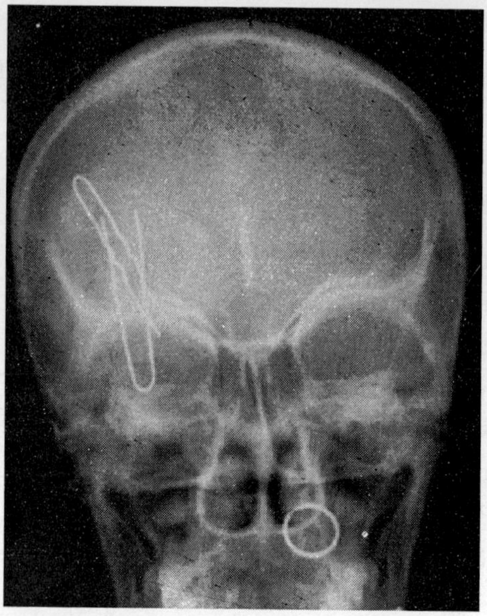

Fig. 103.2: Plain radiograph of the skull shows falcine calcification

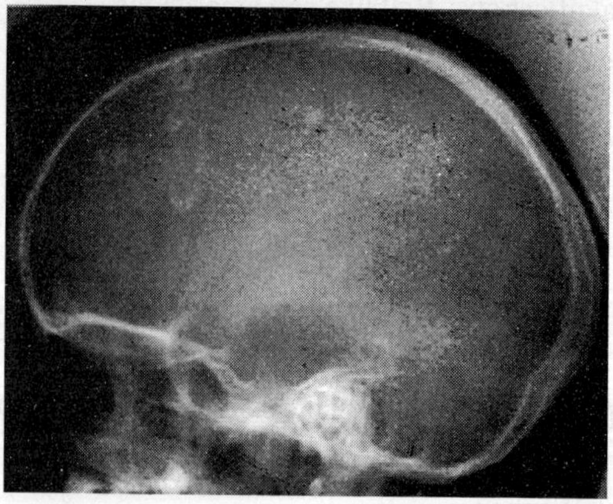

Fig. 103.3: Radiograph of the skull shows multiple calcified lesions corresponding to large intraparenchymal calcified granulomata

Angiomas

- Can diagnostic calficiation, scattered specks of calcium associated with presence or one or more ring or arc shadows.

Chronic Sudural Hematoma

Occasionally slow calcification.

- Characteristic position.

Atheromas

- Linear flecks are common in carotid siphons and can be quite extensive.

INFECTIONS AND INFESTATIONS

Tuberculomas

- Rare on plain film, may be seen in treated patients, small nodules in healed basal exudates and occasionally intracerebral lesion.

Toxoplasmosis

- Congenital toxoplasmosis show characteristic calcification, multiple scattered flecks of calcification in cortex and linear streaks in the basal ganglia.

CMV

- Characteristic widespread periventricular calcification may outline the dilated ventricles.
- Stippled, bilateral and symmetrical microcephaly.

Cysticercosis

- Scattered calcified nodules (not oat shaped) as only scolex calcifies (2-3 mm).

Metabolic and Miscellaneous

Basal ganglia calcification – usually a chance finding.

Bilateral and symmetrical and commences in the region of head of the caudate nucleus.

- The dentate nucleus in posterior fossa can also be affected without supra territorial calcification.

  Most cases idiopathic, related to age.
- Secondary causes, hypoparathyroidism, pseudo HPT.

  Fahn's syndrome, Cockayne's syndrome, lead and carbon monoxide poisoning, γ– radiation.

10 Section

Hyperparathyroidism

- Extremely rare falx and tentorium in CRF patients.

MF

- Extensive calcification of choroid plexus of 3rd and 4th ventricle.

Tuberous Sclerosis

- Multiple areas of dysplasia may contain calcification.
- Discrete nodules of varying sizes.
  Sturge-Weber syndrome, unilateral, occipital cortical calcification typically streamlines.
- May be bilateral and extensive.

Lissencephaly

- Characteristic small-calcified nodule in the septum pellucidum and just behind the foramen of Monro.

Abnormal Vascular Markings

Meningioma

- Most common of pathological vascular markings in the skull vault.
- In addition to middle meningeal vessels diploic vascular markings and emissary venous making may be increased in the region.

Angiomatous Malformation

- Sometimes supplied by the meningeal arteries as well as by the ICA resulting in hypertrophied meningeal vessels and markings.
- Prominent emissary venous markings – dural AV fistula.

LUCENCY IN THE SKULL VAULT WITH SURROUNDING SCLEROSIS

Neoplastic – Multiple Myeloma

- Involves cancellous and both tables of cortical bone (punctured appearance). It can affect the mandible.
- Skull may be normal even with widespread lesions elsewhere.

Metastasis

- Usually irregular and ill defined.
- Breast, kidney and thyroid – common.
- Children – neuroblastoma and leukaemia.

Hemangioma

- Soap bubble appearance can cause “Hair on end” appearance.

Langerhan Cell Histiocytosis

- Eosinophilic granuloma usually produces solitary lesions, bevelled edges due to partial destruction, and no sclerosis until healing.
- Neurofibroma – May characteristically cause a lucent defect in occipital bone usually adjacent to left lambdoid suture.
- May also involve temporal bone or great wing of sphenoid.

Adjacent Malignancy

- Carcinoma of ear, rodent ulcer.
- Paget’s sarcoma.

Traumatic

Burr hole – very well defined—when recent.

- Leptomeningeal cyst – if the dura is torn, the arachnoid membrane can prolapse and the pulsations of CSF – progressive widening and scalloping of the fracture line.
- May persist into adult life.

Idiopathic

Osteogenesis Circumscripta

- Occurs in the active lytic phase of Paget’s

disease. Starts in the lower part of frontal and occipital regions, can cross suture lines to involve large areas.

Metabolic

Hyperparathyroidism (Pepper Pot Skull)

- Rarely severe enough to cause overt lytic lesions.
- The calvarium is affected in approx 20% of primary HPT.
- Mandible common site of brown tumors, loss of lamina dura around teeth, basilar invagination.

Infective

- Tuberculosis may produce a localized rounded destructive lesion, often associated with a soft tissue mass.
- Hydatid—multilocular mass expanding the bone and bulging it outward.
- Syphilis—rare moth eaten appearance.
- Pyogenic osteomyelitis – usually direct infection from adjacent frontal sinus or secondary to compound fracture and to surgery.

Lucency in the Skull Vault with Surrounding Sclerosis

Fibrous Dysplasia

Developmental

1. Epidermoid – scalloped appearance with thin sclerotic margin. Intramedullary can expand both inner and outer tables.
    - Common in sq. portion of occipital and temporal bones.
    - Meningocele – large midline detects and has a smooth sclerotic margin with an overlying soft tissue.

Neoplasia

- Hemangioma – Early rarely has a sclerotic margin.
- Radiating spicules of bone within it.
- LCH—sclerotic margin if in the healing phase.

Infective

- Sclerosis dominates with only few cystic areas.

GENERALISED HYPEROSTOSIS OF SKULL

Paget's Disease

- Multiple islands of dense bone.
- Later difference between outer and inner table is lost and the skull vault is thickened (2-5 times).
- Basilar invagination.
- Loss of lamina dura may occur.

Fibrous Dysplasias

- If the lesions are widespread throughout skeleton, skull always affected.

Dystrophica Myotonica

- Small pituitary fossa may also be seen.

Acromegaly

- Enlarged frontal sinuses, prognathism, enlarged sella, thick vault.

Renal Osteodystrophy

- Osteo sclerosis occurs in 25% skull and spine commonly involved.

Sclerotic Metastasis

- Fluorosis – Calvarium rare site.

Chronic Hemolytic Anemia

- Widening of diploe, bone texture also abnormal with linear radiating spicules.

Congenital

- Pyknodystosis.

- Osteopetrosis.
- Pyle's disease – metaphyseal spraying of long bones.

LOCALISED HYPEROSTOSIS OF SKULL

Meningiomas

- Commonly invade the bony skull and produce localized hyperostotic reaction.
- Initially confined to inner table, then spreads.
- When protruding externally, sun ray appearance.

Primary Osteosarcoma

- Rare, often with "sunray spicules" in Paget's disease.

Osteoma

- Dense flat ivory nodules growing from the surface. More commonly chance finding.
- Usually 1 cm in size, large osteomas peforate through the sinus produce pneumocephalus.

Fibrous Dysplasia

- May involve vault, skull base or facial bones.
- Leontiasis ossea – hyperostosis affecting frontal bones and facial bones.
- Hyperostosis frontalis interna – In adult patients, post menopausal women.
- Irregular modular thickening of inner table of frontal region.

Craniovertebral Junction and Its Anomalies

- CVJ includes paired atlanto-occipital joint, the ligaments connecting the axis and occipital bone as well as the atlantoaxial joints.
- Anterior atlanto-occipital membrane – upper aspect of anterior arch of C1 to foramen magnum.
- Posterior atlanto-occipital membrane – posterior arch of C1 to foramen magnum.
- Atlanto-occipital ligaments – external to capsule of lateral atlanto-occipital joint.
- Anterior atlantoaxial ligament – anterior midportion of dens to the inferior aspect of anterior arch of C1.

Internal Craniocervical Ligament

- Tentorial membrane – Superior extension of posterior longitudinal ligament and attaches to the anterolateral aspect of foramen magnum.
- Transverse ligament – Thick band oriented in coronal plane extending from the tubercle on the inner aspect on one side of atlas to a tubercle in the opposite side – superior fasciculi, inferior fasciculi.
- Apical ligament – Apex of the dens to occipital bone.
- Alar ligament – Superior and lateral aspect of dens to the medial aspect of occipital condyle.

Landmarks on Plain Radiography

Mc Gregor's Line: From the postero superior margin of the hard palate to the most inferior surface of the occipital bone.

Normal odontoid apex should not lie 8 mm in males and 10 mm in female above this line.

Significant – Abnormal superior position of odontoid is indicative of basilar impression. Common association include platybasia, atlas occipitalization, Paget's disease, osteomalacia and FD.

CHAMBERLAIN'S LINE/PALATO-OCCIPITAL LINE

A line is continued from the posterior margin of the hard palate to the posterior aspect of the foramen magnum.

Normally the tip of the odontoid process should not project above this line, a variation of 3 mm above this line may occur. A measurement of 7 mm or more is abnormal.

MACRAE'S LINE

Landmarks – A line is drawn between the anterior (basion) to the posterior (opisthion) margins of the foramen magnum.

Normal – The inferior margin of the occipital bone should lie at or below this line.

- A perpendicular line drawn through the odontoid apex should intersect these line anterior quarters.

  Significance: If the inferior margin of the occipital bone in convex in a superior direction and/or lies above this line, basilar impression is present. Predisposing causes include platybasia, occipitalization, RA, Paget's disease, osteomalacia and FD.

- If the odontoid apex does not lie in the ventral quarter of this line, a dislocation of the atlanto-occipital joint or a fracture of dysplasia of the dens may be present.

DIGASTRIC LINE/BIVENTOR LINE

Studied on a open mouth projection of CVJ.

Landmarks–The digastric groove radial to the base of the mastoid process is located on each side and a line is drawn between them. The vertical distance to the odontoid apex and atlanto-occipital joints is then measured.

Normal–The digastric line odontoid apex average measurement is 11mm.

The digastric line atlanto-occipital joint average measures is 12 mm.

HEIGHT INDEX OF KLAUS

Projection – Lateral skull.

Landmarks – A line is drawn from the tuberculum sellae to the internal occipital protuberance. The vertical distance between this and odontoid apex is then measured.

Significance – A measurement of less than 30 mm indicates basilar insufficiency.

BOOGARD'S LINE AND ANGLE

Projection – Lateral skull, lateral cervical spine.

Boogard's line – A line is drawn connecting the nasion to the opisthion.

Boogard's angle – A line is drawn between the lesion and opisthion (Maclae's angle) a second line is drawn from the dorsum sellae to the basion along the plane of the clivus.

Normal Measurement

Boogard's line – The basion should lie below this angle.

Boogard's angle – Normal angle of 135°.

Significance – Basion will be above Boogard's line and the angle will be greater than 135°.

POWER'S INDEX

Projection – Lateral cervical spine, lateral skull.

Landmarks – Four osseous landmark are located – the basion, opisthion and the ant and posterior arches of the atlas. Two measurements are then made.

1. The distance between the basion and the posterior arch at the spinolaminar junction (B-P).
2. The distance between the opisthion and the posterior margin of the anterior arch (O-A).

The ratio of these two measurements is then calculated.

Normally the ratio is always less than one.

Significance: When the ratio is equal to or greater than one, then an anterior atlanto-occipital dislocation exists.

ATLANTODENTAL INTERSPACE

Landmarks: The distance is measured between the posterior margins of the anterior tubercle and the anterior surface of the odontoid.

Normal measurement: Adults - 2 mm.
Children - 5 mm.

Flexion—V Configuration.

Extension—Inverted pattern.

Significance—Decreased space is seen in degenerative joint disease of the atlantoaxial joint.

Increased space is seen in the following conditions:

- Trauma.
- Occipitalization.
- Down's syndrome.
- Pharyngeal infections.
- Inflammatory arthropathies:
  - Ankylosing spondylitis.
  - RA.
  - Reiter's syndrome.

ATLANTO AXIAL ALIGNMENT

Projection: AP open mouth, cervical spine.

Landmarks: The lateral margins of the atlas lateral masses are compared to the opposing lateral corner of the axis articular surface.

Normal: These two landmarks should be in vertical alignments.

Significance: If the lateral margin of the atlas lies lateral to the lateral axis margin, this is a sign of Jefferson's fracture, odontoid fracture, alar ligament instability, rotatory atlantoaxial subluxation.

CONGENITAL ANOMALIES OF CRANIOVERTEBRAL JUNCTION (Table 104.1)

Table 104.1: Differentiating features between congenital and acquired conditions

Primary Congenital	Secondary Acquired Condition
e.g. occipitalization of C1	e.g. Paget's disease
Spina bifida occult a of atlas	Fibrous dysplasia
Anomalies of odontoid	HPT, OI, RA
Agenesis or hypoplasia of atlas	Rickets/osteomalacia
Down's syndrome	Hurler's syndrome
Syringomyelia-Chiari malformation	Post traumatic
Klippel-Feil syndrome	

Occipitalisation of Atlas/Assimilation of CI:

- Fusion of atlas to the base of occiput.
- Most cephalic blocked vertebra.
- Embryologically there is lack of segmentation and separation of the most caudal occipital sclerotome during the first few weeks of life.
- Association is with platybasia, basilar impression, Arnold Chiari malformation (type I), atlantoaxial dislocation or instability, Sturge Weber's syndrome and Klippel-Feil syndrome.

Radiologic Features

Lateral view shows increased or non-existent space between the post arch of C1 and base of occiput.

Frontal view with head in optimal position shows non-visualization of atlanto-occipital joint due to relative basilar impression.

Flexion and extension view—absence of motion between the posterior arch of C1 and lower margin of occiput.

CT—Osseous anomalies.

MRI—Neural anomalies.

Occipital Vertebrae

- This is a developmental anomaly due to the failure of fusion of the terminal segments of the base occiput.
- If the defect is anterior, it leads to the 3rd condyle.
- Laterally placed anomalies are termed paracondyle, paramastoid or epitransverse process.

Third Condyle/Condylus Tertius

- Results from a failure of fusion of the most caudal occipitoblast, near the midline resulting in a small bony ossicle near the antero inferior margin of the foramen magnum.

Radiological Features

- Lateral view – Small 3rd condyle are impossible due to superimposed mastoid and petrous portion of the temporal bone.

- Large 3rd condyle as oval or round bone densities equal in size or smaller than the anterior arch of atlas.

Epitransverse/Paracondylar Process

- It is a broadbased, cone shaped osseous mass projecting from the lateral aspect of the occipital condyle towards the transverse process of CI.
- The process is in the location of insertion of the lateral rectus capitis muscle.

Radiologic Features

It requires the case of supportive tomography as the teeth of the maxilla often obstructs the view of this area on well position open mouth view.

Table 104.2: Different lines and their measurements (Fig. 104.1)

Synonyms	Definition	Normal measurement	Implications
1. Wackeheim's line (Clivus canal line)	Line drawn along Clivus into cervical canal	Odontoid tip is ventral and tangential to this line	Odontoid process transects the line in basilar invagination
2. Height index of Klauss	Distance between tip of dens and tuberculum-torcula line	40-41mm	<30 mm in basilar invagination
3. McGregor's line (basal line)	Hard palate to most inferior surface of occipital bone	Odontoid apex should not lie above this line >8 mm in males and > 10 mm in females	Abn superior position of odontoid indicates basilar impression
4. Chamberlain's line (palato occipital line)	Line from post margin of hard palate to opisthion	In majority of patients the tip of dens should not project above this line, however, variation of 3 mm above this line may occur	Measurement of ≥7mm is definitely abnormal and suggestive of basilar impression
5. Macrae's line (foramen magnum line)	Joins basion to opisthion	• Inf margin of occipital bone should lie at or below this line • A perpendicular line through odontoid should intersect this line in its ant 1/4	• If inferior margin of occipital bone is above this line or convex sup. → basilar impression • If odontoid does not lie in ventral quarter dislocation of atlanto occipital joint or fracture or dysplasia of dens
6. Basilar angle	Angle between the lines drawn from basion to tuberculum sella and t sella to basion	123-152°	> 152° → platybasia
7. Boogard's line and angle	Line →drawn connecting basion to opsithion Angle triangle between Marcrae's line and line drawn from dorsum sella to basion along Clivus	Basion should lie below this line 119-135°	Basion above this line & >135° →basilar impression
8. Diagastric line (Biventer line) (AP open mouth view)	Line →connecting two diagastric groove med to base of mastoid process	—Diagastric line-odontoid apex measurement ang 11mm (1-21mm) odontoid should not project above this line —Diagastric line—A-O joint avg measurement 12 mm (4-20 mm)	Both measurement will decrease in basilar impression

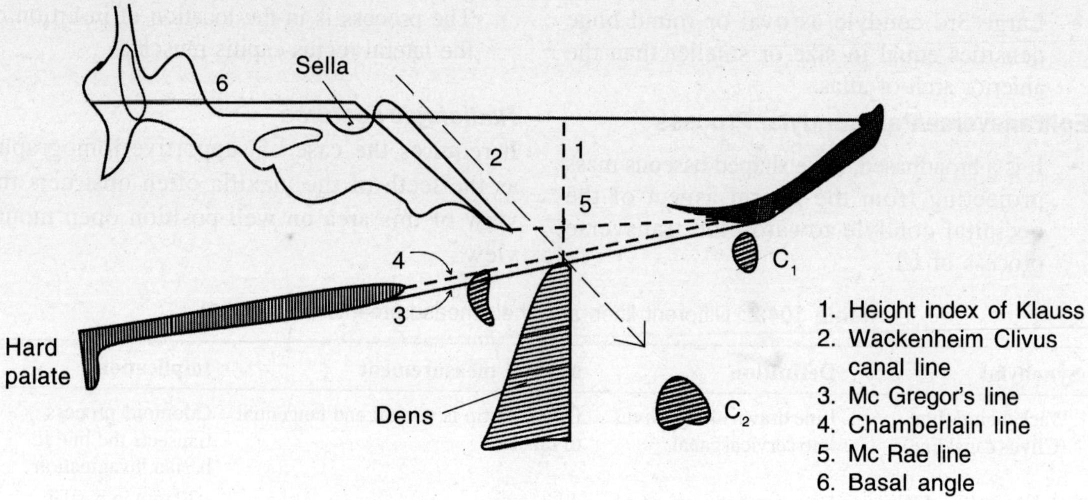

Fig. 104.1: Figure shows various lines and angles

- A slightly rotated open mouth view will shift the molar on the side opposite the direction of head rotation away from the area of interest so that the bony connection between the occiput and transverse process is seen.

  CT Scan: It helps to differentiate smaller process from traumatic changes.
- Larger processes may need CT scan to differentiate between fusion and articulation with the transverse process of the atlas.
- The paracondylar power usually has a broad base and can be the shape of a cone. A cortical layer with a centre of spongy bone borders the process (Table 104.2).

PLATYBASIA/BASILAR INVAGINATION

Platybasia: It means broadbase:

- It is the result of congenital maldevelopment of the sphenoid and/or occipital bones.
- Martin's basilar angle (angle formed by the clival line and a line drawn along the floor of anterior cranial fosse). If this angle is more than 152° platybasia exists.
- It is often associated with occipitalization of C1 and Klippel-Feil syndrome.

Basilar impression/invagination – It is defined as upward displacement of vertebral column. Elements into the foramen magnum with platybasia.

OS Odontoideum

- It describes a condition in which the dens is separated from the axis body.
- It is usually discovered by the principle of "traumatic determination" i.e. the underlying condition preceded the injury and it is not caused by current trauma.

Congenital failure of fusion of dens to axis

↓

Mobile or insufficient dens

↓

Incompetent TAL

↓

Ineffective translation of atlas on axis

↓

Upper cervical cord or vertebral artery

Impingement (+)

- The odontoid usually fused to the C2 body by 5-7 years.

- Associated conditions – Morquis syndrome, multiple epiphyseal dysplasia, Klippel-Feil syndrome and Down syndrome.

Radiological Features

X-ray smooth, wide lucent defect separating the odontoid proven from C2 body at the level of the superior articular possess and there is an associated stress hypertrophy of ant tubercle of atlas (Table 104.3).

Table 104.3: OS odontoideum fracture

Zone of separation	Wide	Narrow
Odontoid orientation	Round, smooth sclerotic	Irregular
Posterior Interrupted cervical line	Normal	
Anterior tubercle size/density	Increased	Normal
Anterior tubercle – posterior margin	Angular	Straight

OS TERMINALE PERSISTENS OF BERGMAN

- The cephalic portion of the odontoid process develop on secondary growth centre from the 1st occipital sclerotome that appear about the 2nd year and usually unites at 10 to 12 years of age.
- On this secondary growth centre does not unite with the subjacent odontoid process and remain as a separate ossicle.

X-ray – Discrete, round oval or diamond shaped piece of bone at the most cephalic portion of the dens in a patient over the age of 12 years.

HYPOPLASTIC OR AGENETIC ODONTOID PROCESS

- Extremely rare.
- On an open mouth view, a hypoplastic odontoid process is seen as an abbreviated stump of bone projecting slightly above the C1-C2 articulation.
- This anomaly should be diagnosed at the time of birth through open mouth view, as the ossification centre for the odontoid process should positive.

FRACTURES OF THE CERVICAL SPINE

Fractures of the Atlas

Jefferson's Fracture (Burst Fracture of the Atlas)

- It is a compression injury created by a forceful blow upon the skull vertex, which is transmitted through the occipital condyles to the lateral masses of the atlas.
- The force displaces the lateral masses lateral classically producing the fracture on each side of the anterior and posterior arches of the atlas.

At open mouth X-ray: Spreading apart of the lateral masses, creating a ↓ed periodontal space laterally.

FRACTURES OF THE AXIS

Hangman's fracture (Traumatic spondyloliothesis):

- The fracture occurs as a bilateral disruption through the pedicles, sometimes referred to as pars interarticularis.

CT/LAT VIEW

- Bilateral disruption through the pedicles. The fracture line is seen just anterior to the inferior facet in association with anterior displacement of C2 upon C3.

↑ed retropharyngeal interspaces.

ODONTOID PROCESS FRACTURE

Type	Location	Stability
I	Odontoid tip	(+) union
II	Odontoid base	Unstable (non union)
III	Extension into body	(+) (union)

Plain Film Radiography

Lateral projection
- Fracture line.
- Odontoid displacement.
- Disrupted axis ring.
- Enlargement of C2 body.
- Retropharyngeal swelling.

Frontal projection
- Fracture line.
- Filled odontoid process (>5).

Osteolysis of the odontoid.

CT (Figure 104.2)

Axial and reconstructed image.

- Displacement of odontoid.
- Comminution of axis.
- Prevertebral swelling.
- Central canal compromise.
- Intraspinal hematoma.

MRI: T1 and T2 weighted sagittal and coronal.

Images

- Vertebral marrow signal change.
- Spinal canal and cord integrity.
- Intraspinal hematoma.

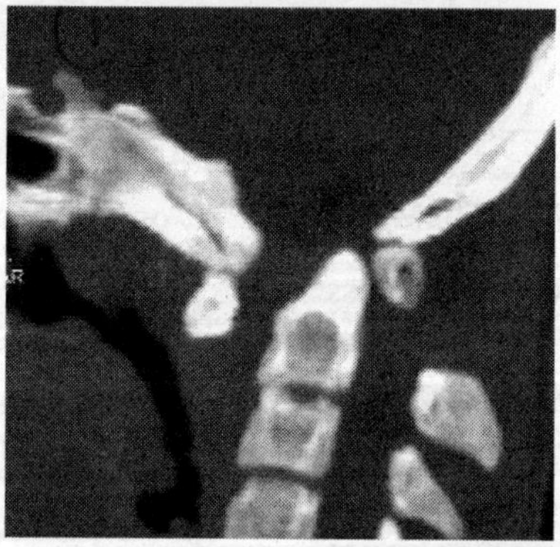

Fig. 104.2: Sagittal MIP CT image shows atlanto-axial dislocation

Spinal Dysraphism

Abnormal or incomplete fusion of midline embryologic mesenchymal, neurologic, bony structures. External signs may be seen in roughly 50% of cases:

- Subcutaneous lipoma.
- Hypertrichosis.
- Pigmented nevi.
- Skin dimple.
- Bladder + Bowel dysfunction.
- Pathologic plantar response.
- Spastic gait disturbance.
- Foot deformities.
- Absent tendon reflexes.
- Sinus tract.

Spina Bifida: Incomplete closure of bony elements of the spine (lamina+spinous process) posteriorly.

Spina bifida occulta (Occult spinal dysraphism): It is a skin covered defect and constitutes 15% of Dysraphism and rarely leads to neurologic deficit in itself. It may be associated with:

- Vertebral defects (85-90%).
- Lumbosacral dermal lesions (80%) like hair tuft, dimple, sinus, nevi, hyperpigmentation, hemangioma and subcutaneous mass.
- Diastematomyelia.
- Lipomeningocele.
- Tethered cord syndrome.
- Filum terminale lipoma.
- Intraspinal dermoid.
- Epidermoid cyst.
- Myelocystocele.
- Split notochord syndrome.
- Meningocele.
- Dorsal dermal sinus.
- Tight filum terminale syndrome.

Spina bifida Aperta (Spina bifida cystica): There is posterior protrusion of all/part of the contents of the spinal canal through a bony spina bifida and constitutes 85% of the cases of dysraphism and is associated with neurologic deficit in > 90% of cases. It is of four types:

- Simple meningocele.
- Myelocele.
- Myelomeningocele.
- Myeloschisis.

Meningocele

- Relatively rare congenital anomaly.
- There is herniation of CSF filled sac without neural elements.There is a dorsal spinal defect.
- Patient presents with a subcutaneous mass

that charges size on valsalva, neurologic deficit is uncommon with simple meningocele.

- More than 80% are located in lumbosacral spine.
- Imaging shows spina bifida with a narrow focal defect or broader lesion with thinned dorsally everted flared laminae.
- A sharply demarcated fluid filled sac that is isodense or isointense with CSF and devoid of neural tissue is present.
- The overlying skin is typically intact.
- Simple meningocele are rarely associated with other spine or spinal cord anomalies.

Dorsal Dermal Sinus

- It is an elongated epithelium lined tube connecting the spinal cord with skin.
- Seen in early childhood to 3rd decade with a M:F of I.
- Clinically there is a midline dimple or pin point ostium.
- Hyperpigmented patch, hairy nevus or capillary angioma may be seen.
- Lumbosacral location is the most common but it can be seen any where from occipital location to rarely ventral.
- CT myelography is by far the best modality to define the intraspinal anatomy. The findings including those of NECT.
  1. Grove in upper surface of spinous. process + lamina of vertebra, with a hyperdense sinus tract in subcutaneous fat passing through a dysraphic or dysplastic lamina.
  2. Hypoplastic spinous process.
  3. Single bifid spinous process.
  4. Focal multilevel spina bifida.
  5. Laminar defect.
  6. Dorsal tenting of dura and arachnoid.
  7. Sinus may terminate in conus medullaris/ filum terminale/nerve root fibrous nodule in dorsal aspect of cord/dermoid/ epidermoid.
  8. Nerve roots bound down to capsule of dermoid or epidermoid cyst.
  9. Displacement or compression of cord by extra medullary dermoid or epidermoid.
  10. Expansion of cord by intramedullary dermoid or epidermoid.
  11. Clumping of nerve roots by adhesive arachnoiditis.
  12. 50% of dermal sinuses end in a dermoid or epidermoid cyst.
- MRI has an advantage over CT that it can show the subcutaneous portion of the sinus tract to best advantage, however the intraspinal. segments may be difficult to delineate unless they are lined by fat.

Spinal Lipomas

- It is the most frequently associated malformation with all types of occult dysraphism.
- These are masses of mature fat and fibrous tissue that are connected with leptomeninges or spinal cord.
- It is divided into three principal categories.
- Lipomyelomeningocele.
- It is a lipoma tightly attached to exposed dorsal surface of neural placode blending with subcutaneous fat.
- Most commonly located at lumbosacral location and may have longitudinal extension, along the whole length of spinal cord.
- Lipoma may enter central canal and extend rostrally (intradural, intramedullary lipoma).
- Lipoma may extend within spinal canal external to dura (epidural lipoma).
- Tethered cord.

10 Section

- Radiologically there is an enlarged spinal canal with erosion of vertebral, body and pedicles and posterior scalloping with focal spina bifida. There may be segmental anomalies like butterfly vertebra and partial sacral agenesis may be present.
- MR scans disclose a low lying spinal cord that continuous dorsally with the neural placode and the nerve root arise from the placode not the lipoma. The lipoma usually lies outside the dura and is contiguous with the subcutaneous fat. Syringohydromyelia is present in 25% of cases.
- **Filum terminale fibro lipoma:**
  - Usually asymptomatic but has the potential of development of tethered cord.
  - Small lipomas occur in the filum itself whereas larger lipomas are usually found at the lower dorsal dural attachment.
  - They are seen as thin linear high signal areas on T1 weighted MR scans.
- **Intradural lipomas:**
  - They may be intradural, subpial or juxtamedullary lesions.
  - Overlying skin is most often normal.
  - Spinal cord is open in midline dorsally.
  - Lipoma in opening in between lips of placode.
  - Exophytic component at upper/lower pole of lipoma.
  - Syringohydromyelia in 2%.
  - Focal enlargement of spinal canal with or without that of adjacent neural foramina.
  - Narrow localized spina bifida.

Diastematomyelia

- There is a sagittal division of cord into two hemicords each of which contains a central canal one dorsal and one ventral horn.
- Usually associated with myelomeningocele.
- There is congenital scoliosis.
- Spina bifida over multiple levels.
- Antero posterior narrowing of vertebral bodies.
- Widening of interpedicular distance.
- Narrowed disk space with hemivertebra, butterfly vertebra, block vertebra.
- Fusion of adjacent laminae.
- Bony-spur through centre of spinal canal arising from posterior aspect of center.
- Thickened filum terminale.
- Tethered cord.
- Low conus medullaris.
- The 2 hemicords usually unite caudal to cleft.

Split Notochord Syndrome

- Spectrum of anomalies with persistent connection between gut and dorsal ectoderm. Types include:
- Dorsal enteric fistula is a connection between intestinal cavity and dorsal midline skin traversing pre vertebral soft tissue, vertebral body, spinal canal and posterior elements of spine. The opening passes meconium and feces.
- Dorsal enteric sinus is a blind remnant of posterior part of tract with midline opening to dorsal external skin surface.
- Enterogenous cyst is either prevertebral, postvertebral or intraspinal enteric lined cyst. The spinal canal is enlarged at the site of cyst with MR and CT depicting the full anatomy.
- Dorsal enteric diverticulum is a tubular or spherical diverticulum arising from dorsal mesenteric border of bowel.
- Dorsal enteric cyst is due to involution of a part of diverticulum near gut.

Myelocystocele (Syringocoele)

- There is hydromelic spinal cord with arachnoid herniation through posterior spina bifida and is the least common form of dysraphism.

- There is a cystic skin covered mass over spine.
- Cloacal exstrophy is frequent.
- On imaging it presents as a direct continuity of meningocele with subarachnoid space with a cyst communicating with widened central canal of spinal cord typically posteriorly and inferiorly to meningocele.
- Lordosis, scoliosis and partial sacral agenesis is common.

Myelomeningocele

- Sac covered by leptomeninges containing CSF and variable amount of neural tissue herniated through a defect in the posterior/anterior elements of spine.
- It may be associated with hydrocephalus, Chiari II malformations, congenital kyphoscoliosis, vertebral anomalies, diastematomyelia, hydromyelia.
- Dorsal meningocele is most commonly lumbosacral.
- Anterior sacral meningocele is a prolapse through anterior sacral bony defect and is occasionally associated with NF I, more fans and partial sacral agenesis.
- Lateral thoracic meningocele is through enlarged intervertebral foramen into extra pleural aspect of thorax and right is more common than left.
- Lateral lumbar meningocele is through enlarged foramen into subcutaneous tissue.
- Cranial meningocele also known as encephalocele.
- Obstetric USG findings:
  - Detection rate of 85-90% are seen, best results are seen if scanning is done after 16-20 weeks of GA.
  - Spinal level is estimated by counting up from last sacral ossification centre i.e. S4 in 2nd trimester and S5 in 3rd trimester.
  - A soft tissue mass is seen protruding posteriorly.
  - Widening of lumbar spine with fusion enlargement of spinal canal.
  - Splaying of ossification centres of laminae with cup or wedge shaped pattern in transverse plane.
  - Absence of posterior line in sagittal plane.
  - Gross irregularity in parallelisms of lines.
  - Head may show lemon sign concave or linear frontal contour or banana sign, due to obliteration of cisterna magna with cerebellum wrapped around posterior brain stem secondary to downward traction of spinal cord.
  - There can be non visualization of cerebellum.
  - Ventriculomegaly.
- Plain films may show bony defect in neural arches.
- CT and MR may be used in cases presenting late and for accurate depiction.

Section 10—Musculoskeletal System

Chapter 106

Pott's Spine

POTT'S SPINE

- Spinal TB 50% of skeletal TB.
- Lumbar (45%) lower thoracic (32%).

  Young adults, <30 years.

  Imaging findings vary depending on the initial focus.

  - Paradiscal – marginal demineralisation.
  - Central disc space either not affected or minimally.
  - Anterior subperiosteal disc – destruction late—Aneurysmal effect.
  - Neural arch—pedicular and laminar involvement.

CT: Four patterns of bone destruction (Figure 106.1).

- Fragmentary, osteolytic, subperiosteal and well-defined lytic lesions with sclerotic margins.
- Disc space narrowing, multilevel involvement and kyphosis.
- Associated soft tissue abscess are usually larger than the extent of bone destruction. Calcification – pathognomonic.

MRI: T1W–↓ signal within the affected vertebral marrow.

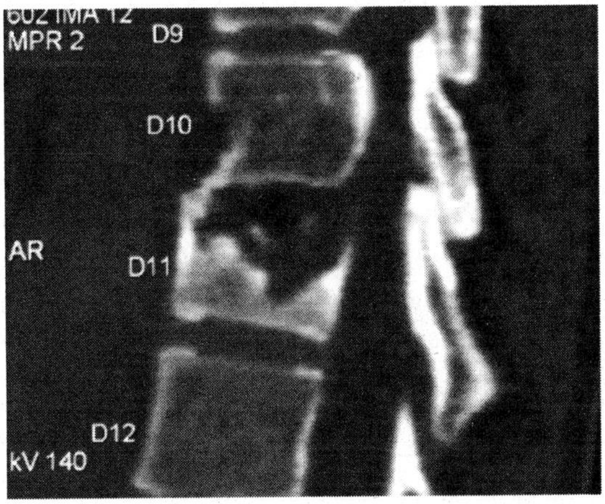

Fig. 106.1: Sagittal MPR CT image shows tubercular spondylitis (Pott's disease)

T2W: Relative increase in signal intensity in vertebral bodies and discs.

DIFFERENTIAL DIAGNOSIS

Hydatid Cyst

Spine involvement begins in the vertebral body where the parasite develops in multiple small cysts. Then spread to pedicles, lamina and paravertebral soft tissues.

X-ray can reveal a widened spinal canal with non-specific osseous destruction.

CT – Intra or extradural multiloculated cystic mass, extension into soft tissue mass and calcification.

MRI– Primary radiological investigation – in myelo-radiculopathy.

- Confirms cystic nature.
- High signal on T2W.

Pyogenic Spondylitis

- Most often effects of vertebral bodies.
- Usually homogeneous – S. aureus, 6-7th decade lumbar spine.

Plain film – Normal for first 8-10 days, ↓ disc space and end plate erosions.

CT – May also be normal in early disease,—disc space, cortical bone loss and paraspinous soft tissues.

MRI–T1W low signal intensity in the adjacent vertebral bodies of—disc space.

- Subligamentous or epidural soft tissue masses.
- Paraspinous abscess, epidural extension and meningeal inflammation.

T2WI show-signal in infected disc and vertebral bodies.

MULTIPLE MYELOMA/PLASMACYTOMA

- Often disseminated, may be localized primarily to spine.
- Thoracic and lumbar regions most commonly involved.

  50% develop neurologic symptoms.

CT – Very sensitive for detecting and confirming myeloma lesions— the typical CT appearance are punched out lesions.

CT – Diffuse osteopenia.

MRI – T1 W1 Hypointense T2W – hyperintense.

METASTASIS

- Adults mostly breast, lung or prostate, Children – Ewing's sarcoma and neuroblastoma.
- Most commonly seen in middle aged and elderly.
- Paediatric – neural foramen, adults – vertebral body, typically the posterior aspect (lower thoracic and lumbar).
- Mostly osteolytic, pedicle destruction is the most common plain film finding.
- Bone scintigraphy – sensitive.

NECT – Readily defines osteolytic or osteoblastic lesion, intrathecal contrast for precise extent.

MRI – More sensitive, also delineates epidural and paraspinous soft tissue involvement.

Form patterns:

1. Focal lytic.
2. Focal sclerotic.
3. Diffuse inhomogeneous.
4. Diffuse homogeneous.

OSTEOBLASTOMA

- Typically =2 cm in size, smaller lesions – osteoid osteoma.
- 5-50 years (20 years) – M: F – 2.5:1.
- 40% occur in spine, 40% in C. spine, 2/3rd are confined to posterior elements.

Imaging: Plain films and CT – shown well defined scalloped, or lobulated lytic expensile mass arising from neural arch.

- Half of spinal lesions – are mainly lytic.
- A thin bony or sclerotic rim with soft tissue extension is a common appearance.

MRI – Intermediate signal intensity on T1WI and with mixed high signal foci on T2WI.

Section 10

CHORDOMA

- Arise from intraosseous notochord elements.
  - Rare tumors.
  - Most common primary sacral neoplasm.
- Peak age – Six decade, M: F 2:1.
- From clivus to coccyx in midline.

Imaging – CT shows lytic, destructive skull base or spinal lesion.
– Mixed solid and cystic components.
– Calcification in 30% - 70%, soft tissue mass.

MRI – T1WI – Low signal intensity, in homogeneously.
T2WI – Equal or exceed CSF intensity (on PD also).

HEMANGIOMA

- Slow growing benign neoplasm, dilated vessels are interspersed among sparse thick trabeculae.
- 75% occur in spine, lower thoracic and lumbar, multiple 25-30%.
- Discovered incidentally, acute cord compression or progressive deficit.

Plain film – Lytic foci with honeycomb trabeculation or thick vertical striations giving rise to 'corduroy appearance'.

NECT – Lucent lesion with typical 'polka dot' densities in the medullary space.

ANEURYSMAL BONE CYST (ABC)

Etiology and Pathology – Benign, non-neoplastic lesion of unknown etiology.

- 30-50% associated with a pre-existing osseous lesion such as chondroblastoma, GCT, osteoblastoma, NOF or FD.
- Trauma or hemorrhagic infarction.

Age/Sex—80% is <20 years, slightly more in females.

Site—20% in spine (Cervical and thoracic), typically occur in the posterior elements; secondarily involve pedicles and vertebral body.

C/F—Pain and swelling, spinal – Pathological fracture and cord compression.

Imaging: Plain films and NECT show an osteolytic lesion surrounded by expanded, thinned eggshell like cortical bone.

Soft tissues usually present, matrix calcification – absent.

MRI – Lobulated, multiseptated lesion with fluid-fluid levels and blood degradation products.

GIANT CELL TUMOR

- Grossly, lytic, expansile locally aggressive bone tumors extend to cortex but rarely transgress the periosteum.
- Peak age, 3rd decade.
- Occur at end of long bone in spine mostly sacrum.
- Pain and neurological deficits, recurrence is common.

Imaging: Plain film radiograph and CT – typically disclose a lytic expansile, destructive sacral or vertebral mass.

- In sacral region, near SI joint.

MR – Low intermediate signal intensity on T1W.

- Heterogeneous intermediate intensity on T2W.
- Enhance brilliantly on gadolinium administration.

Section 10—Musculoskeletal System

Chapter 107

Rickets

- Rickets is a metabolic disease of childhood in which the osteoid i.e. the organic matrix of bone fails to mineralise due to interference with calcification mechanism which is seen prominently at the growth plates, resulting in softening of the bowels and development of deformities.

PHYSIOLOGY AND METABOLISM OF VIT D

- Vitamin D is a fat-soluble vitamin, which exerts its physiological effects on bone, intestine, kidney and the parathyroid gland to modulate calcium and phosphorous metabolism.
- The active principle of vitamin D is synthesized under metabolic control via successive hydroxylations in liver and kidney and is then transported through blood to the target tissue (i.e. the intestine and bone), where it regulates calcium homeostasis.
- Vitamin D is synthesized as follows:

7-deoxyhydrocholysterol $\xrightarrow{\text{UV light}}$ cholecalciferol (vit D3) 25(OH) D3 1-2(OH) ase in kidney

$\xrightarrow[\text{in liver}]{\text{25 (OH) asc}}$ 1,25 (OH) D3 and (1,25 – DHCC).

- Action of vitamin D is:
  1. In intestine—it enhances absorption of Cr L^+ and PO_3^{3-}.
  2. In bone – appears to help bone mineralization indirectly by maintaining normal plasma Ca^{3+} and Pa^{3-} conc.
  3. In kidney – It enhances prox. tubular reabsorption of Ca^{2+} and PO_4^{3-}.

PATHOGENESIS OF RICKETS

Vit. D (deficiency)

↓Ed Ca^{2+} resorption from intestine — ↓Ed Ca^{2+} deposition in bone

↓Sr.Ca^{2+}.

↑Ed PTH

↑Ed Ca^{2+} absorption From kidney — ↑ Ca^{2+} resorption from bone — ↑Ed PO_4^{3-} excretion

↓

Compensatory attempts At the bone formation — Phosphatemia and by phosphatemia

↓

↑ALP levels.

CAUSES OF RICKETS

1. Nutrition deficiency of vitamin D:
   - It occurs when both a deficient diet and lack of adequate exposure to UV light co-exist.
   - It classically becomes apparent a clinically in infants between the age of approx. 10-15 months.
   - It is more commonly seen in black tinned immigrants who make these homes in colder and less sunny areas of Northern Europe and have maintained their original borderline diet.
2. Disorders of absorption due to GI cases:
   - Any malabsorption state will result in vitamin D deficiency like:
   - Crohn's disease, celiac disease, lymphoma, amyloidosis, small bowel fistula, bowel resection and hepatobiliary disease.
   - Rickets also may occur, rarely, in neonates as a vessel of hepatitis and biliary atresia. Both 25 HCC and 1,25- OHCC probably have an enterohepatic circulation, which may be disturbed in these cases.
3. Defects in metabolism of vitamin D.
   a. Renal mechanisms:

   CRF: This is due to renal parenchymal disease; there is osteomalacia (rickets in children), secondary hyperparathyroidism and osteosclerosis. This combination is process as "renal osteodystrophy". There is impairing of (OH) later of 25-HCC to 1,25 – DHCC due to ↓ ed renal mass.

Familial Hypophosphatemia

Is a most common form of renal tubular rickets traditionally known as vitamin D resistant rickets.

- Hyperphosphaturia, hypophosphatemia, normal S. Ca^{2+} levels and failure to respond to high doses of vitamin D is characteristics.
- X-linked dominant disorder though recessive transmission is also reported.
- Presents usually between the age of 12-18 months.
- In this, serum levels of 1, 25-DHCC are low or even normal, but considering the degree of hypophosphatemia these levels are relatively low suggested an inadequate response of the renal enzyme system.

Cystinosis

- It's a disease of childhood previously termed on FANCONI'S SYNDROME.
- Inherited as AUTOSOMAL RECESSIVE TRAIT.
- Hence, there is deposition of cystine crystals in many organ including renal tubules; this leads to reduced renal tubular resorption of phosphorous.

Oncogenic Osteomalacia/Rickets

- In a vitamin D resistant/refractory evaluation.
- It occurs usually due to highly vascular mesenchymal tumor, 90% of which are benign and most are found in the extremities or maxillofacial region.
- Hypophosphatemia secondary to renal phosphate wasting and low levels of 1,25-DHCC are major biochemical abnormalities.
- S. Ca^{2+} and PTH levels are normal.
- It appears that tumor produces a humoral agent named as PHOSPHATONIN that reduces proximal tubular PO_4^{3-} reabsorption and 1-a(OH)ase activity.
- Resolution occurs when tumor is removed completely.

Cadmium Poisoning

- Due to inhalation and ingestion of cadmium oxide in the preparation of akaline carcinoma batteries, which cause renal tubular damage.
- Associated with ITAI disease.

Neurofibromatosis

- Occurs due to 2 reasons:
  a. Renal stenosis with pseudoaneurysms and resulting in loss of renal mass.
  b. Renal tubular distress.
  c. Hepatic mechanisms
     - It occurs due to malabsorption of vitamin D due to lack of bile salts in the gut, which is required for absorption of fat-soluble vitamin D.
     - Drugs implicated in vitamin D deficiency viz. phenytoin, phenobarbitone, act by inducing hepatic enzymes which degrade vitamin to less active metabolites. Other drugs indicated are glutethimide and Rcin.

Other Causes

- Consumption of Al $(OH)_3$ and $MgSO_4$, which cause deficiency of phosphorous.
- Congenital rickets (mature with osteomalacia).
- Temporary neonatal rickets (enzyme immaturity (liver).
- Associated with Wilson's disease.

CLINICAL FEATURES OF RICKETS

- Clinical manifestations of rickets are the result of skeletal deformities, susceptibility to fractures, weakness and hypotonia and disturbance of growth.
- In first 6 months of life, mostly infants with rickets present with tetany of confusion and only minor skeleton changes. After 6 months, tender enlargement of the bone ends, specially consists, ankles and knee age observed.
- Manifestations are:
  - CRANIOTABES: Pressure over the soft membraneous bones of the skull is felt like a ping-pong ball.
  - ANTERIOR FONTANELLE: Is large and its closure is delayed beyond 18 months.
  - FRONTAL BOSSING: Evident >6 months of age.
  - RACHITC ROSARY: Costochondral junction becomes prominent.
  - HARRISON'S GROOVE: Indentation of lower ribs at the site of attachment of diaphragm.
  - DELAYED ERUPTION OF PRIMARY DENTITION.
  - KYPHOSIS, SCOLIOSIS OR LORDOSIS MAY OCCUR.
  - BROADENING OF WRIST: Around 6-9 months of age.
  - ANTERIOR BOWING OF LEGS, KNOCK KNEES, COXA VERA: Are usual deformities that occur when the child starts bearing weight.
  - POT BELLY: Because of hypotonia.

RADIOLOGICAL FEATURES

- The earliest radiological finding is slight axial widening of the growth plate because of the increased osteocartilagenous mass. As disease progress, there is further widening (Figure 107.1).
- There is loss of definition of zone of provisional calcification adjacent to metaphysis. This begins with an indistinctness of the metaphyseal margin, progressing to a FRAYED appearance.
- Weight bearing and stress on the calcified bone

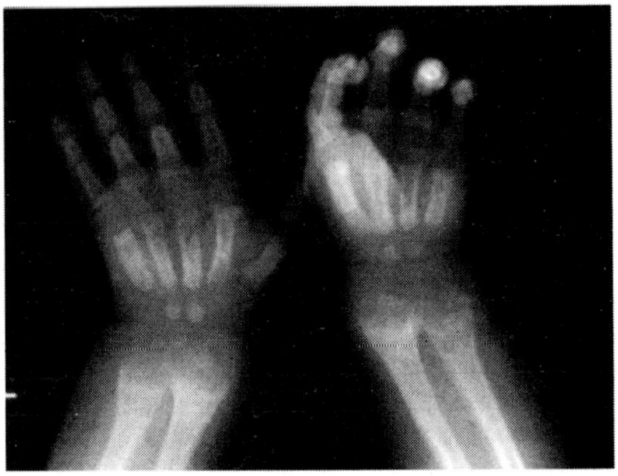

Fig. 107.1: Radiographs of the wrists show features of rickets

gives rise to CUPPING and SPLAYING of the metaphysis.

- Such evidences occur in different sites maximally at different age i.e. changes occur marginally at the wrist upon the age of 5-6 years, at the KNEE between 5-10 years and at the iliac crest between 12-18 years.
- Also there is thinning of the cortex due to impaired Ca^{2+} deposition in the sub-periosteal region.
- The cartilaginous cells of epiphysis are also affected. The bony epiphysis shows poor definition of its normal dense rim, with decrease in density of its centre and blurring of trabecular components.
- Costochondral junction enlarge to produce swelling described as rachitic rosary.

DIFFERENTIAL DIAGNOSIS OF RICKETS

- Radiological diagnosis of rickets is not usually difficult, but it's often impossible to suggest the cause of vitamin D deficiency.
- In hypophosphatemic rickets, change at the growth plate is not severe and the abnormalities at the knee are more often greater than at the wrist.
- Bow legs or knock knees, are found particularly in nutritional rickets and familial hypophosphatemia as these patients remain ambulatory.

Table 107.1: Types of rickets

	Type I (Calcium deficit)	**Type II (Phosphate deficit)**	**Type III (End organ resistance to 1,25-DHCC)**
S Ca^{2+}	(n) or ↓	(n)	Low
S PO_4^{3-}	Usually low	Low	(n)
ALP	↑ ↑	↑	
Secondary hyper-parathyroidism	(+)	(-)	–
Causes	• Def. of vit. D • Malabsorption • Liver disease • Anticonvulsant therapy • Renal osteosdystrophy • Vit.D dependent rickets type I	• Phosphophatemia • Fancoi syndrome —cystinosis • Type II proximal RTA • Dot of PO_4^{3-} or malabsorption	Vit. D dependent rickets type II

These two signs are not seen in patients with cystinosis, RTA, renal osteodystrophy, as they often are too ill to subject their limbs to continued stress of weight bearing.

- Another important and main differential diagnosis is SCHMID type of metaphyseal osteochrondrodysplasia. In this not only the metaphyseal irregularity and widening of plate is less severe but also, these changes do not respond to administration of 1,25-DHCC.
- In contrast to rickets, metabolically active growth plates are less severely affected, so that, in metaphysical dysplasia, greater abnormality is seen may be shown by proximal rather than distal femoral growth plates.

Differential Diagnosis

- Fraying of metaphyses.
- Rickets.
- Hypophosphatasia.
- Chronic stress (e.g. gymnasts).
- Cu. deficiency.
- Metaphyseal dysplasia.

Cupping of Metaphysis

- **Normal:** Esp. distal ulna and prox. fibula of young children (no fraying).
- **Rickets:** With fraying and widening of growth plate.
- **Trauma:** To growth plate and/or metaphysis.
- **Bone dysplasia:** Achondroplasia, pseudochondroplasia, dysplasia, diastrophic dwarfism, metaphyseal chondrodysplasia and hypophosphatasia.
- Scurvy.
- Metaphyseal dysplasia.

Rib Lesions

1. Neoplastic

Secondary tumors more common than primary. Primary malignant tumors more common than benign tumors.

A. **Metastases**

B. **Primary malignant tumors**

- Multiple myeloma/plasmacytoma.
- Chondrosarcoma.
- Ewing's sarcoma.
- Osteosarcoma (rare).
- Fibrosarcoma.

C. **Benign tumors**

- Osteochondroma.
- Enchondroma.
- Eosinophilic granuloma.
- Hemangioma.
- Giant cell tumor.
- Aneurysmal bone cyst.

2. Non-Neoplastic

A. Healed rib fracture.

B. Fibrous dysplasia.

C. Osteomyelitis – Bacterial, tuberculous, fungal.

D. Brown tumor of hyperparathyroidism.

Rib Metastasis

- Both lytic and blastic lesions are encountered.
- Common primary sits are carcinoma bronchus, kidney or prostate in males, carcinoma breast in females.
- Metastatic neuroblastoma is common in children.
- Radiologically there may be:
  – Partial or complete destruction.
- Well defined lytic holes.
- Multiple cortical breaks and pathological fracture.
- Extrapleural sign: Due to associated soft tissue mass with sharp margins convex towards lung fields with peripheral tapering margins along the chest wall.
- Metastatic neuroblastoma causes extensive destruction with multiple fairly symmetric lesions. Sunburst periosteal reaction may be positive.

Multiple Myeloma

- Multiple osteolytic lesions in ribs, associated with lesions in skull, vertebrae, pelvis.
- Lesions are characteristically punched out with a sharp margin, and are almost uniform in size.

- In ribs the cortex eventually may be eroded, may expand causing lytic expansile lesions.
- Pathological fracture may occur.

Plasmacytoma

- Represents a localised form of plasma cell proliferation.
- 50% patients present before age 50.
- Radiographically a highly expansile lytic lesion producing ballooning of bone is seen in the bone and may break through the cortex.
- Residual strands of destroyed bone may give soap bubble appearance.
- Large extra pleural mass can be associated.

Ewing's Sarcoma

- It is the most common malignancy of chest wall in children.
- Children normally present with a palpable mass that may mimic infection.
- Radiologically, there is permeative type of bone destruction with periosteal reaction, which may be lamellated or sun burst.

  There is also reactive new bone formation resulting in increase in bone density and trabecular prominence especially in flat bones.

Chondrosarcoma

- Occurs in 40-60 years of age.
- Radiologically – Large radiolucent poorly defined lesion with destruction of cortex, and foci of irregularly scattered calcifications within the tumor matrix (Fig. 108.1).
- Calcifications are stippled, fluffy typical of chondroid calcification.
- Eventually a large soft tissue mass may be present along with bone lesion.

Osteosarcoma

- Rarely occurs in ribs. Patients 10-25 years.
- Permeative type of bone destruction with cortical destruction, reactive new bone formation seen as periosteal reaction, calcifications within soft tissue components.

Fibrosarcoma

- Occurs in older patients.
- Typically a lytic lesion causing cortical thinning and endosteal erosion.
- No matrix calcification.
- Large associated soft tissue mass.

Osteochondroma

- Occurs in ribs in 3% cases.
- It is the most common benign chest wall bone tumor.

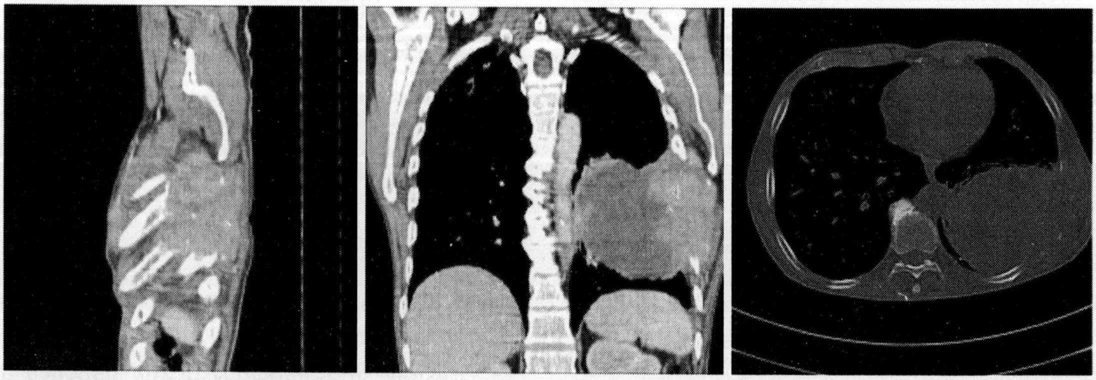

Fig. 108.1: Sagittal and coronal MPR and axial CT images in the soft tissue and bone window settings show chondrosarcoma of the ribs on the left side

- Most cases occur under 20 years of age.
- Patients present with a slowly growing painless mass.
- These are pedunculated or sessile outgrowth with a cartilaginous cap showing spotty calcification.
- The distinguishing feature is the continuity of the bone cortex between normal bone and cortex of lesion and similarly the continuity of bone spongiosa.

Enchondroma (Figures 108.2 and 108.3)

- Ribs affected in 13% cases.
- Well-defined, lytic expansile lesion with ground glass haziness and small punctate calcifications, usually eccentric.
- Cortex is preserved although may be extremely thinned out.

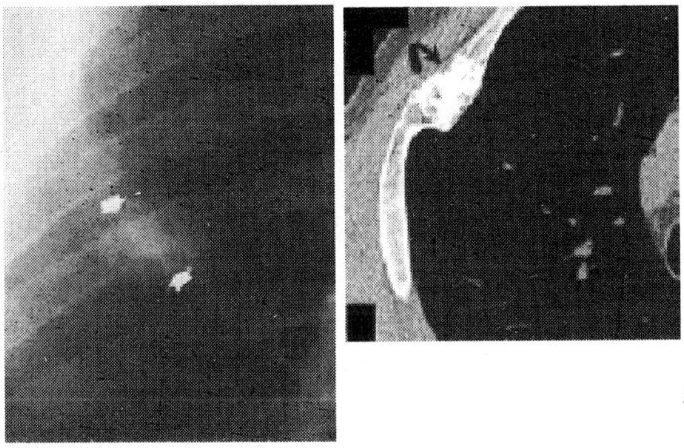

Fig. 108.2: On standard radiograph, sclerotic lesion is seen to involve anterior aspect of fourth right rib (*arrows*). Helical CT image shows expansile tumor of rib that contains multiple foci of calcification (*arrow*). Biopsy was consistent with enchondroma

Hemangioma

- Rare in ribs and are usually capillary in type.
- Expansile, well-demarcated, lytic lesions with thin cortices and fine lacy trabecular pattern.
- The radiating coarse linear strands diverging from the center also occur giving sunray appearance.
- An adjacent soft tissue mass may be seen.

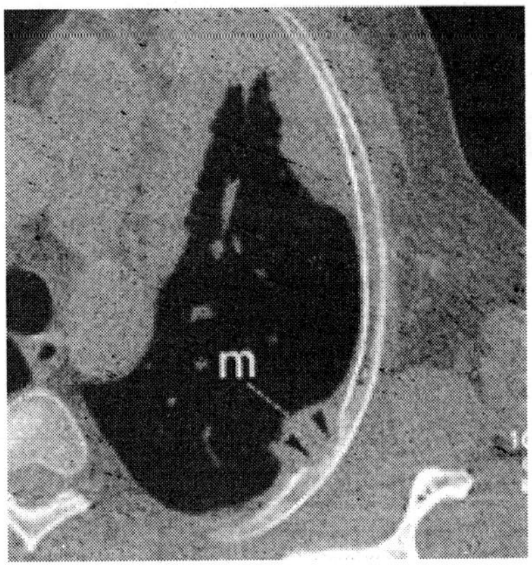

Fig. 108.3: CT image shows osteolysis of inner rib cortex of third rib (*arrowheads*). m = mesothelioma

Aneurysmal Bone Cysts

- Lytic expansile lesion, with sharp scalloped borders and a thin sub periosteal shell.
- On CT and MRI fluid-fluid level may be seen.

GIANT CELL TUMOR

- Presents as expanding, radiolucent soap bubble lesion.
- No periosteal reaction occurs.

Fibrous Dysplasia

- It is the most common benign rib lesion, more commonly monostatic.
- Usually >4 cm in length.
- Lesions are radiolucent, with ground glass opacity, and have a thick sclerotic border.
- There is widening of medullary canal with thinned scalloped endosteum.

Osteomyelitis

- May be tubecular, bacterial or fungal.
- Patients present with fever, pain and minor skin changes.
- There is bone destruction with periosteal reaction and associated abscess formation.

- Underlying pleural and pulmonary involvement may be seen.

Healed Rib Fractures

If callus has begun to form, there will be localized increase in density with bulbous expansion at fracture site.

Tietze's syndrome (Costochondritis)

(2-4th ribs on (L) side)

- Hypertrophy of costochondral junction with pain without any soft tissue mass.
- Previously calcified costal cartilage may show dissolution of calcium.

Section 10—Musculoskeletal System

Chapter 109

Achondroplasia

Synonyms

- Chondrodystrophia fetalis.
- Chondrodystrophic dwarfism.

Features

- Most common congenital dwarfism (1 in 25,000 births).
- Hereditary autosomal dominate in epiphyseal chondroblastic growth and maturation.
- Sporadic mutations account for 80% of achondroblastic birth.
- Homozygous – a lethal condition.

  Gene FGFRR3 is the only gene associated.

CLINICAL FEATURES

- Characteristic facies with frontal bossing and midface hypoplasia.
- Contracted skull base.
- Adult male height – 131 cm.
- Adult female height – 124 cm.
- Normal trunk length with rhizomelic shortening of limbs.
- Trident hand and brachydactyly.
- Thoracolumbar gibbus in infancy, which usually disappears with walking and is replaced by exaggerated lumbar lordosis.
- Genu varum, limited elbow extension.
- Ear infections – narrow passages.
- Crowded and malaligned teeth.
- Low back and leg pain.
- Cesarian section is recommended to reduce the CNS complications like IVH.
- Chronic hypoventilation – apnea and sudden death.

Radiological Features

Skull

- Receding bridge of nose.
- Brachycephaly with enlarged bulging forehead.
- Relative pragmatism (normal mandible).
- Small foramen magnum.
- Communicating hydrocephalus - obstruction of basal cisterns + aqueduct.

Chest and Spine

- Squaring of inferior scapular margin.
- Narrrow chest – short ribs, not extended around the thorax.

- Mild platyspondyly, amount of disc cartilage ↑.
- Interpedicular spaces decrease caudally in the lumbar region with exaggerated lordosis.
- Pedicles are short and thick.
- Posterior scalloping.
- Angular kyphosis – at thoracolumbar junction due to ballet nosed vert.

Pelvis

- Square shaped flat non-flared pelvic bones.
- Flattened iliac wings (Champagne glass).
- Horizontal acetabuli.
- Small sacrosciatic notch.
- Backward tilt of pelvis and hip joints.

Extremities

- Trident hand separation of 2nd and 3rd finger.
- Rhizomelic shortening of long bones, may not be observed until 3rd trimester.
- Ball in socket "epiphysis" (Chevron deformity).
- High position of fibular head, short ulna brachydactyly, divergent fingers.
- Carpal and tarsal normal.

Neurologic Symptoms

Factors

- Decreased interpedicular distance and short and thick pedicles.
- Stenosis of nerve root canal (L5-S1) (lateral entrapment syndrome).
- Narrow foramen magnum.
- CT and MRI – particularly useful.

Four Clinical Syndromes

- Nerve root compression by disc herniation.
- Transverse myelopathy gradually induced by severe kyphosis.
- Acute traumatic transverse myelopathy with sudden paraplegia.
- Intermittent claudication of the cauda equina.

In Utero

US

- May be normal till late 2nd trimester.
- Shortening of proximal long bones.
- Increased BPD, HC and HC: AC ratio.
- Decreased FL: BPD ratio.
- Normal mineralization, no fractures.
- Normal cardio thoracic ratio.

Differential Diagnosis

Hypochondroplasia (AD) separated from classical achondroplasia.

- Skull is never affected.
- Usually normal in height.
- Rhizomelia with short broad femoral neck.
- Overgrown fibula, absent trident hand.
- Mental retardation in 10-20%, neurology component not seen.

Pseudochondroplasia

- Both recessive and dominant forms.
- Skull normal.
- No changes seen in 1st year.

Spine

- Vertebral bodies flat/irregular with central anterior tongues.

Long Bones

- Delayed in appearance and markedly irregular.
- Epiphyseal dysplasia.

Pelvis

- Acetabulum is irregular and premature OA.
- Ilia large, pubis and ischia short.

Hand

- Tubular bones short, stubby with delay in ossification of irregular epiphysis and carpal bones.
- Shortening of ulna and radius – 'v' at wrist.

Thanatophoric Dwarfism

- Recently separated from achondroplasia and is the most common fatal neonatal dysplasia.
- Large head, short base, occasional clover – leaf skull.
- Narrow chest and short ribs (pulmonary hypoplasia).
- Platyspondyly – H shaped vertebrae.
- Last few vertebrae show—interpedicular distance.
- Severe micromelia, metaphyseal flaring (telephone-handle).

Asphyxiating Thoracic Dysplasia (Jeune's Disease)

- Autosomal recessive disorder.
- Narrow, elongated cylindrical chest with flared base.
- Normal sized heart.
- Horizontal clavicles and ribs.
- Skull and spine – normal.
- Trident pelvis – spurs from acetabular roof.
- Wine glass pelvis
  - Cephalocaudal shortening.
  - Flared small iliac bone.
- Postaxial hexadactly, cone shaped epiphysis in feet.
- Rhizomelic brachymelia.

Kidney

- Enlarged kidneys with linear streaking on nephrogram.

Spondyloepiphyseal Dysplasia (Congenita)

- Ossification is delayed – pubic bone, proximal femur.
- Femoral head – severely affected, coxa vera—OA.
- Horizontal acetabular roofs, short iliac roofs.
- PEAR-shaped vertebrae – bulbous anteriorly.
- With age—platyspondyly—extreme short.
- Odontoid hypoplasia.
- Rhizomelic shortening.

Osteogenesis Imperfecta

- Blue sclerae, joint laxity.
- Shortened broad, crumpled bones.
- Bone angulations, bowing and demineralization.
- Thin poorly ossified skull.
- Thin beaded ribs

Mucopolysaccharidosis

- Mucopolysaccharides are widely distributed tissue structural component consisting of a protein core from which polysaccharide chain arises. These side chains are composed of repeated disaccharide units each consisting of a URONIC ACID and a SULPHATED HEXOSAMINE RESIDUE.
- Mucopolysaccharides are normally excreted in the urine in amounts <15 mg/24 hours. In genetic mucopolysaccharidoses, patient often excrete >100 mg/24 hours.
- Each disease is characterised by a predominant urinary MPD (mucopolysaccharidase).
- The BASIC EFFECT is the impairment of breakdown of the side chains owing to specific enzyme defects.
- The disease is classified on the basis of CLINICAL FEATURES and predominantly excreted MPD (Table 110.1).

HURLER'S SYNDROME

- Also known as gargoylism, dysostoses multiplex, lipochondro dystrophy, Hurler-Faundler syndrome.
- In this disease patients secrete heparin and dermation SO_4 in urine.
- AR transmission presents usually at the end of the 1st year but never at birth, rarely presents as early as 2 months of age.

CLINICAL FEATURES

- Dwarfism, infantilism, MR, coarse facial features.
- Large buldging head, flat bridge of the nose, flared nostrils.
- Large tongue and lips, hypertelorism, corneal opacities.
- Deformed tooth, HSM, short neck.
- KYPHOSIS with DL gibbus, limited extension of joints.
- Severe respiratory infection and cardiac failure usually causes death within 1st decade.

Radiologically

- Marked variation is seen in involvement of extremities – long bones show thickening and sclerosis; however, an osteoporotic type of variation may be present. Upper extremities lower extremities, either end of the long bone show involvement. Principle change is thickening of shafts and tapering towards the end. Diaphysis has irregular wavy contour.
- Cortex may be thickened or thinned. There is angulated obliquity of the growth plates.

Table 110.1: Types of mucopolysaccharidosis

Disorder	Stored material	Inheritance	Neurologic	Skeletal disease	Ophthalmologic	Clinical features
MPS 1H, Hurler	Dermatan SO_4 Heparin SO_4	AR	Mental retardation	++++	Corneal clouding	Coarse facial features, CVS involvement, Joint stiffness, HSM etc.
MPS IH/S, Hurler/ scheie	Dermatan SO_4 Heparin SO_4	AR	Mental retardation	++++	Corneal clouding	Coarse facial features, CVS involvement, Joint stiffness, HSM etc.
MPSIS, scheie	Heparin SO_4	AR	None	++++	Corneal clouding	Coarse facial features, CVS involvement, Joint stiffness, HSM etc.
MPS II, Hunter	Dermatan SO_4 Heparin SO_4	XLR	Mental retardation	++++	No corneal clouding retinal degeneration+	Course facial features, CVS involvement, Joint stiffness, distinctive possibly skin lesions
MPS IIA, sanfilipo A	Heparin SO_4	AR	Severe MR	+	None	Mild coarse facies
MPS IIIB, sanfilippo B	Heparin SO_4	AR	Severe MR	+	None	Mild coarse facies
MPS III, sanfilipo C	Heparin SO_4	AR	Severe MR	+	None	Mild coarse facies
MPS IIID, sanfillip D	Heparin SO_4	AR	Severe MR	+	None	Mild coarse facies
MPS IV, morqui	Keratin SO_4 Chondroitin- 6-SO_4	AR	None	++++	Corneal clouding	Distinctive skeletal deformities, odotoid, hypoplasia, aortic valvular disease
MPV VI, maronterx lamy	Dermatan SO_4	R	None	++++	Corneal clouding	Coarse facies, valvular heart disease
MPV VII sly	Dermatan/oleporton	AR	None	+++	Corneal clouding	- do -
MPS VIII Dyggve melchior clausen	Heparin SO_4 Altered hyaluronic acid	AR	Mental reticulation	+++	Corneal clouding	Coarse facial features, valvular involvement, hydrops, fetalis in neonatal form.

Radius and ulna may be tipped towards each other. Dorsal angulation of proximal. Humerus may be seen causing limited motion of the shoulder.

- Hands are trident and shows coarse trabeculation. Most characteristic changes in the hands are the PROXIMAL TAPERING OF THE METACARPALS and the phalanges do not have a normal diaphyseal constriction.
- Skull is large and is dolichocephalic because of premature fusion of sagittal sutures. Frontal bones are prominent.
- A 'J' shaped sella turcica is characteristic.
- Mandible is broad with poor developed dentition and widely separated teeth. Mandibular condyles show flattening/ concavity of the articular surface.
- Ribs, widened at the shafts, causing decrease in intercostal space. There is a 'spatula like' narrow origin and a bullet nose appearance of the termination resulting in CANOE PADDLE ribs.
- Pelvis shows flaring of iliac wings and tapering or constriction of the ilia near the acetabulum. There may be shallow acetabular or acetabular protrusion.
- SPINE shows distinctive changes. Oval centera with anterior inferior beak are present. Such hypolastic 'sail' vertebra in the lumbar with inferior. Beaking cause Sharpe angular kyphosis.
- There is hypoplasia and demineralization of pedicles with widening of inter pedicular spaces giving a false impression of intraspinal mass.

SCHEIE'S SYNDROME (TYPE I)

- Manifestations are variable.
- Corneal clouding occurs at about 6 years of age, but the range in from infancy to adolescence.
- MR is positive.
- Mild visceral and skeletal abnormalities are seen.
- Aortic regurgitation may occur.
- Patients may survive till adulthood.

HUNTER'S SYNDROME (TYPE II)

- Similar clinically as well as radiologically to Hurler's but has a slower rate of progression.
- Usually detected between 2 to 6 years of age.
- MR is present.
- Corneal clouding is absent.
- Transmitted as XLR.
- Death occurs in the 2nd and 3rd decade.

SANFILIPPO'S SYNDROME (TYPE III)

- Sign of MR occurs towards the end of the 2nd year of life.
- There is mild but progressive coarsening of facial features and hypertrichosis.
- Dwarfism does not occur and skeletal abnormalities are minimal.
- Significant heart disease is rare.
- Progressive spastic paraparesis occur resulting in death in 1st or 2nd decade.

MORQUIO'S SYNDROME (TYPE IV) (Figure 110.1)

- Clinical manifestations are seen during the 2nd year of life with slowing of linear growth and progressive skeletal deformity.
- Corneal opacities are present.
- Hepatomegaly, cardiac lesions and deafness may occur.
- Body proportions are opposite to that of achondroplasia i.e. it has short trunk and relatively normal length of the extremities.
- Head is of normal shape, facies are normal.
- No MR is seen.

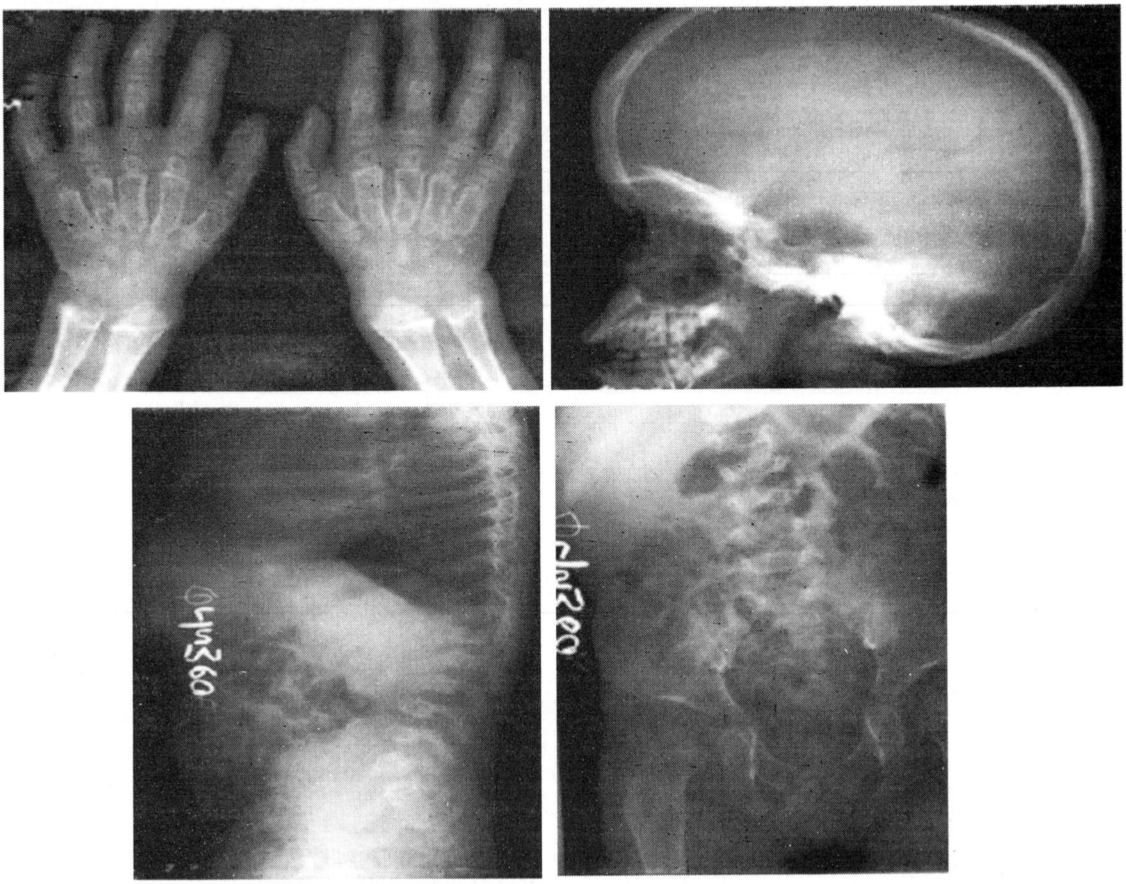

Fig. 110.1: Radiographs of the hands, skull, spine and pelvis show features of Morquio's disease

- There is dorsolumbar kyphosis and multiple deformities of extremities with flexion deformity of both hips and knees resulting in a semi crouching stance, knock knees, swelling of knees and elbows and flat feet.
- Chest shows pigeon chest deformity.
- Weakness of the extremities is associated with clumpsy gate.
- Death may occur in 1st or 2nd decade.

Radiologically

- Most important changes are seen in spine and consist of universal vertebra plana, which is the cause of loss of stature.
- Dense is hypoplastic, which may cause neurological symptoms.
- Vertebral bodies show a central anterior beak in contrast to antero inferior beak seen in Hurler's syndrome.
- IV disc space are initially normal but later gets narrowed.
- There is shortening of neck, dorsal scoliosis and dorso lumbar kyphosis.
- Wide intrapendiculate distance is seen.
- There is defective and irregular ossification of femoral capital epiphyses with flattening. Femoral neck is short, thick and there may be varus/valgus deformity.
- There is delayed appearance the epiphyseal centres and carpal and torsal bones.

- Metacarpal ends have an irregular conical appearance.
- Appearance of long bones are variable, some may resemble rickets with metaphyseal flaring.
- Skull and facial bones are normal.
- Mandible and teeth are normal.
- Ribs may be thickened or thinned and is often associated with a barrel chest.
- Pelvis shows rounding of iliac crests with tapering of distal ilia, acetabulum is deep, enlarged and has irregular contour.
- Sacrum may be small and may articulate low on the ilia.
- There may be wide pubic synchondrosis.
- There is marked degeneration involving all the articular surfaces.
- Wrists and ankles develop irregularity and amputation.
- Hyperlaxity is present which progress to limitation of motion.

MAROTEAUX – LAMY SYNDROME (TYPE VI)

- Skeletal dysplasia occurs between the ages of 2 to 5 years.
- Corneal clouding is seen.
- Intellect in normal, no MR is seen.
- Progressive bony changes similar to Hurler's syndrome ensue, leading to dwarfism and flexion contracture of joints.
- Macrocrania and hydrocephalus may occur.
- Hepatomegaly is positive, cardiac lesions are frequent.
- Hearing loss is also present.

MARDYGGUEMELCHIOR – CLAUSEN SYNDROME (TYPE VII)

- Rare syndrome with MR.
- Dwarfism is said to occur.
- Radiologically, spine shows platyspondyly (i.e. flatness of vertebral bodies) with relatively wide IV disc space.
- No irregularity or central 'tongue' pattern of vertebral bodies is present.
- Anterior ribs are flared.
- Pelvis shows irregular radiolucencies at the iliac crests with narrow sclerotic margins. Similar changes are seen at the inferior margin of the scapulae.
- Irregularity at the metaphyses may be noted which may be confused with that of rickets.

Differential Diagnosis of Morquio's Syndrome

- Spondyloepiphyseal dysplasia congenital.
- Spondyloepiphyseal dysplasia – tarda.
- Metatropic dwarfism.
- Parastemmatic dwarfism.
- Kniest's dwarfism.
- Diastrophic dwarfism.

SPONDYLOEPIPHYSEAL DYSPLASIA CONGENITA

It is to be differentiated from Morquio's by:

1. Absence of corneal clouding and mucopoly-sachariduria.
2. Presentation at birth.
3. Unlike this condition, Morquio's shows severe changes in hand and feet.

Other Features

- AD transmission.
- Flattening of vertebral bodies, odontoid hypoplasia.
- Horizontal deep acetabulum.
- Shortening of long bones with rhizomelic distribution.
- Hand feet are normal.

SPONDYLOEPIPHYSEAL DYSPLASIA TARDA

Differentiated from Morquio's by:

- XLR inheritance, only male affected.
- Rarely seen <10 years of age.
- Deep and narrow pelvic configuration which later progress to osteoarthritis of hips.

Also there is platy spondyly and a hump shaped mound on the superior and inferior surfaces of lumbar vertebra may be seen.

METATROPIC DWARFISM

Differentiating from Morquio's by:

- No corneal opacity, no mucopolysacchariduria.
- Tubular bones are shortened, thickened and DUMBELL shaped due to hyperplastic metaphysic but seen at lesser trochanter.
- Interpediculate distance is normal; base of the skull is also normal.

Other Features

- Short limb dwarfism with rhizomelic distribution.
- Initially changes of achondroplasia are seen to the maximum proportion resembling Morquio's.

PARASTEMMATIC DWARFISM

- Small iliac wings with dysplastic acetabuli.
- Platyspondyly with biconcave deformity.
- Decreased bone density.
- Short hands and thin and bowed tubular bones.

KNIEST'S DWARFISM

Differentiating features from Morquio's are:

- Short arms and legs at birth.
- Fusiform swelling of joints.
- Abnormal large skull with large head.
- Craniofacial disproportions, severe platyspondyly.
- Narrow interpediculate distance.
- Pelvic bones are small with large dislocated femoral head and neck.

Others

- Hypoplasia of odontoid process.
- Shortening of long bones with metaphysial flaring.

DIASTROPHIC DWARFISM

Features include:

- Talipes equino varus deformity seen which resists correction.
- Long bones are shortened, more pronounced at forearm.
- Femoral heads are larger than acetabuli; metaphysis are wide and flared with cupping.
- Brachydactyly with abducted thumb known as 'HITCHHIKER' thumbs is seen.
- Narrow interpedicute distance, body of vertebra is normal.

Section 10—Musculoskeletal System

Chapter 111

Differential Diagnosis of Dwarfism

1. SHORT LIMB SKELETAL DYSPLASIA

Rhizomelic (Proximal Limb Shortening)

Achondroplasia

- ↓ Intrapedicular distance in lumbar spine caudally.
- Squared iliac wings with small sciatic notch.
- Flat acetabular roof.
- V shaped notch in growth plate (Cherion deformity).

Hypochondroplasia

- No normal widening of interpediculate distance in spine caudally.
- Variable brachydactyly.
- Elongation of distal fistula and ulnar styloid process.

Pseudochondroplasia

- Platyspondyly with tongues like anterior protrusion of vertebral bodies.
- Biconcave configuration of upper and lower vertebral end plates.
- Atlanto axial dislocation.
- Irregular acetabulum.

Chondrodysplasia Punctata

- Strippled calcification in cartilage, particularly around joints and in laryngeal and tracheal cartilages.
- Shortening of long bones.
- Vertebral bodies show coronal clefting.

Mesomelic (Middle Segment Limb Shortening)

- Dyschondrosteosis (Leri-Weil disease).
- Shortening and bowing of radius.
- Madelung's deformity.
- Dislocated distal ulna and radius head.

Mesomelic Dysplasia

a. Type Langer.

b. Type Reinhandt-Pfeiffer.

Acromesomelic (Middle and Distal Limb Shortening)

Chondroectodermal dysplasia (Ellis-van Creveld syndrome):

- Short iliac wings and horizontal acetabulum.
- Premature ossification of femoral capital epiphysis.

- Exostosis of medial and upper tibial shaft.
- Carpal fusion, polydactyly of hand and feet.

Acromesomelic Dysplasia

- Short tubular bones especially the radius and ulna.
- Platyspondyly with anterior beaking and posterior wedging of vertebrae.
- Lumbar intrapediculate distance is narrow.

Mesomelic Dysplasia

a. Type Nieweigelt.
b. Type Rowbinow.
c. Type Wegner.

Acromelic (Distal Limb Shortening)

- Asphyxiating thoracic dysplasia (Jeune's syndrome):
  - Small thoracic with short rib, horizontally oriented.
  - Wide costochondral junction.
  - High clavicles.
  - Iliac bones short, horizontal acetabulum.
  - Polydactyly.
- Peripheral dysostosis.

2. PLATYSPONDYLY (UNUSUAL VERTEBRA PLANA)

Congenital

- Thanatophoric dwarfism:
  - Irregular metaphysis, epiphysis of knee absent at birth.
  - Platyspondyly with normal post element causing 'H' shaped vertebra on anterior view.
  - Widened disc spaces – Trunk height – normal.
  - Skull shows lateral temporal bulging (clove leaf skull).
- Metatropic dwarfism
  - Tubular bones shortened, thickened and dumbbell shaped due to hyperplastic metaphysis.
  - Inter padiculate distance is normal.
- Osteogenesis Imperfecta IIA
  - Long bone short, broad and bowed with numerous fractures.
  - Ribs broad with continuous beading.
- Platyspondyly in late childhood
  - Morquio's disease.
  - Spondyloepiphyseal dysplasia congenita.
  - Spondyloepiphyseal dysplasia tarda.
  - Kniest's dwarfism.

Acquired Platyspondyly

- Osteoporosis.
- Trauma.
- Infection.
- Sickle cell anemia.
- Neoplastic disease.
- Scheurmann's disease.
- Langerhans cell histiocytosis.

3. ANTERIOR VERTEBRAL BODY BEAKS

- Central.
- Morquio's syndrome–described lat.
- Lower third.
- Hurler's syndrome.

Spindle Shaped

- Diaphysis may have irregular wavy contours.
- Proximal tapering of metacarpals.
- J shaped sella.
- Broad mandible with flat or concave mandible condyle.

- Widened intrapediculate distance.
- Achondrosplasia – discussed before.
- Pseudoachondroplasia – discussed before.
- Cretinism.
- Wormian bones in the skull.

Bilateral Symmetrical ← Epiphysis Appears Late and are Fragmented

Bowl shaped sella or cherry sella, scalloping:

- Down syndrome.
- Neuromuscular disease.
- Hypotonia is one of the causes.
- ↑ed thoracolumbar kyphosis.

4. WIDENED INTERPEDICULAR DISTANCE

- Meningomyelocoele.
- Fusiform distribution with greatest separation at the midpoint of the involved segment.
- Disc space narrowed, body appears widened.
- Scoliosis seen in 50-70% cases ± kyphosis.
- Intraspinal mass
  - Specially ependymomas.
- Diastematomyelia
  - 50% seen between L1 to L3; 25% between T7 to T12.
  - Spine visible only in 33% cases.
  - Spine extends from neural arch forwards.

5. ODONTOID HYPOPLASIA

- Morquio's syndrome.

Stippled Epiphysis

- Vertebra plana/platyspondyly.
- Central anterior beaking.
- Femoral neck short and thick.
- Acetablum, enlarged with irregular contour.
- Hands and feet develop irregularities.

Spondyloepiphyseal Dysplasia Congenita

- Deep horizontal acetabulum ↑ed acetabular angle.
- Hand and feet are spared.
- Low square ilium.

Spondyloepiphyseal Dysplasia Tarda

- Deep and narrow pelvic configuration which later on causes osteoarthritis of hip.
- Hump shaped round on superior and inferior surface of lumbar vertebral bodies.
- Kniest's dwarfism
  - Narrow interpediculate distance.
  - Craniofacial disproportions.

6. IRREGULAR EPIPHYSIS

Normal

- Specially in distal femur.
- Avascular necrosis
  - Single – Perthes disease, usually unilateral, if bilateral-asymmetrical.
  - Multiple – sickle cell anemia.

Congenital Hypothyroidism – Bilateral Symmetrical

- Not present at birth.
- Delayed appearance and growth of ossification centres.

Morquio's Disease

- Irregular ossification of the femoral capital epiphysis.

Multiple Epiphyseal Dysplasia (MED)

- Onset 5-14 years.
- Delayed appearance and growth but time of fusion is normal.

10 Section

- Carpals, tarsals, hip and knee affected most commonly.

Meyer's Dysplasia

- Resembles MED but localized to femoral heads only.

Chondro Dysplasia Punctata

- Stippled calcification in cartilages.
- Vertebral bodies show coronal clefting.
- Shortening of long bones.

Trisomy

Prenatal infection.

Warfarin's embryopathy.

- Stippled uncalcified epiphysis particularly of axial skeleton, prox. femur.
- Disappearance by 1st year.
- Zellweger syndrome.
- Fetal alcohol syndrome.

7. CUPPING OF METAPHYSIS

Normal

- Of distal ulna and proximal fIbula of young children.
- No fraying.

Rickets

- Widening of growth plate.
- Loss of zone of provisional calcification.
- Fraying +, splaying +.
- Thinning of the cortex.

Trauma

- To growth plate/metaphysis.
- Localized changes.

Scurvy

- Pelican spur.
- Wimberger's sign.
- Usually after fracture.
- Trumsfield zone.
- White line of frankel.
- Pencil thin cortex.

Bony Dysplasia

- Viz Achondroplasia, Pseudoachondroplasia, metatropic and diastrophic dwarfism and hypophosphotasia.

8. FRAYING OF METAPHYSIS

Rickets

Cupping + widening of growth plates.

- Already described.

Hypophosphatasia

- Similar to rickets but refractory to vitamin D therapy.

Chronic Stress

- With wide irregular, assymetrical widening or the distal radial growth plate and metaphyseal sclerosis.

Copper Deficiency

- ↑ed bone density, cortical thinning with delayed maturation.
- Unlike rickets, zone of provisional calcification is preserved.

Metaphyseal Chondrodysplasia (Schmid Variety)

- It is similar to rickets in all aspects except that the metaphysis do not appear to be demineralised and looser's zone not typically seen.

Section 10—Musculoskeletal System

Chapter 112

Radiograph of Hand as An Indicator of Systemic Disease

Several systemic diseases manifest on the radiograph of hand.

- Congenital/developmental.
- Inflammatory.
- Infective.
- Nutritional/metabolic.
- Hemopoietic.
- Neoplastic.
- Miscellaneous.

CONGENITAL DEVELOPMENTAL DYSPLASIAS

Osteopoikilosis

- Presence of multiple, dense, radio opaque islands of the cortical bone noted in the spongy bone, end of long bones and around joints.

D/D—Tuberous sclerosis.

- Mets.
- Carpal/tarsal bones.
- Pelvis.

Osteopetrosis

- Generalized ↑ in bone density.
- Bone within bone appearance.
- Modelling deformities.
- Obliteration of marrow cavity.

Pyknodysostosis

- Increased bone density.
- Acroosteolysis.
- Obtuse angle of mandible.
- Open fontanels and sutures.

Melorrheostosis

- Multiple areas of hyperosteosis with segmental distribution (Dermatome).
- Sclerosis of phalanges and metacarpal.

Achondroplasia

- Shortening of tubular bone of hand and feet.
- Trident hand – separation of middle and ring fingers.
- Occasionally polydactyly.
- Shortening of ulna.
- Cheveron deformity.

Spondyloepiphyseal Dysplasia Congenita

- Mainly spinal involvement with severe platyspondyly.

- Irregularity of epiphysis with small epiphysis.
- Acetabular dysplasia.

Spondyloepiphyseal Dysplasia Tarda

- Shortening of 3rd and 5th metacarpals.
- Short terminal phalanges.
- Small carpals.
- Platyspondyly with posterior hump.
- Dysplasia of hip and shoulder joints.

Multiple Epiphysial Dysplasia

- Bilateral symmetrical epiphyseal irregularities and hypoplasia and sclerosis.
- Small bones of hand and feet are short and broad but relative length are maintained.
- Tibio-talar slant.

Dysplasias Epiphyseal Punctata

- Stippled epiphysis with increased density.

Dysplasias Epiphyseal Hemimelica

- Enlarged scaphoid and trapezium, which are partially fused.
- Multiple calcified loose bodies.
- Deformity of distal radial epiphysea.

Cleidocranial Dysplasia

- Acroosteolysis
  - Craniosynostosis, wormian bones.
- Clavicles hypoplasia.
- Widening of pubic symphysis.

Diaphyseal Aclasia

- Multiple exostoses.
- Medelung's deformity.

Olliers' Disease

- Multiple enchrondromatosis.
- Multiple lytic lesions with thinning of cortex with areas of calcification.

Maffuci's Syndrome

- Multiple chondromas with hemangioma.
- Soft tissue swelling with phleboliths.

Pathology

- Preaxial – Holt-Oram, Fanconi's.
- Postaxial – Ellis-von Creveld syndrome.
- Lawrence Moon Biedl (polydactyly, MR, obesity, retinitis pigmentosa).
- Trisomy 13.

  ATID.

Syndactyly

- Apert's syndrome with craniostenosis.
- Fanconi's.
- Lawrence Moon Biedel.
- Trisomy 13, 18.

Polysyndactyly with Craniostenosis

- Acrocephalosyndatyly.

Radial Defects

- Hypoplastic thumb to complete absence of radius, scaphoid, trapezium and thumb – radial club hand.
- Ectodermal dysplasia.
- TAR.
- Halt Oram – absent radius with ASD.
- Ectopic rudimentary thumb.
- Trisomy—18.
- Thalidomide embryopathy.
- Renal and esophageal anomalies.
- Harris Osborn disease – absent radius on either side with (ventricular radial dysplasia) V.S.D.

Carpal Fusion

- Transverse – isolated.
  - Lunar, triquetral.
  - Capitate, hamate.

May be

  - Post traumatic.
  - Post infective.
  - In rheumatoid arthritis.

Down's Syndrome

- Clinodactyly.
- Hypoplastic and triangular middle and distal phalanges of 5th finger.
- Pseudoepiphysis of 1st and 2nd metacarpals.
- Associated – hip dysplasia.
- Endocardial cushion defects.

Conida de Large Syndrome

- Short 1st metacarpal.
- Poximally placed thumb.
- Phocomalia.

Turner's Syndrome

- Short 4th and 5th metacarpals (+ve metacarpal sign).
- Shortening of middle phalanges of 2nd and 5th finger.
- Phalanges have slender shaft with large head "drumstick appearance".
- Madelung's deformity.

Ellis-van Creveld Syndrome

- Polydactyly, syndactyly, syncarpus, mesomelic dwarfism.

MPS

- Stippled epiphysis.
- Short broad and small tubular bones (undertubulation).
- Proximal tapering of metacarpals.
- Distal ends of radius and ulna slope towards each other.

Rheumatoid Arthritis

- Bilateral symmetrical juxta articular osteoporosis.
- Bare area erosions → MPJ, PIPJ all wrist compartments.
- Soft tissue swelling.
- Geodes.
- Carpal fusion.
- Subluxation with ulnar dislocation.
- Boutonniere and swan neck deformity.
- Periostitis along mid shaft of phalanges and metacarpals.

Osteoarthritis

- Target areas include – 1st MP joint and trapezio-scaphoid joint.

  Involvement of distal I.P. joints with swelling —Heberden nodes.

  With osteophytosis PIP—Bouchard's nodes.

  - Relative lack of osteoporosis.
  - Geodes – joint narrowing.

Psoriasis

- DIP involvement.
- Articular surface erosion – Gull's wing appearance.
- Joint space narrowing may occur.
- Periosteitis with soft tissue swelling "sausage digit".

Neuropatheic changes may occur in middle and distal phalanges with longitudinal and concentric bone resorption leading to "licked candy stick appearance".

- Bone density relatively preserved.

Gout

- Punched out peri articular erosions – classical site 1st metatarsophalangeal joint.
- Osteoporosis usually not seen.
- Joint space preserved.
- Eccenteric soft tissue swelling with or without calcified tophi.

Collagen Vascular Disorder

- Acrosteolysis.
- Osteoporosis.
- Subcutaneous soft tissue calcification with soft tissue atrophy.
- ± Erosions with joint space narrowing.
- ± Joint subluxations.

Congenital Syphilis

- Periostitis.
- Syphilic dactylitis – bone widening due to cortical thickening – cortical new bone formation.
- Metaphysitis.
- Osteitis.
- Hot cross bun skull.

Tuberculosis

- Spina vintosa – phalangeal widening due to medullary expansion.
- Lytic areas in midshaft of short tubules bones of hand and feet.
- Periosteal reaction.
- Periarticular osteoporosis.

Leprosy

- Mainly neuropathic changes – acrosteolysis.
- Licked candy stick appearance.
- Specific changes of osteitis leprosa (15%) granuloma course area/focal articular or medullary.
- Bone loss.
- Round or infiltrative lesions with lace like pattern of destruction.
- Widening of nutrient foramen (May be seen in sarcoidosis).
- Diffuse osteoporosis.

Sarcoidosis

- Idiopathic, non-caseating granulomatous disorder.
- Young adult.
- Hand and feet must commonly affected.
  - Punched out areas of lucency in phalanges.
- Enlarged nutrient foramen.
- A more diffuse reticular lace like pattern of distinction.
- Sclerosis, which may be widely disseminated.
- Periosteal reaction.
- Periarticular calcification.
- Soft tissue nodules (more common than bony changes).

NUTRITIONAL DISORDERS/METABOLIC DISORDERS

Rickets

- Cupping, fraying, spraying of metaphysis.
- Physis widening.
- Osteopenia.

Osteomalacia

- Reduced bone density with lack of cortical and trabecular differentiation.
- Looser's zones.

Endocrinal

- Hypothyroidism.
- Delayed bone age.
- Stippled epiphysis.

Hyperthyroidism

- Accelerated skeletal maturation.
- Osteopenia.
- Subtle periosteal new bone formation along shaft of 2nd metacarpal is seen in thyroid acropathy.

Pseudohypo/Pseudohypoparathyroidism

- Shortening of metacarpals and metatarsals.

Hyperparathyroidism

- Diffuse osteopenia.
- Subperiosteal bone resorption – classically radial side of middle phalanx of index finger and middle finger.
- Intracortical bone resorption.
- Brown tumors may be seen in phalanges, metacarpals and metatarsals.
- Acro osteolysis.
- Cartilage calcification (articular cartilage calcification of hip joints) more common with secondary hypertension.

Acromegaly

- Hands show enlargement of bones with soft tissue with spade like terminal tufts or arrowhead distal phalanges.

Hemopoietic Disorders

Thalassemia

- Coarsening of trabecular pattern.
- Medullary expansion.
- Shafts of phalanges and metacarpals becomes biconvex.
- Osteoporosis.

Sickle Cell Anaemia

- Osteosclerosis due to endosteal apposition of new bone.
- Shortening of metacarpals, metatarsals and phalanges due to premature fusion.
- Multiple bone infarcts in long and short bones.
- Dactylitis due to superimposed infarction.

Neoplastic Disorders

- Systemic
  - Leukemia - Periosteal reaction.
  - Lymphoma - Metaphyseal lucencies in leukemia.
  - Metastasis - Uncommon.
    - Rarely lung mets may cause lytic lesions.

Miscellaneous

- Hypertrophic osteoarthropathy
  - Diffuse periosteal reaction of metacarpals and metatarsals with clubbing of phalanges.
  - Painful.
  - Spare epiphysis.
  - Clinical features differentiates it from polydermoperiosteitis.
- Localized gigantism
  - Macrodystrophia lipomatosa - Overgrowth of soft tissue and bone.
  - Neurofibromatosis - Most severe involvement of distal phalanges.
    - Median nerve distribution.
    - Clinodactyly/ polysyndactyly.
  - Occurs due to plexiform neurofibroma with hemangioma and lymphangioma with mesenchymal dysplasia.
  - Usually bilateral - may not be contiguous involvement.
  - Premature fusion of growth plate.
- Distal phalanges are not most severely affected.

Section 10

Section 10—Musculoskeletal System

Chapter 113

Fluorosis

FINDINGS

- Generalized increase in bone density (sclerosis).
- Interosseous membrane calcification.
- Calcification at the insertion of the iliopsoas muscle at the lesser trochanter.
- Osteophyte formation seen in the lumbar vertebra.

The above findings are suggestive of FLUOROSIS.

FLUOROSIS

- Chronic ingestion of excessive amounts of fluoride results in fluorosis.
- Osteosclerosis occurs with a concentration of: 8 ppm in the drinking water.
- Maturity can occur at levels = 100 ppm.
- Mottling of the dental enamel: Aprox 2 ppm.

Paradoxically, a level of 1 ppm desires the prevalence of dental caries.

PATHOPHYSIOLOGY

- Alteration in the bone metabolism is most clearly understood but seems to be multifactorial.
- Fluorapetite crystals get deposited in the bone which appear to be less prone to surface exchange.

RADIOLOGICAL FEATURES

Osteosclerosis (Figure 113.1)

- Is generalized, but occurs predominantly

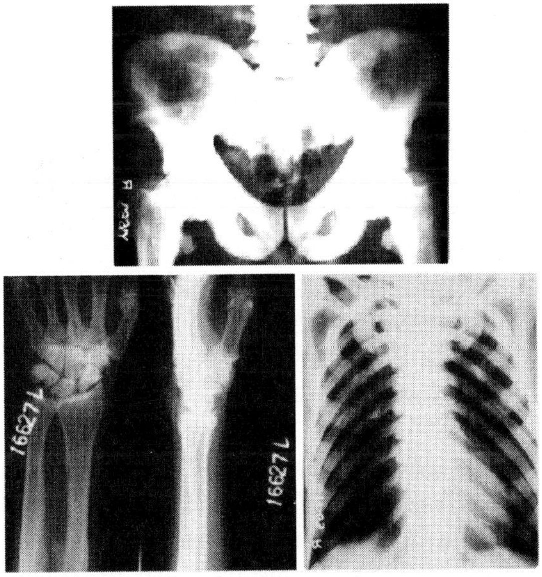

Fig. 113.1: Radiographs of the pelvis, chest and forearm show features of fluorosis

trabecular bone and characteristically seen in the axial skeleton.

Vertebral Osteophytosis

- Vertebral osteophytes may be seen which can be severe and at times encroaches the spinal canal.

Calcification/Ossification of Ligaments

- Soon characteristically in paraspinous, sacrotuberous and iliolumbar ligaments.

ENTHESOPATHY

- Calcification/ossification is seen at the fusation of the ligaments and tendons to the bone.

DIFFERENTIAL DIAGNOSIS

Generalized/Diffuse Osteosclerosis in Adults

Hematological Causes

- Include sickle cell disease, mastocytosis, myelofibrosis, polycythemia rubra vera.
- These diseases are characterized by sequential development of reactive marrow hyperplasia, atrophy fibrosis and finally reactive osteostenosis.
- Sickle cell disorder can be easily distinguished by presence of diffuse medullary bone infarct, ischemic necrosis, 'H' shaped or biconcave vertebral bodies and "hair on end" appearance of skull.
- Mastocytosis: Diffuse trabecular thickening accounts for generalized osteolesion. Typically seen in vertebrae, skull, ribs and pelvis. Superimposed on this there may be reticular or modular sclerosis.

Metabolic Causes

Renal Osteodystrophy

- Associated with stenosis of the spongiosa of the axial and appendicular skeleton.
- Cortical bones frequently become angular resorbed and striated.
- Thickening of trabecular bone is most strikingly seen in ribs, pelvis, spine, skull and metaphysis of lung bones.

Primary Hyperparathyroidism

- Scoliosis with lytic areas in the skull is seen (salt and pepper skull).
- Sclerosis of vertebral end plates.
- Diffuse osteosclerosis involving axial skeleton more than appendicular skeleton.

X-Linked Hypophophatemic Osteomalacia

- Mild generalized osteosclerosis is common.
- There is diffuse stenosis of trabecular bone, bowel, and shortened/thickened long bones.
- Peculiar intra articular accessory ossification at the wrist and elbow.

Hypoparathyroidism, Pseudohypoparathyroidism and Pseudohypoparathyroidism

- Calvarial thickening, basal ganglia and metacarpal/metatarsal, shortening and exostosis.
- Soft tissue calcification.
- Premature closure of epiphysis.

Neoplastic Causes

- Include prostate carcinoma, breast carcinoma, GI adenocarcinoma, carcinoid tumor, transitional cell carcinoma, bladder, myeloma, leukemia and lymphoma.

PAGET'S DISEASE

- There is dense expanded bone with thickened trabecular and flare shaped leading edge aids in establishing the diagnosis.
- An early change is a spotty cotton wool pledged insizure in density of bone.
- Spine may show characteristics, though infrequent, picture frame appearance with condensed and thickened end plates and vertebral margins enclosing a cystic spongiosa.

GENERALIZED OSTEOSCLEROSIS IN CHILDREN

Osteopetrosis

- Bone becomes very fragile and may present as fractures.
- Abnormal modelling of the metaphysis, which are widened with alternating band of radiolucency and sclerosis.
- Bone within bone appearance.
- Ricket and basal ganglia calcification may be seen in autosomal recessive form.

Pyknodysostosis

- Wormian bone are seen.
- Delayed closure of fontanelles.
- Generalized increase in density of the skeleton.
- Straight mandible, prognathism.
- Reabsorption of lateral and of clavicles.
- Hypoplastic terminal phalanges.

Renal Osteodystrophy

- Discussed earlier.
- Feature of rickets may also be seen.

Lead Poisoning

- Dense metaphyseal bands.
- Severe modelling defect are seen e.g. plastic shaped femora.
- Typically involves the knee with involvement of proximal rubella being especially characteristics.

Fluorosis

- Discussed previously.
- Usually seen in adults.

Hypervitaminosis D

- Metaphyseal band of increased density, cortical thickening and widespread osteosclerosis.
- Focal or generalized osteoporosis (in adults).
- Periarticular lobulated calcification.
- Metastatic soft tissue calcifications (children and adults).

Chronic Hypervitaminosis A

- Metaphysis and ulnar hyperostosis.
- Cupping and splaying of metaphyses.
- Widening of cranial sutures.
- Vertebral osteophytosis (particularly) cervical spine (more common in adults).
- Mild appendicular enteropathic changes (adults).
- Mandible not involved.

CAFEY'S DISEASE (INFANTILE CORTICAL HYPEROSTOSIS)

- Involvement of mandible, clavicles, ribs and ulnar.
- Periosteal new bone formation and cortical thickening is limited to the diphyseal region; epiphyses and metaphyses are spared.
- Involvement is asymmetric.

- Mandible involvement is the key in separating this entity from hypervitaminosis A (in which mandible is spared).

IDIOPATHIC HYPERCALCEMIA OF INFANCY

- Probably a manifestation of hypervitaminosis D.
- There is generalized - bone densities and dense metaphyseal bowels.
- Also, there is increased density of the skull bone.

LOCALIZED INCREASE IN BONE DENSITY

Metaphyseal transverse bands of increased radiodensity.

Normal Variant

- In young children, metaphyses appear dense and yet be normal.
- Transverse growth arrest lines are seen in cases of past episodes of stress when growth temporarily halted.

Scurvy

- Other change of scurvy differentiates it from other differentials.
- Pelkan spin: Marginal fraction.
- Winbuger's law: None of increased density around the epiphyses.
- White line of fronkel ↑ed density and widening of zone of proximal calcification.

Treated Rickets

- Due to calcification of the non-calcified bone of provisional calcification.

Heavy Metal (Pb, Bi) Poisoning

- Transverse radiodense metaphyseal bands.
- Failure of normal modelling of tubular bones.

Hypervitaminosis D

- Soft tissue calcification.
- Lobulated periarticular calcification.

Hypothyroidism

- Retarded skeletal maturation.
- Bilateral symmetrical epiphyseal dizziness (Fragmented epiphyses).
- Wormian bones.
- Bullet shaped vertebral bodies.

Disorders Associated with Hyperostosis of Cortical Bone

Progressive Diaphyseal Dysplasia

- Also known as CAMURATI-ENGELMANN DISEASE.
- Progressive, bilateral symmetrical, diaphyseal sclerosis of the long bones from endosteal and periosteal new bone formation.

Endosteal Hyperostosis

- It's a feature of Van Buchem's disease.
- Lung bones as well as the skull and facial bones are affected.

Pachydermoperiotosis

- Periosteal and endosteal new bone formation in the entire length of the bone.
- Rest similar to hypertrophic osteoarthropathy.

Hypertrophic Osteoarthropathy

- Perosteal and endosteal new bone formation seen in forearm bone and lower leg bone and later on hand and feet.
- Insulin diaphysis and metaphysic, epiphysis is characteristically spared.

Hypervitaminosis A

- Periosteal new bone formation of ulna and metatarsal.

- Widening of cranial sutures.
- Vertebral osteophytosis (particularly ex spine).

Thyroid Acropachy

- Periosteal reaction predominantly in metacarpals, metatarsals and paralysis (proximal and middle) is characteristically diaphyseal in location and asymmetrical with radial side being more involved.
- Clustering and soft tissue swelling of objects.
- Pretibial myxedema.

PAGET'S DISEASE

- Discussed earlier.

CAFEY'S DISEASE (INFANTILE CORTICAL HYPEROSTOSIS)

- Discussed earlier.

FOCAL OSTEOSCLEROTIC DISORDERS AFFECTING THE TRABECULAR BONE

Osteopoikilosis

- Associated with subcutaneous fibrous nodules.
- Small round or oval areas of sclerosis particularly in the pelvis and epiphysis and metaphysis of long bone.

Melorheostosis

- Dense cortical longitudinal hyperostosis of the bones.
- Appearance is like WAX running down the side of a candle.
- Particularly involves the long bones.

Osteopathia Striata

- Fine dense linear striation, most usually noted at the end of the long bones.

Section 10—Musculoskeletal System

Chapter 114

Expansile Lytic Lesions or Bubbly Lesions of Bones

CAUSES

1. Neoplastic

Benign

- Giant cell tumor (Figure 114.1).

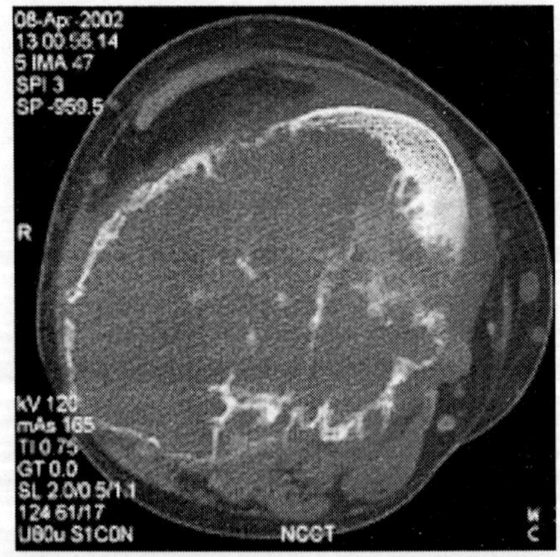

Fig. 114.1: Axial CT images show a large giant cell tumor of the upper end of tibia

- Chondromyxoid fibroma.
  - Enchondroma.
- Plasmacytoma.

Malignant

- Giant cell tumor.
- Osteoblastoma.

Angiosarcoma

- Metastasis.

2. Infection

- Echinococcus.

3. Endocrinal

- Hyperparathyroidism.

4. Tumor like Lesions

- Non-ossifying fibroma.
- Aneurysmal bone cyst (Figures 114.2 and 114.3).
- Simple cyst (Figure 114.4).
- Hemophilic pseudotumor.

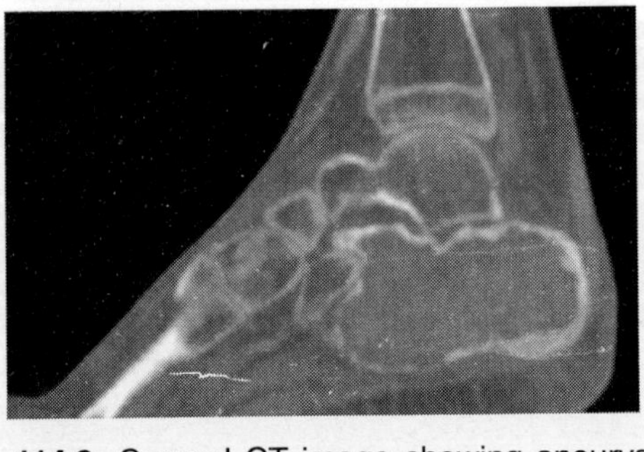

Fig. 114.2: Coronal CT image showing aneurysmal bone cyst of the calcaneum

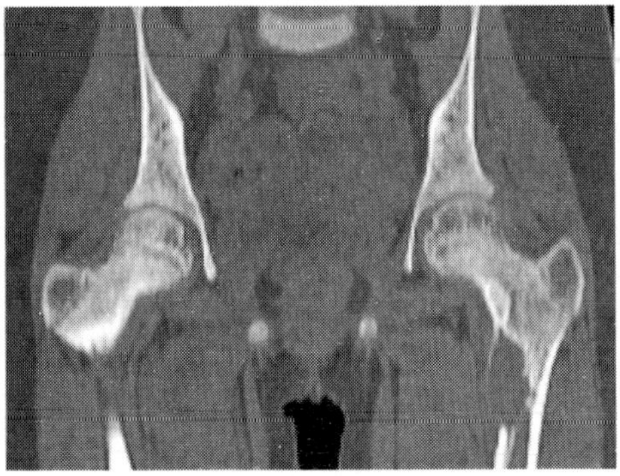

Fig. 114.3: Coronal MPR CT image shows a fibrous cortical defect in the medial cortex of the left femur in the proximal third shaft region

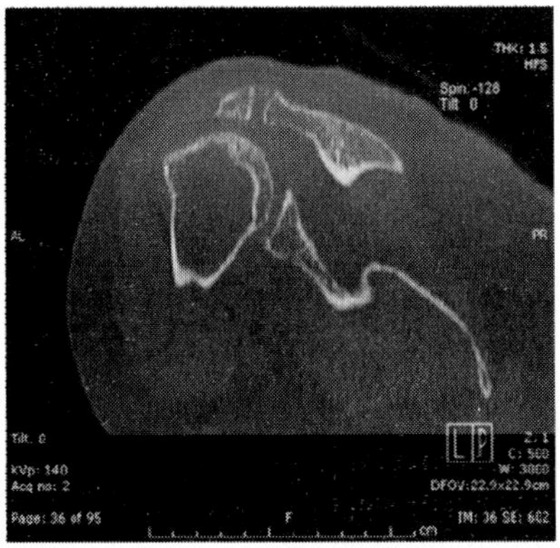

Fig. 114.4: CT coronal MPR image of shoulder showing a lytic lesion involving head of humerus

5. Idiopathic

- Fibrous dysplasia.

Enchondroma

Solitary enchondroma is found incidentally or present as painless bony swelling in 3rd or 4th decade. Found most frequently in bones of hands and less frequently in feet, long bones are not exempted.

Located centrally in metaphysis of long bones or diaphysis of short tubular bones.

Radiographic findings of the lesion in hand/foot is characteristic well defined lobulated lesions causing endosteal scalloping is positive in the medullary cavity. Cortical expansion, thickening or a pathological fracture is seen.

In the long bones, the radiological appearance is similar and less diagnostic in flat bones. However, its differentiation from low-grade chondrosarcoma is difficult radiographically. Extensive endosteal scalloping and less prominent matrix calcification with periosteal reaction, cortical destruction, soft tissue mass suggest the possibility of chondrosarcoma.

- On MR examination enchondroma appears as a well circumscribed, lobulated lesions of low signal intensity on T1W1 and high signal intensity on T2W1. Calcification appears as regions of low signal intensity.

Osteochondroma: This rare primary bone tumor affects mostly males of less than 30 years.

- Local pain is the usual presenting feature.
- Most commonly affects the flat bones or vertebrae (post elements). In a long tubular bone, lesion is present in the diaphysis in the 3/4th cases and in the metaphysis in the remainder.
- Radiographic features are nondiagnostic-osteolytic,osteosclerotic or mixed lytic-sclerotic lesions are observed.Cortical thickening,bony expansion an soft tissue extension may accompany.
- In long bones it appears as medullary/cortical/subperiosteal, mixed oval predominantly osteolytic well defined expansile lesions with areas of calcification. Extensive sclerosis and periosteitis may be seen.
- In the spine especially thoracic or lumber segments—well defined expansile osteolytic lesions with partial or extensive calcification present in the post elements suggest the diagnosis of osteoblastoma.
- Radionucleide studies shows increased uptake of radioactive tracer at the site of lesions.
- ... shows the full extent of the lesions an... tissue involvement in aggressive o...blastoma. Fluid level may be seen in osteoblastomas.

Metastasis

Expansile metastasis arise from renal cell carcinoma, thyroid and hepatoma. Expanded lytic bony contour is evident. Mets from RCC give a septated appearance. Large expansile osteoblastic metastasis may be seen from carcinoma of prostate.

Infective-Echinococcus

Caused by larval stage of E. granulosis humens are intermediate hosts is infected by ingestion of the eggs contained in the faeces of dogs, sheep, cattle. Osseous involvement occurs in 1-2% of cases as a primary infection.

Vertebral column is involved in 50% of cases, other bones to be involved are pelvis, long bones and skull.

Radiologically, single/multiple expansile osteolytic lesions containing trabeculae. Cortex may be destroyed with evidence of soft tissue mass.

CT shows the soft tissue mass (center has a fuid of water attenuation) clearly in relation to the bony lesions. MR also shows the cystic lesions in the bone and adjacent soft tissues. Numerous cystic lesions of high signal intensity in T2 weighted images. Thus MR images appears to be diagnostic.

Plasmocytoma

Myeloma occurring as a solitary bony lesions.

- In comparison to multiple myeloma it is rare, affects relatively younger (middle aged, elderly) patients,commonly accompanied with neurological manifestation and radiologically resembles GCT.

  Spine is most commonly involved—thoracic and lumbar segments followed by pelvis.
- Radiologically, it appears as a osteolytic, expansile , trabeculated lesions. In the vertebral involement lesions may cross the intervertebral disc and invade the adjacent vertebrae.The vertebrae may collapse and disappear completely (Table 114.1).

Table 114.1: Differentiating features of giant cell tumour from aneurysmal bone cyst

Giant cell tumor	Aneurysmal bone cyst
Points favouring	**Points favouring**
• Eccentric, expansile cystic lesion	• Expansile lytic lesion
• Medullary origin	• Medullary origin
• Wide zone of transition	• Thin cortex, no periosteal mass, no sub periosteal new bone premation
• Cortical thinning, no periosteal reaction, no sub periosteal new bone formation	• Joint not involved
• Ill defined endosteal margins	• No surrounding sclerosis
• No surrounding sclerosis	• No soft tissue extension
	• Eccentric lytic lesion
Points against	**Points against**
• 97% are seen after fusion of epiphysis, at the epiphysis and are subarticular (i.e. juxtaepiphyseal location) only 3% seen at metaphysic and before fusion	• Narrow zone of transition (wide in this case)
• Joint nearby is usually involved	• Well defined endosteal margin (ill defined in this case)

GIANT CELL TUMOR (OSTEOCLASTOMA)

- Presents as pain or swelling, or sometimes following trauma or as an incidental finding.
- Histologically, rich vascular tissue containing plump spindle cells and numerous giant cells containing 50-100 nuclei.
- Tumor produces near bone nor cartilage.
- Usually presents between the age of 20-40 years.
- Only 3% arise in immature skeletons, distinguishing this entity from ABC in whom tumor maximally occurs before epiphyseal fusion.

- GCT's are multifocal in just 0.5% cases.
- Solitary lesion shows a predilection for bones adjacent to knee joints and the distal end of radius.

RADIOLOGICAL FEATURES

- Zone of translucency seen typically beneath the articular cortex.
- Sited eccentrically at the end of lower bone.
- Lesion shows no calcification/ossification unless complicated by a fracture.
- 40% cases may be characterized by a 'soap bubble' pattern of trabeculation.
- Margins purely osteolytic, sclerotic margin rarely evident.
- Characteristically margins are hazy and ill defined with no bone reaction. Endosteal margins are also illdefined.
- More aggressive lesion shows widening of zone of transition.
- Tumor may produce well-defined extension into the adjacent soft tissue but without any evidence of calcification or new bone formation.
- Angiographically and blood pool phase of bone scan, vascularity is markedly increased, with increase in number of vessels, AV shunting and tumor stenting.
- Delayed phase of bone scan is usually normal.
- CT and MRI may be necessary to delineate fully the soft tissue extension of the tumor.
- Tumor has tendency to recur even after successful curettage and packing.
- Secondary sarcomatous changes may also occur following radiotherapy after interval of several years.

ANEURYSMAL BONE CYST

- It's a blood filled, expansile, sponge like tumor containing numerous giant cells.
- Presents in childhood or early adolescence.
- Predilection for long bones and spine. Those arising in spine occur slightly later in life between 10-20 years of age.
- Prognosis is entirely benign apart from secondary neurological lesion due to spinal canal compression.

RADIOLOGICAL FEATURES

- Typically area of bone resorption occurs with slight/marked expansion.
- Overlying cortex is thinned.
- Endosteum is well defined against the cortex.
- Ill defined zone of transition is seen between the lesion and medulla.
- Angiographically, similar to GCT, in particular a rich increased in vessels with diffuse opacification and early venous filling.
- CT and MRI may show fluid levels in vascular spaces.

Differentiated from GCT by:

- 3/4th of ABC's occur before epiphyseal fusion.
- Widespread anatomical distribution contrasts with the majority of GCT's occur around knee and wrist.
- ABC's rarely extend to the articular surface.
- ABC is a good example of the importance of radiological investigation being complete before biopsy is undertaken, because these lesions, not surprisingly, bleed considerating and pre-operative demonstration of its vascular nature can prevent profuse bleeding.

Treatment

- Treated by curettage or radiotherapy, the latter being used in spinal lesions when surgery is hazardous.

- There is an increasing only of transcatheter embolization in the minimizing the size and vascularity of these tumors.

FIBROUS CORTICAL DEFECT

- These are very common, seen between ages of 2-15 years.
- Characteristically seen around the knee, especially in the distal posteromedial femoral cortex.
- Discovered by chance, not known to be symptomatic.

Radiologically

- Blister like expansions of cortex with a thin shell of covering bone.
- Very sharply defined.
- Have a fine sclerotic margins.
- With increasing skeletal maturity, the lesion may appear to migrate towards diaphysis.
- Becomes progressive sclerotic and involution completely.
- Bone scan, is unremarkable, shows minimal increase in activity on delayed phase in proportion to the size of the lesion.

Differential Diagnosis

- Cortical desmoid/cortical avulsion syndromes.
- In a chronic low grade fracture resulting in irregularity of the cortex, some time with radiolucency with angular calcification at the insertion of adductor magnus muscle or the origin of medial head of gastrocnemius.
- These lesions are traumatic in origin.

Bone Scans

- Shows abnormal increase in activity and angiogram shows slight increase in vascularity.

NON-OSSIFYING FIBROMA

- Similar to fibrous corticle defect except it is larger and occur in slightly older age between 10-20 years.
- Mostly seen around the knee joint, most common location is distal end of femur.
- Usually asymptomatic, occasionally presents as pathological fracture.

Radiologically

- Increased radiolucency which is sharply defined at metadiaphysis.
- Margins are smooth and sharp.
- There is a thin zone of reactive sclerosis.
- Larger bone like fibula, whole width is involved. In tibia lesions may be eccentric. The outer margin of the cortex is usually slightly expanded but remains intact and thinned.
- Bone scan, minimal increase in activity on delayed phase scan.
- It resolves spontaneously, initially with increased sclerosis and later replaced by normal bone.

Differential Diagnosis

1. Simple bone cyst:

   Very difficult to differentiate on radiological grounds.
2. Monostotic fibrous dysplasia:

   Differentiated by its avidity of bone seeking radiopharmaceuticals.

CHONDROMYXOID FIBROMA

- Is predominantly a chrondroid tumor, but contain myxomatous tissue and giant cells.
- Non-specific presentation, usually localized pain and swelling.

- Peak incidence is between 20-30 years, no sex predilection.
- Most common site: Around the knee joint (in 2/3rd cross) with special affinity for proximal end of tibia.

Radiological Features

- Radiolucent, eccentric, SOL at the metaphysis.
- Well defined margins with surrounding sclerosis.
- Sharpens of the margin between the lesion of sclerosis.Which CONTRASTS with the rather ill defined margin between the sclerosis and normal bone.
- Calcification is very uncommon.
- Bone scan and angiography: Reveal slight increase in perfusion of the lesion.

Brown Tumors

Though characteristics of primary hyperpara-thyroidism, these lesions are now also seen with increasing frequency on secondary HPT.

- Brown tumors are localized collection of fibrous tissue and giant cells which may undergo necrosis and cyst formation.

  Radiographically they are single/multiple well defined lytic lesions of axial/appendicular skeleton. They may produce bony expansion and are more commonly located eccentrically or in the cortex.
- Facial bones, pelvis, ribs and femur are the common sites of involvement.
- Other manifestations of hyperparathyroidism.

Hemophilic Pseudotumor

Intraosseous hemorrhage in cases of hemophilia produce a lytic expansile medullary lesions indistinguishable from primary bone tumor. A well demarcated, eccenteric/cortical radiolucent lesions with trabeculation and sclerosis of surrounding bone. Subperiosteal bleeding produce periosteitis.

Other Features—Joint contraction, intraarticular destruction, soft tissue mass/ hemorrhage/calcification and history suggestive of hemophilia is the key to reach the diagnosis.

Fibrous Dysplasia

A developemental anomaly in which the round marrow and cancellous bones are replaced by immature bones and dense fibrous tissue.

- May occur as metastatic or polystotic variety.
- 70%-80% are monostotic and affects ribs, femur tibia, jaw bone, calvaria and humerus. Polystotic form more commonly involve skull, facial bones, pelvis and shoulder girdle and spine.
- The degree of bony involvement, linear growth disparities and clinical symptoms of pain, hip deformity and fracture are more in the polyostotic variety. Hazy ground glass well defined radiolucent lesions causing expansion of bone is seen. Lesions in long bones are intramedullary, predominantly diaphyseal, and eccentric/central and may show endosteal scalloping.
- A bony deformity and fractures may be evident.

Section 10—Musculoskeletal System

Chapter 115

Imaging in Arthritis

Athritis may result from or be associated with a number of conditions including connective tissue diseases; trauma; congenital disorders, inflammatory diseases, hematological and neoplastic diseases. The role of imaging is:

- To diagnose.
- To evaluate the activity of the disease; and
- To monitor the effect of therapy.

Plain Radiographs of the affected joint(s) remains the primary modality of diagnosis and follow-up of joint disease especially in the peripheral skeleton. Moreover, it may, visualize early changes of arthritis such as soft-tissue swelling, periarticular osteoporosis, and periostitis and accelerated maturation of the epiphysis. In younger children, growth disturbances secondary to the hyperemia of the inflammatory process may be seen after a few months. Accelerated maturation of the local epiphyseal ossification centers, round bones and sesamoids, together with widening and elongation of the bone ends near the joints may be seen. A bulbous appearance of the distal portion of the proximal phalanges is a typical finding. In the knee the distal femoral epiphysis or the patella may be enlarged. In cases of unilateral affection, radiograph of bilateral joints are mandatory to detect subtle differences.

Ultrasound (US) is the method of choice in detection of joint effusion and may also differentiate between fluid and a thickened synovia. With high frequency linear probes, it is possible to roughly estimate the amount of fluid and to measure the thickness of the synovia, and hence to evaluate activity of the disease. Moreover, ultrasound may facilitate diagnostic aspiration if indicated, and also guide the injection of steroids.

Computed Tomography (CT) (Figures 115.1 and 115.2) provides greater details than conventional radiographs especially in the central skeleton but is equally useful at the peripheral joints. With good multiplanar reconstruction images and

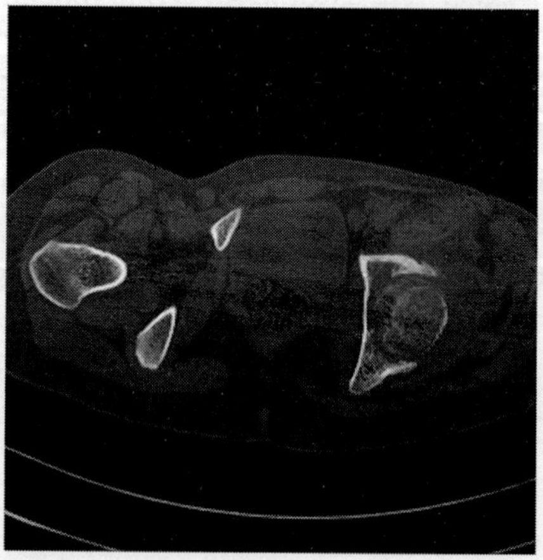

Fig. 115.1: Axial CT image shows tubercular arthritis of the left hip with joint effusion

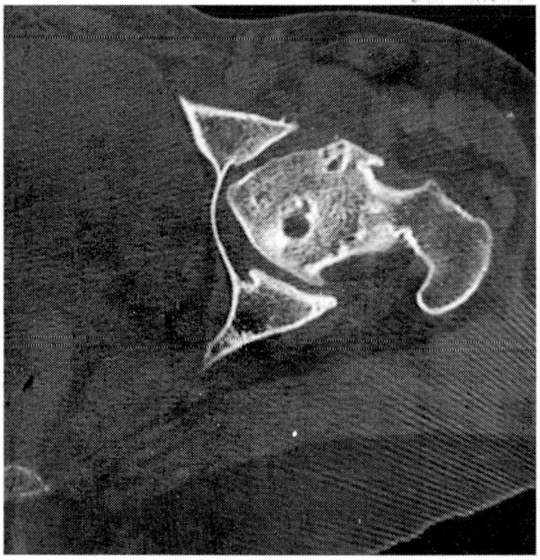

Fig. 115.2: Axial CT image shows secondary osteoarthritis in a case of AVN of the left femoral head

MSCT, it can provide greater overview of the joint diseases in all the three dimensions.

Magnetic Resonance Imaging (MRI) is superior to other modalities, in showing subtle cartilage and soft-tissue changes and joint effusions in the early stages of the disease, when, radiographs are still normal. It can demonstrate the vascularity in and around the joint as well as the effect of arthritis on the nerves especially in arthritis involving the spine. Synovitis is seen as areas of low signal intensity on T1 weighted images. Opposite to fluid, a hypervascular synovia enhances after administration of intravenous contrast. Today, however, the majority of children up to 4-5 years of age need sedation, which limits the use of the method.

Bone Scintigraphy may be useful in evaluating the activity of the disease, however, the method is flawed with both false positives and false negatives.

Classification of Joints

The structure of the joint determines their reaction to various disease processes. There are three types of joints based on their structure:

- Fibrous joints or synarthroses are immobile, e.g. cranial sutures.
- Cartilaginous joints or amphiarthroses contain fibrous cartilage and allow limited movement e.g. intervertebral disks, symphysis pubis.
- Synovial joints or diarthroses are covered by hyaline cartilage and a capsule surrounds the joint. These joints allow free movement. The outer layer of the capsule is fibrous. The inner layer is composed of the vascularised connective tissue called the synovium, which does not cover the articular cartilage it merges with the periosteum, covering the intracapsular portion of the joint, except for marginal bare areas. The synovium secretes fluid that lubricates and nourishes the articular cartilage. The joints of the extremities and the apophyseal joints, of the spine are the examples. Only synovial joints are affected by inflammatory arthritis.

The basic parameters that are of significance in interpreting the images in arthritis are as follows:

- Patterns of osteopenia.
- Joint effusion and joint space narrowing.
- Erosions, cysts, geodes and bone resorption.
- Changes in the ossification centers and small bones.
- Periosteal new bone formation.
- Malalignment, subluxation, dislocation.
- Disorganizaion.
- Ankylosis.
- Soft tissue welling, atrophy and calcification.
- In the spine features are noted in the:
  - Vertebral body.
  - Intervertebral disks.
  - Apophyseal joints.
  - Atlanto-axial joint.
  - Paravertebral region.

OSTEOPENIA

It is associated with several arthritides. In inflammatory arthritis, synovial hyperemia leads, to early periarticular osteopenia. Others like Neuropathic arthropathy and dialysis arthritis are also associated with osteoporosis. In chronic arthritis, osteoporosis proceeds to uniform bone atrophy, with a thin, sharp cortex. Subchondral osteoporosis occurs in rapidly developing processes such as septic arthritis. Arthritides like gout, psoriatic arthritis, Reiter's arthritis and pigmented villonodular synovitis are characterised by lack of osteporosis.

JOINT EFFUSION

It occurs in early synovial disease. MRI can demonstrate small effusions at the earliest. Large effusions usually can be seen well on conventional radiographs.

Effusions at the PIP and MCP joints are typical of rheumatoid arthritis of the hands. The signs of knee effusion are the fullness of the suprapatellar pouch seen on lateral view, and curved, displaced radiolucent fat planes medial and lateral to the distal femur in the suprapatellar region, seen on AP radiographs. Posterior displacement of the fabella also indicated effusion. In the elbow, effusion and hemorrhage is indicated by displacement of the fat planes, particularly posteriorly. This is called the fat pad sign. Haziness is another characteristic of joint effusion, causing a loss of the sharp, white, subchondral cortical line.

Hip effusion in an inflammatory process in children may be detected by displacement of the fat line at the obturator internis muscle medially. This is due to adjacent muscular edema. However, ultrasound is the investigation of choice.

If the amount of fluid increases, joint space widening will occur, if fluid further accumulates, particularly in the hip and shoulder in children, dislocation will follow.

JOINT SPACE NARROWING

It is caused by cartilage atrophy or destruction. Cartilage atrophy may result from disuse. Normal cartilage nutrition is by diffusion of synovial fluid driven by pressure from joint motion. Atrophy may also follow surgical procedure.

Rheumatoid arthritis typically results in uniform joint space narrowing whereas, osteoarthritis shows narrowing, and that is most marked in the weight bearing areas, which is the medial compartment in the knee joint and superiorly in the hip. All the three compartments are uniformly narrowed in the rheumatoid arthritis and the Paget's disease also shows uniform joint space narrowing.

EROSIONS, CYSTS, GEODES, BONE RESORPTION

These characterize some arthritides, whereas some are typically non-erosive. The absence of erosions in the hands is typical of Jaccoud's arthritis, Reiter's syndrome and SLE.

Rheumatoid erosions tend to be fuzzily marginated without a sclerotic margin. Erosions are initially located at the bare areas. There may be compression erosions resulting in ball in socket configuration. Erosions may occur at the tendinous insertions.

Later in the chronic disease, the articular cartilage is destroyed and the subchondral bone is eroded and destroyed. Sarcoidosis can also result in bony erosions in the vicinity of the joint. The margins are poorly defined and there is an increased trabecular pattern of the bone.

In infectious arthritis, erosions occur in contact areas. Hemophilia in the knee is characterised by large erosion in the intercondylar notch of the femur, as well as along the articular surface, owing to hemorrhage.

Gouty erosions tend to have a well-defined sclerotic margin with a characteristic, overhanging edge. They can be expansile; the first MTP joint is a typical location.

Erosions in osteoarthritis also have well-defined margins and appear cystic when viewed en-face. Synovial fluid is forced through a defect in the articular cartilage to form a cyst. A cyst-like appearance may also be caused by growth of the granulation tissue into bone. These may enlarge and rarely result in expansion of the cortex. Large cysts are known as geodes. Osteoarthritis in the hands shows central erosions in the DIP joints. A small pit in the femoral neck is a normal variant. Fungal infections also cause erosions in joints without any other obvious changes on conventional radiographs. Irregularities of the articular surface can also be caused by osteochondritis dissecans. Pigmented villonodular synovitis results in well-marginated erosions on both sides of the joint, with preservation, of joint cartilage and bone density.

Resorption of hone is seen in various conditions especially in collagen diseases. It is characteristic of the neuropathic arthropathy. Resorption of part or entire humeral head may occur. Tapering of one side of joint is seen in the hands and feet, along with exaggerated concavity of the opposite side, giving pencil in cup appearance. Resorption and dislocation at multiple joints of the hand cause shortening and deformity of the fingers, resulting in the main-en-lorgnette or opera glass hand of end-stage rheumatoid arthritis.

Resorption of the distal end of the clavicle may occur following trauma or in hyperparathyroidism and rheumatoid arthritis. Terminal phalangeal tuft resorption occurs in several conditions including scleroderma and hyperparathyroidism.

CHANGES IN THE OSSIFICATION CENTER AND THE SMALL BONES

Such changes are seen in JRA, juvenile articular infections and hemophilia, with changes in the time of appearance and fusion of the epiphyseal ossification centers. A characteristic appearance includes enlargement, irregularity of contour squaring, osteoporosis and coarsening of the trabecular pattern of the epiphysis. In addition, alteration in the length of the extremity may occur.

Tibiotalar slant is characteristic in JRA, hemophilia and multiple dysplasias. Hemophilia also shows squaring of the inferior margin of the patella. Bony proliferation of the epiphyseal ossification centers is seen in dysplasia epiphysealis hemimelica, or Trevor's disease.

AVN of the epiphyses may begin as a subchondral radiolucent fracture line. It then proceeds to sclerosis and deformity. MRI can demonstrate this with better detail. Later collapse and cyst formation may occur. Legg Perthes disease is a specific type of AVN that occurs in childhood. AVN of the small bones occurs frequently, and various eponyms have been used. For example, Koehler's disease is AVN of the navicular bone.

SUBCHONDRAL SCLEROSIS AND OSTEOPHYTES

It is characteristic of osteoarthritis. Rheumatoid arthritis in the weight bearing areas develops secondary OA with subchondral sclerosis after cartilage destruction. Friction of the apposing bone ends leads to osteosclerosis. Reactive osteitis of the sesamoid bone may be a cause of pain. Rarely, osteoblastic metastases may involve a peripheral small bone. Sclerosis around a joint may also be seen in melorheostosis.

Osteophytes at joint margins are a characteristic feature of OA. They extend horizontally from the articular margins. The cortex of the osteophyte is continuous with that of the adjacent bone. The interior of the spur consists of trabeculae and fatty marrow, often covered with cartilage or periosteum. They represent reactive bone formation. Hook-like osteophytes is characteristic of hemochromatosis and CPPD.

PERIOSTEAL NEW BONE FORMATION

It may be seen in the reactive inflammatory arthritides. It is rare in adult-onset RA (5%) but in JRA it is typical. Reiter's syndrome also characteristically exhibits thick, fluffy periosteal new bone. Septic arthritis and osteomyelitis also exhibits periosteal reaction. Ankylosing spondylitis may be associated with irregular new bone formation at entheses. Fluffy periosteal new bone formation at the base of the distal phalanx of the great toe can be seen in Reiter's syndrome and psoriatic arthritis. Periosteal reaction is a characteristic feature of pulmonary hypertrophic osteoarthropathy. This has a characteristic appearance on radioscintigraphy with increased activity on both sides of the bone, the double rail sign. Various tumors in the vicinity of the joints are also associated with periosteal new bone formation like osteoid osteoma.

MALALIGNMENT, SUBLUXATION, DISLOCATION

Malalignment may be seen as deviation, flexion or hyperextension. Deviation is caused by muscular imbalance. Ulnar deviation of the fingers at the MCP joints is typically seen in rheumatoid arthritis, SLE and Jaccouds arthritis. In RA, ulnar deviation is irreversible and is associated with erosions. In the last two conditions, the reverse is true.

Deformities of flexion and hyperextension include the boutonnière (flexion at the PIP and hyperextension at the DIP joint) and swan-neck deformity (hyperextension at PIP and flexion at the DIP joint). The former is seen in RA, SLE and Jaccoud's arthritis. Interference with the growth plate from injury or a disease process results in deformities.

Subluxation and dislocation result from progression of malalignment, from large effusions, pyogenic arthritis or erosions and destruction of the bone ends. Large effusions of the shoulder or hip in infants result in dislocations. Carpal malpositions occur in RA and JRA. Elevation of the humeral head owing to the erosion of the rotator cuff tendon occurs in RA. Displacement can also occur at the epiphyseal cartilage plate, as in slipped capital-femoral epiphysis.

DISORGANISATION

Disorganisation of a large joint is typically seen in neurotrophic arthropathy. Fragmentation of bone, dislocation and soft tissue debris occur. The fragments may later fuse into a bony mass. Arthritis mutilans refers to destructive end-stage arthritis of the hands and feet. It may result from RA, IRA, psoriatic arthritis, leprosy and diabetes mellitus.

ANKYLOSIS

It has a different distribution and frequency pattern in the various arthritides. Interphalangeal bony ankylosis is more common in JRA and in psoriatic arthritis. It is rare in adult-onset RA. Carpal and tarsal fusion can be seen in adult and juvenile RA. Ankylosis of the hip and knee is most commonly seen in JRA. In the sacroiliac joints, the inflammatory arthritides can ankylose the synovial-lined lower two-thirds, whereas in DISH, ligamentous ossification can fuse the upper third.

DISTRIBUTION AND SEQUENCE OF CHANGES

The distribution of joint involvement is significant in diagnosis because sites of predilection of the various arthritides differ in the hands. The DIP joints are often initially involved in primary OA and psoriatic arthritis. The PIP joints are typically involved with RA. CPPD has a tendency to involve the radiocarpal compartment of the wrist, whereas gout tends to involve the carpometacarpal compartment.

Primary OA often involves the first CMC joint. Bilateral symmetrical involvement is characteristic of RA whereas gout is sporadically distributed. Bilateral symmetrical involvement of the SI joints is typical of ankylosing spondylitis. However, the typical distribution does not occur in every case.

The time and sequence of events are important for the diagnosis and management of the arthritis. Demonstration of early erosions is an indication to change therapy. The evolution of changes is important, for example, in pyogenic arthritis with rapid progress, destruction precedes osteoporosis, whereas in tuberculous arthritis, the reverse is true.

SOFT TISSUE SWELLING, ATROPHY AND CALCIFICATION

Soft tissue debris is characteristic of a neuropathic joint. Clubbing of the terminal phalanges is seen in hypertrophic osteoarthropathy, acromegaly and hyperparathyroidism. Soft tissue swelling representing tophi is seen in gout. Soft tissue nodules may be seen in RA, amyloidosis, thyroid acropachy and xanthoma. Diffuse swelling of the entire digit (Sausage digit) can be seen in psoriatic and infectious arthritis as well as in macrodactyly diffuse soft tissue enlargement of the entire limb may be seen in plexiform, neurofibromatosis. Soft tissue prominence with calcification may be seen in vascular malformations and hemangiomas. Rheumatoid arthritis has a typical early distribution of soft tissue swelling about the ulnar styloid process and the PIP joints, and later at the MCP joints. Soft tissue mass in the popliteal fossa may represent Baker's cyst, tumors and aneurysms of the popliteal artery.

Soft tissue atrophy is seen at the terminal phalanges in scleroderma. Atrophy of the thenar and hypothenar muscles, giving a concave rather than convex hypothenar border is seen in SLE.

Soft tissue calcification may be metabolic calcifications, calcinosis (subcutaneous calcification) or dystrophic calcification. They may be paraarticular in vessels, tendons, bursa, the joint capsule, articular cartilage or fibrocartilage. Metabolic calcifications are seen in CRF, hypo and hyperparathyroidism. Calcinosis is seen in scleroderma and CREST syndrome. Dystrophic calcification is seen in gouty and tumoral calcinosis.

Hydroxyapatite deposition disease (HADD) is a cause of calcific tendonitis, bursitis and periarticular calcification. Vascular calcification occurs most frequently in atherosclerosis, DM and renal osteodystrophy. Hyaline articular cartilage and meniscal calcification is characteristic of chondrocalcinosis (CPPD). Synovial osteochondromatosis is a condition of intraarticular calcific bodies resulting from synovial chondrometaplasia.

SPINE

The vertebral margin can characterize several processes. Marginal osteophytes are mechanical reactive proliferation of the cortical bone, with a medulla and cartilaginous cap. They have a horizontal take off as compared to syndesmophytes, which have a vertical orientation. CT shows osteophytes as linear osseous structures adjacent to the vertebral body. Posterior osteophytes may encroach on the intervertebral foramina, and may cause radiculopathy. They may even encroach on the spinal canal. Some osteophytes are 1 mm removed from the actual vertebral corner and are termed as traction spurs and indicate segmental instability.

Thin marginal syndesmophytes are calcification of the outer fibers of the annulus fibrosus and the inner fibers of the longitudinal ligament. They are characteristic of AS and reactive spondylitis. They can be seen on CT as a thin line adjacent to the vertebral body. Thicker marginal syndesmophytes may also occur in the above conditions.

Thick non-marginal syndesmophytes are seen in psoriatic arthritis and Reiter's syndrome. They extend from the midvertebral bodies.

DISH has a characteristic appearance of ossification of the anterior longitudinal ligament with a thin radiolucent line of separation from the vertebral body margin. Rarely, the posterior longitudinal ligament may also calcify.

Changes in the shape and density of the vertebral bodies occur in various conditions. A specific appearance seen in AS is squaring of the vertebral bodies in late. AS, squaring of the entire vertebra and syndesmophytes formation produccs a bamboo-spine. Biconcavity of the vertebral bodies is seen in sickle cell disease and homocystinuria. Collapse of vertebral bodies can occur from osteoporosis and tumor metastases. Wedge-like collapse can be caused by trauma and metastases. Wafer-like collapse can be caused by metastases or eosinophilic granuloma.

Osteopenia can be seen in metabolic bone disease, along with flattening of the vertebral bodies. Focal end-plate depressions are seen due to Schmorl's nodes.

Osteosclerosis can occur in various forms as rugger jersey spine of renal osteodystrophy, the picture frame appearance of Paget's disease and bone in bone appearance of osteopetrosis tarda. Diffuse sclerosis is seen in osteoblastic metastases Hodgkin's disease and third stage Paget's disease.

The intervertebral disk may show loss of height, contain gas or calcification. Localized narrowing at one or more spaces may be caused by herniation of the nucleosus pulposus, disk degeneration, infection, congenital anomaly or atrophy accompanying fusion of the segmental apophyseal joints chronic diskitis and tuberculosis also result in reactive sclerosis. Generalized disk space narrowing with associated diskal calcification is suggestive of ochronosis. Localized calcification of a disk may be idiopathic, post-traumatic or infectious. The presence of air in the disk vacuum phenomenonis a sign of disk degeneration.

The apophyseal joints of the spine may show narrowing and erosions in RA and AS, which progress to fusion. AS involves the lower spine, whereas RA predilects the cervical spine. Apophyseal joint fusion is accompanied by atrophy of the corresponding intervertebral disk. OA of the facet joints cause spur formation and hypertrophy, which can encroach the intervertebral foramina and lateral recesses—best seen on MR imaging. Vacuum sign can be seen on CT.

The atlantoaxial articulation is a critical area because of the subluxation occurring in several conditions. The most common cause is RA and is also commonly seen in Down's syndrome. In RA and IRA, erosions destruction, and fractures of the odontoid process may occur, as well as a large mass of pannus may form that encroaches the neural canal. MRI best demonstrates this region. Lateral radiography of the neck in flexion and extension can demonstrate atlantoaxial instabilty.

The paravertebral area can be involved by thick syndesmophytes in psoriatic. Arthritis and Reiter's syndrome. A soft tissue mass can occur in association with various diseases, including inflammatory and extramedullary hematopoiesis. A calcified paravertebral mass is typical of the tuberculous spondylitis or Pott's disease.

Section 10—Musculoskeletal System

Chapter 116

Muscle Tumors

1. Desmoids (Figure 116.1).
2. Rhabdomyoma.
3. Leiomyoma.
4. Rhabdomyosarcoma.
5. Leiomyosarcoma.

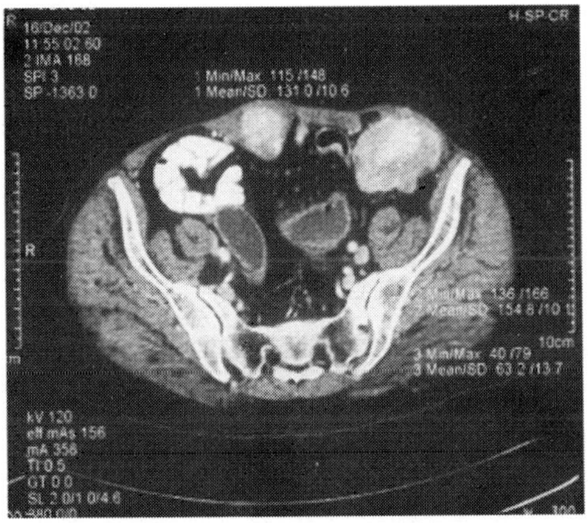

Fig. 116.1: Axial CT image shows multiple abdominal wall desmoid tumor

Desmoid

- Uncommon benign tumor but is locally aggressive and infiltrates contiguous structures and has a strong tendency to recur after resection.
- The most common location being mesentery, may also have a musculoaponeurotic origin especially from that of either the recti or internal and less commonly external oblique muscles.
- Peak incidence is in 3rd decade and is three times more common in females.
- Pathologically it is poorly defined and usually confined to musculature or its aponeurosis.
- Clinically it is a firm slowly growing deep-seated mass.
- May cause retraction, distortion, compression and kinking of bowel loops.
- On USG it may be hypo, iso or hyperechoic and is sharply defined and smoothly marginated.
- On CT it appears as an ill-defined or well-circumscribed mass and usually has attenuation higher than muscle. It may show enhancement on post contrast images.
- On MRI it is hypo intense to muscle on Tl weighted images and variable in intensity on T2 weighted images.

Rhabdomyoma and Rhabdomyosarcoma

- Seen usually in pediatric age group.
- Usually presents as a large mass in the retroperitoneum or muscles.
- Infiltrates the surrounding structures and may

also present with metastasis, usually blood borne.

- Lymph nodal metastasis may also occur.
- Very heterogeneous in appearance on imaging studies and may have areas of necrosis.
- Some post contrast enhancement is seen on CECT.

Leiomyoma and Leiomyosarcoma

- Usually presents as a moderately sized to large mass arising from the smooth muscles of the gut.
- Benign tumor, which may degenerate into malignant form especially in the retroperitoneum.
- On imaging studies it usually presents as a homogenous well-defined tumor showing diffuse contrast enhancement.
- The malignant form however may present with heterogeneous appearance with areas of necrosis and hemorrhage.

Soft Tissue Tumors

CLINICAL INFORMATION REQUIRED IN THE ASSESSMENT OF A SOFT TISSUE TUMOR

- Is the lesion painful?
- Is there a history of trauma?
- Has the lesion remained stable for long?
- Is there a history of a previous lesion or malignancy?
- Is the lesion solitary or multiple?

PURPOSE OF IMAGING

- Confirm the presence of the lesion.
- Precise site.
- Extent of the tumor.
- Detect neurovascular invasion.
- Cortical infiltration.
- Regional nodal metastasis.
- To aid biopsy.

CLASSIFICATION OF SOFT TISSUE TUMORS (Table 117.1)

IMAGING IN SOFT TISSUE TUMORS

- **Plain radiography**
  - Soft tissue swelling.
  - Displaced/hazy fat planes.
  - Calcification.
  - Phleboliths.
  - Bone involvement.
- **Computed tomography**
  - Size.
  - Site.
  - Extent.
  - Fat/calcific density.
  - Fibrous/neural tumors.
  - Contrast enhancement.
  - Necrosis and hemorrhage.
  - Radiotherapy treatment and planning.
- **Magnetic resonance imaging**
  - Exact size.
  - Location.
  - Compartment spread.
  - Tumor margin.
  - Signal intensity.
  - Enhancement characteristics.
  - Neurovascular invasion.
  - Bone infiltration/destruction.
  - Adjacent soft tissue.
  - Signal intensity.

Table 117.1: Different types of tumors

Presumed origin	Benign	Locally aggressive	Malignant tumors
Fibrocytes	Keloid	Desmoid tumor	Fibrosarcoma
Fibroblasts	Fibrous histiocytomas	Dermatofibrosa protuberans (DFSP)	Malignant fibrous histiocytoma (MFH) 1
Smooth muscle	Leiomyoma	-	Leiomyosarcoma
Striated muscle	Rhabdomyoma	-	Rhabdomyosarcoma
Fat cells	Lipoma Lipoblastoma Hibernoma	Well differentiated liposarcoma	Liposarcoma
Endothelial cells	Hemangioma	-	Angiosarcoma Kaposi's sarcoma
Nerves	Neural sheath tumors (Neurofibroma, schawannoma, granular cell tumor)	-	MPNST (Malignant peripheral nerve sheath tumor)
Neuronal cells	-	-	PNET's
Unknown	-	-	Synovial sarcoma

- US.
- Bone scintigraphy.
- Angiography.

PLAIN X-RAY IN SOFT TISSUE TUMORS

1. **Calcification** – Seen in:
   - Myositis ossificans – more at periphery, lacy pattern.
   - Hemangioma – Phlebothis.
   - Liposarcoma.
   - Soft tissue osteosarcoma.
   - Synovial sarcoma.
   - Soft tissue chondrosarcomas.
   - Fibroma.
   - MFH.
2. **Fatty component characteristic of LIPOMA.**
3. **Soft tissue swelling with well-defined margins** (Figures 117.1 and 117.2).

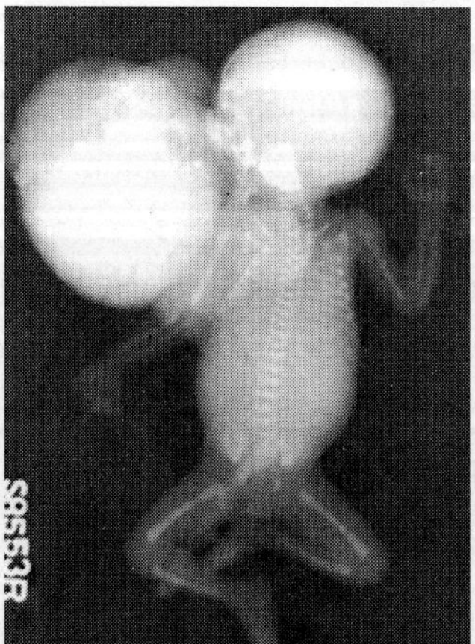

Fig. 117.1: Radiograph of the baby shows a large cystic hygroma

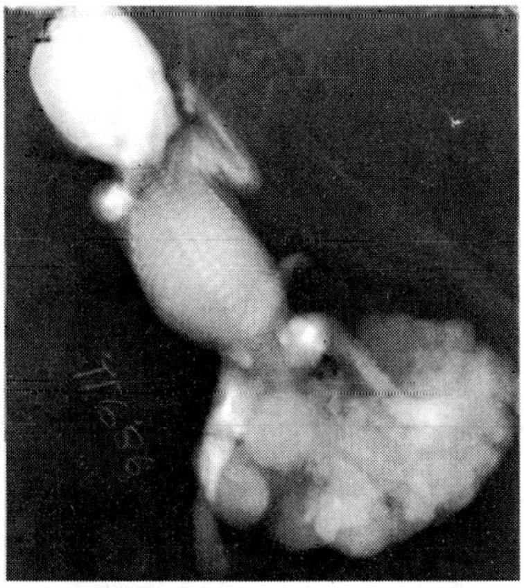

Fig. 117.2: Radiograph of the baby shows a large sacrococcygeal tumor

4. Bone involvement – as

Erosion and/or saucerisation.

- Extra osseous Ewing's sarcoma.
- Fibrosarcoma.
- MFH.
- PNET's.
- MPNST's.

US Findings

- Can tell the relation of a mass to adjacent nerves, vessel and bone.

  CT in soft tissue masses.

Lipoma

- Characteristic fatty component.
- Thin soft tissue capsule.
- Homogenous fatty density with few septae.
- Positive in subcutaneous fat.

Hemangioma

- Phleboliths.

  Areas of fatty tissue between and around the blood vessels with post contrast enhancement.

Neurofibroma

- Soft tissue density lower than the muscle.
- Well-defined oval/rounded masses.

DESMOID TUMOR

- CT attenuation higher than soft tissues 100-200 HU.

MALIGNANT SOFT TISSUE MASSES

- Lobulated, heterogenous density soft tissue masses with variable contrast uptake and areas of necrosis and hemorrhage being more common.

MRI IN SOFT TISSUE TUMOR

- Signal intensity pattern on T1W images.

1. Homogenous Low Signal Intensity (SI)

- Cyst.
- Ganglion.
- Lymphocele.
- Cystic hygroma.
- Myxoma.
- Myxoid sarcoma.

2. Moderate to High SI

- Lipoma.
- Subacute hematoma.
- Well differentiation liposarcoma.
- Lipoma arborescens.
- Elastofibroma.
- Intralesional hemorrhage.
- Fibro lipo hematoma.
- Melanoma.

3. Slight Increased SI

- Neurofibroma.
- Hemangioma.
- Abscess.
- Solid malignancies.

Low SI on T2W Image

- Fibrous lesions
  - Plantar fibroma.
  - Morton's neuroma.
  - Fibromatosis.
- MFH.
- MPNST.
- PVNS.
- GCT's of tendon sheath.
- AVM's.
- Chronic hematoma.
- Amyloid.
- Gouty trophus.

Peripheral N. Tumors are:

- Fusiform in shape.
- Decreased echogenicity than the normal nerve.
- Increased through transmission.
- Pseduocapsule in malignant forms.

SYNOVIAL SARCOMA AND MYXOID LIPOSARCOMA APPEAR

- Cyst like.
- Hypoechoic masses.

PVNS

- Typically hypoechoic.
- Very vascular.

Lipoma

- Hyperechoic/hypoechoic/isoechoic/mixed.
- Elongated shape.
- Oriented parallel to skin.
- Well marginated, rarely poorly defined.

Hemangioma

- On CDFI – feeder/draining vessels.
- Phleboliths.

MALIGNANT SOFT TISSUE TUMOR (Figures 117.3 and 117.4)

- Typically ill marginated.
- Hypoechoic necrotic areas.
- Peripheral vascularity; calcification; +/-.

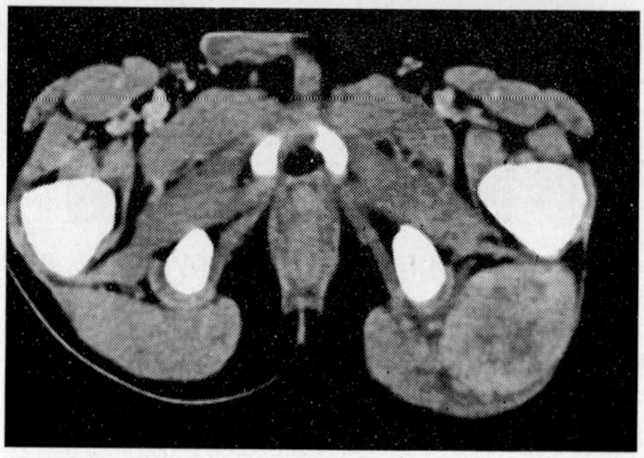

Fig. 117.3: Axial CT image showing a well defined, enhancing soft tissue tumor in the left gluteal region

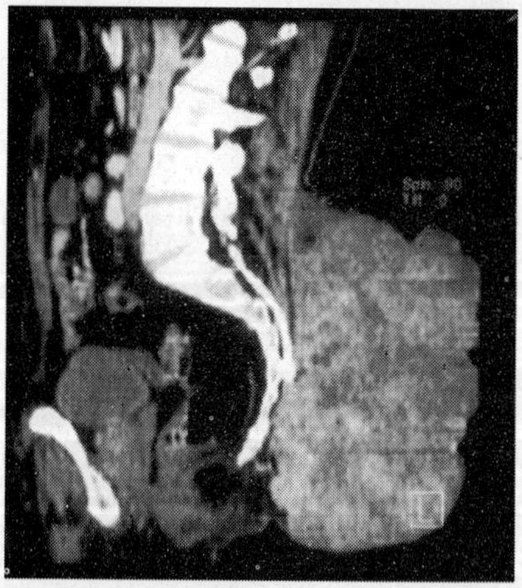

Fig. 117.4: Sagittal MPR CT image shows a large soft tissue tumor in the sacrococcygeal region

Sarcomas (Figure 117.5)

- Comprise most pediatric solid tumors.
- Infiltrate and invade surround tissues.
- Capacity to metastasize.
- Are originated from more primitive precursor cells.

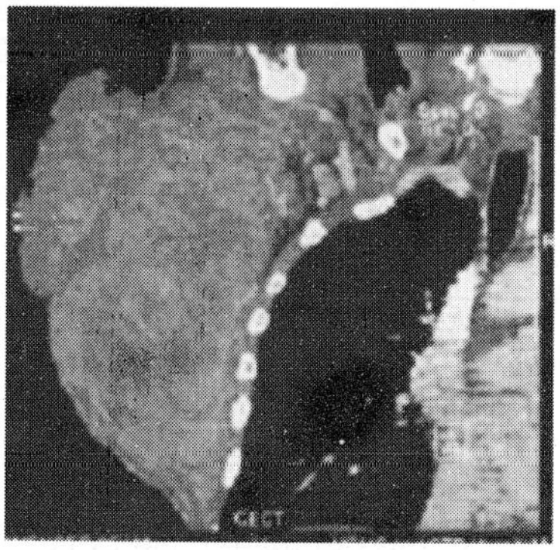

Fig. 117.5: Coronal MPR CT image shows a large soft tissue sarcoma in the right shoulder region

- 3 broad categories:
  1. Round cell sarcoma
     - Common in childhood.
     - Rapid growth rate.
     - E.g. rhabdomyosarcoma.
       PNET's.
       Extra osseous Ewing's sarcoma.
  2. Spindle cell sarcomas
     - Common in adulthood.
     - Slower growth rate.
     - E.g. leiomyosarcoma.
       MPNST's.
       MFH.
  3. ODD sarcoma types
     - Idiosyncratic types.
     - Indecent course often deadly.
     - E.g. angiosarcoma.
       Kaposi's sarcoma.

SPINDLE CELL SARCOMAS

Malignant Fibrous Histiocytoma

- Male: Female=1.5:1.
- 2-8th decades.
- Most common malignant soft tissue tumor seen in adults.
- 5-year survival rate 60-70%.
- Histologically contains both histiocytic and fibroblastic cells.
- Usually – large.
  Necrosis and hemorrhage are common.

Leiomyosarcoma

- Smooth muscle origin.
- Sites – uterus.
  GIT.
  - Retroperitoneum.
  - Extremity.
  - Size – small to very large.

MALIGNANT PERIPHERAL NERVE SHEATH TUMORS

- Also known as – neurofibrosarcomas.
  - Malignant schwannomas.
- 4-5% of patients with neurofibromatosis have MPNST's.
- Highly malignant tumors.
- 5-year survival rate – 50-70%.
- Extremity tumors have favorable prognosis than those on the trunk retroperitoneum/ mesentry.

ODD SARCOMA TYPES

Liposarcoma

- Common in adults; very rare in children.
- Large bulky masses.
- Sites – thigh/retroperitoneum.
- Histo types:
  - Myxoid.
  - Non-myxoid /round cells and pleomorphic types.

Synovial Sarcoma

- Mostly present in young individuals.

- Misnomer – do not arise from synovial cells.
- Tendons, joints or bursae.
- Small or large.
- Calcification common.
- Prognosis poor – hemat. metastasis.
- Known as carcinosarcoma of soft tissues.

Epitheloid Sarcoma

- Arise in distal portions of the extremities.
- Slow growing.
- Along the length of the tendon.
- Dermatofibrosarcoma protuberans.
- Fibrosarcoma.
- Angiosarcoma.
- Kaposi's sarcoma.

PROGNOSIS OF SARCOMAS

Prognosis depends on:

1. Histologic subtype grade I-III.
2. Staging of tumor I-III.
3. Depth.
4. Size.

SARCOMAS TYPICALLY METASTASIZE HEMATOGENOUSLY

Nodes involvement is seen in:

- Synovial sarcoma.
- MFH.
- Round cell sarcomas.

Rhabdomyosarcoma

- Most common childhood sarcoma.
- Histologic subtypes:
  - Embryonal RMS < 6 years.
  - Sarcoma boryroides – very young.
  - Alveolar RMS – 10-25 years.
  - RMS in older adults – 4-7th dec.
- Bimodal age distribution.

PNET's /Neuroepithelioma

- On chest wall known as a skin tumors.
- Age between 5-15 years.

Extra Osseous Ewing's Sarcoma

- Resembles PNET's.

Section 11—Miscellaneous

Chapter 118

Splenic Lesions

CYSTS

1. Infective.
2. Primary congenital cysts.
3. Post traumatic.
4. Intrasplenic pancreatic pseudocyst.

Splenic Tumors

I. Benign

1. Hemangioma.
2. Lymphangioma.
3. Splenic hamartomas.

II. Malignant

1. Lymphoma.
2. Fibrosarcoma.
3. Angiosarcoma/hemangioendothelioma.
4. Leiomyosarcoma.
5. Malignant teratoma.
6. Malignant fibrous histocytoma.

III. Metastasis.

Splenic Infections

- Solid nodular masses.
- Splenic abscess.
- Splenic trauma
  - Intraparenchymal hematoma.
  - Subcapsular hematoma.
  - Pericapsular hematoma.

Misc.

- Sarcoidosis.
- Hemochromatosis.
- Amyloidosis.
- Splenic involvement in pancreatitis.

Commonly pseudocyst following old hematoma or infarcts.

INFECTIVE CYSTS

- Usually hydatid though spleen is least common site.
- 2/3rd of all splenic cysts.
- In 75% of cases have foci of infection elsewhere.
- Symptom is related to large size and complications.

U/S

- Large multiloculated cystic mass, solid central nidus and thick ectocyst wall.

- Detachment of germinal layer may produce floating membrane.
- Superinfected or partially treated hydatid appear solid.
- Long-standing cyst may calcify.

CT

- Well-circumscribed non-enhancing low density lesions.
- Cyst wall calcification better appreciated.

MRI

- T1W1 – hypointense.
- T2W1 – hyperintense - to liver parenchyma.
- 75% cases heterogeneous SI.
- Daughter cyst give slightly—SI than parent cyst on T1W1.
- A continuous 4-5 mm thick low intensity rim surrounding the cyst.

CONGENITAL EPITHELIAL CYST (EPIDERMOID, MESOTHELIAL)

- Thought to arise from embryonic rests of primitive mesothelial cells.
- 20% of non-parasitic cyst.
- Childhood or in early adult life, >common in male.
- 80% solitary and unilocular.

U/S

- Epithelial cysts often have uniform echogenic fluid content from secretions and exfoliation of lining membrane.

CT

- Spherical sharply circumscribed water density lesion without any central/rim enhancement after contrast.
- Cyst wall trabeculation or peripheral septatations.
- Cyst wall occasionally calcify.

POST TRAUMATIC CYSTS (Figure 118.1)

- Represent the final stage in cases of splenic hematoma.
- Not lined by epithelium referred to pseudocyst.
- On CT appear as sharpy demarcated lesion, are unilocular, show no enhancement and certain fluid of density similar to slightly above that of water.
- Non-parasitic cyst may present as LUQ mass, sense of epigastric fullness of intermittent dull pain.

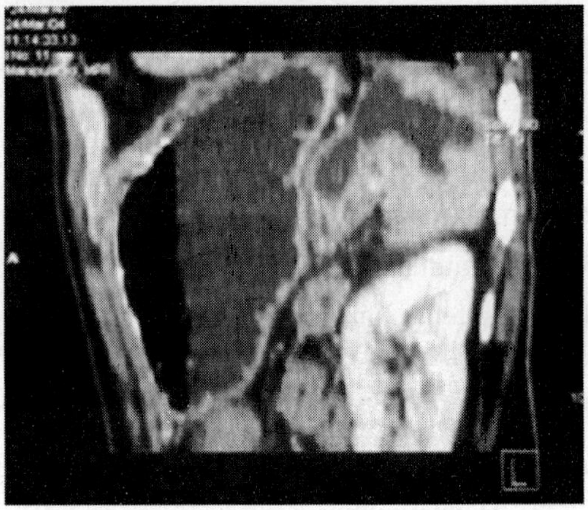

Fig. 118.1: Sagittal MPR CT image shows splenic pseudocyst secondary to pancreatitis

D/D

Abscess, acute hematoma, intrasplenic pancreatic pseudocysts, cystic neoplasm, lymphangioma.

SPLENIC TUMORS

Lymphomas

- Most common primary malignancy.
- Rare, 1 to 2% of all lymphoma.
- Usually NHL small cell type B cell origin.
- Secondary splenic involvement in HD and NHL is frequent with lymphoma, most common splenic malignancy.

- At time of diagnosis 1/3 to 1/4 of patients of HD and NHL present with splenic involvement.
- In NHL associated paraortic node infiltration seen in 70% cases.

VARIOUS FORMS OF INVOLVEMENT

a. Homogeneous enlargement – low-grade lymphomas.
b. Miliary nodules – small cleaved, mixed cell types, lymphocytic lymphomas.
c. Multifocal lesions of size 1-10 cm.
d. Solitary mass
   - Large cell lymphoma produces either solitary or multiple masses.
   - HD can cause solitary or multiple mass or miliary pattern.
   - Necrosis of large lesion can give cystic appearance.
   - Calcifcation reported in aggressive lesions and after treatment.

U/S

Focal lesions are well-defined rounded poorly echogenic with occasional focal echogenic areas.

Diffuse involvement difficult to detect.

CT

- Focal lesions show ↓ attenuation than normal splenic parenchyma.

MR

- Unenhanced – no significant change on T1 and T2 valves.
- Post contrast T1 and T2 WI – lesions isointense with splenic parenchyma.
- Assess of - and ↓ SI may be due to necrosis, hemorrhage, fibrosis or edema.
- IV contrast MR improve detectability of focal lesions.
- Agents specific for RE tissue (SPIO) improve ability of MR normal spleen from diffuse splenic lymphoma.
- Markedly enlarged spleen (weight - than 400-500 kg) almost always shows lymphomatous involvement.

OTHER PRIMARY SPLENIC MALIGNANCY: VASCULAR TUMORS MOST COMMON OF MESENCHYMAL TUMORS

Angiosarcoma

- Cause by exposure of thorotrast.
- Symptoms include abdominal pain, LUQ mass, fever, weight loss, anemia and consumptive coagulopathy.

CT

- Focal rounded or irregular areas of heterogenous ↓ attenuation.
- Cystic and necrotic areas are evident.

Angiography

- Multiple vascular lakes observed mimicking cavernous hemangioma.

MALIGNANT FIBROUS HISTOCYTOMA

- Described as large mass with extensive areas of necrosis.

BENIGN TUMORS

Hemangioma

- Reported in 14% patient undergoing autopsy.
- Cavernous type more common.
- Usually isolated but may occur in association with stigmata of KTWS.
- Usually asymptomatic, less commonly present as abdominal pain and mass.
- Rupture and hemorrhagic 25% cases.

- Anemia, thrombocytopenic and consumptive coagulopathy (Kesalback Merrette syndrome) have been noted.

U/S

Variable

The lesion has well defined echogenic appearance, however lesions of mixed echogenicity with cystic spaces are also noted.

CT

NECT: Well defined hypodense mass that may contain cystic components.

CECT: Lesions may remain hypodense or show peripheral enhancement though centripetal filling may not be seen on delayed scan.

Calcification occur as scattered punctatic curvilinear densities or dense rays from central portion.

MR

T1W1 – Hypo to isointense with respect to spleen.

T2WI – Hyperintense.

Heterogeneous SI reflecting presence of cystic or solid component with varying amount of fibrosis, necrosis and hemorrhage is noted.

Lymphangioma

- Single or multiple.
- Asymptomatic or discovered as LUQ mass.

U/S Features same as hemangioma.

CT Well marginated cysts often subcapsular.

No enhancement noted with CT attenuation 15-35 HU curvilinear calcification noted.

Hamartoma

- Rare benign lesions, reported as rare manifestation of TS.
- Composed of anomalous mixture of normal splenic elements with predominance of red pulp.
- Single or multiple, size ranging <1 to >15 cm.
- Detected incidentally or because of mass symptoms.

CT

NECT: Iso to hypodense occasionally showing cystic components.

CECT: Show enhancement with prolong enhancement similar to that of hemangioma.

MR

T1W1: Isointense.

T2W1: Hyperintense.

INFLAMMATORY PSEUDO TUMOR

- Rare benign lesions consisting of polymorphs inflammatory cell infiltrate with varying amount of granulomatous reaction fibrosis to necrosis.
- Asymptomatic or present as more accompanied by vague constant symp.
- Etiology uncertain. Infection/autoimmune origin is speculated.

CT

- Well-circumscribed heterogenously hypodense encapsulated mass. They range 1.5-14 cm in diameter.
- Usually solitary but can be multiple.
- Progressive enhancement after IV contrast is noted although persistent cases of hypodensity due to fibrosis noted.
- Pressure of central stellate area of hypodensity (scar) is suggestive.

MR

- T1W1 – Slight hyperintense.

  T2WI – More marked hyperintense with mild to mod enhancement after contrast.

Metastases

- Unusual and generally occur as a late phenomenon rather presenting feature.
- Most common route hematogenous with most common primary breast and lung.
- Melanomer highest frequency of splenic involvement or per primary basis with 34% of melanoma patients showing splenic mets on autopsy.
- Most common occur as multiple nodule although diffuse unit in 8-10%.
- Usually asymptomatic.

U/S: Usually hypoechoic but may be echogenic or have mixed echogenicity.

CT: Nodular mets rounded hypodense lesions.

- Cystic lesion occur from ovary, breast, endometrium and melanoma.
- Peritoneal implant in case of ovarian carcinoma, GIT or pancreatic carcinoma cause scalloping of capsular surace of spleen.
- Direct spread rare, primary in stomach, colon, pancreas and kidney.

SPLENIC INFECTION

- Occur as a single focus or a part of a diffuse or miliary process. There are increased number of cases as a result of increased prevalence of immunosuppression in cancer patients, transplantation patients and AIDS.
- Hematogenous dissemination with predisposing primary infection like endocarditis, UTI, surgical wound infection, appendicitis and pneumoni.
- Direct spread – Carcinoma descending colon and penhepatic abscess.
- Non-infections predisposing factors include diabetes, SCA, immunosuppression.

SPLENIC ABSCESS

- Present clinically with fever and pain in either LUQ or (L) chest or referral pain.
- Most common presentation is splenomegaly.
- Most common organism staph and strepto (10-20%), salmonella and E. coli also common anaerobic—5-17%.
- Mycobacteria, candida, P. carinii also occur with prevalence of immunosuppression, fungal infection more frequent (25%).

US

- Appearance similar to simple cyst but clinical findings aid in diagnosis.
- Gas is present frequently within abscess cavity which appear as PAS/Ring down artifacts.

MULTIPLE NODULES

- Also found in patients with splenic infection ESP in immunocompromised.

U/S

- Hepatosplenic candidasis present as 'WHEEL within WHEEL' appearance but nodule may have bull eye appearance or many by hypo/hyperchoic.
- TB present as solid focal hyperechoic lesions with or without shadowing.
- Miliary TB appears as tiny echogenic foci diffusely scattered.
- In active TB hypoechoic or cystic lesions representing TB abscess is noted.
- Fungal infection due to HISTOPLASMOSIS have similar appearance as TB but lesions have miliary multifocal and multiloculated.

CT

- Splenic abscess appear as non enhanching area of ↓ attenuation.

- Rim of abscess is iso dense and enhance after contrast.
- In miliary abscess typical of fungal pre and post contrast images preferred.
- 64% of multilocular abscess have fungal etiology and unilocular bact (99%).

Calcification (Figure 118.2)

- Noted in treated candida microabscess and lesion caused by other fungi, mycobact and p. carinii infection.

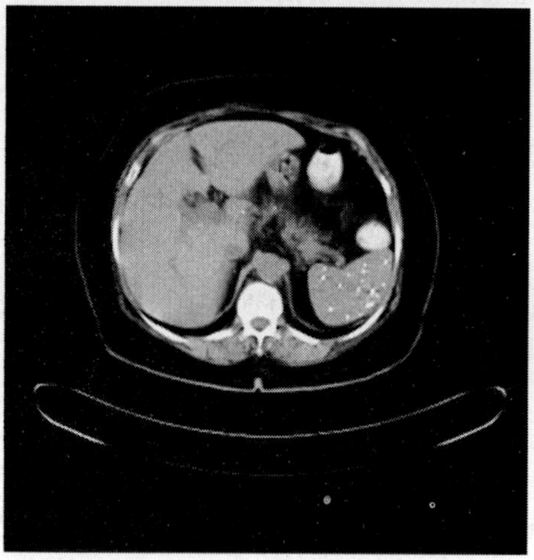

Fig. 118.2: Axial CT image shows multiple fccus of calcification in the splenic parenchyma

MR

- Splenic candidiasis → Low SI on T1W1.
  High SI on T2W1.
- No enhancement after gadolinium. Early post contrast T1W1 of spoled GE imaging is most sensitive.

SPLENIC INFARCTION

- One of the most common causes of focal splenic lesion.
- Occur as a result of embolic disease of cardiac and atherosclerotic origin and in patients with arteritis; myeloproliferative disease; pancreatitis; SCA.
- Small infants asymptomatic. However large infarct cause LUQ pain, fever and diaphragmatic irritation.

U/S

- Typical wedge shaped hypoechoic lesion byt may have nodular appearance or appear hyperechoic as fibrosis progresses.

CT

- Most commonly sharply marginated hypodense wedge shaped region with the base at splenic capsule and apex at hilum. They may be poorly marginal.
- With infarction of entire spleen i.e. after avulsion or occlusion of splenic artery, there is failure of contrast enhancement of all but parenchyma subadjacent to capsule called 'RIM SIGN' and is due to arterial supply from capsular vessels.
- Lack of splenic parenchyma enhancement without infarction occurs in setting of profound hypotension.
- In massive splenic infarction gas bubbles appear in uninfected parenchyma confusing with abscess.

MR

- Hemorrhagic infarct high SI on T1 and T2 WI.

  In SCA patients have repeated episodes of infarction with acute splenic sequestration crisis is characterised sudden massive splenomegaly.

SPLENIC TRAUMA

- Most common injured abdominal organ.
- Injury occur as a result of blunt or penetrating injury.
- Take in form of laceration, intrasplenic hematoma, subcapsular hematoma or infarction.

U/S

- Very useful and highly accurate in diagnosis of subcapsular and pericapsular hematoma and also intrasplenic hematoma.
- Timing of sonographic examination result of trauma is important.
- Immediately – hematoma is liquid so easily differentiated.
- After blood clots and for 24-48 hours – echogenicity of perisplenic clot similar to spleen parenchyma.
- Subsequently – blood liquefaction appear as irregularly marginated echogenic mass.
- Subcapsular hematoma – cresenteric and conforms contour of spleen while perisplenic hematoma appear as irregularly shaped collection.
- Intrasplenic hematoma – initially heterogenous area, subsequently hematoma may resolve and repeat scan show cyst at the site.

CT

- Splenic laceration – irregular linear area of hypodensity on CECT.
- Intrasplenic hematoma – Border area of hypodense non perfused splenic parenchyma on CECT and may appear hyperdense on NECT.
- Subcapsular hematoma – appears as crescent collection of fluid that indent or flatten underlying splenic parenchyma.

SPLENIC INFARCTS

- May appear as wedge shaped non perfused area extending to capsule.

MIRIVI'S CLASSIFICATION

Grade I	Capsular avulsion, superficial laceration(s) or subcap. hematoma <1cm.
Grade II	Parenchymal laceration(s) 1-3 cm deep central/subcap hematoma <3 cm.
Grade III	Lacerations >3 cm deep central/subcap hematoma (s) > 3 cm.
Grade IV	Fragmentation of 1 or more sections, devascularized spleen.

Miscellaneous.

AMYLOIDOSIS

- Result from deposits of extracellular fibrillar material in wide rarity of tissues and organs.
- Usually multisystem involvement, localized form reported.
- Splenic involvement common in both primary and secondary systemic disease with diffuse and homogenous enlargement (most common) however focal tumor like lesion is reported.

CT

- Reduced attenuation with focal or diffuse enhancement on contrast extensive splenic calcifications.
- MR ↓SI on T2WI.

PELIOSIS

- Rare condition associated with OCP's and anabolic steroids and also in patients with HIV infection.
- Blood filled spaces in spleen.

NECT – Hypodense lesions, may coalesce to form large multilocular mass with well-defined septae enhancement variable.

MR – SI varies depending on the state of contained blood.

Section 11—Miscellaneous

Chapter 119

Radiology of Adrenal Masses

Anatomy

- **Right:** Triangular, medial ring is largest superiorly and may be absent inferiorly, may be shaped like inverted V or Y. Relation – immediately posterior to IVC. It lies between crus of diaphragm and posteromedial margin of right lobe of liver.
- **Left:** More crescentic. Its anteromedial ridge is slightly convex that right.
  - Wings are shorter than right.
  - **Position:** Lateral or slightly post to aorta and lateral to left crus of diaphragm. It is posterior to lesser sac superiorly and posterior to pancreas inferiorly.

Average size

- l: 3-6 cm.
- b: 2-3 cm.

  Wt: 3-5 cm.

  Thickness: 2-6 mm.

  90% contributed by cortex.

In **USG:** Used most common in children therefore with high-resolution real time scanners. Right gland is demonstrated in 92%.

Left gland is demonstrated in 71%.

- **Cortex:** Echo poor.
- **Medulla:** Thin reflective structure in centre of cortex in 13% of adults.
- Neonatal adrenal is larger = 1/3 of kidney.

  ↓

  Due to thick cortex.

In **CT:** Left gland is more easily identical.

CLASSIFICATION OF ADRENAL MASSES

(Figures 119.1, 119.2 and 119.3)

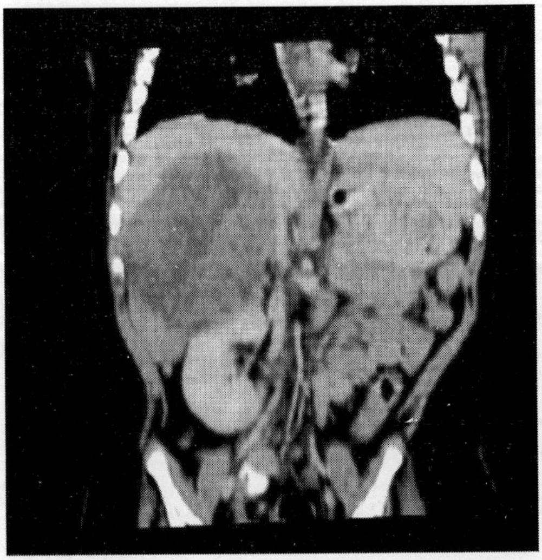

Fig. 119.1: Coronal MPR CT image shows a large right adrenal mass

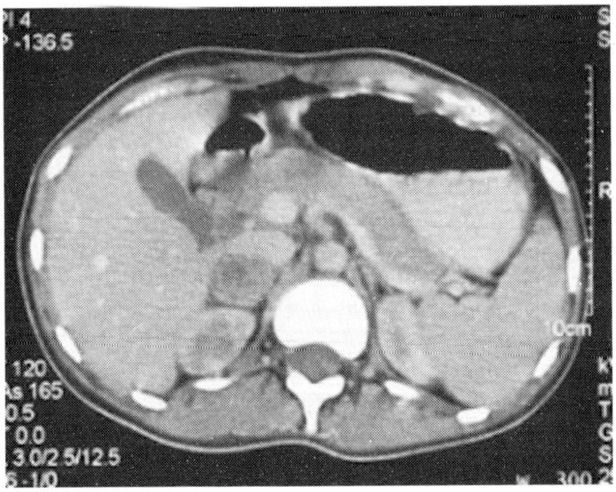

Fig. 119.2: Axial CT image shows adrenal adenoma on right side

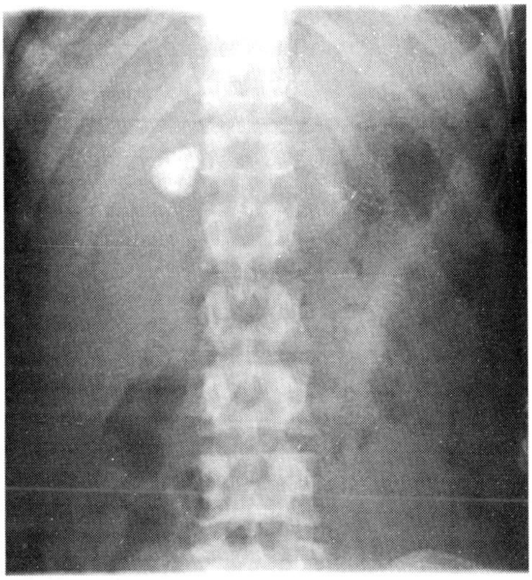

Fig. 119.3: Plain radiograph of the abdomen shows a calcified adrenal gland on right side

A. Neoplasm

- Cortical
  - Adenoma usually unilateral.
  - Carcinoma (±pd).
- Medullary
  - Neuroblastoma.
  - Phaechromocytoma.
  - Ganglioneuroma.
- Stromal
  - Lipoma.
  - Myolipomy.
- Metastasis
  - Most common with lung and breast 30-40%.
  - 10-20% melanoma.
    - GIT.
    - Lymphoma.
    - RCC.
- Other has:
  - Hemangioma.
  - Angiosarcoma.
  - Pre malignant melanoma.

B. Infection

Acute: Meningococcal or other forms of septicemia of little radiological importance.

Chronic: Granulomas.

- T.B.
- Histoplasmosis.
- Blastomycosis.

C. Hyperplasia

- Wolman disease (AR).
- Congenital adrenal hyperplasia (ped).
- Due to Conn's syndrome.
- Due to Cushing (hypercortisolim).

D. Cyst 'v' Unilateral

E. Hematoma/hemorrhage (uni or bilateral (+pd)

Adrenal pseudomas (E. simulate adrenal mass).

- Thickened diaphragmatic crus.
- Accessory spleen.

- Gastric fundus.
- Gastric diverticulum.
- Renal vein.
- Retrocrural and retroperitoneal adenopathy.
- Upper pole renal cyst and tumors.
- Pancreatic tumors.
- Hypertrophied caudate lobe of liver.
- Fluid filled colon interposed between stomach and kidney.

Investigations

MRI and CT: IOC.

Plain X-ray: Mass effect seen, displacing kidney (large mass).

- <5 cm mass not usually visualized.
- D/D renal cystic, accessory spleen, pancreatic mass.
- Liver mass, para aortic glands.
- IVP, retroperitoneal air insufflation, arteriography are now obsolete.
- Selective adrenal vein phlebography in both sides is very reliable method for demonstrating small tumors as occur in adrenal.

Pri: Hyperaldosteronism.

Complication: Adrenal infarction.

So occassionaly used for:

- Deliberate infarction of adrenal or small tumors.
- For venous hormone assay.

USG

For large tumors.

For infants + children.

And for pregnant women.

Small tumors or ectopic tumors can be missed.

CT

- IOC for small tumors even <1 cm and ectopic tumors as phaechromocytoma can be identified.
- Lipoma, myolipoma, adenoma, adenoma have higher lipid content (Low HU) so can be D/D from metas.

MRI

T1W1: Normal gland and tumors are hypointense.

T2W2: High signal intensity of tumors.

Contrast enhanced MR and chemical shift MR can differentiate adenomas and metastasis.

Adrenal Scintigraphy

Provide both anatomic localization and in vivo functional characterization of adrenal glands and masses due to accumulation with radiolabelled analogues of cholesterol e.g. 75 Se sclenomethyl nor cholesterol, NP-59 beta iodomethyl-19-nor cholesterol by function adrenal cortical tissue.

NP-59 is highly accurate in characterization by adrenal masses as adenomas vs non adenomas.

- Hyper secretory as well as non hyper secretory adenoma demonstrate NP-59 accumulation and scintigraphic visualization on side of CT scan detected adenomas greater than that seen in contralateral normal adrenal gland (cordant imaging pattern).
- PRI and mets. Tumors typically show declared a distorted or absent radio cholesterol uptake by the affected adrenal compared with contralateral normal adrenal gland (discordant imaging pattern). For setting of normal biochemical evaluation.
- NP-59 is 100% accurate predictor of adrenal adenoma whereas discordant imaging has been 100% accurate predictor of absence of simple non hyper secretory adrenal adenoma. Thus suggesting possibility of malignancy.

  (Demonstration of autonomously functioning adrenal (cortical) adenoma improved by dexamethasone suppression of residual normal cortex to increase tumor/background ratio).

- For adrenal medulla: Iodine 131 Meta iodobenzylguamidine (m1BG) is NA precursor analogue used in imaging adrenal medullary lesions especially in detection and characterization of phaechromocytoma and neuroblastoma and their metastasis.

Percutaneous biopsy: For histological confirmation.

A. Specific tumors

Approach to adrenal mass.

Mass is:

- Suspicious for malignancy.
- Pheochromocytoma.
- Inflammatory.

Rather than benign if following criteria are present.

Large = 5 cm Inhomogeneous ↑ed signal on T2W mass.

Intermediate Mass

= 3 cm: Follow up at 3/6/12 months.

Adenoma: 10% bilateral ↑ with age.

- Hyperfunctioning → Conn's segment and Cushing syndrome.
- Non-hyper functioning.

USG: If a larger size can be assessed by USG, particularly in right upper quadrant, causes retroperitoneal fat reflection displacement anteriorly (cap. hepatic and sub hepatic mass which displace it posteriorly.

CT: Typical features of benign adenoma:

1. Smooth contour.
2. Homogenous sharp margins.
3. Usually <3 cm.
4. <5 cm.

When these are to normal biochemical studies serial imaging with CT at 6 months interval for upto 2 years is often recommended.

Adenoma compsed of lipid rich cells, so unenhanced.

CT densitometry is very helpful in D/D adenoma with non-adenomas.

There is 73% sensitivity and 96% specificity for the diagnosis of adenoma using threshold of 10 HU as HU falls towards zero specificity increases reaching 100% at 2 HU.

- There is also role of "delayed contrast enhanced CT" to differentiate benign adenoma from non-adenoma washout of contrast material at the delayed times is assessed which shows loss of contrast enhancement and its relative percentage is greater for adenomas than non-adenomas.
- **Hyperfunctioning adenomas:** In Conn's syndrome are small, <2 cm, and low-density lesions frequently eccentric within gland.
- Hyperplasia as a cause of Conn's syndrome shows bilateral enlarged irregular adrenal glands.
- For equivocal loses 'adrenal venous sampling' is performed to aid in diagnosing a localization of disease process.
- 20% of Cushing syndrome is due to adenoma. These are larger (2-4 cm) than tumors of Conn's syndrome but giving same low density signal.

MRI

- In MRI most promising approach now is chemical shift imaging. Significant amount of lipid often present in adenomas and typically – present in most metastasis and other non-adenomas so there is decrease signal intensity of adenomas.
- In MR imaging adrenal SI normalized to that of spleen is used to calculate adrenal spleen ratio (ASR). This is used to combine the accuracies of unenhanced CT scan densitometry and chemical shift MR in D/D benign from malignant mass.

In this approach:

CT

- = 0 HU Benign.
- > 20 HU Likely malignant.

Intermediate 0-20 HU → for this gap ASR done gap.

ASR <70	ASR >70
Benign mass	Biopsy to rule out mets.

Adrenal cortical carcinoma:

- 4th decade
  - In 50% cases non-functional.
  - Left adrenal mass commonly involved.
  - Often large.

USG: **Hyperfunctioning tumor:** Smaller and homogenous, renal, similar to cortex.

Non-functioning – Large 'U; > 6 cm.

- More heterogenous.
- Areas of central necrosis.

4th decade

- In 50% cases non-functional.
- Left adrenal mass commonly involved.
- Often large.

USG: **Hyperfunctioning tumor:** Smaller and homogenous.

Renal.

Similar to cortex.

Non-functioning.

- Larger U >6 cm.
- More heterogenous.
- Areas of central necrosis, hg.
- 20% calcification.
- 27% echogenic thin zise seen.

CT: Large mass that usually envelops much of area surrounding the involved adrenal gland ± degeneration, cystic changes, 30% calcification.

CECT: Relatively vascular in certain areas.

MR: T1: ↓ S.I.

T2: ↑ S.I.

Adrenal Metastases

- Unilateral.
- Bilateral.

Adrenal very common site for metastases involved in lung 30-40% breast carcinoma, melanoma, GIT, renal and lymphoma 20%. Most are clinically silent necrosis. Hg± calcification is rare. Smaller <8 mm lesions can be missed in cross-sectional imaging.

In MR: Seen as high SI lesion in T2WI.

Staging of carcinoma – TNM.

T1 < 5 cm.

T2 5 cm.

T3 Tumor extending beyond gland not involving adjacent organ.

T4 Tumor extending beyond gland and involving adjacent organ.

NO Nodal.

N1 Local nodes involved.

Mo No mets.

M1 Metastases.

Lipoma and M: Benign

Rare non-functioning tumors (0.1-0.2%) composed mainly of fat cells ± myeloid tissue.

USG: Highly echogenic, bright hyper choice.

CT: Seen as fatty density.

MR: T1 is diagnostic with fat suppression sequences.

Phechromocytoma: 4-6 m decade (C-cells of chromatin cell of medulla).

Most common adrenal tumor observed clinically.

90% scene catecholamines (other Herman also PTH calcitron gastrin secretion ACTH).

(R) More involved.

The role of 10 consist of 10% cases are:

- Familial.
- Bilateral.
- Multiple.
- Extra adrenal most common site organ Zuckerkandal at Ao bifurcation.
- Children.
- Malignant.

Avg size: 7 cm (2-20 cm) well marginated.

- Calcification very rare, if very large undergo cystic necrosis, and cystic changes, which is well seen at USG/CT.

CT: Enhances uniformly after contrast administration (low osmolar contrast should be used to avoid hypertensive crises).

MR: Usually bilateral. These tumors are usually larger (>5 c), poor resolution not a problem.

T1: Iso to Hypo T2 with: ↑ SI.

MIBG scanning – Complementary in evaluating intra adrenal pathology, but extremely valuable in extra adrenal and recurrent phechromocytoma. MIBG is actively taken up in these catecholamine-secreting tumors.

Neuroblastoma: One of the most common tumors of childhood 82% <5 years of age and 1/3rd <2 years of age.

30% can arise from extra renal site as organ of zuckerkandl, thorac and neck.

MSG: Most commonly used as primary investigation.

Typically heterogenous with areas of high reflectivity which may represent calcification which is present in over > 50% of cases.

- It often cross midline, major vessels aorta and IVC may be surrounded and narrowed as well as elevated by tumor mass.

CT: Helps in staging by confirming local invasion liver metastases, spread to para aortic nodes.

MIBG scanning: Can show both primary tumors and metastases, which can be seen in bones, liver and orbits.

Ganglioneuroma is mature form of neurogenic tumor.

- Can arise from adrenal as well as extra adrenal from parasympathetic system elsewhere along spine.
- More common in children (<20 years).
- May show calcification, invade spinal canal.
- If the lesion present in child + calcification present in paraspinal mass and it should always be considered.

CT: Hypodense with punctate calcification.

Enhancement +ve.

MR:

T1WI.

T2WI - Intermediate.

Granuloma (Infection)

- Other than granulomas/TB/histoplasmosis/blastomycosis) are CMV, herpes, echinococcus, pneumocystis also infect adrenal gland.

TB: USG

Has a variable appearance, depending on stage of infection. Acutely there is bilateral diffuse enlargement often in homogenous ± punctate calcification chronically – gland become atrophic and calcified.

CT: Non-specific

Includes soft tissue masses, cystic changes/ irregular amorphous calcification.

C. Cysts: Rare, incidental findings, unilateral mostly.

- Endothelial in 45% (angiomatous, lymphangiomatous, hemastomatous).
- Pseudocyst 40% (clinically encountered most common).
- Epithelial 10%.
- Parasitic 5% (mostly echinococcal).

- Endothelial cysts are most often lymphangiomatous and contain clear fluid.
- Pseudocyst sac to hemorrhage into a normal adrenal gland/tumor.

USG: Same characteristic as cysts elsewhere in body with good through transmission. 15% display peripheral curvilinear calcification usually in pseudocyst and parasitic cyst.

Hemorrhage

- Acute Hg can follow overwhelming septicemia, in bleeding diasthesis, pregnancy, severe HT, in-patient with ACTH treatment, stress.

  Neonatal due to birth trauma, coagulation disorders and acute septicemia.

USG: In acute Hg bright echogenic masses in adrenal bed which become smaller and anechoic with time.

- It is one of the causes of enlarged adrenal in infancy with resolution focal areas of calcification will develop.
- In post traumatic (R) affected more than (L).

CT: Depending on the duration time between Hg and CT scan examination acute/sub-acute process may be seen, characteristic by regions of high attenuation (50 – 50 HU) within hematoma.

Streaky infiltration of periadrenal fat may also present.

Hyperplasia

- Congenital adrenal HP: Ar, due to in born error of metals in enzymatic production of cortisol or aldosterone.
- Infants born with ambiguous genitalated.

USG – Assess adrenal size as well as genital abnormalities.

Bilateral diffuses enlarged adrenal seen.

- Wolman disease – AR lipid storage disease.
- Characteristic by hepato splenomegaly and massive adrenal enlargement. Adrenal demonstrate diffuse calcification.

Section 11—Miscellaneous

Chapter 120

Intrauterine Growth Retardation (IUGR)

- IUGR is a common diagnosis is obstetrics and carries on ↑ed risk of perinatal mortality and morbidity.
- Identification of IUGR is crucial because proper evaluation and finally management can result in favourable outcome.

DEFINITION

- Most widely used definition of IUGR is "fetal weight below the 10th percentile of its gestational age". The cut off birth weight is 2500 grams.

Other definitions used in recent literatures are:

- AC <2nd, 3rd, 5th or 10th percentile or standardized growth charts.
- No increase in AC/HC on two consecutive scans done at least 2 weeks apart.
- HC: AC ratio > 2 SD.
- Fetal growth rates <10h percentile of an appropriate reference population.

PREVALENCE

- The overall prevalence of IUGR is 10%, however, it is not uniform. Population group in which mothers are healthy and well nourished have prevalence of 3-5% whereas in women with hypotension or a previous growth restricted fetus, the prevalence is 25% or higher.

INCIDENCE

- It varies depending upon the population.
- 4-8% of all infants born in developed countries and 6-10% in developing countries are growth restricted.

CAUSES OF IUGR

1. Fetal Factors

- Chromosomal abnormalities
  - Trisomy, 13, 18, 21.
  - Deletions.
  - Confirmed placental mosaicism.
- Congenital malformations
  - Absence of fetal pancreas.
  - Anecephaly.
  - Diaphragmatic hernia.
  - Omphalocele.
  - Gastrochisis.
  - Renal agenesis/dysplasia.
  - Multiple malformations.

- Multiple gestations
  - Monochorionic twins.
  - One fetus with malformation.
  - Twin-twin transfusion.
  - Discordant twices.
  - Triplets.

2. Placemental Factors

- Abnormal trophoblastic invasion.
- Multiple placental infarction (Chronic abruption).
- Umbilical-placental vascular anomalies.
- Abnormal cord insertion.
- Placenta pravia.
- Circumvallate placenta.
- Chorioangiomata.

3. Maternal Factors

- Genetic/constitutional.
- Nutrition/starvation
  - Inflammatory bowel disease.
  - Iliojejunal bypass.
  - Chronic pancreatitis.
  - Chronic pre pregnancy weight.
  - Poor pregnancy weight gain, 2nd and 3rd trimester.
- Hypoxic
  - Severe lung disease.
  - Cyanotic hem disease.
  - Sickle cell anemia.
- Vascular

  Chronic hypertension- Preeclampsia.
  - Collagen vascular disease—Type1 DM.
- Renal
  - Glomerunephritis—Lipid nephrosis.
  - Arteriolar Nephrosclerosis—Renal transplantation.
- Antiphospholipid albumin.
- Environment and drugs.
  - High altitude—Emotional stress – Physical stress.
  - Cigarette smoking –Alcohol abuse – Substance abuse (Heroin, cocaine).
  - Therapeutic drugs (antimetabolites, anti implants, anticonvulsants).
  - Pour obstetric history:
    - Previous stillbirths.
    - Previous IUGR birth.
    - Recurrent abortions.
    - Previous preterm birth.
- Of all the above-mentioned causes primary placental insufficiency is the most common cause of IUGR.
- 2 types of IUGR have been described:
  - Asymmetric.
  - Symmetric.

A. *Asymmetric IUGR*

- In this, not all fetal parts are decreased in size.
- Fetal abdomen is small due to ↑ fetal cellular hypertrophy and possibly of decreased glycogen storage in the liver. Head and extremities are normal or near normal in size (known as) head sparing type of IUGR.
- Common type among the two types and IUGR.
- Mostly caused by primary or secondary placental insufficiency.

B. *Symmetric IUGR*

- In severe and early onset cases, the fetal

is symmetrically small (including the head and extremities).

- Less common type.
- Results from an early insult such as a chromosomal anomaly or infection early in pregnancy.

These two can be differentiated using HC/AR ratio:

HC/AR Ratio

- Normal in symmetric IUGR.
- ↑ed in asymmetric IUGR.

Diagnosis

- One of the major requirements of accurate diagnosis of IUGR is an accurate calculation of gestational age. Assuming that data can be determined from LMP or early 1st trimester USG, the following are the ways to diagnose IUGR.

1. CLINICAL

- Maternal weight gain and fundal height may be used but there are not very sensitive and have a low positive predictive value.
- IUGR should be suspected if the maternal weight is inadequate or is decreasing.
- Height of fundal height of 4 cm or more? Strongly suggest IUGR.

2. ULTRASOUND/SONOGRAPHY

- Diagnose IUGR if the sonographically estimated weight falls below the 10th percentile for the gestational age. This requires 3 steps:
  - A gestational age is assigned to the fetus.
  - Fetal weight is estimated.
  - Weight percentile is calculated from estimated weight and gestational age.

This is known as straightforward approach.

GESTATIONAL AGE

Should be assigned at the time of 1st sonogram during the pregnancy. Thereafter, the gestational age should be assigned on the basis of the initial sonographic examination as the age at the 1st examination plus the number of weeks elapsed since.

- Gestational age is assessed by using:

  —CRL →T1.

  —HC, corrected BPD → T2 (corrected BPD) =

$$\sqrt{\frac{BPD \times OFD}{1.265}}$$

  —HC, corrected BPD, FL → T3.

- Accuracy of age assignment becomes progressively worse as pregnancy proceeds, from ± 0.7 weeks in T1 to ± 3 weeks in late T3. It has been suggested that the most accurate dating method is USG examination at 8-13 weeks.
- FETAL WEIGHT can be estimated by using measurements of a variety of fetal body parts. The overall accuracy improves with increasing number of body parts upto 3. No further improvement occurs adding 4th or 5th body part to the weight formula. The accuracy is such that the predicted weight will within 15-18% of the actual weight in 95% of cases.
- Once the gestational age and fetal weight have been estimated, the two values are assessed in relation to one another to determine the weight percentile for gestational age (Table 120.1).
- If an earlier sonographic examination was not performed, and the patient is fairly certain of 1st day of her last normal menstrual period, it is preferable to use this gestational age for determining weight percentile.

Table 120.1: IUGR as per percentile criteria

Gestational age	Weight percentile (10th)
25	490
26	568
27	660
28	765
29	880
30	1020
31	1171
32	1338
33	1519
34	1714
35	1919
36	2129
37	2340
38	2544
39	2735
40	2904
41	3042
42	3142
43	3195

ADDITIONAL SONOGRAPHIC CRITERIA FOR DIAGNOSING IUGR

These includes:

- HC/AC ratio:
  - It normally exceeds 1<32 weeks, is approx, 1 at 32-34 weeks and <1.0 after 34 weeks.
  - Not useful in symmetric IUGR as both HC and AC decreases.
- FL/AC ratio:

  FL/AC ratio >23.5 from 21 weeks onwards suggest the presence of IUGR.

Table 120.2: Sensitivity and specificity of different measurements

	Sensitivity	Specificity	PPV	NPV
↑HC/AC ratio	82%	94%	62%	98%
↑FL/AC ratio	34-49%	78-83%	18-20%	92-93%
↓AFV	24%	98%	55%	92%
Advanced placental grade	62%	64%	16%	94%

- Oligohydraminous without ruptured membranes:
  - Amniotic fluid index of <5 cm or a single vertical pocket of amniotic fluid <1cm is suggestive of IUGR.
  - Presence of advanced placental grade.
  - All the above parameters have low PPV but high NPV. This is due to low prevalence, not due to the excellence of the criteria for excluding IUGR.
  - Overall no single non-Doppler sonographic parameter permit confidant diagnosis of IUGR.

DOPPLER CRITERIA FOR DIAGNOSING IUGR

- Fetal, placental and uterus vasculature is assessed.
- In umbilical artery, rising ratio of systolic/ diastolic frequency reflects and increasing amount of impedance/resistance to the flow to placenta. This is due to ↑ed resistance as a result of reduced number of tertiary villous arteries, mostly resulting from material vascular disease such as hypertension. Decreased, absent or reverse diastolic flow are signs of worsening IUGR and has a very poor outcome.
- In uterine artery, an abnormal flow velocity waveform demonstrating a persistent diastolic notch beyond 24 weeks of gestation reflects

abnormal resistance downstream i.e. in the ultra placental vascular bed. Persistent abnormalities in those uterine artery waveforms have been seen with IUGR and are predictive of pre-eclampsia.

- In extreme cases of fetal hypoxia, a phenomenon known as 'brain sparing' is seen with dilatation of the fetal intracranial vessels, namely, MCA that provides protected blood flow to the brain at the expense of other organs. The presence of such compensation suggests a compromised fetus.
- Together, those three arteries have provided best Doppler information in the assessment of fetal IUGR and should become a routine part of IUGR assessment. However, the overall, sensitivity for DOPPLER prediction of IUGR tends to low (~ 40-80%).
- One additional vessel that may be informative in the presence of IUGR is the DUCTUS VENOSUS. The waveforms encountered in that vessels include 2 peaks, 1st and 2nd peak coinciding with ventricular systole and early diastole, when there is passive filling of ventricles. Following this 2nd peak is the "nidus" before the onset of next systole. This "nidus" of brief diminished forward flow coincides with atrial contractions during late diastole. Ductus venosus is identified in a sagittal/oblique sector through the upper fetal abdomen. It is seen as a continuation of the intra abdominal umbilical vein with a narrow inlet and wider outlet and connects to the IVC. Blood flow velocity recording is done with gate placed above the inlet of the ductus venosus.

In IUGR → when there is progressive hypoxia.

↓

Worsening of contractility of ventricles and atria.

↓

↓In the forward flow in ventricle and atria.

↓

In the size of the 1st and 2nd peak and ↓ or absent or reverse flows during atrial contractions i.e the nadir.

DIAGNOSIS OF IUGR USING MULTIPLE PARAMETERS

- With this technique, IUGR can be diagnosed most accurately using combination of 3 parameters:
  - Estimated weight percentile.
  - Amniotic fluid volume.
  - Material BP status (hypertension labelled when diastolic BP is = 90 mmHg or systolic BP= 140 mmHg or a rise in form of at least 15 or in latter of at least 30 mmHg).

DETERMINING THE CAUSE OF IUGR

- This includes assessment of both mother and father.

Material Evaluation

- History.
- Physical examination.
- Appropriate blood or other tests.

  (i.e. uncover causes of IUGR such as WT/T1 renal disease, collagen vascular disease.
- Previous viral illness or exposure to infectious agent during pregnancy.

Fetal Evaluation

- This is done by careful sonographic examination.
- If onset is IUGR is before T3 → chromosomal anamoly are suspected.
- Echogenic bowel, choroid plasma cyst or other structure anomalies.

  → Associated with anencephaly.
- Holoprosencephaly, omphalocele, polycystic kidney, congenital heart disease.

  → Trisomy 13.
- Clenched hand with overlapping index finger, rocker bottom foot, micrognathia, choroid

plexus cyst, diaphragmatic lesions, congenital Heart disease → Trisomy 18.

- Severe T2 IUGR + oligohydramnios – Triploidy.
- Hydrocephalus or microcephaly with intracranial calcification → Toxoplasmosis or CMV infection.
- If chromosomal cause is suspected, weight can be confirmed/excluded by determining the fetal karyotype vs USG guided amniocentesis or umbilical cord blood sampling. An infection origin can be compound by testing for immunoglobin is an umbilical cord blood sample.

MONITORING THE GROWTH RESTRICTED FETUS

- IUGR fetus should be delivered before term if risks associated with remaining in utero are greater than outside the uterus.
- If IUGR is diagnosed and lethal cause is excluded, fetus is monitored closely with sonography for remainder of pregnancy.
- Timing of USG depends upon severity and gestational age. Weekly or biweekly scans are done in T3 IUGRs.
- Sonographic features to be monitored include:
  - Fetal growth.
  - Biophysical profile score.
  - Amniotic fluid volume.
  - Spectral Doppler waveforms.
- Fetal measurements are taken not more than once a week.
- Biophysical profile induced test fetal hypoxia.

  Ac. hypoxia: Fetal gross body measurement, fetal breathing measurement, fetal tone and fetal heart rate.
- **Chr. hypoxia:** Amniotic fluid volume.

  Data suggests that biophysical profile surveillance of IUGR fetuses and prompt delivery when the profile score is low decreases the perinatal morbidity and mortality rates.
- Doppler imaging is of value for monitoring the pregnancy because it can provide evidence of fetal compromise. Elevation of umbilical artery S: D ratio or pulsatility index is a moderately accurate predictor or adverse outcome in IUGR fetuses. Decreased S: D ratio or pulsatility index of fetal MCA suggests fetal hypoxia because the fetal response to hypoxia is to decrease resistance which leads to increased blood flow to brain.

  Absent/reverse flow in umbilical artery suggests poor outcome and have prompt delivery must be seriously considered.

BIOPHYSICAL PROFILE

Non Stress Test

2 (NST2): 5 or more fetal heart rate acceleration of at least 15 bpm in amplitude and at least 153 cc duration associated with fetal measurements in a domain period.

1 (NST1): 2 to 4 accleration of a least 15 bpm and at least for 15 second in domain period.

0 (NST0): 1 or less acceleration in domain period.

Fetal Movements

2 (FM2): At least three gross (truck and limbs) episodes of fetal movements within 30 min; simultaneous limb and trunk movements were counted as a single movement.

1 (FM1): One or two movement in 30 min.

0 (FMO): Absence of fetal movement in 30 min.

Fetal Breathing Movements

2 (FBM2): At least one episode of fetal breathing

11

Section

movements at least 60 sec duration with 30 minutes observation periods.

1 (FBM1): At least one episode of fetal breathing lasting for 30 to 60 seconds within 30 minutes.

0 (FBM0): Absence of septal breathing or breathing <30 seconds within 30 minutes.

Fetal Tone

2 (FT2): At least one episode of extension of extremities with return to primary and also one episode of extension of spine with retention to flexion.

1 (FT1): At least one episode of extension of extremities with return to flexion or one episode of extension of spine to flexion.

0 (FTO): Extremities in extension, fetal movements not followed by return to flaxion; open hand.

Amniotic Fluid Volume

2 (AF2): Fluid evident throughout the uterine cavity; a pocket that measures 2 cm or more in vertical diameter.

1 (AF1): A pocket that measurres <2 cm but more than 1 cm vertical diameter.

0 (AF0): Crowding of fetal small parts; largest > pocket <1 cm in vertical diameter.

Doppler USG Examinations

Uterine Arteries

- The major arterial supply to uterus is through the uterine artery, a branch of anterior division of internal iliac artery.
- Doppler volumetry is done, where the cross-over between the large iliac vessels and the uterine artery can be easily visualized in real time colour imaging.
- In pregnant uterus, a progressive transition from a low volume high resistance to high volume low resistance circulation becomes established by the 1st trimester.
- Apart from changes of vascular impedance and flow, a very important change seen in uterus the disappearance of an early diastolic notch during early T2.
- Presence of diastolic notch and ↑ed RI or PI with advancing gestation are indicator of ↑ed uterine resistance and impaired uterine blood flow.
- The reference range of PI and RI are as follows:

GRAPH OF UTERINE ARTERY P1 AND UTERINE ARTERY R1

Umbilical Arteries (UA)

- The volume flow in the uterine artery's ↑es the high vascular impedance, ↑es gradually with advancing gestation.
- A substantial—in the existence of feto placental unit lead in—in EDY or its absence. Those changes determines the transplacental O_2 transfer to fetal and leads to IUGR.
- Index like S/D ratio, RI and PI have been used to assess UA flow velocity.

S/D ratio was abandoned, given absent EDV; S/D ratio will not be measurable. However, S/D ratio should be <3 in normal fetuses. With absent EDV, RI value will become maximum i.e. 1. So, PI seems to be the most clinically relevant index to use.

GRAPH SHOWING UMBILICAL ARTERY PI

Middle Cerebral Artery (MCA)

- The PI in MCA disease during the latter weeks of gestation.

GRAPH SHOWING MCA PI

- In response to hyperemia on fetus, there is redistribution of flow which favours the brain, myocardium, and adrenal gland at the expense of viscera.
- During the pregnancy, there is continuous flow in all the cerebral arteries throughout the cardiac cycle.
- In SGA foetuses, hence the PI is lower and mean systolic velocity is higher as compared to normal foetuses. However this is transitory with worsening of hypoxemia. PI tend to rise which may be attributable to development of brain edema.
- Transition from low impedes to high impedance flow with reverse diastolic component may precede IUD.

Section 11—Miscellaneous

Chapter 121

Tissue Harmonic Imaging

INTRODUCTION

It is a well-known phenomenon that in tissue ultrasound imaging suffers from significant, lateral and contrast resolution losses due to the defocusing (or phase aberration) effects, produce (by inhomogenities in the tissue. The decrease of lateral and contrast resolution is associated with the increase in the width of the main beam and the increase in side lobe levels, respectively. This loss of resolution has represented a significant hurdle to improving the clinical utility of ultrasound images.

A new approach, Tissue Harmonic Imaging (THI), uses the nonlinearity of the propagating beam in tissue, making it possible to correct these defocusing effects. In combination with advanced signal processing techniques, the ultrasound image is based on the received nonlinearly generated higher harmonics associated with the transmitted signal. Harmonic imaging was first developed to further enhance the blood flow detection sensitivity in color and power doppler applications using echo enhancing contrast agents. Based on research results using Contrast Harmonic Imaging (CHI) the possibility was investigated that harmonic imaging would also improve B mode imaging without the use of a contrast agent, particularly in difficult-to-image patients. Since the introduction of Tissue Harmonic Imaging it has become apparent, that this new technology can increase spatial and contrast resolution over conventional B-mode imaging not only on obese patients but also in many other applications.

Physical and Technical Principles (Figure 121.1)

Harmonic imaging is based on the fact that echo signals received from structures in the body carry not only the frequencies of the original transmit pulse, but also include multiples, or harmonics of these frequencies. Echoes from tissue as have predominantly linear components, i.e. the echo frequencies are the same as the transmit frequencies. These linear components are used in conventional, fundamental D-mode imaging.

(A) (B)

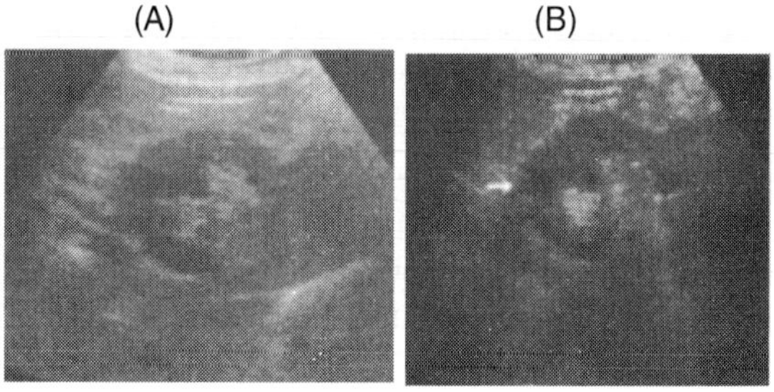

Fig. 121.1: (A) Small hemorrhagic cyst of left kidney. Fundamental B-mode sonogram shows hypoechoic lesion. (B) Tissue harmonic image is better quality overall than A and has fewer scattering artifacts. Solid portion of lesion can be differentiated from fluid-filled part (*arrow*) with higher diagnostic confidence. Distinct distal acoustic enhancement is visible

So in linear imaging:

F receives = f transmits.

Non-linear effects cause harmonic echo frequencies during the propagation of ultrasound in tissue. Therefore in non-linear imaging:

F receives = f transmits + f2 transmit + f3 transmit.

Where:

F2 = 2nd harmonic.

F3 = 3rd harmcnic frequency.

THI is based on the effect that ultrasound signals are distorted while propagating through tissue with varying acoustic properties. A sound wave propagating through the body is in fact a pressure wave. This pressure wave compresses and relaxes the tissue. As the pulse propogates through the target media, a fundamental change occurs in the shape and therefore the frequency of the transmitted signal. This distortion of the waveform causes harmonics to be generated. The harmonic effect in tissue is accumulative and builds up with increasing penetration depth, i.e. the harmonic amplitudes increase with depth. For this reason THI will be most efficient in the mid to far range before absorption limits its penetration. In tissue harmonic imaging, second harmonic is the frequency used.

There are two harmonic imaging methods. In conventional frequency-based 2nd harmonic imaging the receive frequencies are selected to be twice the transmit - frequencies. The frequency spectrum of an echo from a narrow band transmits. In addition to the fundamental echo frequency (centered at on a relative scale) 2nd and 3rd harmonics are generated at relative frequencies 2 and 3, but with lower amplitudes. In order to separate the fundamental from the harmonic efficiently, a narrow transmit frequency bandwidth must be selected. This will reduce spatial resolution. A high pass or narrow band pass filter must also be used to separate the strong fundamental echo components from the harmonic components. This results in a loss of contrast resolution due to the inherent overlap of the fundamental echo with the harmonic signal. The conventional method therefore has the shortcoming of both, reduced spatial resolution and contrast resolution.

Unlike such a conventional method, a new Wide Band Harmonic Imaging method, which is based on a patented phase inversion technique. With this method the full bandwidth of the transducer is utilized to receive all echo signals dynamically optimized for best image quality at each imaging depth. The Phase Inversion technique is based on the digital signal processing capabilities of the ultrasound system two consecutive pulses are transmitted into the body, with the phase of the second inverted relative to the phase of the first. When the echoes from these transmitted pulses are added together, the echoes from linear body structures effectively cancel each other, whereas echoes from non-linear structures do not. The result of adding the echoes is illustrated by the spectral representation. As a result of the 180 degree phase difference, the fundamental and odd harmonic signal components are effectively suppressed, whereas the even harmonic components, in particular the second harmonic component, are amplified. The result is B-mode images with superior contrast and spatial resolution, exceeding the performance of conventional imaging.

The impact of this technique on the imaging performance which compares the relative lateral beam profiles of the fundamental and the harmonic signals. Side lobes, which are responsible for artifacts affecting image quality particularly in obese patients, and in other difficult imaging conditions are significantly reduced compared to conventional imaging. The narrower beam width results in better lateral resolution. In addition, the wide band technique ensures that axial resolution is maintained. Images appear sharper and crisper, with less noise and with higher contrast resolution.

Tissue Harmonic Imaging also Relies on Two Other Basic Concepts

Time and Distance Travelled

Time is the critical factor in that the signal pulse must travel (propagate), a certain distance for the physical change in the sound wave (frequency) to occur. This time elapsed and the distance results in a sweet spot in the image at which the harmonic generation will be optimal. Therefore in most of the cases the near and the far fields of an image are less affected by the harmonic than the sweet spot.

Filtration of the Unwanted Frequencies

Filtration of the unwanted frequencies must be done to return the precise harmonic frequency necessary for the optimal image quality. However, filtration has its own disadvantages. This results in a narrow band harmonic which can reduce the effectiveness of the returning signal. This in turn limits signal penetration and the image resolution.

CODED HARMONICS

This provides solution to the filtration problem by substracting rather that filtering the fundamental transmit frequency from the returning harmonic. This subtraction is possible through the use of DIGITAL ENCODED ULTRASOUND. This technology transforms conventional sound waves to digital codes. This process provides precision transmission, reception and the signal processing techniques. The use of codes also provides the patterns that the receiver uses to decode the returning signal so specific, unwanted frequencies may be substracted. This provides exceptionally clear images with increased sensitivity.

Echo frequency response from a narrow band transmits pulse using a high pass filter or narrow.

Band filter (filter A) cannot effectively separate the fundamental from the harmonic signal due to the overlap of the signals.

After phase inversion, the summing of the even harmonic components results in greater harmonic signal amplitude. Wider band pass filtering can now be applied more effectively (filter B). The result is improved contrast and spatial resolution.

Present Status of Tissue Harmonic Imaging

Since its introduction in 1998, THI has become a clinical standard in many ultrasound departments. THI has been applied across a range of transducer transmit frequencies from 1.8 MHz to 7 MHz. This has enabled its use in a wide range of clinical applications, from low frequency transcranial and abdominal imaging, to high frequency breast and endovaginal applications.

CONCLUSION

The technique of tissue harmonic imaging provides imaging with better resolution. Tissue harmonics provide:

- Reduced reverberations.
- Reduced beam aberration.
- Reduced beam side lobes.
- Reduced haze.
- Improved cystic clearing.

Coded harmonics prove:

- Reduced haze.
- Improved resolution and sensitivity.

Section 11—Miscellaneous

Chapter 122

Positron Emission Tomography

Positron – Emitting radionuclides – 1940.

PET imaging – first developed in 1970 – molecular imaging technique provides images of physiological processes.

Positron Physics

- Detection of the two annihilation photons produced when a positron is emitted from a radioisotope.
- PET radiotracers may be labelled with any positron emitting radionuclide.

Radionuclide	Half-life.
Fluorine 18 k	110 min.
Carbon 11	20 min.
Nitrogen 13	10 min.
Oxygen 15	122 sec.
Rubidium 82	75 sec.

Deoxyglucose labelled with fluorine 18 – mainly used (^{18}FDG).

Malignant cells → ↑ Glucose metabolism.
↑ Glucose receptors.
↑ Hexokinase mediated glycosis.
↓ Dephosphorylation by G.6 phosphate.

FDG → slow dephosphorylation, accumulator equilibrium in 45-60 min.

- Absolute measurement of glucose uptake into lesions or specific organs difficult.
- Standardized uptake value (SUV) – estimate in comparison mean uptake in rest of body.

Instrumentation for PET

- Simultaneous detection of 511 Kev photons.
- Since no collimotors used → increased efficiency.
- Either multihead gamma camera or a dedicated PET camera.
- PET camera → thicker and more crystals, more photomultiplier → increased resolution and sensitivity (lesions <2 cm).
- Bismuth germinate (BGO) – high stopping power for energy photons.
- PET images need to be interpreted in conjunction with CT or MR anatomy, especially in oncology.
- Mounting spiral CT and part ring PET on same gantry – functional and anatomical data in single examination.

PET APPLICATIONS

Lung Tumors

- Non-small cell lung carcinoma – amenable to surgery.

FDG-PET

- Highly accurate in staging mediastinal notices.
- At least as accurate as CT and scintigraphy for abdomen, pelvis and bone not brain.
- Fall in FDG uptake response to treatment.

Solitary Pulmonary Nodule

- 95% sensitivity.
- >80% specificity.
- Lesions <1 cm.

Colorectal Cancer

- Margin use – local recurrence after treatment and metastatic disease.
- Most accurate modality for distinguishing fibrosis from tumor → 90%.
- PET superior to CT for detecting extrahepatic metastasis.
- Response to treatment – baseline uptake by 6 months.

Lymphoma

- Most types of lymphoma show ↑ed uptake.
- Most intense uptake – worst prognosis.
- More accurate than CT for staging.
- Fall in FDG uptake seen after 1-2 cycles of chemotherapy.

Head and Neck Cancer

- Majority show ↑ed uptake of FDG.
- Advantage over CT/MRI.
- Equivalent to CT/MRI for staging with over primary or secondary.
- Recurrence after treatment.

Breast Cancer (Figure 122.1)

- Early detection of breast tumors, useful addition to mammography particularly in patients with dense breasts, fibroystic disease, previous surgery or radiotherapy, breast implants.

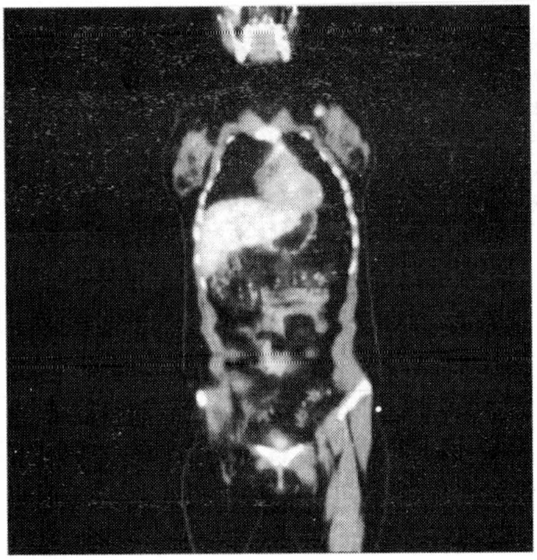

Fig. 122.1: PET-CT image shows a hot spot in the left breast

- PET for detecting distant metastasis.
- Body metastasis – lytic lesions—more.
  Sclerotic lesions—less.

Other Tumors

- Malignant melanoma - Highly effective for distant mets.
- Oesophageal tumors - Superior to CT for distant mets.
  - Locally also probably better.

Other Applications

- Refractory epilepsy – where surgical excision of temporal lobe lesion is indicated.
- SPECT – if radiopharmaceutical injection during seizures.
- Metabolic brain imaging using PET – more sensitive.
- Myocardial viability in patients with inconclusive studies on SPECT.

Section 11—Miscellaneous

Chapter 123

Radiation Hazards and Protection

- Radiation is defined as that form of energy, which can travel from one place to another in vacuum i.e. without any medium.
- The radiation such as X-ray cannot be felt by our senses. Therefore no immediate pain is felt with overexposure to radiation like X-rays.
- The radiation like X-rays have the property of creating ionisation of matter which means creating positive and negative ions. Henceforth the term ionizing radiation is used.
- The substances like radium emits +vely charged helium nuclei called γ particles and neutral but penetrating radiation called γ-radiation.
- γ-radiation is electromagnetic radiation like X-rays but are more energetic compared to X-rays produced by X-ray machine.
- The present philosophy for radiation protection is that the exposure be reduced to as low as possible but kept within 20 mS (r Rem) per year for radiation workers and 1mSU (0.1 Rem) per year for member of public. The high exposure should be avoided. This is known as the principle of ALARA (as low as reasonably achievable).

RADIATION HAZARDS

- The net injury depends upon the energy imparted per unit length. Thus greater the energy.

Absorbed Per Unit Length, Greater will be the Damage to the Body

- Since the alpha particles have the least range compared to beta or gamma particles of the same energy, alpha particles will be most hazardous in case of internally located isotopes and gamma will be least hazardous.
- In case of externally located source or externally falling beam, the gammas are most hazardous because they are most penetrating and they can impart maximum energy to the whole body while alpha are least penetrating and absorbed in the uppermost layer of the body. Hence if the alpha beam is strong, it may cause to skin only.
- The net biological effect is therefore maximum in case of alpha particles and minimum in case of X or gamma rays of the same energy. Beta lie between. Thus the net effect is expressed in terms of energy of the radiation and the type of particles. It is defined as the product of absorbed energy and the quality factor, which is dependent on type of particle. The unit of combined effect is sievert (SU) which was earlier REM.

Table 123.1: Whole body exposure

Dose	Immediate effect
100mSV (10 REM)	None detectable
01. SV to 02.5 SV (10 REM to 25 REM)	Chromosome aberration detectable
0.2 SV to 1.0 SV (25 REM to 100 REM)	Change in blood picture, decrease in blood counts, non-lethal, and 100% recovery.
15SV to 3SV (100 REM to 300 REM)	Vomiting, diarrhoea etc. death possible in few people.
3 SV to 5 SV (300 REM to 500 REM)	Severe radiation sickness (loss of weight appetite etc) Death may occur to 50% of people exposed.
Above 5SV (500 REM)	All above effect and death within few days.

Table 123.2: Local irradiation

Region	Dose	Effect
Skin	3 SV to 2O SV	Epilation and erythema to ulceration and necrosis (over a period of 30 days)
Eye lens	5 SV too 8 SV	Cataract (within 5-10 years)
Ovary	1 SV to 4 SV	Temporary to permanent sterility
Testis	0.25 SV to 4 SV	Temporary to permanent sterility

RADIATION PROTECTION

Units

Units are necessary for quantitative description of any physical concept. In radiation physics, the internation commission on radiation units and measurements defines units.

The Units of Interest are as follows:

1. Activity.
2. Exposure.
3. Dose.
4. Equivalent dose.
5. Effective dose.

Activity

- The activity of a radiation source (radioisotope signifies the output of radiation from the source. The activity of a source is defined in terms of disintegration per second it undergoes. The unit is Becquerel (Bq) one by corresponds to one disintegration per second. Formerly the unit of activity was termed curia (Ci) corresponding to 3.7×10^{10} disintegration per second.

Exposure and Dose

- The unit of exposure has been named, as Roentgen "One Roentgen" is an exposure dose of X- or gamma radiation such that the associated corpuscular emission per 0.001293 gm of air, produces in air ions carrying out electrostatic unit of quantity of charge of either sign. The associated corpuscular emission produced by X- or X-radiation in primary ionisation may have very long ranges so it is difficult to measure directly the ionisation produced by the electrons that are produced in 0.001293 gm of air because these electrons produce ionisation beyond 0.001293 gm. Hence the compensate that this volume is surrounded by equal range of these electrons so that the secondary electron generated in that regions produce ionisation in 0.001293 gms of air. This is called electronic equilibrium conditions roentgen in S.1 system is to be replaced by coulombs per kg (1R J 2.53×10^{-4} ckg $^{-1}$).

Dose

- Also called absorbed dose. The dose from ionisation radiation is the energy imparted to matter by ionisation radiation per unit mass of the steadiated material at the phase of interest. Earlier unit of dose was rad. One rad is equal to 100 ra per gram. The present unit is gray (Gy). One gray is equal to one Joule of energy imparted to q kg of any material. Gray = 100 rad = 1 joule per kg.

Equivalent dose (HT): Equivalent dose is the product of dose averaged over the tissue or organ and radiation weighing factor WR.

For a tissue or organ HT=absorbed dose × WR.

Radiation weight WR – This is the factor by which absorbed dose is weighted for radiation quality.

Rem = absorbed dose in rad X radiation weighing factor (WR).

UNIT-SIEVERT (SU) —Effective dose: For a given equivalent dose, the probability of stochastic effect depends on the organ/tissue irradiated. When several tissues are irradiated to different doses, the equivalent dose to a tissue is weighted by the factor was called the tissue weighing factor for that tissue. This weighted dose is called the effective dose. It is the sum of weighted equivalent doses in all the tissues and organ of the body.

Effective dose = absorbed dose × WR × WT.

Occupational Exposure of Women

- The basis for control of occupational exposure of women who are not pregnant is the same as that for men. However, once pregnancy has been declared, the conceptus should be pre tested by applying a supplementary equivalent dose limit to the surface of the women's abdomen by ImSv for remainder of the pregnancy and by limiting intake by radio nuclides to 1/20 of ALI.
- **Principles of protection:** There are three ways by which the exposure can be reduced to desired levels. They are as follows:
    1. By ↑ing distance between source and area under consideration.
    2. By providing shielding.
    3. By reducing the duration of exposure.

1. **Distance:** The intensity of radiation varies inversely as the square of distance. This means:

   $I \times 1/d^2\ (C^{-1})$

   $I = k \times 1/d^2$

2. **Shielding:** The radiation, when they pass matters losses and energy by intracting with matter. When I_o in the incident intensity and I the emergent unattenuated base added.

   I=Io –ux not emerged out. This is valid only if the scattered photons do not emerge out i.e. for a narrow beam. It is known that if the beam is broad, the intensity will be more than what is represented by the above equation, the intensity in this case is given by I=D Io-ux where D is called units, X=thickness of the material. Attenuation curves are plotted between fractional transmission (I/Io) and 'x' the thickness.

Time

The total dose is the product of exposure rate and duration of exposure. This can be shown as follows:

Dx = Dr x t.

D_t = Total dose.

D_r = Dose rate.

T = Duration of exposure.

- Hence to reduce the exposure, duration of exposure should be minimized.
- The atoms of the medium x and y radiation is interact with matter in three main process namely:
    1. Photoelectric process in which the protons are absorbed by bound electrons and electron is liberated.
    2. Compton effect in which the photons interact with free electron and photons

get scattered and free electron is liberated.

3. Pair production in which the photon is absorbed in the nuclear field and a pair of positron and neutron is produced. This pair after loosing energy again combines to form a gamma proton.

- The probability of these processes depends upon the energy of photon and the atomic number of absorbing medium.
- In general probability decreases as energy increases.
- At sufficient lower energies protoelectric effect is predominant.
- In medium energy range the Compton effect is predominant.

METHODS OF PROTECTION

The protection is achieved by ensuring that:

1. The installation is adequate.
2. Proper protection devices are used.
3. The equipment is satisfactory.
4. The work practices are satisfactory.

DIAGNOSTIC X-RAY INSTALLATION

Use of Protective Devices

Protective Barrier

- In case of diagnostic tubes operating at 110 KV and above, the control panel should be located in a separate room and the technician should position himself inside the control room whenever the tube is energized.
- In case of diagnostic tubes operating at 100 KV, the control panel should be located either in a separate room or behind a mobile protective barrier of 1.5 mm lead equivalence or a partition wall with a viewing window of lead glass of 1.5 mm lead equivalence as far away as possible but not less than 2 meters from the tube. The technician should position himself behind the protective shielding.
- If the unit is located in a separate room the means of communication between the patients and operator at the control panel should be provided.
- In cases of radiography the vertical cassette holder (chest stand) should have a backing of at least 1.5 mm thick lead.
- Using gonadal shields should reduce the dose to gonads of the patients.
- Some sort of shielding devices having lead equivalence of not less than 0.5 mm should cover buckeye.
- In case of fluoroscopy machines, the shutter control should be shielded as to provide adequate protection for the hands of radiologist.
- The screened should be backed by lead glass having lead equivalence of 1.5 mm lead up to 70 kv and 2 mm between 70 kV and 100 kV.
- Above 100 kV, the thickness should be increased by 0.01 mm for each kv increase.
- Protective glass (visual lead compound) of at least 0.25 mm lead equivalence should be used during vertical fluoroscopy. This helps in further reduction of dose to the radiologist.
- The protective flaps of 0.55 mm lead equivalence, if attached to the gonads of the radiologists. These flaps of size 45 cm × 45 cm should be hung from the bottom of the screen. In case of vertical fluoroscopy, these flaps overlap the fluoroscopy chair. In case of horizontal fluoroscopy, these flaps should be hung from the edge of screen such that flap extends down to the tabletop. Vertical fluoroscopy means the patient is standing and beam is horizontal. Horizontal fluoroscopy means the patient is in lying position and the beam is vertical.
- The radiologist or technician should wear a protection apron of at least 0.25 mm lead equivalence.
- In cases, CT machine the control panel is located in separate room, the viewing window

should have the lead equivalence such that it may offer the same protection as the rest of the wall. It may be between 2-3 mm lead equivalence.

Work Practices

- The protective devices should be regularly checked for their protective adequacy, the beam-limiting diaphragm should be checked periodically to ensure that radiation and light beam fields coincide and they define the beam correctly.
- It should also be ensured periodically that the primary beam does not escape through the diaphragm due to wear and tear.
- To avoid unnecessary exposure it should be ensured that the red light warning signal is made "on" before giving the exposures.
- There should not be any person other than those required for the examination inside the X-ray room and two machines are not installed in the same room.
- The beam-limited diaphragm should be used to limit the diaphragm.
- Special care taken for X-ray examination of persons of reproductive age specially women. The X-ray examination of pelvis and abdomen of a lady of reproductive age group should be done during first ten days from the first day of the menstrual period.
- The X-ray examination of pregnant lady should be avoided specially when they are in 3-15 weeks period. If the exposure is given during this period, there are chances of mental retardation.
- Radiation worker should not hold children or infant patients. In unavoidable cases, if they have to hold or any of the relative holds, the protective apron must be worn and he or she should stand by the side of the patient. The proper distance between focus to the patient or cassette should be kept so that the divergence of the beam in passing through the body is minimum and the dose to the patient is within limit for example in the fluoroscopy work, the patient to focus distance should not be less than 45 cms.
- In case of radiography the distance between patient and cassette should be about 72 inches.
- In case of screening, palpation should not be done by bare or even gloved hands. A palpation spoon should be used. It may be noted that gloves or aprons offer protection against secondary radiation and not against primary radiation.
- The dose to the patient can be reduced by:
  a. Low tube current.
  b. Use of fast screen.
  c. Use of image intensifier coherence possible. If image intensifier is used, the machine can be operated at low currents and hence exposure can be reduced.
  d. Limiting beam size.
  e. Using proper filtration – this will cut off software components, which do not give any information.
  f. The eyes of the radiologist should be dark adapted by pulling on the red goggles before starting the examination. Red goggles are removed after the eyes have been dark-adapted.
  g. By reducing the time of examination. This is possible, if experienced and qualified doctors are available.
- The operator should stand as far as possible away from the patient's machine and the useful beam. For their purpose maximum length of cable must be used. The beam should not be directed towards door window and occupied areas. The film cassettes should not be held by hand.

- In special examination like photofluorography the high efficiency optical system should be used to reduce the dose to the patient.
- To reduce the radiation doses the patient, the no. of radiographs during a particular examination must be reduced.
- Facilitating the free movement of radiographs from one hospital to another can minimize the frequency of such examination.
- The special examination like mammograph should be carried out on special equipments because they do not need high potentials as available in normal machine.
- Similarly where high doses such as in case of tomography are involved, proper care should be taken. In such cases or in case of CT machines, where dynamic studies are undertaken, the proper mapping of doses should be done so that the portion of standing for giving injection can be chosen.
- Personal monitoring badge before starting work should be put on and kept back in the storage area after finishing work.
- Films should be kept in radiation free area.
- Control film should also be kept in the storage area, which should be radiation free, such office etc.

Index

Index

R

Index